COMPREHENSIVE
DENTAL HYGIENE CARE

COMPREHENSIVE
DENTAL HYGIENE
CARE

SECOND EDITION

Irene R. Woodall
R.D.H., M.A., Ph.D.

Clinical Associate Professor, Department of Dental Care Systems, University of Pennsylvania School of Dental Medicine, Philadelphia, Pennsylvania

Bonnie R. Dafoe
R.D.H., B.S.

Clinical Instructor, School of Dental Hygiene, University of Michigan, Ann Arbor, Michigan

Nancy Stutsman Young
R.D.H., M.Ed.

Assistant Professor, Department of Dental Hygiene, Indiana University School of Dentistry, Indianapolis, Indiana

Leslie Weed-Fonner
R.D.H., M.Ed., M.S.W.

Formerly adjunct instructor, Department of Dental Hygiene, Fairleigh Dickinson School of Dentistry, Hackensack, New Jersey

Samuel L. Yankell
Ph.D., R.D.H.

Research Professor, Department of Periodontics, University of Pennsylvania School of Dental Medicine, Philadelphia, Pennsylvania

with 694 illustrations and 4 color plates

The C. V. Mosby Company

ST. LOUIS • TORONTO • PRINCETON   1985

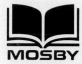

MOSBY

A TRADITION OF PUBLISHING EXCELLENCE

Editor: Darlene Warfel
Assistant editor: Melba Steube
Manuscript editor: Judith Bange
Book design: Jeanne Genz
Cover design: Nancy Steinmeyer
Production: Carol O'Leary, Mary Stueck, Barbara Merritt

SECOND EDITION

The C.V. Mosby Company
11830 Westline Industrial Drive, St. Louis, Missouri 63146

Library of Congress Cataloging in Publication Data

Main entry under title:
Comprehensive dental hygiene care.

    Bibliography: p.
    Includes index.
    1. Dental hygiene. I. Woodall, Irene R., 1946-
[DNLM: 1. Dental Prophylaxis. WU C737]
RK60.7.C65   1985   617.6'01   84-14805
ISBN 0 8016-5700-8

GW/VH/VH 9 8 7 6 5 4   02/D/261

BIOGRAPHICAL DATA

Irene R. Woodall was awarded a certificate in dental hygiene from the University of Detroit, a bachelor of science degree in social sciences and philosophy from Grand Valley State College, and a master of arts degree in communications from Western Michigan University. She holds a doctorate in organizational development from Temple University.

During the first 12 years of her career in dental hygiene, she practiced in general and periodontics practices, held a variety of offices in the Michigan and American Dental Hygienists' Associations, taught in both university and community and junior college programs, and directed the dental hygiene program at Kalamazoo Valley Community College from 1971 to 1976. She developed and chaired the program for the Third International Symposium on Dental Hygiene in 1973.

In 1976 she was appointed Assistant Professor and Chairperson of the Department of Dental Hygiene at the University of Pennsylvania and in 1977 authored her first book, *Leadership, Management, and Role Delineation: Issues for the Dental Team.* She is the author of many articles and learning packages and has taught a variety of continuing education courses and workshops, ranging from clinical instrumentation to communications skills and peer review mechanisms. Currently she owns a consulting firm and teaches behavioral sciences. She is Senior Editor of *RDH* magazine.

She is married and has two daughters.

Bonnie R. Dafoe received her diploma in dental hygiene from the Madison Area Technical College, Madison, Wisconsin, in 1970. She was employed for 5 years as a clinical practitioner for a general dentist and for 1 year as a clinical practitioner for a pedodontist.

In 1974 she spent the summer as a clinical instructor with the Dental Hygiene Department of Guy's Hospital in London, England. In 1975, as a clinical instructor at the University of Pennsylvania, she acquired expanded function skills in periodontics, anesthesia, restorative procedures, and intraoral photography. After taking her bachelor of science degree as a summa cum laude graduate of West Chester State College in 1976, she joined the University of Pennsylvania faculty to teach local anesthesia, dental health education, preclinic, periodontics, and intraoral photography in addition to clinical instruction.

Bonnie has given continuing education courses for the University of Pennsylvania and the Philadelphia component of the American Dental Hygienists' Association.

Bonnie has recently been employed in private practice and is a member of the editorial board of *RDH* magazine. Currently she is a clinical instructor at the University of Michigan, School of Dental Hygiene.

She is married and has one daughter and one son.

Nancy Stutsman Young earned an associate degree in dental hygiene and a bachelor of science degree in dental public health from Indiana University. She received her master of education degree from Temple University.

As a full-time faculty member of the Department of Dental Hygiene at the University of Pennsylvania from 1974 to 1979, she directed a wide variety of courses and prepared numerous learning packages and related audiovisual software. She served as clinic supervisor for 2 years. She is acknowledged among the faculty members as an outstanding teacher and one who is able to integrate inquiry learning into both didactic and clinical teaching.

Nancy has also taught in a community college program and has participated in research projects at the Oral Health Research Institute, Indianapolis, Indiana. She has practiced dental hygiene in the states of Indiana, Pennsylvania, and North Carolina. She has also been active in professional associations and held office in the Philadelphia component of the American Dental Hygienists' Association. She has given a number of continuing education courses.

Nancy is currently a full-time member of the Dental Hygiene Department at the Indiana University School of Dentistry. In addition to clinical teaching, she carries major responsibility for the public health dental hygiene course in the associate degree curriculum and for a research-oriented course in advanced dental science within the bachelor of science degree curriculum.

Leslie Weed-Fonner graduated from Temple University's dental hygiene program and earned her bachelor of science degree from Columbia University and her master of education degree from Temple University.

She has had a variety of clinical experiences in pedodontic, general, and periodontic practices, performing both traditional dental hygiene procedures and restorative, periodontal, and local anesthesia expanded functions. As a faculty member of the Department of Dental Hygiene at the University of Pennsylvania, she taught this wide range of skills to dental hygiene students for 4 years. In 1979 Lesliie coordinated the Penn-EFDA Faculty Institute I: Periodontics/Anesthesia and taught dental hygiene faculty members from a variety of institutions how to perform and teach expanded functions to their students.

She has been able to combine her interests in clinical practice and teaching with her interest (and graduate degree) in group process by team teaching courses in practice management, communications, and community dentistry externships.

After participating in a Peace Corps program in the Philippines, Leslie taught in the Department of Dental Hygiene at Fairleigh Dickinson. She has further pursued her interests in group process, developed in the Philippines, by earning a master of

social work degree with a major in group process from Hunter College in New York City.

Leslie is married to Michael Fonner, they have one child, Zachary Nathaneal Weed-Fonner. The three have moved to Bangkok, Thailand, where Michael is teaching.

Samuel L. Yankell received his bachelor of science degree in biology from Ursinus College and attended Rutgers University to obtain a master of science degree in physiology and a doctorate in biochemistry. He received his certificate in dental hygiene from the University of Pennsylvania. Most of his career has been in industry, beginning with a position as a senior biochemist at Colgate Palmolive. He then went to Smith, Miller and Patch as Department Head of Pharmacology and Biochemistry and then to Menley & James Laboratories, a division of SmithKline Beckman Corp., as Department Head of Biological Sciences. Since 1975 he has been at the University of Pennsylvania in the Department of Periodontics. Although his primary efforts have been in research, he has lectured in biochemistry and nutrition in the dental hygiene program and is responsible for the graduate dental education course on new advances in cariology.

He is a member of many scientific organizations, including the American Association for the Advancement of Science, the American Chemical Society, the American Society for Pharmacology and Experimental Therapeutics, the European Organization for Caries Research, the International Association for Dental Research, the Society of Toxicology, and Sigma Xi. He has authored more than 150 publications in the scientific literature.

He is married and has two sons and a daughter.

TO

My brothers, **Richard D.** and **William R. Zimmerman,** who taught me about competition and to have high expectations of myself; my mother, **Augusta V. Doktor,** who taught me how to respect my womanhood in a man's world; and my father, **William W. Zimmerman,** who taught me how to throw a ball and how to care.

IRW

My teachers, professional colleagues, students, and patients who have made providing dental care a satisfying career; and to **Don, Erin,** and **Andrew** for their love and support.

BRD

Phil, with all my love, for his patience, endurance, support, and love during this project.

NSY

My favorite two loved ones, **Michael** and **Zachary;** and to my loving, and loved, cohorts: **Bonnie, Irene, Nancy,** and **Sam.**

LWF

Kuna for her patience, understanding, and help; and to **Sandra Scott** and the general office staff and **Catherine Reddon** and the word processing team for their continued cooperation and friendship.

SLY

FOREWORD

This text lives up to its title of being the most comprehensive volume in the practice of dental hygiene in the United States to date. The authors have gone to meticulous detail to describe the scope of dental hygiene as it is currently, with prognostications as to the future of this important health care profession. As the functions of the hygienist broaden to be more inclusive, the need for this edition becomes more critical, since it represents a thorough review of the literature and includes some important reports published in 1984 that should influence clinical practice. The recent Consensus Conference held by the National Institute for Dental Research on the use of sealants in the prevention of dental caries places a greater responsibility on the dental hygienist in delivering this preventive measure to children.

The role of the dental hygienist in detecting dental caries and periodontal disease is well covered in this text, and I consider the description of examination and documentation of oral tissues by means of study models, intraoral photography, and oral cancer examination to be the finest in any single publication.

The authors have been able to bring together the various skills necessary for the master clinician to deliver optimum care in a fashion that is easy to follow and read. The sequence of chapters is designed to acquaint the therapist with the fundamentals of the environment in which one practices, the total evaluation of the patient, and the basic techniques of treatment. The chapters on treatment planning, planning for the control of dental disease, nutrition, and root planing are particularly valuable, since they are not usually covered as well in other volumes. Root planing has been demonstrated to be one of the most important procedures in the treatment of plaque-induced periodontal disease and in many practices this technique is best delivered by the dental hygienist.

The review questions are appreciated by the reader, as well as the objectives that precede each of the 38 chapters. It is clear that this edition should prove valuable to the potential applicant to dental hygiene programs interested in learning about the practice in the 1980s, as well as the hygiene student anxious to learn the various aspects of hygiene care. It should be particularly helpful to the dental hygienist who may have taken a leave from the field and is desirous of being updated in the current practices before returning to the profession.

It has been a privilege to read this text, and I compliment the authors for an exemplary contribution to the oral health profession.

D. Walter Cohen
Dean Emeritus and
Professor of Periodontics,
University of Pennsylvania

PREFACE

We originally prepared this text to bring together our collective experiences and philosophies with regard to teaching and learning clinical dental hygiene in the hope that dental hygiene can continue to grow in degree of responsibility and participation among the health care professions. The scope of the text; the emphasis on goal orientation, mastery learning, and the use of a variety of learning strategies; the sequence of skill development; the integration of behavioral and basic science principles with clinical skill development; the overlay of a program of care for individual patients using the theme of assessment-planning-implementation-evaluation; and the focus on the patient as a partner in care are the unique elements of the text and represent our collective teaching experiences over the past two decades.

This second edition is enhanced by our collective growth over the past 5 years—as practitioners, educators, writers, researchers, social scientists, and as people. We have, of course, updated the content and philosophy to reflect new research findings. We have added to or expanded most chapters and have included new chapters on instrument sharpening and care of appliances. The chapters on the guided oral assessment and the oral cancer self-examination have been combined to enhance the flow between those two components of care. The chapter introducing medical emergencies has been moved forward to ensure its inclusion prior to the students' entering the clinic to care for patients. The color plates have been added to enhance learning about hard and soft tissue characteristics and to emphasize the importance of the dental hygienist as a diagnostician of patient needs that can be met through dental hygiene care. We listened carefully to review comments from the many faculty members who use this text. We hope the changes will help you teach and learn together.

A review of the table of contents should reveal that some elements of clinical practice either not typically included or not extensively developed in other texts receive considerable attention in *Comprehensive Dental Hygiene Care*. Examples are the chapters relating to comprehensive periodontal assessment, involving the patient in learning self-assessment of oral health, planning for care, ultrasonic scaling devices, intraoral photography, pain control in dental hygiene care, case documentation, and integrating dental hygiene principles in dental practice. The content of this text reflects a substantial reliance on basic and behavioral science research as it relates to dentistry in particular and health care in general.

In addition to the content, which should support both the needs of preclinical courses and the various stages of advanced clinical learning, the *sequence* of material can be readily adapted to preclinical and subsequent courses. This sequence was developed to facilitate the use of goal orientation—for the students to begin to feel participation in and ownership of the goals of the course. The constant theme or goal of the early chapters is preparation for competent and confident clinical practice. The target or goal is the "first day" of clinic when a trusting patient appears for care. The faculty member's function is to present that day as the reason for preclinical learning and to present each chapter as one means, in tandem with classroom and clinical activities, for mastering each step along the way toward *providing the care appropriate for the patient*. Thus the first chapters are devoted to "preparing the site" so that students can operate and maintain the equipment that supports the delivery of care. The student is also prepared with an introduction to sterilization and to the prevention of cross-contamination. Later chapters introduce the student to the care of the patient, beginning with the health history and including identifying and responding to medical emergencies. Time is set aside to learn positioning at the chair and basic principles of instrumentation to facilitate sit-down, four-handed procedures and to enable students to perform the subsequent assessment steps of intraoral and extraoral examinations and chartings. Rather than teach instrumentation skills as a separate, parallel laboratory experience, we recommend teaching these techniques as a part of the material in each chapter. Once the students have gained basic competence in position, grasp, stroke, and wrist motion, they can refine and develop those skills while actually observing and recording clinical data for student partners (or patients of more advanced students). The purposeful, goal-directed use of probes and explorers seems to hasten the development of basic skills. The significance of acquiring good instrumentation skills cannot easily escape the awareness of a student who is learning to use instruments to prepare a pocket depth or caries charting.

As basic skills develop, instruments with contra-angles, blades, and other features requiring greater skill development in line angle adaptation, insertion, angulation, and working stroke are introduced for continued practice. Student partners can serve an important role in developing these skills in instrumentation but cannot in many instances satisfy the need for students to find a deep pocket; observe varieties of calculus; compare tissue color, texture, shape, and consistency; and remove deposits. For those students whose partners exhibit high levels of oral health, it is particularly helpful to be paired with an advanced student who is providing care for patients with evidence of disease. An important phase of development is to see the range of cases, from health through subtle change to advanced disease.

Depending on the philosophy of the dental hygiene program, the teaching of some chapters may be delayed until the student is further along in training. Examples are ultrasonic instrumentation, curettage, and periodontal dressings. Generally speaking, the transition from preclinical to advanced clinical skill development occurs in the move to the chapters dealing with occlusion and chemical agents.

Thus one important theme is the preparation for the "first day" of clinic as a confident and competent clinician. As each chapter is concluded, the students should ask themselves if they are ready to perform the newly acquired skills as an entry-level clinician. While some anxiousness may be felt by the students, they should begin to feel that they *can* perform basic skills safely, particularly as they practice and use each skill during preclinical education and later during "in clinic" sessions where

basic skills can be developed into varying degrees of refined expertise.

A second goal orientation of preclinical learning integrated in the text that tends to increase the interest of students in their learning is that many chapters prepare the student not only for clinic, but also for additional course work in the program. The chapter on emergencies, for example, serves as an introduction to complete courses in cardiopulmonary resuscitation, first aid, and pharmacology. The chapter on health histories is a prelude to pathology and many of the basic sciences. The sequences on examination and periodontal care prepare the student for periodontics, pathology, and chemistry courses. Pointing out their relevance can facilitate positive anticipation of later course work.

The structure of each chapter makes it possible to develop shorter-range goal achievement as well. A list of suggested objectives is provided, which may be discussed with the students. They may be altered, deleted, or expanded on as a result of the discussion. In inquiry learning, the faculty member may ask the students to develop their own objectives. Comparing their objectives with the chapters' may stimulate discussion and problem-solving sessions. Content in a narrative format follows the objectives. Suggested activities and review questions follow the content. It should not be necessary to conduct formal lectures or presentations for each chapter if the students have sound reading comprehension skills. Other than a few points of clarification being offered or a piece of recent research being explained, the lecture can be replaced by class activities that tend to develop a higher level of cognitive and affective learning. Search and discovery, problem solving, case analysis, values clarification, small-group tasks, role play, inquiry, and guided discussion should be useful techniques for maximizing the opportunity for growth that is available when a class of students is together. Active involvement of the students with each other as they *use* the content of the chapters enhances their acceptance of the basic principles of dental hygiene as their own and stimulates their ability to think, create, and investigate.

In addition to its broad scope of content and its goal orientation approach, *Comprehensive Dental Hygiene Care* is organized around the program development model of assessment-planning-implementation-evaluation. Although this model has been employed in community program development for years, its usefulness in clinical, one-to-one health care designs is not widely reflected in clinical dental hygiene references. We believe this model has great relevance in providing individual patient care and that its application in clinical care ensures a well-informed, logical approach to improving health status and to preserving the challenge and stimulation, as well as the gratification, of being a practicing dental hygienist.

One additional theme that is constant in the text is that of the patient as a partner in care—as a person involved in care. We believe that care is not done *to* the patient or *on* the patient but rather *for* and *with* the patient. This stance is based on a wealth of behavioral science research and on personal humanistic philosophies that identify the need for active, rewarding involvement as a corequisite for positive, long-term change. The current emphasis on prevention and self-care models in health care draws on these principles of human behavior. In addition, we believe that a major source of satisfaction in health care delivery is the warmth and caring that emanates from an accepting, egalitarian relationship between the helper and the helped.

Our best wishes are yours as you teach and learn together as the helper and the helped. We welcome your responses and your suggestions.

Irene R. Woodall
Bonnie R. Dafoe
Nancy Stutsman Young
Leslie Weed-Fonner
Samuel L. Yankell

ACKNOWLEDGMENTS
for first edition

Many people contributed their efforts to make the final preparation of the manuscript possible. Conrad Woodall, Phil Young, and Kuna Yankell were invaluable in our times of greatest need, not only with their support, but also with their willingness to type, duplicate, collate, proofread, and visit the post office and the office supply and photographic stores. Don Dafoe was especially helpful in his review of the chapters on health history and emergency procedures. Sally Verity's review of the chapters on comprehensive charting was also particularly helpful. Jane Griffin and Susan Muhler deserve a thank you for finding rare equipment items for our use.

The word processing staff, Catherine Redden, Delores DiCocco, Patricia DeVuono, and Julia Marguilles, were invaluable in their preparation of the final manuscript, especially in May and June, 1979. Emily Mintz deserves a thank you for her contribution in typing tables and letters for us.

We also wish to thank Michael Schwager for his advice and efforts in meeting our most critical photographic needs. We wish to acknowledge the case documentation prepared by Deborah Drazek while she was a student at the University of Pennsylvania and the role she, Diana Mumma, and Sharon Herr played in photograph preparation. Rosemarie Valentine's leadership and efforts in developing learning materials for the department are also gratefully acknowledged. Slides prepared by Mary Robb Gross and Catherine Schifter were especially helpful in showing the use of Gracey instruments, and we thank our colleagues for sharing them with us.

Elissa Berardi, our medical illustrator, worked long and hard to prepare the many detailed drawings for the text. Her work is beautifully done and reflects a great deal of caring for the quality of the project.

We also owe thanks to all the participants in the Penn-EFDA Faculty Institute I: Periodontics/Anesthesia for their continuous support and for sharing in the excitement during the final weeks of our efforts. We shall never forget Sue Agostini, Regina Byrne, Sue Colangelo, Sue Daniel, Kandie Dautel, Mary Ann Haag, Gwen Hlava, Joyce Jenzano, JoAnne Karr, Jane Emerson Knight, Joan Madden, Pat Mulford, Lin Nassar, Joan Gluch-Scranton, Maureen Pratt Smith, and Debbie Vlanis.

ACKNOWLEDGMENTS
for second edition

Once again, many people helped us in preparing the manuscript and in ensuring that the time and moral support were there when we needed them most. We offer our heartfelt thanks and appreciation.

For their reviews of the first edition—Phyllis Beemsterboer, Debbie Brown, Sherry Castle Harfst, Ralph Lobene, Hunter Rackley, Patricia Randolph, Karen Ridley, Ellen Rogo, and Joan Gluch Scranton.

For his review of the intraoral photography chapter—Clifford L. Freehe; and for his review of the medical history and emergencies chapters—Donald C. Dafoe.

For their assistance in locating references—Sue Seeger and Ruth Cressman at the University of Michigan dental library and Kathy Marousek, Helen Itkin, and Dorothea Colburn at the Fairleigh Dickinson dental library.

For their outstanding photographic assistance—Bonnie Dafoe, William Prior, Catherine Schifter, David Sullivan, and Robert Benedon; and for the beautiful new illustrations—Elissa Berardi.

For giving permission to use the Fairleigh Dickinson School of Dentistry facilities—Richard Oglesby.

For the index preparation and service as a photographic model—Conrad Woodall.

For the much needed time to write—Michael Fonner and Dani Kazista.

For continuing support during the project—the dental hygiene faculty at the Fairleigh Dickinson University (especially Ellen Rogo and Cheryl Westphal) and at the University of Pennsylvania (Catherine Schifter, Kate Fitzgerald, Jean Byrnes, Charlotte Hangorsky, Roberta Throne, Joyce Levy, and Joanne Prifti, and Janet Yellowitz).

For their consistent, helpful presence and support in every way during this project—Conrad Woodall, Kuna Yankell, and Phil Young.

CONTENTS

PART ONE
PREPARATION

1 Dental hygiene practice, 3

2 Preparing the site: operation and maintenance of equipment, 11

3 Disease transmission theory and control of contamination, 22

4 The complete dental record, 56

5 Basic instrumentation and positioning, 63

6 Instrument sharpening, 95

PART TWO
ASSESSMENT

7 The patient's perceptions, 109

8 The comprehensive health history, 117

9 General physical evaluation and the extraoral and intraoral examination, 135

10 Basic emergency procedures, 164

11 Comprehensive caries, restorative, tooth characteristic, and radiographic charting, 177

12 Calculus detection, 196

13 Plaque and gingival indices, 204

14 Periodontal examination and charting, 217

15 Preparation of study models, 238

16 Intraoral photography, 271

PART THREE

PLANNING

17 Planning for the control of dental disease, 295

18 Formulating a treatment plan, case presentation, and appointment plan, 330

19 Guided self-assessment of oral conditions and oral cancer self-examination, 345

20 Nutritional self-assessment and modifications, 361

PART FOUR

IMPLEMENTATION

21 Removing heavy deposits: hand scaling, 377

22 Removing heavy deposits: ultrasonic instruments, 393

23 Removing fine deposits and root planing, 410

24 Soft tissue curettage, 430

25 Periodontal dressings and suture removal, 443

26 Polishing the teeth, 464

27 Care of removable dental appliances, 477

28 The role of occlusion in dental health and disease, 483

29 Fluoride therapy, 499

30 Pit and fissure sealants, 522

31 Control of tooth hypersensitivity, 535

32 Pain and pain control: topical and local anesthesia, 541

33 Nitrous oxide and oxygen conscious sedation, 561

34 Modification of dental hygiene care for patients with special needs, 574

35 Restorative procedures, 597

PART FIVE
EVALUATION

36 Case documentation, 651

37 Evaluating success of dental hygiene care, 665

38 Integrating dental hygiene procedures into a practice setting, 671

Suggested responses, 676

Color plates

1 PBI scores, 216

2 Variations in gingival form and color, 216

3 Complete intraoral photographic series, 281

4 Treatment sequence for soft tissue curettage, 442

COMPREHENSIVE
DENTAL HYGIENE CARE

PART ONE

PREPARATION

Before a clinician greets a patient, determines that person's needs, or delivers any preventive or therapeutic care, he/she should be fully aware of how to operate the equipment and ensure that the clinical area is free from hazards. The clinician should know how to interpret a dental record and use correct positioning at the dental unit to maximize access and to minimize stress and strain. In addition, the clinician should know how to select and use basic dental instruments and ensure that they are properly cared for.

The first six chapters in this text address these preparatory functions, giving the rationale and the procedures to be followed.

The first chapter introduces the student to what dental hygiene has been, what it is today, and what it could be. It also lays out the components of the comprehensive dental hygiene appointment and discusses the array of settings in which hygienists can provide care. The subsequent chapters introduce the dental operatory and support equipment, control of microbial contamination, the components of the dental record, basic instrumentation and positioning at the chair, and instrument sharpening.

Once this preparation is mastered, the student is ready to greet a patient and begin assessing that person's individual needs—procedures that are addressed in detail in Part Two.

1 DENTAL HYGIENE PRACTICE

OBJECTIVES: *The reader will be able to*

1. Define a philosophy of patient-centered care.
2. Identify examples of patient-hygienist interactions that reflect the philosophy of patient-centered care.
3. Identify his/her own reasons for selecting dental hygiene as a profession.
4. Define his/her own entering expectations of dental hygiene education and of dental hygiene practice.
5. Explain why the perceptions and expectations of faculty members may differ from those of students.
6. Identify changes that occurred in the 1960s and 1970s that had a major impact on the scope of dental hygiene practice.
7. Describe the impact of state dental practice acts on the scope of practice and educational programs.
8. Given the four phases of program development, identify all the procedures a dental hygienist may perform in helping meet patient needs.

This text was written to prepare dental hygiene students for clinical practice. Its primary goals are to help students feel confident and competent on their first day of clinical practice and gain personal satisfaction from having an understanding of how dental hygiene care contributes to the well-being of the people they serve.

The early chapters introduce the student, step-by-step, to the sequence of procedures typically followed in the comprehensive dental hygiene appointment plan. Later chapters address more advanced clinical skills and provide guidelines for integrating ideal principles of care into a realistic practice environment.

The philosophy of patient-centered care is integrated into each phase of care. The patient is viewed as the partner in care, involved extensively in decision making and in the self-care components necessary for restoring and maintaining the patient's oral health. The mastery of technical procedures is emphasized in the individual chapters to ensure safe and effective therapy. But in each instance the *need* for the procedure and the *way* in which the *patient* is involved in the procedure are critical components of developing the relative role of technical skill in dental hygiene care.

Many beginning students see the profession of dental hygiene as being founded on this service orientation, which is the philosophic basis for patient-centered care. For those students, the text should enhance that approach to learning dental hygiene care. Other new students, whose exposure to the profession has been somewhat limited, may focus largely on the technical components of dental hygiene practice. For those, the text should help develop a more comprehensive approach to dental hygiene care.

Additionally, this book was written to help prepare students for future roles in health care delivery by introducing a flexible approach to patient care and by introducing controversies regarding the efficacy of time-honored practice procedures.

MOTIVATIONS FOR SELECTING DENTAL HYGIENE

Persons select dental hygiene as a career for many different reasons. The initial interest of some students is derived from their own encounters with dentistry and dental hygiene. As patients they may have learned to respect and enjoy the people in the dental office. Some students may see the traditional white uniform and gown as a sign of status and achievement. In selecting a career, students may consider the clean, reasonably relaxed atmosphere to be an attractive working environment. Students who were visited by the school dental hygienist each year may identify with the relative independence of the person who travels from school to school helping young people improve their oral health. As with most professions, a family tradition in dentistry or dental hygiene may be a major determining factor. Growing up around a dental office can have a significant impact on a person's career awareness and interest. For some students, careful career counseling and information programs may be the reason for selecting dental hygiene.

EXPECTATIONS FOR PRACTICE

However, most applicants have a few common needs or expectations. When asked what special characteristics a dental hygienist should have to function well, most students identify the ability to work well with people and the ability to use their hands. They expect to earn a reasonable income, to work in pleasant surroundings, to have flexibility in scheduling, to have the respect of the patient, and to help people. When the functional role of the dental hygienist is addressed, most see the primary duties to be "cleaning teeth" and "teaching people how to care for their teeth." Most applicants expect to work with a dentist in private practice.

There are, of course, a few students whose expectations are quite different from the ones described. Varying perceptions may be due to a quite different exposure to the profession or perhaps due to misinformation.

However, it is critical that any incoming student clarify specifically what expectations and perceptions he/she has of the profession and of his/her expected performance in the educational program. Sharing these perceptions with each other and exchanging perceptions with the faculty members can be an enlightening experience and one that can prevent or at least reduce conflict. A student who expects to learn one thing, but who is constantly expected to learn another, can experience anxiety. The knowledge that different people can have widely varying expectations can help reduce the frustrations for a student.

Usually the more extensive exposure of dental hygiene faculty to the profession has altered their initial perceptions of dental hygiene. A faculty member has had an opportunity to compare expectations with reality and to develop an educational approach that blends the ideal with the real. Faculty members may vary greatly with regard to their respective perceptions. Whereas one faculty member may relate to practical applications of skill, another may strive to preserve ideal, conceptual approaches to patient care with a strong basic and behavioral science foundation. Still other faculty members may see their role as one of preparing hygienists for the future—dental hygiene as it "ought" to be rather than as it is.

CHANGES IN THE PROFESSION
Legal and educational changes

Many of these varying perceptions, whether among faculty or students, are due to the rapid changes that have taken place in the profession since the early 1960s. After several decades of slow, at times imperceptible, change the profession encountered the era of "expanded functions" and the challenge of defining how its members could maintain or alter their role.

Prior to the flurry of debate of the 1960s, dental hygiene, for the most part, was practiced in solo dental practices. The role of the dental hygienist was largely defined as oral prophylaxis, patient education, and the exposing of radiographs. Particularly in the East, hygienists were employed in school systems providing dental health education, prophylaxis, and fluoride treatments. (See Fig. 1-1 for a view of a school-based clinic in the early days of dental hygiene.)

The events of the 1960s and 1970s helped revise that relatively narrow scope of practice. In *Survey of Dentistry,* Hollinshead (1961) describes the deplorable state of our nation's oral health. Many wondered how a country that was a world leader and that was investing in a major space program and providing millions of dollars in aid to foreign countries could allow its own people to have such limited access to quality dental care. President Lyndon Johnson launched his War on Poverty in the mid 1960s with a call for legislation to provide comprehensive federally funded medical care for the elderly and other needy persons. Under Medicaid, states would provide dental benefits to qualified, financially handicapped persons. In addition, numerous proposals for federally supported health care for all persons were introduced in the federal

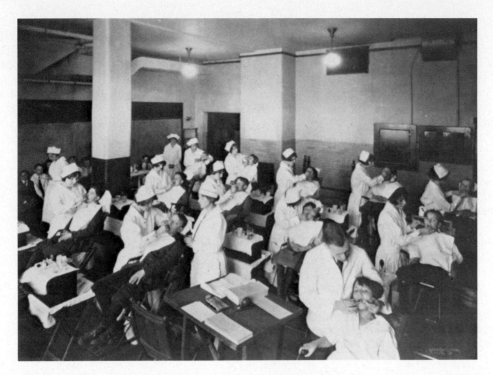

Fig. 1-1. Students in early 1900s of the Department of Oral Hygiene, University of Pennsylvania Holding Clinic in the S. Weir Mitchell School, 50th and Kingsessing Ave., Philadelphia.

legislature, some of which included dental benefits. It seemed imminent that people previously denied medical and dental care because of financial barriers would soon be flooding the health care delivery system.

The 1970 Carnegie Commission report stated that there would soon be a great shortage of physicians and dentists. "With the advent of national health insurance, the shortcomings in our methods of health care delivery and the critical shortages of our health manpower and facilities will become even more glaringly apparent." The Carnegie Commission's recommendation for dentistry was that "progress could be achieved through more extensive use of dentist's assistants and dental hygienists and through greater emphasis on preventive programs."

Several plans developed from this recommendation, including the allocation of federal funds to increase the numbers of dentists, physicians, nurses, and other health care providers being prepared in educational programs. Experiments to evaluate the delegation of functions to dental assistants and dental hygienists were conducted to determine whether the dentist could be relieved of some of the clinical functions he/she typically provided. In many states, as the results of the research proved to be positive, laws were debated and changed to permit auxiliary personnel to perform additional services. Curricula in dental assisting and dental hygiene programs were altered to include the new skills and knowledge required to provide these additional services.

Although dental and medical programs expanded and support personnel for dentistry and medicine increased in number and variety, national health insurance still had not been enacted by 1984. In 1976 the Carnegie Council (formerly the Carnegie Commission) revised its recommendations to state that increased numbers of physicians and dentists were not needed but that the number of support personnel should continue to grow and be used to provide greater varieties of health care service.

Along with deciding which skills should be

added to practice, there was considerable discussion among dental hygienists regarding increasing the variety of settings and the range of responsibility and decision making a hygienist might assume. In the early 1970s the American Dental Hygienists' Association defined practice sites including hospitals, geriatric centers, penal institutions, and centers for the physically and mentally handicapped as appropriate and desirable locations for serving the public. Programs of care, whether for individuals or for groups, were identified as the function of the hygienist; these were programs in which a great deal more expertise and responsibility would be required of the hygienist (ADHA Resolutions 1971, 1973, 1975, and 1976).

The number of programs rose from 70 in 1967 (ADA annual report, 1969) to 187 in 1978. The number of graduates increased from 1739 to 4847 per year between 1967 and 1977 (ADA annual report, 1978). The range of functions taught in various programs now varies from the most limited scope to a full range of procedures.

Bachelor's and master's degree programs available to dental hygienists increased in number and variety. In addition to the several long-standing bachelor of science programs in which clinical dental hygiene training followed previous college education in the sciences and liberal arts, newer programs offered the dental hygienist with a certificate or associate (2-year) degree the opportunity to add new skills and knowledge and earn a bachelor of science degree. (Just as the 2-year basic preparation in dental hygiene varies greatly from state to state and from program to program, the content and emphasis of the bachelor's and master's degree programs vary greatly. These degree programs may focus on teacher education, public health, oral medicine, expanded functions, research, administration, biocommunications, or any combination of these elements.)

Thus the 1960s and 1970s marked a period when the definition of legally allowable clinical skills for dental hygienists changed in a variety of ways, depending on the state. It was also a time when sites and roles were reevaluated and new emphases on comprehensive care were developed that decreased the dichotomy between the interests of the "clinician hygienist" and the "community dentistry hygienist." Conceptually, at least, dental hygiene grew in scope and responsibility, but also in complexity.

Practice roles

Dental hygiene is not what it was in 1960, or so it would seem from all this discussion of changed laws, functions, education, responsibilities, and practice sites. Yet, most entering students describe the dental hygienist in terms reminiscent of the pre-1960s evolution.

After 25 years of debate and attempts at regional and national planning, each state still has its own definition of dental hygiene and assisting practice with some duties disallowed and others permitted under varying degrees of supervision. The practice of dental hygiene differs from state to state (Table 1-1).

Educational programs differ with regard to what the students learn according to the legal definition of practice in the state in which the program is located (Deuben et al., 1981). Therefore a program located in a state where no change in the law has occurred or where the expansion of duties is limited may include only the traditional functions of scaling, polishing, fluoride treatments, exposing radiographs, and recording the medical history and intraoral findings. In another state students may learn local anesthesia, curettage, placement of restorations, and physical evaluation.

The following list of functions includes those aspects of care that have been shown to be both efficacious and safely delegable to dental hygienists. The percentage listed next to each reports the percentage of programs that actually were teaching those functions in 1977 to 1978.

Application of pit and fissure sealants	77%
Root planing and soft tissue curettage	74%
Advanced periodontal procedures	63%
Suture placement and removal	54%
Amalgam placement and finishing	52%
Silicate cement, composite resin restorations, placement, and finishing	49%
Injection of local anesthetic	36%
Biopsy procedures	34%
Preparation for placement of temporary crowns or bridges	34%
Cavity preparation	12%

Programs responding to the Deuben survey cited a lack of resources along with opposition from the dental profession and legal barriers as reasons for not including these functions in their curricula (Deuben et al., 1981).

Many graduates who learned expanded functions

Table 1-1. Number of states with expanded function training and examination requirements for delegating specific expanded functions to dental assistants (DA) and/or hygienists (DH) as of Spring, 1980

	Formal training in expanded function*		State board examination required (DA)*
	DA	DH	
Make radiographs	15/50	NA	8/50
Take impressions for study casts	8/34	3/41	4/34
Place periodontal dressings	5/19	6/30	1/19
Remove periodontal and surgical dressings	9/35	5/44	2/35
Remove sutures	8/36	6/42	2/36
Apply topical anesthetic agents	6/32	NA	1/32
Inspect oral cavity	4/19	NA	1/19
Polish coronal surfaces of teeth	7/19	NA	3/19
Apply anticariogenic agents topically (i.e., fluoride)	7/32	NA	2/32
Administer local anesthetic agents	0/0	6/9	0/0
Place rubber dam	11/43	5/45	2/43
Remove rubber dam	11/43	4/45	2/43
Place matrix	7/33	3/33	1/33
Remove matrix	6/30	4/32	1/31
Place temporary restorations	8/22	5/33	3/22
Remove temporary restorations	6/20	3/28	3/20
Place amalgam restorations	3/7	4/9	2/7
Carve amalgam restorations	3/8	4/10	2/8
Polish amalgam restorations	9/19	5/42	4/19
Place and finish composite, resin, or silicate cement restorations	3/6	4/9	2/6
Remove excess cement from coronal surfaces of teeth	7/33	NA	2/33
Apply pit and fissure sealants	3/12	6/30	1/12
Applying cavity liners and bases	4/13	4/21	2/13
Root plane	NA	6/40	NA
Do closed soft tissue curettage	NA	6/32	NA
Administer nitrous oxide	2/5†	3/9	1/5

From Legal provisions for delegating expanded functions to dental hygienists and dental assistants. 1981. Chicago: American Dental Association, Division of Educational Measurements, Council on Dental Education.
*The number on the right of the / is the number of jurisdictions that permit delegation of the functions.
NA, Not applicable as an expanded function.
†Monitoring.

have found that they cannot use those skills even in states where they are legally allowed. Respondents to surveys of dental hygienists show that there is a gap between the functions they learned in dental hygiene school and those they perform routinely (Heine et al., 1983; Minervini et al., 1981).

Even in the 1980s most graduates seek employment in private practice (ADHA, 1982). Employers still expect prophylaxis and associated traditional functions to be the role of the dental hygienist. This, in addition to the hesitancy to delegate functions when dentists are not overly busy themselves, explains in part the reason why practice has not kept up with research findings regarding delegation

nor with the skills many graduate hygienists possess. Thus the idealism of the educational world is slow in altering the postgraduate practice world.

In addition, hygienists educated 15 or more years ago may have had no exposure to potential additional skills and may have little opportunity to master new clinical functions that require extensive laboratory and clinical education and practice. Ironically, the skills and expectations of many women hygienists returning to practice after a so-called family sabbatical may be more compatible with those of the employer than are the skills and expectations of current graduates.

As a result, the bulk (76.7%) of a dental hygienist's time is spent on the traditional preventive services of prophylaxis, patient education, and fluoride treatments. An additional 11.8% is spent performing diagnostic procedures. Thus minimal time is spent on the expanded functions many hygienists learned (Douglass et al., 1982).

Scope of practice

The scope of practice of dental hygiene continues to be defined by what actually occurs in practice, regardless of the idealistic, futuristic definitions of dental hygiene and, in many cases, regardless of the legal scope of practice or the educational preparation of dental hygienists.

Opportunities for practice are dependent on the law, on the state board of dentistry's interpretation of the law and published rules and regulations, on the willingness of dentists to hire hygienists, and, as indicated earlier, on the employer's expectations.

In each licensing jurisdiction the legislative body enacts the dental practice act, usually with the counsel of the state board of dentistry and after having heard testimony from dental-related associations, such as the state dental and dental hygienists' associations. On enactment, the state board is empowered to enforce the law. It has the power to grant and revoke licenses to practice and has certain police powers with regard to violations of the law. In many jurisdictions the state board has authority to prescribe rules and regulations interpreting the law, which more specifically define the scope of practice and which offer an avenue of revision of practice that may not necessitate the revision of the entire practice act, a very lengthy and complicated process.

Future changes

Some people believe that the laws will continue to be revised to expand the scope of practice but at a slower pace than that experienced in the 1960s and 1970s. They see changes tied in part to nationwide economic recovery and to the resultant increased demand for care (and thus, busy dentists interested in maximizing output through delegation). Employment opportunities in a variety of settings are projected by others as being a critical source of change in responsibilities. Yet others project that research findings for the control or elimination of dental disease (such as a vaccine or rinse) will drastically change the profession. Additionally, studies that prove or disprove the efficacy of scaling, polishing, and periodontal procedures in controlling disease may affect dental hygiene practice. The advent of a national health insurance program may have a major impact on both the scope of practice and employment opportunities.

Perhaps the most wide-sweeping impact on dental hygiene practice would be the legalization of independent practice. Hygienists are now required in all states to be supervised by a dentist. Many require that a dentist be on site any time a dental hygienist is performing services for patients. If this restriction were successfully challenged, either as a restraint of trade or as an anachronism for a fully licensed profession, hygienists would control the scope of practice they provide. The services they provide patients could more closely approximate the skills they have learned in school in accordance with their state's practice acts. Independent practice would open opportunities for entrepreneurial hygienists, who currently are required to function as employees. Since only 42% of solo-practice dentists employ hygienists (Douglass et al., 1982), which severely limits the market of available positions for dental hygienists, the possibility of independent practice would open numerous employment opportunities for hygienists. It could extend care to a segment of the population that is willing to seek relatively nonthreatening dental hygiene care but that is afraid of dentistry. Hygienists earning the confidence of such patients could provide a pool of patients for dentists seeking to build their practices and who are willing to provide care for apprehensive people.

Thus it is important for the beginning dental hygiene student to learn the ideal, the conceptual, and the futuristic models as well as the realistic, immediately applicable models of dental hygiene. Graduates may need to be able to function within delivery systems of the past, present, and future. For this reason, the scope of practice is broadly defined as *dental hygiene care*.

THE DENTAL HYGIENE APPOINTMENT

One way to define dental hygiene clinical practice is to review the procedures of the dental hygiene appointment that are implemented by providers of care who are involved in all four phases of a program of care: assessment, planning, implementation, and evaluation.

I. Assessment
   A. Comprehensive health history
   B. General physical evaluation
      1. Vital signs
      2. Extraoral examination
      3. Intraoral examination
   C. Comprehensive charting of hard and soft tissues
      1. Comprehensive caries, restorative, and tooth characteristic charting, including radiographic findings
      2. Plaque and gingival indices
      3. Calculus charting
      4. Periodontal charting
II. Planning
   A. Planning for control of disease
   B. Formulating a treatment plan
   C. Case presentation
   D. Appointment planning
III. Implementation
   A. Patient self-assessment of needs
   B. Periodontal care
      1. Scaling
      2. Root planing
      3. Curettage
   C. Topical and systemic agents for control of caries and tooth hypersensitivity
   D. Local anesthesia and nitrous oxide–oxygen conscious sedation
   E. Restorative procedures
IV. Evaluation
   A. Case documentation
   B. Success of therapy and control
   C. Cost-effectiveness

Associated with these procedures are the support functions of preparing the clinical site, maintaining contamination control, anticipating and responding to emergencies, meeting legal and ethical responsibilities, developing a practice philosophy, and adapting all phases of care to patients with special needs.

This text is designed to prepare students for entry into a clinical practice that will require the performance of these functions and the assumption of these responsibilities.

ACTIVITIES

1. Divide the class into groups of three, and appoint a recorder for each small group. Have each person share his/her definitions and expected functions of the dental hygienist with the other two members of the group. The recorder lists all the definitions and functions given by the group and presents these to the entire class. Finally, the faculty member identifies his/her definitions and list of functions. Center group discussion on differences of expectations among students and between students and faculty, and the possible problems and/or benefits in the educational process that may result from the differences and similarities. The faculty member collects and retains the reports for redistribution to the students during their final week in the program so that students may identify the changes in their perceptions.
2. Have each student ask a dentist what he/she believes are the functions of a hygienist. Compare replies in class and see how accurately they reflect the skills the student will learn.
3. Discuss each of the phases of the dental hygiene appointment, using the program model of assessment, planning, implementation, and evaluation.
4. Review functions that are legally allowable in a variety of states. Summarize the variety of ways in which *supervision* is defined in a number of states. Students should select those states in which they plan to seek licensure. This information can be found in the American Dental Association's most recent edition of *Legal Provisions for Delegating Expanded Functions to Dental Hygienists and Dental Assistants.*
5. Review publications written by hygienists about their practice sites, particularly those that differ from traditional solo and group practices. Discuss the advantages and disadvantages of each and what special skills or interests a hygienist would need to fulfill each role.

REVIEW QUESTIONS

1. Briefly define a philosophy of patient-centered care.
2. Why may faculty members' perceptions of dental hygiene education and practice differ from students' perceptions?
3. What impact do dental practice acts have
   a. On the scope of practice?
   b. On educational programs?
4. What impact might the legalization of independent practice have on dental hygiene?

REFERENCES

American Dental Hygienists Association. 1982. Who we are: a report on the "Survey of Dental Hygiene Issues: Attitudes, Perceptions, and Preferences." Dent. Hyg. **56**(12):13.

American Dental Hygienists' Association Resolutions SR-45-71; R-17-Am-73-H; SR-18-73-H; R-30-73-H; R-10-Am-75; SR-36-Am-76; and R-56-1976-H.

Annual report on dental auxiliary education, 1968-1969. 1969. Chicago: American Dental Association, Division of Educational Measurements, Council on Dental Education.

Annual report on dental auxiliary education, 1976-1977. Suppl. 2. Employment of 1976 graduates of auxiliary programs. 1977. Chicago: American Dental Association, Division of Educational Measurements, Council on Dental Education.

Annual report on dental auxiliary education, 1977-1978. 1978. Chicago: American Dental Association, Division of Educational Measurements, Council on Dental Education.

The Carnegie Commission on Higher Education. 1970. Higher education and the nation's health: policies for medical and dental education. New York: McGraw-Hill Book Co.

The Carnegie Council on Policy Studies in Higher Education. 1976. Progress and problems in medical and dental education: federal support versus federal control. San Francisco: Jossey-Bass, Inc., Publishers.

Deuben, C.J., et al. 1981. Survey of expanded functions included within dental hygiene curricula. Educ. Dir. Dent. Aux. **6**(3):22.

Douglass, C.W., et al. 1982. Dental hygienists' services: a study of group and solo dental practices. Dent. Hyg. **56**(10):17.

Heine, C.S., et al. 1983. Dimensions of career satisfaction for the dental hygienist. Dent. Hyg. **57**(3):22.

Hollinshead, B.S. 1961. Survey of dentistry. Washington, D.C.: American Council on Education.

Legal provisions for delegating expanded functions to dental hygienists and dental assistants. 1981. Chicago: American Dental Association, Division of Educational Measurements, Council on Dental Education.

Malvitz, D.M., et al. 1982. Comparison of Michigan dental hygiene surveys. Dent. Hyg. **56**(1):27.

Malvitz, D.M., et al. 1982. Profile of dental hygienists licensed in the United States. J. Public Health Dent. **42**(1):54.

Minervini, R., et al. 1981. Assessing expanded functions performed by hygienists in Missouri. Dent. Hyg. **55**(5):36.

Sodano, V.L. 1980. Attrition for dental hygiene: fact or fiction? Dent. Hyg. **54**:562.

2 PREPARING THE SITE: OPERATION AND MAINTENANCE OF EQUIPMENT

OBJECTIVES: *The reader will be able to*

1. Identify and operate and/or adjust the following operatory equipment:
   a. Dental chair, including lowering, raising, tilting, and lowering back; rotating chair; and adjusting headrest
   b. Dental unit, including operating tri-syringe, handpiece, prophylaxis angle, high-volume suction, and cuspidor (if applicable)
   c. Overhead light
   d. Clinician's and assistant's stools
   e. Sink and soap dispenser
2. Given any of the common components of the dental operatory, identify basic maintenance procedures to improve its longevity and ensure its cleanliness and satisfactory appearance.
3. Given a series of mechanical or cleanliness problems associated with equipment, identify how the problem could have been prevented.

The provision of most dental services is more easily accomplished with dental equipment specifically designed for patient, clinician, and assistant comfort and for housing special electrically powered or air-powered equipment. This includes a dental chair; a dental unit with overhead intraoral illumination, air, water, high- and slow-speed rotary engines, and high-volume evacuation equipment to remove fluids from the patient's mouth; and stools for the clinician and the assistant (Richardson and Barton, 1978; Snyder and Domer, 1983).

It is helpful to be completely familiar with the dental equipment and its function prior to seating a patient. Therefore this section presents the operation and control of various pieces of equipment. Although every operatory is different, there are many principles of operation and maintenance that are common to most models. In addition to the generally applicable guidelines presented, a maxim to follow is to *read the directions* provided by the manufacturer. Once the directions have been reviewed, it is wise to follow suggestions for cleaning, lubricating, and securing periodic maintenance evaluations and to retain the brochures, warranties, and instructions for future reference.

Properly maintained equipment will break down less often and require replacement less frequently. Considering the cost of dental equipment and the importance of productive hours of "chair time," care in using and maintaining equipment results in less frustration and is an important cost-effective measure (Richardson and Barton, 1978).

THE DENTAL CHAIR

Most modern dental chairs provide for four or five basic adjustments. There usually are three controls located on the side of the chair back or on the back of the chair directly below the headrest. One button or switch will *raise* or *lower the entire chair*. A second will *raise* or *lower the back* of the chair, and a third will *tilt* the entire chair back so that the footrest rises and the headrest is lowered without changing the angle between the back of the chair and the seat of the chair (Figs. 2-1 to 2-3).

With these three basic controls it is possible to (1) seat the patient in an upright position, (2) tilt the chair back so that the patient's hips are well seated at the angle of the chair, (3) lower the back of the chair so that the patient is in the supine position, and (4) raise or lower the entire chair to the correct height for the clinician.

11

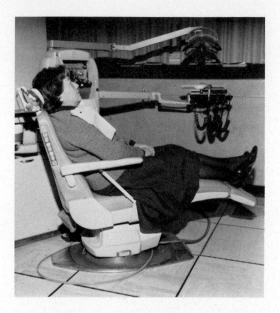

Fig. 2-1. Dental lounge chair positioned with back upright. Patient should be seated with the chair in this position as the first step in attaining the supine position.

Some dental chairs, designed with economy in mind, omit the tilt control, and the patient must reposition his/her hips after the back is lowered to ensure that he/she is not suspended between the backrest and a point somewhere on the seat. The patient's back should receive full support from the chair.

Most models allow for *rotating* the chair on its axis. This control is usually located at the base of the chair and allows the clinician to seat the patient with maximum space available for the patient's maneuvering and then (5) rotate the chair to approximate other stationary equipment and to best facilitate the seating of the clinician and assistant. This is particularly useful for left-handed clinicians who function best with the chair in a position different from that which may provide best patient access to the chair.

Although some chairs are secured to the floor, many others can be moved with a few hefty pushes. A few models allow for easy movement by literally floating on a cushion of air when the appropriate control is activated.

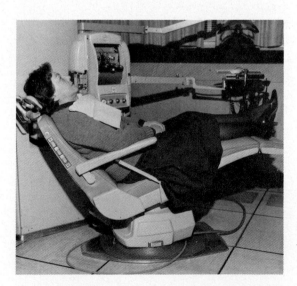

Fig. 2-2. Second step in placing patient in supine position. Chair is tilted backward so that patient's hips are well seated in angle of chair.

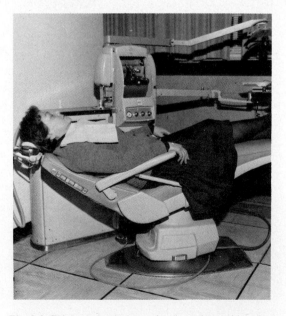

Fig. 2-3. Third step in placing patient in supine position. Back of chair is lowered until patient is in full supine position with toes and chin at approximately the same height. Overall height of chair can then be adjusted to position of seated clinician.

It is helpful to identify what capacity for adjustment each particular chair has. This is helpful in obtaining optimal patient positioning and saves the clinician the embarrassment of running the chair up and down when it is obvious that it is supposed to tilt back. Some chairs have locking devices, and one press of a button will move the patient to a full reclining position. The clinician who intends only a minor chair adjustment may find this runaway chair quite unexpected (Weinert, 1971).

Headrest adjustments also vary from chair to chair. Historically, they have presented the greatest challenge to dental personnel because of their several hinges and multitude of possible positions, with only one or two variations offering comfort to the patient.

Fortunately for the patient, most modern equipment uses a ring- or horseshoe-shaped pillow-style headrest that is easily adjusted and attached with adhesive material to the underside of the chair back. It can be removed entirely with the chair back, providing support for very tall patients or small children (Weinert, 1971).

For those chairs with the multijointed headrest,

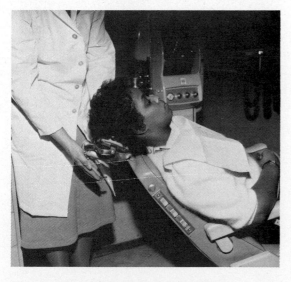

Fig. 2-4. Adjust hinged headrest so that occipital bone at base of skull is resting on padding and neck is in same plane as patient's back. When these criteria are met and patient is comfortable, lock headrest in place by pushing up on lever.

the best rule to follow in positioning the headrest is to seat the patient in the fully supine position and then adjust the headrest so that the pads or bowl of the headrest is located behind the occipital bone. With the patient's head resting in the headrest, the clinician can then raise or lower the whole unit (head and headrest) until the patient's neck is in the same plane with the spine (Fig. 2-4).

THE DENTAL UNIT

Frequently, the electrical circuitry for chairs is connected to the master switches for the dental unit. On some models the master switch is marked clearly, but on other models the switches are located in obscure, unmarked places. Again, it is wise to locate this switch prior to the arrival of the patient. If a modular cart is connected to the main circuitry to ensure remote air and water flow, high-volume suction, and other systems, often there will be a second master switch on the cart itself.

Once the master switches are activated, the following pieces of equipment should be tested for their proper function:

Tri-syringe

Frequently referred to as an *air-water syringe* or *triplex syringe* (Fig. 2-5), the tri-syringe enables the clinician or assistant to direct a stream of water, air, or an air-water spray onto the operative site (Richardson and Barton, 1978). Usually there is one button for air and one for water, with spray resulting with both buttons are pushed simultaneously. Most quality syringes contain a heater to ensure that air and water temperatures are comfortable for the patient.

The syringe has outdated the cup of water that for decades was the primary means available for rinsing. Current practices include irrigating the oral cavity with an air-water spray, with the resultant fluid and debris being evacuated by high-volume suction. "Cuspidor calisthenics" throughout the appointment are no longer necessary.

Many units no longer include the flushing bowl of water. Provided instead is a funnel with a paper liner (Fig. 2-6). The funnel connects to the high-volume suction system. This provision is useful at the conclusion of the appointment when the patient may be given the opportunity to swish and empty as a conclusive gesture.

If a cuspidor is included with the unit and is used

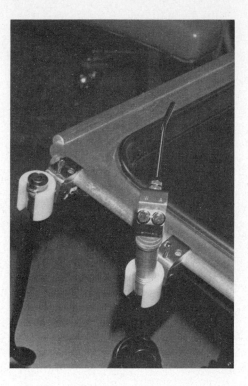

Fig. 2-5. Tri-syringe (or triplex or air-water syringe) includes a button for water and a button for air; activating both buttons results in air-water spray that is ideal for flushing oral cavity. Routine use of this device eliminates need for frequent rinsing with a cup of water.

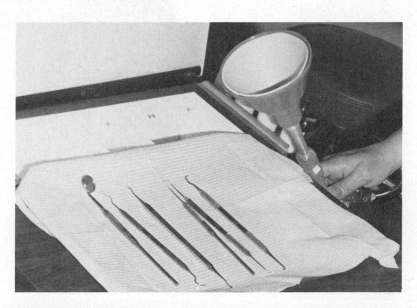

Fig. 2-6. Funnel attachment with disposable paper liner is used as a "cuspidor" and is inserted into hosing of high-volume evacuation system.

by the patients, it is important to locate the controls for the volume of water. It is possible to overflow a cuspidor if the volume of water flow is too great. Conversely, a mere trickle is inadequate to clear away debris. Usually the spout from which the water emerges swivels. The spout should be positioned so that water flows around the bowl. The trap in the cuspidor should be removed at the completion of each appointment and freed of debris to ensure proper drainage (Richardson and Barton, 1978). This task may be another reason for the growing popularity of high-volume suction. The system should be flushed with a warm solution of bleach (one part bleach to six parts water) weekly. Some other disinfectant solution should be used if the piping is of cast aluminum (Williams and Williams, 1982).

Older models provide a place for a cup of water to rest and to be refilled. On most, there is a single control to fill the cup; some have temperature controls as well. A few models have a weight-sensitive cup rest that senses when the cup should be refilled. When the cup is replaced by the patient, the water automatically fills the cup until it reaches the predetermined optimal weight. Generally, the convenience of the cup of water adds considerably to chair time because of the time it takes to reach for the cup, swish, empty into the cuspidor, replace the cup, fill it, and resettle in the chair. Most clinicians ignore the gadget on the unit entirely, opting for the water syringe and suction instead.

Many modern units have more than one trisyringe for use by the clinician and assistant.

High-volume suction

The high-volume suction system replaces the passive gurgling of the saliva ejector. It was introduced to dental practice to enable rapid removal of the coolant water that accompanies the high-speed drill (Richardson and Barton, 1978). It is also useful in removing the water used with the ultrasonic scaler and in evacuating the mouth with frequent use of an air-water spray. In dental hygiene procedures in which loosened deposits, polishing pastes, and necrotic tissue need to be flushed from the sulcus surrounding each tooth, the air-water spray and the high-volume suction are close companions. Evacuation is, of course, useful for restorative procedures as well and for helping remove saliva during fluoride and sealant applications.

After each patient, the line should be flushed by sucking a pint of clean water through the hosing. Tips used intraorally should be autoclaved or discarded if disposable.

Rotary engine equipment

A complete dental operatory includes slow- and high-speed rotary equipment powered by electricity (electrotorque) or compressed air (air torque, air rotor). A slow-speed handpiece is used for finishing and polishing restorations, for some steps in cavity preparation, and for polishing teeth. It operates at approximately 6000 revolutions per minute (rpm) and offers sufficient torque power to facilitate removal of stains when an abrasive agent is applied to the tooth with a rubber cup or brush attachment. High-speed handpieces operate at over 100,000 rpm (Sockwell, 1971).

The handpieces are activated by a foot pedal, called a *rheostat*. Depending on the design, the pedal can be activated by pressing down, by moving a lever to the side, or by rotating a disk. Pushing the lever or disk in one direction causes the handpiece to move forward; moving it in the opposite

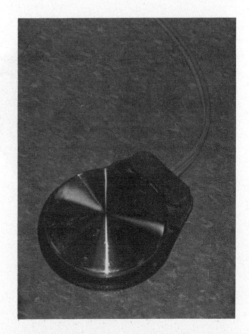

Fig. 2-7. Foot pedal adjusts speed of operation of handpiece. This style requires downward foot pressure. Other styles have a pedal that rotates with a push of the foot.

direction runs it backward. There are often buttons on the rheostat to cause water to flow through the hose (intended as a coolant for high-speed cutting). Therefore if a stream of water is running out of the handpiece at its base, stepping on the water control on the rheostat may stop it. Also, the switch for low or high speed may be on the rheostat. Fig. 2-7 shows one type of rheostat, which is activated by downward foot pressure.

It is important to know which hoses are for high speed, which hoses are for low speed, and which handpieces are intended for each. Hoses should be wiped clean with disinfectant; those covered with cloth usually require regular wiping with a dressing to keep them flexible. Hoses on retractable reels should be gently withdrawn from storage and carefully replaced. They should not be stuffed back into their compartments.

Older equipment may still rely on the belt-driven engine for slow-speed needs. Since an occasion to use this equipment may arise, a few precautions should be kept in mind:

1. Be certain that the belt is not frayed; change it if there is any possibility of its breaking during use.
2. Position the arm of the belt-driven engine so that it will not entangle hair (a knot of hair becoming firmly attached to the belt-driven engine is embarrassing and painful).
3. Ensure that the handpiece will reach to all areas of the dentition when the patient is in the supine position. This may require moving the entire dental chair closer to the engine, since relative positions for equipment were at one time defined by the limits of stand-up dentistry rather than sit-down dentistry.

Handpieces, whether for electric, air, or belt-driven engines, require regular cleaning. It is imperative to follow manufacturer's directions for each handpiece, since some require disassembling and thorough cleaning and lubricating and others are *not* to be dismantled and require only a blast of a canned cleaning/lubricating fluid especially developed for this purpose. Some handpieces should be autoclaved; others would rust and should be disinfected or dry heat sterilized (Sockwell, 1971).

The prophylaxis angle is attached to the slow-speed handpiece. This angle adapts the torque power of the handpiece to the specific purpose of polishing teeth or restorations. In almost all instances the angle needs complete disassembling and cleaning after each polishing procedure, since the abrasive polishing paste easily enters the gears of the device, wearing the gears away and usually clogging the mechanism so that it freezes shut. A few brands are sealed so that entry of contaminants is reduced or eliminated. These brands are accompanied by specific maintenance directions that must be followed carefully to ensure longevity of the angle.

There are a variety of methods for attaching rubber cups or brushes to prophylaxis angles to hold the polishing paste against the tooth. (For discussion of these methods, see Chapter 26).

The prophylaxis angle typically presents the greatest mechanical problems for the dental hygienist. It tends to freeze when not carefully cleaned and lubricated, and it is a weak link in the control of cross-contamination. Its working parts can easily harbor debris and microorganisms; yet few are designed for the autoclave. In the best interests of controlling the spread of disease, only angles that can be cleaned and autoclaved should be used. They are more expensive than others, but some carry guarantees and offer replacement kits for worn parts.

Overhead light

Once all the unit controls are identified and found to be functional, it is appropriate to locate and turn on the overhead, intraoral light. Usually there is a single switch on the light itself. A special high-intensity lamp shines out onto a highly reflective concave surface that focuses the light rays so that they may be directed to illuminate the oral cavity. The reflective surface should be polished at least daily to ensure brightness. This should be done at the start of the day when the lamp is cool (Williams and Williams, 1982a).

The lamp should be allowed to cool before a burned-out bulb is replaced. Since lights often fail when they are first switched on, the lamp may still be cool to the touch and not cause a schedule delay. If the dental light has a quartz halogen bulb, only the sleeve should be handled, since fingerprints can cause the bulb to explode or to burn out more quickly. Sealed-beam bulbs require that the entire unit containing the bulb be replaced. A spare bulb or unit should be kept available for replacement and reordered according to specifications on the package as soon as a bulb is used. In some units a fuse in the dental lamp will blow at the same time that the bulb fails. Extra fuses should be kept for this purpose (Williams and Williams, 1982a).

Many overhead lights are covered by a plastic shield as a safety precaution against an exploding lamp or shattering reflector. A piece of metal flung from rotary equipment could easily trigger such an accident.

To diminish wear on the switch and the lamp, the overhead light should be turned on at the beginning of the appointment and left on for the duration of the visit. When not in use, it can be directed down from the patient's face. Turning the lamp on and off causes it to burn out more rapidly than when it is left on. As with any mechanical switch, each use causes wear. Many clinicians leave the overhead light on all day if a succession of patients is to receive care, turning it off only during extended periods of nonuse, such as during the lunch period. It should, of course, be turned off at the end of the day, as should all switches on the unit. Leaving a dental unit on for extended periods of nonuse will burn out its electrical components.

Another precaution is to shut off the water supply so that pressure is not exerted against the tubing in the unit. Rises in water pressure occur most often at night; thus so do floods in operatories where water pressure is left on overnight (Williams and Williams, 1982b).

Bunsen burner

Dental units often include a small Bunsen burner to provide a source of natural gas that can be used for annealing gold foil or for softening waxes. If the odor of gas is detected when the burner is not in use, the control for the burner should be checked to ensure that it is off. Hoses should be checked and replaced as they show wear. This piece of equipment is rarely used for dental hygiene care.

CLINICIAN'S AND ASSISTANT'S STOOLS

When all main equipment appears to be functional and the hygienist has familiarized himself/ herself with its operation, the clinician's and assistant's stools should be adjusted for their intended occupants. The clinician-hygienist should seat him-

self/herself so that the feet are flat on the floor, the thighs are parallel to the floor, and the abdominal rest is firmly below the rib cage when the clinician inclines forward. A five-castor stool will minimize forward tipping as the clinician inclines toward the work area. Many stools have backrests that should be adjusted to support the lower back.

The height adjustment mechanism for the stool may be a simple screw that moves the seat up or down as the seat is rotated, a foot pedal that releases the seat to rise, or a hand lever that raises the seat as weight is lifted from it and lowers the seat if weight is added to it. Regardless of the mechanism, the stools should be adjusted to proper heights for the clinician and the assistant and kept that way.

The assistant's stool should allow an eye level approximately 4 to 6 inches above that of the clinician. Except in the case of an extremely tall assistant, this will require a ring on the stool for the feet to rest. Neither the clinician nor the assistant should feel the pressure of the stool against the back of the thighs, since that position inhibits blood circulation to the legs (Cooper, 1974; Harris and Crabb, 1978; Richardson and Barton, 1978).

THE SINK

The sink is another essential item of equipment. It should be used for thorough scrubbing at the beginning of a clinical period and for thorough handwashing prior to seeing each patient and whenever an item is touched that may have microorganisms other than those specific to the patient's oral flora (cross-contaminants).

If the sink has no handles, a foot pedal probably controls the water flow. Often a foot pedal also controls the soap dispenser. This obviously decreases the possibility of the sink being a fomite for transferring bacteria from patient to patient.

Towel dispensers should allow the person to grasp and remove a single paper towel without touching the dispenser itself.

STORAGE CABINETRY AND TRAY SYSTEMS

Most operatories allow for some storage of supplies and instruments. The most flexible, of course, is modular or totally movable cabinetry, which can be brought to the operative site. A timesaving and safe (in terms of preventing cross-contamination) method of storing instruments and supplies is the

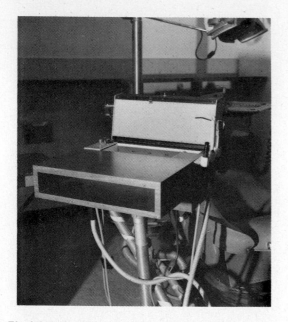

Fig. 2-8. Cart outfitted with tri-syringe, evacuation system, and handpiece for slow- or high-speed use may be all that is needed as a "dental unit" for many intraoral procedures.

tray system. All needed instruments and disposables for a given procedure are stored on a covered tray, which can be pulled for use when that procedure is indicated (Hillborn et al., 1974).

The mobile cart provides an alternative to the traditional over-the-patient instrument tray. The tray of instruments may be placed behind the patient's head for ready access to both the clinician and the assistant. It can hold the tri-syringe, handpiece, and suction equipment also (Hillborn, Campbell, and Hall, 1974). For traditional dental hygiene care the mobile cart may be the only "dental unit" needed (Fig. 2-8).

OTHER DENTAL OPERATORY EQUIPMENT

Other essential dental equipment includes the viewbox for mounting and interpreting radiographic film. It should be located at the chairside so that the exposed films can be readily available throughout a procedure. Likewise, it is convenient to have

x-ray equipment in the operatory (Fig. 2-9) to expose films when such diagnostic aids are indicated. The room must, of course, be lead lined and provide complete protection for the clinician. Because of the cost of lead lining and the amount of room needed to manipulate radiographic equipment, such equipment is usually located in a separate operatory for a number of clinicians to use as needed.

Ultrasonic equipment for removing large calcareous deposits from teeth may be included in the operatory. Generally, there is also an amalgamator for triturating metal alloys for amalgam restorations.

Sterilizing or cleaning equipment may be located in the operatory or in an adjacent central laboratory area. Standard equipment includes an autoclave (Fig. 2-10). Ultrasonic cleaning tanks may be used to remove debris from instruments (Fig. 2-11). Dry heat sterilizing equipment may be available to sterilize items that could be dulled by steam under pressure. Maintenance of the autoclave includes using distilled water, periodically running a cycle with a cleaning agent added to the water, and testing the machine for effectiveness. Rubber seals around the door should be replaced as they show wear. (See Chapter 3 for further discussion of the use of sterilizing equipment.)

The ultrasonic cleaner should be drained when it becomes cloudy (at least once a week). The tank should be washed and fresh solution mixed and added. Proper proportions of solution must be used, and the level of solution must be maintained to ensure proper cavitation and, thus, cleaning.

Hand instruments should be handled carefully. If an instrument is dropped, the working end may bend or break. The ends of instruments should be wrapped for protection during sterilization and storage.

Cutting instruments should be routinely sharpened following autoclaving and during procedures that dull them. An autoclaved stone prevents cross-contamination. As discussed in later chapters, sharpening should maintain the intended shape rather than alter it. Instruments sharpened over a long period of time should be discarded or retipped before structural weakness predisposes them to fracture during use.

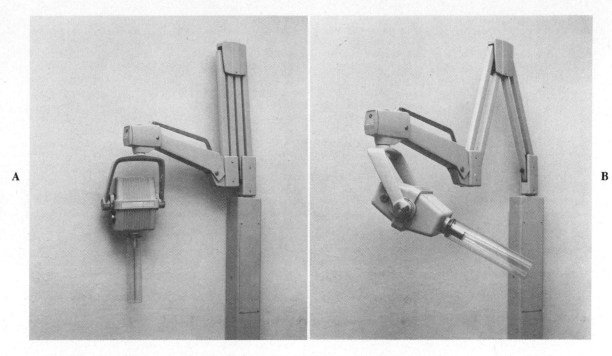

A   B

Fig. 2-9. A, X-ray unit should be stored so that all hinges are closed. This places less stress on hinges and helps prevent eventual "drifting" of head away from patient's face during its use. **B,** Improperly stored x-ray unit.

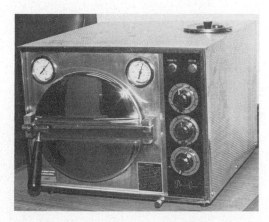

Fig. 2-10. Autoclave provides complete sterilization of instruments and other materials that are able to withstand steam under pressure.

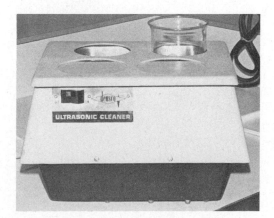

Fig. 2-11. Ultrasonic cleaner removes debris from instruments prior to their being packaged for sterilization.

GENERAL CARE OF EQUIPMENT

Leather and vinyl products should be cleaned regularly with an oil soap that will prevent drying and cracking. The crease where the chair back and seat meet should be cleaned by placing the back of the chair all the way down, and the chair base should be wiped daily to remove dust and debris. The enameled portions of the unit and formica counter tops can be cleaned and polished with glass wax or automobile polish; there are special cleaners for brushed stainless steel. The entire unit should be dusted daily.

The best check of a clean unit is to repose oneself in the dental chair, sit up, and then recline. Looking at the equipment from those perspectives provides the patient's eye view of the otherwise hidden spot of blood, the bespeckled light reflector, the cobweb in the corner, and the red disclosing solution under the lip of the infamous cuspidor.

Patient cancellations and/or an early arrival for the workday provide time for general maintenance of equipment. If these procedures are delegated to another dental team member, the clinician still has the obligation of ensuring that maintenance is carried out thoroughly and regularly.

The benefits include positive patient responses to the general environment; more dependable, functional equipment; improved safety for the patient, clinician, and assistant; and longer-lasting, newer-looking equipment.

• • •

This chapter has addressed some general points concerning cleanliness and prevention of cross-contamination. Chapter 3 focuses on aseptic techniques and control of microorganisms in the dental operatory.

ACTIVITIES

1. In groups of three, use a search and discovery technique to explore a dental operatory in the dental hygiene clinic and elsewhere. (Students should rotate from clinician to patient to assistant roles.) Locate and operate the following items:
   a. Dental chair
      (1) Raise and lower
      (2) Tilt chair back
      (3) Lower back of chair
      (4) Adjust headrest
      (5) Rotate
   b. Dental unit
      (1) Master switch(es)
      (2) Tri-syringe
         (a) Air
         (b) Water
         (c) Air-water spray
      (3) Handpiece
         (a) Mount to hose
         (b) Operate forward and reverse
         (c) Clean and store
         (d) Differentiate high and low speeds
      (4) Prophylaxis angle
         (a) Mount on handpiece
         (b) Attach cup and brush
         (c) Run forward and backward
         (d) Clean and store
      (5) Suction
         (a) Insert tip and funnel
         (b) Activate
         (c) Clean and store
   c. Adjust stool to proper height
      (1) Assistant's stool
      (2) Clinician's stool
   d. Turn on overhead light
      (1) Change lamp in overhead light
      (2) Clean reflector and shield
   e. Identify presence of
      (1) Bunsen burner
      (2) Ultrasonic scaling equipment
      (3) Amalgamator
      (4) Radiographic equipment
   f. Clean the dental chair
   g. Clean the dental unit
   h. Operate sink and soap dispenser
2. Inspect dental equipment for proper function. Discuss how breakage or wear could be prevented.
3. Visit dental offices with modern equipment and offices with older equipment to determine how different models function and how they are maintained.
4. Attend a professional meeting where equipment is displayed. Learn about and report the differences and similarities regarding function and recommended maintenance. Calculate what an operatory of equipment costs, itemizing each essential component.
5. Change a belt on a belt-driven engine.

REVIEW QUESTIONS

1. The overhead light (should/should not) be left on throughout a treatment sequence.
2. The proper sequence for adjusting the dental chair when seating a patient is (five steps).
3. The three functions of the tri-syringe are _____ .
4. Running the prophylaxis angle backward often causes the face of the angle head or the cup/brush to _____ .

5. It is important to know the difference between high- and low-speed hoses and switches because _____ .
6. If a prophylaxis angle "freezes" or will not move, even though the handpiece itself is functional, the probable cause is _____ .
7. The clinician's stool should be adjusted so that _____ .
8. The assistant's stool should be adjusted so that _____ .
9. Leather and vinyl should be cleaned with _____ .
10. Typical equipment used for cleaning and sterilizing instruments includes _____ .

REFERENCES

Carter, L.M., and Yaman, P. 1981. Dental Instruments. St. Louis: The C.V. Mosby Co.

Cooper, T.M. 1974. Four-handed dentistry in the team practice of dentistry. Dent. Clin. North Am. **18:**739.

Harris, N.O., and Crabb, L.J. 1978. Ergonomics: reducing mental and physical fatigue in the dental operatory, Dent. Clin. North Am. **22:**331.

Hillborn, L.B., Campbell, E.M., and Hall, W.R. 1974. Facility design and equipment considerations for the team practice of dentistry. Dent. Clin. North Am. **18:**873.

New dentist buying guide. 1983. Chicago: American Dental Association.

Richardson, R.E., and Barton, R.E. 1978. The dental assistant. ed. 5. New York: McGraw-Hill Book Co.

Snyder, T.L., and Domer, L.R. 1983. Personalized guide to practice evaluation, vol. 1. In Snyder, T.L., and Felmeister, C.J., editors: Mosby's dental practice series. St. Louis: The C.V. Mosby Co.

Sockwell, C.L. 1971. Dental handpieces and rotary cutting instruments. Dent. Clin. North Am. **15:**219.

Weinert, A.M. 1971. An evaluation of the dental lounge chair. Dent. Clin. North Am. **15:**129.

Williams, K.V., and Williams, F.T. 1982. The maintenance of dental equipment. II. Chairs and lights. Br. Dent. J. **153**(2):71 (a).

Williams, K.V., and Williams, F.T. 1982. The maintenance of dental equipment. III. Delivery and disposal systems. Br. Dent. J. **153**(3):113 (b).

3 DISEASE TRANSMISSION THEORY AND CONTROL OF CONTAMINATION

OBJECTIVES: *The reader will be able to*

1. Explain the theory of disease transmission and the necessity for asepsis in dentistry.
2. Identify common pathogenic organisms that may be found in the oral cavity and the disease entities they produce.
3. Define direct and indirect contamination and give examples that illustrate understanding of these terms.
4. Identify precautionary measures that must be taken by dental personnel to prevent disease transfer from patient to patient, patient to clinician, and clinician to patient.
5. Differentiate among the terms sanitation, disinfection, and sterilization.
6. Identify the major sources of contamination in the dental office and describe an effective method of controlling contamination or eliminating it from each source.
7. Discuss five accepted methods of instrument sterilization and identify the advantages and disadvantages of each method.
8. Discuss the choice and use of chemical disinfectants.
9. Describe an effective method of handwashing.
10. Describe the preparation of instruments for sterilization/disinfection.
11. Discuss the operation of the autoclave and the dry heat oven.
12. Discuss indications for the use of gloves, safety glasses, and face masks.

With each educational component of professional preparation, the student hygienist gains a new dimension of respect for the oral environment. This respect should center on the nature of the relationship of the hygienist to the pathogenic (disease-producing) organisms of the oral cavity. Contact with these organisms directly or indirectly occurs practically every minute of the working day. The potential for infection of the clinician, co-workers, and patients is extremely high. Managing disease transmission or, more positively, preserving the health status of patients and dental care providers depends on high standards of asepsis (freedom from pathogenic material) being rigidly applied. In this chapter oral pathogens and modes of microbial transfer are identified. Controlling levels of contamination and procedures for maintaining asepsis are also discussed.

Some professionals may be skeptical about the need for clinician, patient, and environmental protection. Dental treatment may seem benign in comparison with the aseptic and postinfection concerns of the medical-surgical arena. After all, patients are seen for relatively short periods of time, and the treatment in general is superficial. Right?

On the contrary, because the oral cavity supports one of the most concentrated microbial populations of the body, length of time has little significance when procedures (periodontal instrumentation, injection, extraction, endodontics) are performed that expose the underlying tissues to external agents. These procedures cannot be classified as superficial. The main routes for disease transmission occur through contact with the bloodstream and through respiratory nasal/oral secretions. Except for the surgeon, few health professionals come in closer patient contact for longer periods of treatment than the dental team.

For further recognition of the value of rigid aseptic standards, consider the following questions:

How many patients experience (preventable) infection, however minor, because of poor aseptic techniques?

How many professionals suffer eye, skin, or respiratory tract infection or systemic disease because of inadequate self-protection (Hartley, 1978; Miller and Micik, 1978; Rowe and Brooks, 1978; Stortebecker, 1967)?

It is difficult to answer such questions accurately. An awareness of the infectious nature of oral organisms and their potential for transfer is important for the student to master. Beyond developing this conscience about asepsis, maintaining aseptic practices is unquestionably the hygienist's professional responsibility.

MICROFLORA OF THE ORAL CAVITY

The oral cavity represents a host environment possessing features that favor a variety of organisms. These consist of bacteria, yeasts, certain fungi, mycoplasms, protozoa, and viruses (Nolte, 1982). The indigenous resident flora of the oral cavity are listed in Table 3-1. The nature of the oral structures—the mucosa, tongue, and gingival crevice—and the variation in dental anatomy promote the adherence and growth of diverse microbial populations. Salivary components, exudates, and epithelial cells are an abundant intrinsic nutritional source for oral flora. In addition, the foods we ingest are extrinsic nutritional sources. These nutritional sources, ample surfaces to cling to, warmth, and moisture create a comfortable environment for an active microbial community. In

Table 3-1. Microorganisms indigenous to man

Pathogenic staphylococci	Skin, human milk, nasal passages, vagina (during pregnancy), throat, gastrointestinal tract, oral cavity, feces
Micrococci and nonpathogenic staphylococci	Skin, mucous membranes, nose, throat, vagina, postpartum uterus, oral cavity
Anaerobic micrococci	Tonsils, uterus, vagina, respiratory tract
Streptococci	Mucous surfaces, mouth, pharynx, lower intestine, genital tract, vagina
Anaerobic streptococci	Mucous surfaces, vagina, postpartum uterus, oral cavity, human feces
Enterococci	Lower intestine, feces, genitourinary tract, oral cavity, tonsils
Common neisseriae	Oral cavity, nasopharynx, nasal cavity, urethra, vagina
Veillonellae	Oral cavity
Lactobacilli	Oral cavity, gastrointestinal tract, vagina
Actinomyces	Oral cavity, throat
Corynebacteria	Mucous membranes, vagina, skin, conjunctiva, oral cavity, feces
Mycobacteria	Preputial and clitoral secretions, feces, tonsils
Clostridia	Gastrointestinal tract, feces
Enterobacteria	Feces, gastrointestinal tract, vagina, oral cavity, throat
Moraxella, Mima (Herellea) species	Conjunctiva, nose, genitourinary mucous membranes, respiratory tract
Pseudomonas species	Feces, skin, hands, external ear, axilla, perineum
Alcaligenes faecalis	Feces
Haemophilus	Conjunctiva, nose, pharynx, oral cavity, vagina
Bacteroides	Predominant in feces, lower intestine, oral cavity
Fusobacteria	Oral cavity, intestine, throat, genitalia
Anaerobic spirilla and vibrios	Oral cavity
Spirochetes	Oral cavity, genitalia, throat, tonsils, feces, gastrointestinal tract, genitourinary tract
Candida species	Oral cavity, body surfaces, throat, feces, vagina
Pityrosporon ovale	Skin
Torulopsis glabrata	Skin, mucous membranes
Dermatophytes	Skin
Trichomonads	Oral cavity, intestine, genitourinary tract
Amebas	Oral cavity, intestinal tract, vagina, genitourinary tract
Pleuropneumonia-like organisms, L forms, spheroplasts, protoplasts	Vagina, male urethra, oral cavity, throat

From Burnett, G.W., and Schuster, G.S. 1973. Pathogenic microbiology. St. Louis: The C.V. Mosby Co.

fact, the concentration about the gingival sulcus and in plaque approximates 200 billion cells per gram of sample (Burnett and Schuster, 1978).

The normal resident flora and the host generally have a cooperative relationship. Innate bacterial antagonism, salivary lysozyme and peroxidase, and immunoglobulins act to regulate the oral flora and protect the host against visiting pathogens. It is important that the reader understand the body's protective mechanisms before potential pathogens are described. Intact skin and mucous membranes offer a physical barrier against microbial invasion of the bloodstream and deeper tissues. It is interesting to note that the secretions of sweat glands maintain an average dermal pH of 5.2 to 5.8, which is bactericidal and fungicidal (Burnett and Schuster, 1978). To a large extent, once foreign particles enter the oral cavity, they are trapped in the mucus or saliva and are swallowed; gastric acid in the stomach destroys them. In a similar fashion, the respiratory tract has a mucous coat to trap large particles (10 to 50 μg) and a specialized ciliated epithelium that constantly moves the mucus down from the nasopharynx or away from the bronchi of the lungs in order to be swallowed. Smaller particles (0.5 to 5 μg) have the greatest potential for penetration and retention in the lung (Miller and Micik, 1978).

It is the integrity of the individual's innate or acquired immunity, coordinated with the protective physical and chemical factors mentioned, that accounts for blocking disease manifestation.

Tables 3-2 and 3-3 summarize the bacterial and viral pathogens that may be active in the oral cavity or are significant in that they provide a means for transmission by way of the respiratory tract. Hepatitis, tuberculosis, syphilis, herpes simplex infections, and acquired immune deficiency syndrome (AIDS) are discussed in this chapter as contagious diseases that are transmitted via contact with the oral cavity.

PATHWAYS OF DISEASE TRANSMISSION

Diseases are transmitted by inanimate or human sources in a variety of ways.

Direct transmission occurs when organisms are transferred from one host to another, usually by way of the bloodstream, saliva, or respiratory secretions. Entrance to the bloodstream usually oc-

curs when the skin is penetrated by a contaminated instrument or needle or when organisms seep into an open wound such as a cut or torn cuticle on the clinician's hand.

The proximity of the patient and clinician make respiratory sources important. As Tables 3-2 and 3-3 indicate, most of the pathogens inhabit the nasopharynx area (Nolte, 1982). During breathing, conversation, coughing, or sneezing, organisms are sprayed into the environment, producing an aerosol (Johnson and Johnson, 1969; Miller and Micik, 1978). This collection of particles suspended in the air is capable of transmitting pathogens. The organisms may stay suspended for a period of time or may fall rapidly to contaminate the environment and the people in the operatory. Aerosol production is more significant when one considers the equipment and procedures performed by dental clinicians. Handpieces, tri-syringes (air-water syringes), ultrasonic scalers, instrumentation, and even instruction of a patient in toothbrushing are responsible for creating serious aerosols (Williams, 1970). One investigator collected and cultured a sample of air from a carrier that yielded 41 viable colonies of *Mycobacterium tuberculosis*. The highest concentration of microorganisms was found 2 feet in front of the patient where the clinician is usually stationed while an air rotor is being used (Johnson and Johnson, 1969).

Aerosols and organisms carried in the dust make up airborne sources of disease transfer. Patients and workers moving in and out of the treatment area are carriers of pathogens and constantly stir up the airborne dust contaminating the environment. Some organisms (Tables 3-2 and 3-3) are able to survive on inanimate objects—counter tops, sinks, operatory equipment—for extended periods and provide a source of cross-infection. When a pathogen is transferred from one person to another by way of an inanimate source or a source other than the original carrier, indirect transmission has occurred.

As well as being the primary contact between the environment and the patient or between one patient and another, the clinician can be the source of disease. A clinician with an upper respiratory tract infection or, more seriously, a communicable disease such as hepatitis is placing the patient in jeopardy. Wearing a mask and gloves provides pro-

Table 3-2. Summary of bacterial pathogens that may be transmitted by way of the oral cavity during dental treatment

Organism	Bacterial disease	Mode of transmission	Other
Mycobacterium tuberculosis	Tuberculosis of lungs, lymph nodes, meninges, kidneys, bone, skin, oronasopharynx tissues	Organism found in sputum; transmitted by respiratory droplet or contact with contaminated inanimate objects	Microorganisms resist chemicals and survive well on dry surfaces for weeks
Treponema pallidum	Syphilis Primary: chancre of skin, lips, tongue, oral mucosa Secondary: recurrent patch of mucosa Tertiary: gummas of oral cavity, larynx, vocal cords	Contact with oral lesions harboring organism; transmitted by contact with contaminated blood or by penetration of epithelium	Disease is highly contagious in primary and secondary stages; because of nature of symptoms women may be unaware of the disease in early stages; lesions of secondary syphilis may persist or recur for 2 to 3 years
Staphylococcus aureus	Wound infection, abscesses, cellulitis, meningitis, osteomyelitis	Organism found in nose, mouth, skin; transmitted by contact with contaminated blood or inanimate objects	Organism survives well on dry surfaces
Streptococcus pyogenes viridans pneumoniae	Septic sore throat, peritonsillar abscesses, pharyngitis, scarlet fever, rheumatic fever, glomerulonephritis, subacute bacterial endocarditis, pneumonia with secondary septicemia, empyema, pericarditis, and meningitis	Found in saliva, nasopharynx; transmitted by contact with contaminated blood or inanimate objects	Organism survives well on dry surfaces
Pseudomonas aeruginosa	May cause infection in almost all organs, especially in patients with lowered resistance	Lives in water supplies; transmitted through bloodstream by contaminated water supplies	Regular monitoring of water filtering system and maintenance of germ-free lines necessary to prevent transmission of organism
Candida albicans	Adult: candidiasis Child: thrush infection of skin or mucous membrane	Mouth, nails, lungs, skin, gastrointestinal tract, vagina; transmitted by contact with contaminated source	Lesion of the labial commissures occurs similar to lesion of riboflavin deficiency
Actinomyces israelii	Actinomycosis of oral cavity, face, neck, abdominal cavity, lungs	Organism inhabits tonsils, carious teeth, calculus, open wounds, extraction sites, pulp exposures; transmitted through bloodstream and tissue inoculation	Tissue infection usually occurs after repeated exposure to organism following surgery, injury, or chronic irritation
Chlamydia trachomatis	Lymphogranuloma venereum	Oral lesion (primarily tongue) can infect hands of dental personnel	A type of venereal disease seen most often in tropics
Haemophilus influenzae	Pharyngitis, sinusitis, respiratory tract infection, meningitis	Inhabitant of nasopharynx, mucus, sputum; transmitted by respiratory droplet and by contaminated objects	Organism incapsulated and may resist chemicals; organism survives longer on inanimate objects than do other organisms
Bordetella pertussis	Whooping cough	Transmitted by respiratory droplet	Affects 90% of nonimmunized population; vaccine greatly reduces morbidity; incubation 1 to 2 weeks; course of disease runs to 6 weeks
Clostridium tetani	Tetanus	Inhabits soil and intestinal tract; dust-borne spore transmission by spores entering wound site	Spores are highly resistant to physical/chemical agents Protection: DPT vaccine

Table 3-3. Summary of viral pathogens that may be transmitted by way of the oral cavity during dental treatment

Organism	Viral disease	Mode of transmission	Other characteristics
Respiratory virus: adenovirus, coxsackievirus A, echovirus, respiratory syncytial, rhinovirus, poliovirus	Upper respiratory tract infection (sore throat, cough, nasal discharge, fever, chills, muscle aches, fatigue); lower respiratory tract infection; conjunctiva; lesions or oral cavity; meningitis	Organism inhabits nose, mouth, eye; transmitted by respiratory droplet, aerosols, contaminated surfaces	Viruses occur worldwide; peak incidence in fall and winter; asymptomatic carriers and variety of strains make control difficult; all factors of transmission may not be identified as yet
Herpesvirus	Simplex: "cold sores," dermatitis, keratitis (eye infection), whitlow (lesion of fingers); varicella-zoster: chickenpox (child), shingles (adult)	Saliva, direct contact with lesions, respiratory tract transmission	Repeated active phases of herpes simplex may result in chronic problem; chickenpox immunity after childhood episode; only 0.5% to 2% of population may acquire zoster varicellosus
Epstein-Barr (EB) virus	Infectious mononucleosis	Throat-oral respiratory transmission	Incubation period 4 to 49 days; possibility of treating patient in early stages
Hepatitis viruses: A B Other, as yet unidentified viruses	 Infectious hepatitis Serum hepatitis Non-A, non-B hepatitis	Saliva, feces, blood, tears, semen, sweat; transmitted by means of respiratory droplet or contact with contaminated blood	Disease on rise in general population; patient may be a carrier with or without acute episode; incubation period makes treating patient in undiagnosed or carrier state possible; autoclaving instruments necessary to destroy virus
Papilloma virus	Warts	Direct contact or contact with contaminated surface	Patient protection necessary if dental personnel are affected
Mumps virus Rubeola virus Rubella virus	Mumps Measles German measles	Respiratory secretions, saliva, blood, urine, contaminated surfaces	Transfer may occur during incubation phase (18 to 21 days) Vaccine available Rubella is of special concern for pregnant women, since disease may cause congenital defects or death of fetus

tection for both the clinician and the patient. Methods for maintaining asepsis are discussed later in the chapter.

It is also a fact that patients may harbor organisms naturally in the oral cavity that are capable of producing disease if they enter his/her own bloodstream. This resultant condition is referred to as an autogenous infection. The patient is the source of the pathogen (Crawford, 1978). Some of the most prevalent organisms in the oral cavity capable of producing autogenous infection are the various types of streptococci. If during an injection organisms are "seeded" into deep tissues, or if as a result of instrumentation a bacteremia (flood of viable organisms into the bloodstream) occurs, these organisms may cause soft tissue or bone infection. In some patients a serious disease called subacute bacterial endocarditis may result (see Chapter 8).

An awareness of the variety of pathways by which microorganisms, particularly pathogenic ones, may be transmitted in the course of dental treatment is important because all human beings have the potential to contaminate themselves, each

Table 3-4. Comparison of the traditional two types of viral hepatitis

	Infectious hepatitis (A)	*Serum hepatitis (B)*
Virus transmission	Fecal-oral route; also parenteral	From blood and blood products; primarily parenteral; can be by means of oral route and contact with carrier
Incubation period	About 30 days (15 to 50)	30 to 180 days
Age preference	Children, young adults	All ages
Duration of infectious period	Virus in feces and blood 1 to 2 weeks before disease; remains 3 to 4 weeks longer	Virus in blood 3 months before disease; occasional asymptomatic carrier for as long as 5 years
Virus present	Saliva, feces, blood	Blood, feces, saliva
Clinical features*		
Onset	Acute	Slow, usually insidious
Fever	Common before jaundice	Less common
Jaundice	Rare in children, more frequent in adults	Rare in children, more frequent in adults
Severity of disease	Less severe	More severe
Prognosis	Good	Less favorable
Laboratory evaluation		
Thymol turbidity†	Increased	Normal
Abnormal SGOT‡	Transient, 1 to 3 weeks	Prolonged, 1 to 8 months
HAA (Australia antigen) in blood	Not present	Present during incubation period and acute phase; occasionally persists
Prevention and control		
Prophylactic effect of gamma globulin	Good	Possibly beneficial
Dental precautions and control	1. Emergency care during acute phase 2. Mask, gloves, and safety glasses worn 3. Sterilization of contaminated items 4. Disposables used if sterilization is impossible 5. Care with anesthetics (amides) metabolized by liver	1. Emergency care during initial phase 2. Mask gloves, and safety glasses worn 3. Sterilization of contaminated items 4. Disposables used if sterilization is impossible 5. Care with anesthetics (amides) metabolized by liver 6. Update history at every recall visit for carrier status

Modified from Smith, A.L. 1982. Principles of microbiology, ed. 9. St. Louis: The C.V. Mosby Co.
*Many clinical features are the same.
†Test of liver function.
‡The enzyme serum glutamic-oxaloacetic transaminase level is elevated with liver disease.

other, and the environment by direct or indirect transmission. In most cases the exact source of a resulting infection is difficult to identify. This only emphasizes the need for clinics and offices to establish and follow a strict program of asepsis (Crawford, 1978; R.J. Smith, 1968).

Hepatitis

The viral illnesses known as infectious hepatitis, caused by hepatitis A virus, and serum hepatitis, caused by hepatitis.B virus, are of special concern to the dental clinician because they are transmitted by means of the saliva and the blood.

A less common non-A, non-B hepatitis has been diagnosed and is established by exclusion on the basis of the other known hepatitis viruses. In general, the non-A, non-B hepatitis appears to be similar to hepatitis B. It has an incubation period of approximately 7 weeks and a similar clinical course, which may progress to a chronic state (A.L. Smith, 1982).

In all three types of hepatitis, inflammation of the liver occurs. Common signs and symptoms include malaise, fever, loss of appetite, nausea, abdominal discomfort, and vomiting. Jaundice may or may not occur. Arthritis and rash have been noted with hepatitis B. Although the diseases are clinically similar, there are striking differences between them (Table 3-4).

Hepatitis A (infectious hepatitis) has an incubation period of 30 to 50 days after being transmitted predominantly by the oral-fecal route. Parenteral transmission (other than the oral route) is secondary. Approximately 50,000 cases are reported each year in the United States. The disease appears to be acute (having rapid onset) with no residual postrecovery effects noted.

Hepatitis B (serum hepatitis) has an incubation period of 50 to 160 days and is transmitted most frequently by parenteral pathways (intravenously or by a break in the skin).

In the past, controversy existed about the transfer of hepatitis B by means of the saliva. In 1974 Villarejos et al. found hepatitis B antigen in 61% of saliva samples from chronic hepatitis B carriers and in 76% of patients with acute type B hepatitis. Other studies by Ward et al. (1972), MacQuarrie et al. (1974), and Q.T. Smith (1976) indicate the importance of saliva as a nonparenteral route of transmission.

Hepatitis B not only has a lengthy incubation period, but also the actual illness tends to be longer and more debilitating than the infectious type. Host resistance and resilience are factors, but in some cases the disease becomes chronic.

In an informative pamphlet entitled *Hepatitis B and the Dental Profession* (Merck, Sharp & Dohme, 1982), it is stated that there are nearly a million chronic carriers of hepatitis B in the United States, and the pool of carriers is growing by 2% to 3% annually. Exposure to hepatitis may be inevitable as the procedures performed in dental treatment increase the clinician's contact with saliva or blood containing the virus (Kolstad and Crawford, 1978). The health professional's risk of exposure becomes clear in reviewing the following study.

In 1976 Q.T. Smith compared the blood of 6526 first-time blood donors with the blood of volunteer physicians and dentists for the presence of the hepatitis B antibody. The health professionals displayed approximately 3.5-fold greater incidence of hepatitis B antibody than did the first-time blood donors. An increase in prevalence of anti-HBs with age in the health professionals seems to indicate that the longer one is a clinician, the more likely it is that exposure to hepatitis will occur. The result is the development of anti-HBs in a subclinical case or actual manifestation of hepatitis.

Completing a thorough health history will help identify the high-risk patients so that protective measures can be taken. High-risk patients include persons who undergo transfusions frequently (hemophilia patients), those who have impaired immune mechanisms (Down's syndrome, dialysis patients), and those who are drug users and who may be injecting themselves with contaminated needles. The study by Mair et al. (1982) also includes patients reporting a family history (i.e., children of a carrier mother), immunosuppressed patients (organ transplant patients), Southeast Asian immigrants, homosexuals, and prostitutes as part of the high-risk group. Another significant group—health professionals—need to be considered for their potential for transmitting the disease as carriers of the hepatitis B antigen. The incidence of hepatitis B among dentists, physicians, nurses, dental auxiliaries, and laboratory technicians is significantly higher than the incidence in the general population (Rowe and Brooks, 1978).

Some people may be "carriers" of hepatitis. This condition may result after an active illness, or in some cases people harbor the virus without ever having the disease symptoms. These patients transmit the virus as readily as patients with an active case of the virus. To determine whether the antigen has been cleared from the bloodstream, periodic blood tests are recommended for patients with a recent history of the illness. It is also suggested that health professionals be tested occasionally to determine if they are carriers of hepatitis B antibody or antigen.

The risk for the clinician is twofold. Direct transmission of disease can occur through contact with the virus in saliva and blood by means of breaks in the skin around fingernails, etc.; indirect transmission can occur when one is working in a contaminated operatory or accidentally sticks oneself with contaminated needles or instruments.

In addition, the risk of the clinician getting the disease and becoming a carrier puts the patient population at risk. Rimland et al. reported a case in 1977 involving an oral surgeon who was an asymptomatic carrier. Over 4 year's time, 53 cases of hepatitis B were linked to this practitioner. This brings up legal and ethical considerations. Could it be considered negligent behavior not to inform the patient of the risk of hepatitis if a clinician is a known carrier? Sach (1981) implies that courts may view periodic blood tests of dental staff a necessary element of a dentist's standard of care.

Treatment for hepatitis is supportive and includes rest and a balanced diet. The course of the disease and necessary recuperative time will vary from one individual to another. A chronic carrier state develops in approximately 10% of patients, and chronic active hepatitis occurs in about 3% to 5% of cases. It is estimated that 11% of deaths due to cirrhosis are associated with hepatitis B, and the relative risk of primary liver cancer for carriers is 273 times greater than for noncarriers (Merck, Sharp & Dohme, 1982).

Standard measures to prevent hepatitis have included careful history taking prior to treating patients and, once a possible carrier was identified, wearing a mask and gloves, using as many disposable items as possible, and sterilization of all possible equipment. If frank exposure to hepatitis occurred (i.e., penetration by a a needle contaminated by a known carrier), hepatitis B immune globulin was given. Today a vaccine is available to prevent hepatitis B. It will not protect against hepatitis A; non-A, non-B hepatitis; or other viruses that may infect the liver. In light of the seriousness of hepatitis B, health professionals, including dentists, dental hygienists, assistants, and laboratory technicians, need to consider the vaccine for its beneficial protection. The regimen for immunization consists of three injections: two initial injections 1 month apart, followed by a third injection administered 6 months after the first injection (Cooley and Lubow, 1982). Szmuness et al. (1982) had reported on the highly effective nature of the hepatitis B vaccine (Heptavax-B). In a randomized double-blind study of 865 staff members of hemodialysis units, 10% of the subjects receiving placebos contracted hepatitis B infections as compared with 2.2% of the vaccine group. Overall antibodies developed in 92.6% of those who received two injections 1 month apart and in 96% of those who received the third injection at 6 months. Other studies (Frances et al., 1982; Krugman et al., 1981) confirm the high percentage of patients developing antibody to hepatitis B surface antigen after a complete vaccination regimen. Although the specific duration of protection is as yet unknown, available data suggest that immunization will last about 5 years, after which time a single booster of vaccine might be needed to maintain immunity (Merck, Sharp, & Dohme, 1982).

The vaccine is generally well tolerated. The most common complaint reported is injection site soreness. Fever, nausea, headache, and muscle and joint aches have occasionally been reported.

Szmuness (1982) suggests the potential benefits by stating that regular use of the vaccine by groups that are at risk for hepatitis B should cause the incidence of infection to drop appreciably. Furthermore, it should render unnecessary the practice of administering hepatitis B immune globulin after exposure.

Tuberculosis

Tuberculosis is of special concern for dental personnel, since the oral cavity is one of the chief pathways of transmission. Sputum laden with tubercle bacilli presents the most danger for persons contacting the patient. *Mycobacterium tuberculosis* is resistant to many chemical disinfectants and survives well on dry surfaces, making it a matter of concern in maintaining asepsis in the dental environment.

Tuberculosis most often affects the lungs, but other sites of the disease include the mouth (especially a lesion of the tongue), skin, gastrointestinal tract, bone, and salivary glands (Burnett and Schuster, 1978; Rowe and Brooks, 1978).

Urban areas characterized by poor socioeconomic conditions have higher rates of tuberculosis than do areas with high incomes and low population densities (Nolte, 1982).

Effective therapy with medication has significantly reduced the number of deaths due to tuberculosis. Treatment consists of excision of the tubercular lesion and a regimen of medications used in various combinations. Choice of medication is dependent on the antimicrobial sensitivities of the particular strain of organisms involved. Common medications include isoniazid, rifampin, ethambutol, and streptomycin. For those frequently exposed to tuberculosis, such as family members of a tubercular patient or medical personnel working in urban areas or developing countries, a vaccine of attenuated strain is available. Protection may be only temporary with the BCG (bacille Calmette Guérin) vaccine.

Because of the increased opportunity dental personnel have for contracting tuberculosis, periodic skin testing is recommended (Rowe and Brooks, 1978).

Once a tuberculosis patient is treated and

cleared, they are generally followed for a yearly sputum culture and chest x-ray examination to determine any recurrence. A patient who reports a history of tuberculosis but has current medical clearance may be treated as a routine patient.

Syphilis

The incidence of venereal disease is increasing in the United States. The number of cases of gonorrhea is rising more sharply than that of syphilis, but contagious oral lesions associated with the latter disease make if of particular interest to the dental profession.

The organism that causes syphilis is *Treponema pallidum,* a spirochete that enters the body through a break (which need not be obvious) in the skin.

Syphilis has three stages. Each may be characterized by oral manifestations. From 10 days to 3 months after initial contact, a primary stage lesion may occur. This is a chancre and most often occurs on the genitalia, but between 5% and 12% of patients develop extragenital lesions. Greater than 50% of these extragenital chancres occur on the lips, with the tongue and tonsils being other common oral sites. Dental personnel contracting syphilis may develop a chancre of the finger(s). Transmission may occur through mishandling of contaminated dental instruments or inanimate objects such as drinking cups.

After the primary lesion heals, the secondary stage presents. The oral manifestation of this phase is a moist patch on the mucous membrane, occasionally covered by a grey membrane. These lesions are teeming with organisms and are highly infectious. This stage may last as long as 6 weeks and is followed by a nonspecific latent period. Only about one third of persons with untreated syphilis develop destructive lesions of the tertiary stage (Nolte, 1982). Although the occasion for observing a tertiary lesion is rare, tumors of granulomatous tissue, called *gummas,* may appear in the oral cavity. The most common site is the palate.

Treatment with antibiotics is indicated for syphilis. If possible, treatment should begin before the primary lesion occurs. The further along the disease is, the longer antibiotic therapy is necessary.

The dental professional should approach the examination and treatment of each patient carefully. The health history may be helpful in revealing a past episode of syphilis, in which case precautions should be taken by wearing gloves and following strict asepsis. However, some patients may be unaware of having syphilis. Primary stage lesions of the genitalia may go unnoticed, especially in women, and oral lesions may not occur at all. The primary and secondary stages pose the greatest risk for transmitting infection. At any stage, misdiagnosis of oral lesions may occur unless serologic studies are performed. For the added protection of dental personnel, some large clinics, such as those in dental schools, require a blood test as part of the admissions/screening procedure.

To ensure protection during an oral examination, gloves are recommended.

Herpes simplex virus infections

Infections caused by the herpes simplex virus are of particular concern to the dental professional. Transmission of these infections can occur via direct contact with oral herpetic lesions or oral secretions containing the virus, aerosols, or fomites such as dental instruments, handpieces, or impressions (Merchant, 1982). Four diseases caused by herpes simplex viruses are presented here. These are acute gingivostomatitis, recurrent herpes labialis, ocular keratitis, and herpetic whitlow.

Primary herpetic gingivostomatitis is commonly acquired in small children (2 to 3 years of age). Initial symptoms may mimic many acute infections, with generalized malaise, fever, regional lymphadenopathy, headache, pain on swallowing, fretfulness, sleeplessness, and refusal to eat. Within a few days the mouth and gingiva become intensely painful and inflamed. The lips, tongue, buccal mucosa, palate, pharynx, and tonsils may become involved. Scattered aphthouslike lesions appear as crops of small ulcers that coalesce to produce large, shallow, irregular ulcers with surrounding inflammation (Gross, 1981). Merchant (1982) reports that only about 10% of oral infections are clinically apparent, indicating that some children especially may be infectious without usual symptoms or complaints. Within 7 to 14 days the vesicles and ulcers heal spontaneously with no scar formation.

Recurrent oral herpes may appear as herpes labialis or oral herpes simplex. A prodromal itching, tingling, or tenderness may be present in the area 6 to 28 hours before the lesion occurs. The "cold sores" on the lip or at the mucocutaneous junction generally progress from vesicle stage to crusted stage within 1 to 2 days. Discomfort is most severe during the first 24 hours, with the course of the disease running 7 to 10 days. Generally, no scar formation occurs.

The herpes virus may remain latent at the site in the regional nerve ganglia for years. Activation of the virus may be caused by trauma, febrile illness, exposure to sunlight, fatigue, menstruation, pregnancy, allergies, or emotional stress with shedding of the virus as the result. The virus shedding may or may not produce a lesion but may put susceptible individuals who are in contact at risk.

The proof of an antibody titer to herpes simplex virus (HSV-1) does not necessarily protect against reinfection (Merchant, 1982).

The typical features of ocular keratitis include foreign body sensation in the affected eye, followed several hours later by redness, tearing, light sensitivity, and pain. Only one eye is usually involved. Complete recovery occurs within about 3 weeks (Rowe et al., 1982). Ulcers may develop on the cornea, producing ocular damage. The possible debilitation and its effect on employment make recurrent ocular keratitis a serious condition for the clinician.

Herpetic whitlow is a herpes simplex virus of the fingers. Usually the infection follows a puncture wound or a passage of the virus through broken skin around fingernails. The site becomes extremely painful within 3 to 5 days. The digit frequently swells, and one or more vesicles containing clear to turbid, but never purulent, fluid develop. Typically these lesions develop in the areas around the fingernail, although other areas of the finger can be involved as well. The lesion usually resolves within 14 to 21 days, but the clinical course may be prolonged (Merchant, 1982). Rowe et al. (1982) state that the risk of contracting herpes simplex virus infection of the finger or hand for the practicing dental clinician is approximately twice what it would be if he/she were a member of the control population employed in some other field.

Unlike hepatitis B, no vaccine is available to prevent herpes simplex virus infections. As stated above, the proof of an HSV-1 antibody titer does not protect against reinfection. Treatment of herpes simplex is basically supportive in nature, with an emphasis on the prevention of secondary infection.

Topical anesthetics and compounds placed on the lesion to maintain moisture and prevent discomfort have been tried. Gross (1981) reports that topical applications of steroids have been used but have been shown to attenuate the attack and disperse the infection over a larger area. Therefore topical applications of corticosteroid creams should not be used. Compounds such as lysine (Tankersley, 1964) and bioflavonoid ascorbic acid (Terezhalmy et al., 1978) have been cited to accelerate healing time. Currently, acycloguanosine (Acyclovir) has shown promise as a therapeutic agent, and research continues to find other agents to prevent, treat, and diminish recurrences of herpes simplex infections.

Protection and prevention is best obtained by taking a history to identify patients with frequent episodes of herpes. Patients with active oral lesions should not be treated when elective care can be postponed. Wearing protective glasses, a mask, and gloves will reduce the risk of exposure to virus-containing aerosols and saliva.

Acquired immune deficiency syndrome

Acquired immune deficiency syndrome, more commonly known as AIDS, is a disease that causes a breakdown of the body's natural defenses against infections by viruses, fungi, and protozoa. This leaves the patient vulnerable to infections, cancer, or both. A brief description is included because cases of AIDS are being reported more frequently in recent years and there are dental considerations regarding both recognition and transmission of this disease.

The cause of this disease is unknown, but one theory is that it is caused by a virus that is carried in the blood. A prodromal period may last for months, with the patient suffering from fever, chronic diarrhea, weight loss, and general malaise. Oral candidiasis or oral herpes simplex may be present. Lymphadenopathy involving the neck, axilla, and groin areas may occur, followed by skin and ocular lesions of Kaposi's sarcoma. Twenty-eight percent of AIDS patients develop Kaposi's sarcoma, a rare dermal malignancy in which multiple small red-purple to brownish macules/papules from 2 mm to 2 cm appear on the extremities, trunk, and mouth. At this time, no medications are effective against AIDS. The mortality from this disease is 70%. Usually an overwhelming opportunistic infection such as pneumonia is the cause of death.

High-risk patients include homosexual males, intravenous drug users, hemophiliac patients who receive frequent blood plasma, Haitian immigrants, and female prostitutes in contact with other AIDS-susceptible individuals. There is a high incidence of hepatitis B markers in this group. The connection between these two diseases is under current investigation. The evidence that AIDS can be transmitted by blood-borne agents and secretions suggests that the same precautions recommended for hepatitis B protection (wearing gloves, mask, and glasses; use of disposables; and strict sterilization) apply in this situation. The oral appearance of herpes simplex, oral candidiasis, or Kaposi's sarcoma may bring patients with AIDS to the dental office (Cooley, 1983). Although AIDS is not a widespread threat, the seriousness of transmission to dental personnel and other patients and the recognition of the signs and symptoms of this often fatal disease are important.

CONTROL OF MICROORGANISMS

We live in an environment that is filled with microorganisms, including the air we breathe and every surface we touch. In addition, we carry an immense community of bacteria, viruses, and other microorganisms within our own bodies, the richest reservoir of which is the mouth. Many of these microorganisms are harmless to our health, and some are necessary to assist normal functioning of the human body. Others, such as those bacteria and viruses already discussed, are responsible for causing serious communicable diseases. All health professionals are concerned about preventing disease transmission and maintaining an environment where patients can be treated without the risk of contracting infection or debilitating diseases. Optimal safety would require that *all* pathogens be eliminated from the dental office environment, but, of course, this ideal is impossible. It is crucial, however, that dental professionals be aware of the presence of pathogenic microorganisms and their potential for causing and transmitting disease. Furthermore, they must exercise all possible measures to reduce the numbers of pathogens in order to minimize the threat posed to both patients and themselves.

An environment where pathogenic microorganisms are present is called a septic environment; conversely, an aseptic environment would be totally free of microorganisms. Actual asepsis of the dental office is both impractical and impossible, but all attempts toward asepsis improve the likelihood that cross-contamination of pathogens from objects in the dental environment to a person or from one person to another can be prevented. Although achievement of an absolutely sterile office is impossible, providing a safe environment is possible. There are three levels of contamination control that are used to create and maintain a safe dental environment: sanitization, disinfection, and sterilization.

Sanitization

The first level of control is sanitization, which involves the physical removal or cleaning of germ-laden dust and dirt from floors, walls, furniture, and equipment. The elimination of visible soil is the first step in creating a safe environment and must precede all recommended disinfection and sterilization procedures. Sanitization reduces the numbers of microorganisms on surfaces and equipment, thus increasing the effectiveness of disinfection or sterilization procedures that may follow. The presence of excessive numbers of microorganisms, soil, and organic matter (such as blood or saliva) can inhibit or even prevent chemical disinfectants or heat from effectively destroying the target pathogens. For this reason, routine cleaning and scrubbing of all surfaces contacted by patients or clinicians, especially in the dental operatory, is mandatory as the first step in preventing disease transmission.

The general working environment of the dental office should be kept meticulously clean and free of dust. This includes walls, floors, furniture, curtains, cabinets, and counter tops. Daily sanitization of these surfaces is necessary to remove bacteria-laden soil and dust that has entered from the outside environment. Initial cleaning and dusting is best accomplished with a vacuum system that removes the particles rather than a method that pushes them around the room and back into the air. This should be followed by cleaning with a detergent solution. The detergents or soaps used for cleaning not only enhance the ability of water to remove surface dirt and films, but also have mild destructive capabilities against some less-resistant pathogens. In addition, a chemical disinfectant such as a 2% phenol or another hospital-strength disinfectant is recommended to maximize the effects of the sanitization procedures by destroying many of the microbes that might not be removed by mechanical cleaning alone (Crawford, 1978). An especially critical area for contamination control is the lavatory, where pathogens that are spread by means of the oral-fecal route are frequently encountered. Sanitization of lavatories should include not only daily cleaning, but also the use of strong and effective disinfectants that will destroy the large numbers of bacteria found there.

Sanitization of the dental operatory is especially important, since these surfaces are constantly being exposed to oral pathogens during patient treatment. Operatory sinks should be kept clean, and any standing water should be removed from sink counters following handwashing. All disposable refuse should be kept out of sight in trash receptacles that have been lined with disposable bags. Trash containers should be emptied promptly when full.

All surfaces in the dental operatory that would be at or above the eye level of the supine patient should be kept especially clean. Not only will these surfaces be contaminated by aerosols produced during dental procedures, but they are also frequently touched during treatment and are within the viewing range of the patient. To check the effectiveness of operatory sanitization, it is a good idea to recline in the dental chair and take a close look at the dental operatory from where the patient sits. Cobwebs near the ceiling, a spot of blood on the dental unit, or fingerprints on the light shield that may have been undetected from the clinician's vantage point may now be visible. These areas not only indicate inconsistencies or omissions in the cleaning routine, but also affect the patient's opinion of office asepsis. Patients may view these lapses in sanitization as a reflection of a general lack of concern for asepsis and therefore for their own health and well-being. Areas that need special spot cleaning and dusting should be attended to whenever necessary so that visible soil and dust accumulations on surfaces are promptly removed.

Disinfection

Following sanitization, the next level of contamination control is disinfection. Disinfection methods use chemicals or heat to destroy microorganisms or to suppress the growth of microorganisms that remain after sanitization procedures. Disinfec-

tion methods that employ heat as the destructive agent include boiling water and hot oils. These methods are used to treat instruments or other items that are both heat resistant and small enough to be immersed in containers of the hot liquid (see p. 36). A wide variety of chemical agents are also available for use in dentistry as disinfectants. The primary use of chemical solutions is to disinfect surfaces in the dental office that are too large or too fragile to undergo accepted methods of sterilization.

Disinfection methods should be used only to control contamination on surfaces or items within the dental environment that cannot be sterilized. There are instances when instruments or equipment used in patient treatment, such as handpieces, trisyringe tips, or plastic articles, cannot be sterilized by available methods, because they might be damaged by the steam or high temperatures. In these situations high-level disinfection must be used to prevent cross-contamination.

Chemical disinfection. Chemical disinfectants are effective only if a number of critical factors are controlled, including (1) maintenance of optimal chemical concentration, (2) adherence to the recommended exposure time, (3) use prior to expiration of the recommended shelf life, and (4) maintenance of proper temperature of the solution. Specific recommendations for each of these criteria should be followed according to the manufacturer's instructions. In addition, all contaminated surfaces of instruments must be cleaned prior to any disinfection or sterilization process to ensure optimal results. Even under ideal conditions, however, when all these factors are accurately controlled, chemical solutions cannot guarantee complete and consistent control of contamination on all surfaces or instruments. Chemical solutions cannot penetrate into small recesses and destroy pathogens that may lie protected in jointed, hinged, or serrated instruments, or within the cracks and tears in the edge of a previously used rubber polishing cup (Crawford, 1978). Even after recommended exposure to chemical solutions, then, these surfaces may remain contaminated and serve as sources of cross-contamination if reused. Additionally, there are no reliable methods for testing the effectiveness of chemical disinfectants; thus there can be no guarantee that safe levels of protection have actually been achieved. This problem alone should make dental professionals wary of depending on chemical solutions for treatment of instruments or other critical items that could undergo accepted methods of sterilization.

Chemical disinfectants should be chosen according to the range of bacteriostasis or bactericidal activity that is needed. Although some agents can effectively destroy microorganisms, others have only the ability to suppress their growth and multiplication. Those agents that are lethal for bacteria are called *bactericides*. Others, called *viricides*, are effective only against viruses. Similar results are obtained by *fungicides* and *sporicides* (Perkins, 1978). Often the term *germicide* is used to describe an agent that is effective against vegetative bacterial cells but not the more resistant bacteria such as *Mycobacterium tuberculosis* or the virus that causes hepatitis. Even less effective are disinfectants that are described as *bacteriostatic,* which inhibit or suppress future bacterial growth but do not actually destroy all bacteria present on the affected surface.

Only those disinfectants that have a range of destruction that includes all vegetative bacteria, most viruses, and the tubercle bacillus are considered minimally acceptable for use in dentistry (Table 3-5). Higher levels of effectiveness that include destruction of bacterial spores and resistant viruses such as the hepatitis virus are preferred, especially for treatment of critical surfaces and following treatment of high-risk patients.

Surface disinfection. All surfaces or items that are contaminated during patient treatment by either direct or indirect contact with oral pathogens are sources for cross-contamination for patients and dental personnel. Those items that cannot be sterilized and are not disposable must be treated with an effective disinfecting solution following their use.

Since there is such a wide variety of chemical solutions from which to choose when considering appropriate disinfecting procedures, it is helpful to consider the potential for contamination of each surface in the dental office. Any surface or item in the dental environment may be classified in one of three ways:

1. *Critical surfaces* are those that actually enter the mouth (e.g., all dental instruments, dental handpiece, tri-syringe).
2. *Semicritical surfaces* are those that may have frequent contact with aerosols generated during dental treatment or are touched by the patient or the contaminated hands of the clinician or assistant during patient treatment (e.g., chair and unit controls, lamp handle and switch, bases of the tri-syringe and handpiece, chair armrests, drawer pulls, supply container lids, bracket table rims or handles).
3. *Noncritical surfaces* are those that are present in the dental environment but are unlikely to be contaminated by oral pathogens or touched during patient treatment (e.g., floors, walls, furniture, chairs, surfaces outside the dental operatory).

Descriptions of contamination control procedures for each site of frequent contamination in the dental operatory are given starting on p. 47.

After identifying the critical, semicritical, and noncritical items or surfaces in the dental office, one can determine which disinfectant(s) will provide effective and safe levels of contamination control. Chemical disinfectants have been classified as high-, intermediate-, or low-level disinfectants according to their abilities to destroy microorganisms (Bond et al., 1977; Spaulding, 1972). All critical items, especially dental instruments, the handpiece, and the tri-syringe, require sterilization to ensure safe levels of contamination control. Any critical item that cannot undergo sterilization must be treated by a high-level disinfectant under recommended conditions. High-level disinfectants are those that are effective against all vegetative bacteria and viruses, including the tubercle bacillus, bacterial spores, and viruses similar to the hepatitis virus. Intermediate-level disinfectants are effective against all microorganisms except for bacterial spores, and low-level disinfectants are only effective against vegetative bacteria and some viruses (ADA Council on Dental Therapeutics [ADA-CDT], 1982). Semicritical items can be treated by an intermediate-level disinfectant unless there is reason to suspect that they might have been contaminated by the hepatitis virus, in which case high levels of disinfection are required. Noncritical items or surfaces can be safely treated with low-level disinfectants. Table 3-5 lists chemicals that have been recommended for use on instruments and surfaces in dentistry, along with recommendations for their use.

An effective method of disinfecting contami-

Table 3-5. Summary of chemical disinfectants available for use in dentistry

Chemical	Exposure time	Biocidal activity	Limitations
Recommended for instruments and surfaces in dentistry*			
Glutaraldehyde			All glutaraldehydes can cause irritation to
2% alkaline (Cidex)	10 hours	High	skin and eyes; gloves and eyeglasses are
	≥10 minutes	Intermediate	recommended
2% alkaline with phenolic buffer (Sporicidin)	6 3/4 hours	High	After treatment of instruments, rinse in
	≥10 minutes	Intermediate	sterile water or alcohol before use
2% acidic (Wavicide-01)			
Heated (60° C)	1 hour	High	After treatment of surfaces, remove residue
Heated (40°-45° C)	4 hours	High	with an alcohol wipe
Room temperature	≥10 minutes	Intermediate	Overnight immersion can rust some metals
Formaldehyde			All formaldehydes are irritating to skin,
3% aqueous	≥30 minutes	Intermediate	mucous membranes, and eyes; avoid
8% aqueous	10 hours	High	continuous use
8% in alcohol (3-4 g per 100 ml alcohol)	10 hours	High	Unpleasant odor
Chlorine compounds, 1% available chlorine (commercial bleach diluted 1:5)	≥30 minutes	Intermediate	Corrosive to some metals
			May be irritating to skin and eyes; gloves and eyeglasses are recommended
Iodophors, 1% available iodine	≥30 minutes	Intermediate	May stain some nonmetal surfaces
Other disinfectants useful for surface disinfection†			
For routine disinfection of critical and semicritical surfaces:			
1:20 iodophor-alcohol solution (1 part iodophor detergent scrub to 19 parts 70% alcohol)		Intermediate	May stain fabrics (stains can be cleaned using ammonia)
			Residue can be removed by scrubbing for 3-5 minutes with a plain alcohol wipe
For disinfection of critical and semicritical surfaces following treatment of a suspected hepatitis carrier:			
1:1 iodophor-alcohol solution (1 part iodophor detergent scrub to 1 part 70% alcohol)		Intermediate	Surface must remain moist with solution for 30 minutes
Not recommended for instruments and surfaces in dentistry*			
Alcohols		Intermediate	Rapid evaporation does not permit effective
Isopropanol, 90%			exposure of the chemical to microorganisms
Ethanol, 70%			
			Ineffective against hepatitis B and spore-forming bacteria
Phenols, 1%-3%		Intermediate	Same as for alcohols; irregular viricidal activity
Quaternary ammonium compounds		Low	Same as above, also inactivated by soap and other organic materials

*Data from ADA Council on Dental Therapeutics. 1982. Sterilization or disinfection of dental instruments. In Accepted dental therapeutics, ed. 39. Chicago: American Dental Association.
†Data from Crawford, J.J. 1978. Clinical asepsis in dentistry: advanced instruction, ed. 2. Dallas: R.A. Kolstad, Publisher.

nated surfaces includes scrubbing them thoroughly with a 4×4 inch gauze sponge that has been soaked in a disinfecting solution. The term *scrubbing,* rather than *wiping,* is appropriate to describe this procedure in order to emphasize the need to use pressure and repeated strokes of the sponge over the contaminated surface while applying enough disinfectant solution to wet the surface thoroughly for the prescribed amount of time. The actual physical removal of the contaminants increases the effectiveness of the procedure. An effective disinfectant for routine use on surfaces is made from one part iodine surgical scrub (iodophor) mixed with 19 parts isopropyl alcohol. Alcohol used alone is not accepted for use on surfaces or instruments in dentistry, because it evaporates rapidly, does not destroy spores, and is not effective against the hepatitis virus. Its effectiveness, however, is enhanced when it is combined with iodophors. A 1:20 iodophor-alcohol solution provides intermediate-level disinfection, which is superior to the use of iodophor alone. In addition to ADA-recommended high-level disinfectants, a 1:1 solution of iodophor and alcohol is recommended for surface disinfection of critical and semicritical surfaces following treatment of a suspected or known hepatitis carrier. In this situation the surface should be kept wet with the disinfecting solution for a total of 30 minutes to ensure destruction of the hepatitis virus (Crawford, 1978).

Other chemicals recommended for disinfection of critical surfaces include 0.5% sodium hypochlorite (5% hypochlorite laundry bleach diluted 1:10 with water) and 2% glutaraldehyde diluted according to the manufacturer's specifications for high-level disinfection. Sodium hypochlorite can be corrosive to some metals, however, and glutaraldehyde can be irritating to exposed skin. Both the iodine solution and glutaraldehyde may leave a chemical film or residue, which may be removed with an alcohol-soaked sponge.

Practitioners should be aware of the fallacy of the term *cold sterilization* when it is used to describe a chemical method of treating instruments. This term is often used to describe the immersion of instruments between patients; yet most of the solutions that are used are capable of disinfection only and not true sterilization. Therefore cold sterilization is not really sterilization at all, and instruments treated in this way are likely to be sources of contamination when reused. Whenever possible, dental professionals should depend on more effective sterilization methods such as autoclaving, dry heat, or ethylene oxide gas for treatment of all instruments, reusable intraoral supplies, and handpieces.

The use of chemical disinfecting solutions to treat all contaminated dental instruments is not an acceptable procedure by modern standards of safety, with the exception of 2% glutaraldehyde solutions. Many of the chemicals still being used in dental offices do not provide an acceptable level of safety against resistant bacteria, bacterial spores, or the hepatitis virus. Knowing this, dental professionals must consider their legal and ethical responsibilities to the patient before using chemical disinfecting solutions for treatment of instruments and other critical items when more effective and proven methods of sterilization are readily available.

Boiling water and hot oils. Both boiling water and hot oil solutions use heat as the destructive agent. Most vegetative cells are destroyed after being immersed in vigorously boiling water (100° C, 212° F) for 10 minutes. However, since many spores and certain viruses may survive this treatment, boiling cannot be considered a sterilization process. An additional problem with boiling is the corrosive effect of the water on metal. The addition of trisodium phosphate or sodium carbonate to the water will help reduce the corrosion as well as aid in removing debris from the instruments. These additives should not be used for aluminum instruments, which can be corroded by the chemicals (ADA-CDT, 1982).

Immersion of instruments in hot oils or silicone fluids will produce the following effects:

Disinfection: 150° C (300° F) for 15 minutes
125° C (260° F) for 20 to 30 minutes
Sterilization: 160° C (320° F) for 60 minutes minimum

Almost any instrument that can withstand the heat of this process may be treated by this method. A special word of caution: *hypodermic needles and syringes should never be treated with hot oil because of the danger of retained oil being injected into the bloodstream and causing an embolus.* Other disadvantages of this method include cleaning excess oil off items after sterilization or disinfection, difficulty in safely handling the hot oil solutions, and the possibility of unpleasant vapors and fumes from some heated solutions (ADA-CDT, 1982).

Antiseptics. Antiseptics are used in dentistry to reduce the number of microorganisms on living tissues, such as within the mouth or on the clinician's hands (Perkins, 1978). Antiseptics are usually chemical disinfecting solutions that have been diluted so that they will not have a toxic or irritating effect when applied to human tissues. The result of this dilution is that antiseptics have a more limited ability to destroy bacterial cells than do disinfectants used on inanimate objects. Nonetheless, antiseptics can significantly reduce the numbers of microorganisms present and reduce the chances of introducing pathogenic bacteria into the bloodstream during certain procedures. Antiseptics are commonly used before dental injections to cleanse the area so that the needle will not carry a large number of microorganisms deep into the tissue and blood supply. Antiseptics may also be used to clean an area of the mouth prior to a surgical procedure. The use of antiseptic mouthwashes can reduce the numbers of bacteria in the mouth prior to dental treatment (see p. 52). Many clinicians also use some sort of antiseptic as part of their handwashing to enhance the degerming effect that basic handscrubbing has on the destruction and removal of microorganisms. The antiseptic may be contained in the soap or detergent that is used to cleanse the hands, or it may be a separate solution that is applied to the hands after scrubbing. Handwashing is discussed in more detail on pp. 46 and 47.

Sterilization

The highest level of contamination control is *sterilization*. Sterilization results in the total destruction of all forms of microbial life. There are several methods of sterilization (Table 3-6) approved for use by the American Dental Association: steam under pressure (autoclaving), dry heat, ethylene oxide gas, chemical vapor sterilizers, and chemical solutions. Of these methods, the first two, involving heat as the destructive agent, are the preferred methods, with moist heat under pressure considered the most efficient and reliable of all methods (ADA-CDT, 1982).

Autoclaving. Sterilization is accomplished by the action of steam under pressure in a metal chamber called an *autoclave*. The pressure enables the temperature to reach a level high enough to ensure the destruction of even the most heat-resistant bacteria. Water at normal atmospheric pressures cannot be heated to a temperature higher than boiling (100° C, 212° F), but this is not high enough to ensure complete microbial destruction. When water is heated under pressurized conditions, however, its temperature can be elevated beyond the boiling point to produce a super-heated effect that is capable of sterilization. No living thing can survive 10 minutes of direct exposure to saturated steam at 121° C (250° F), which is attained under ideal conditions with 15 pounds of pressure (psi) in an autoclave.

Operation of the autoclave. Preparation of the autoclave should begin by checking the water supply contained in the unit. Steam for sterilization is provided by a supply of distilled water, which may be viewed by lifting the cover at the top of the chamber. The water level must be sufficient to allow for the production of enough steam to fill the chamber completely for each cycle. The tank should be kept filled to the indicator line on the wall of the tank.

Any package, instrument, or container to be autoclaved is loaded onto a metal tray that will be inserted into the chamber. The success of the sterilization procedure is dependent on the ability of the super-heated steam to come in contact with all items; thus they should be packed loosely on the tray to permit an easy flow of steam in and around all materials (Fig. 3-1). If the bags or instruments are jammed tightly against each other, it will be much more difficult for the steam to penetrate through to the innermost layers. Those microorganisms that are insulated or protected from the effects of the moist heat may not be killed during the usual sterilization cycle (Fig. 3-2).

After the trays are properly loaded and placed in the sterilization chamber, the control knob should be turned to the "fill" position. This will allow water, which will later be converted to steam, to enter the chamber. To ensure that a sufficient amount enters the chamber, the metal cover plate at the front of the chamber floor must be completely covered before the knob is turned to the "sterilize" position. At this time the chamber door should be closed and locked into place. All packages should be completely sealed inside the chamber and not caught in the chamber door. If this happens, a com-

Table 3-6. Methods of sterilization

Method	Conditions	Uses	Advantages	Disadvantages
Steam under pressure (autoclave)	Temperature: 121° C (250° F) Pressure: 15 to 20 psi Time: 15 to 20 minutes	All materials except oils, greases, powders, and items that cannot withstand the required temperatures and pressure	Most reliable method Quick and efficient Wide variety of materials can be sterilized	Cannot be used for oils, greases, powders, and heat-sensitive materials May dull cutting edges May rust metal instruments if precautions not taken Metal and glass containers must be open to penetration by steam Failure to follow correct instructions for preparation, packaging, loading, and operating will affect sterilization
Dry heat (dry heat oven)	Temperature: 160° to 170° C (320° to 340° F) Time: 1 hour (plus time required to heat contents to that temperature)	Metal and glass equipment Oils, waxes, greases, powders Needles and other small instruments enclosed in glass or metal	Large capacity Low cost of equipment Does not dull cutting edges Only method for oils, greases, powders Does not erode ground glass surfaces Does not rust or corrode metals Simple to operate Can penetrate glass and metal containers	Requires longer time to sterilize than moist heat Cannot be used on some heat-sensitive materials; temperatures above 170° C (340° F) will disjoin soldered instruments Instruments must be dry before sterilization to prevent rusting
Ethylene oxide gas	Temperature: 120° F Time: 2 to 3 hours or Temperature: room temperature Time: 12 hours	Sterilization of commercial products and items in hospital environments Most dental supplies and instruments	Useful for sterilization of handpieces that cannot be autoclaved Useful for heat-sensitive items	Causes irritation to eyes and nose Inhalation must be avoided Toxic odor may be absorbed by some plastic or rubber items Impractical for routine sterilization between patients Equipment more expensive than other methods
Chemical vapor sterilizers	Temperature: 127° C (260° F) Pressure: 20 to 25 psi Time: 30 minutes	Any item tested for vapor penetration	Does not require high temperatures of dry heat Relatively short cycle useful for handpieces Will not rust instruments	Cannot be used for materials that are sensitive to the necessary temperature or pressure Vapor must penetrate through all materials Some materials may be incompatible with the chemicals used
Chemical solutions (glutaraldehyde)	Temperature: room temperature Time: 6¾ to 10 hours Requires optimal concentration of chemical solution	Plastics and other heat-sensitive materials that cannot withstand heat sterilization	Does not require heat to achieve sterilization Plastics, rubber, and other heat-sensitive materials can be sterilized Good for instruments containing bonded parts (e.g., lenses, mirrors, handpieces) Chemical not affected by soaps and detergents	Requires immersion of objects for minimum of 6¾ to 10 hours to achieve sterilization Destruction of hepatitis virus is probable but not proved Irritates skin and mucous membranes; should be rinsed off instruments before their use May corrode carbon steel after 24 hours of immersion

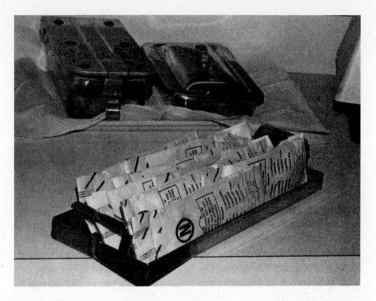

Fig. 3-1. Neat and effective method of arranging instruments on tray. If tray is not overloaded, steam will be able to circulate freely around all packages and complete sterilization should be accomplished. Note also that color indicators on autoclave bags and the sealing tape have changed colors from those in Fig. 3-2. Although this indicates that the load has been heated, it is not a guarantee of sterilization.

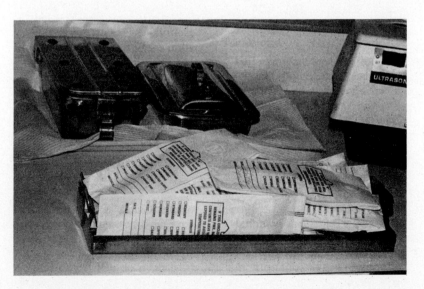

Fig. 3-2. Example of overloaded autoclave tray. If too many items are placed on tray and then crammed into chamber, sterilization may not be achieved. Light shades of sealing tape and color indicators at top of bags indicate that this load has not been heated in sterilizer.

plete seal cannot be achieved within the chamber. As a result, the temperature inside the chamber will not rise high enough to achieve sterilization.

When the knob is turned to the "sterilize" position, water will stop entering the chamber, and the inside temperature of the autoclave will begin to rise. The thermostatic controls on the front of the unit should be set so that when the desired temperature is reached, along with its corresponding pressure, the heat will be maintained at that level for the remainder of the sterilization cycle. Every autoclave should be equipped with a safety valve to prevent the inner chamber from reaching an unnecessarily high temperature or pressure. Once the chamber has reached the appropriate conditions for sterilization, usually 121° C at 15 psi, the timer on the unit should be set for the desired length of time. In most instances this will be 15 to 20 minutes. *It is important to remember that the timing of the sterilization cycle should not begin until the recommended conditions have been reached and the temperature of the contents has reached 121° C.* These conditions must then be maintained for the entire length of the cycle. At the end of this period, as indicated by the timer, the control knob can be turned to the "vent" position. This will allow the steam to escape from the chamber so that the pressure is released, and the chamber will begin to cool. These changes should be indicated by the temperature and pressure gauges as they move slowly toward zero. When both levels have been reduced to zero, the chamber door can be opened. No attempt to open the door should be made until the pressure has subsided within the chamber. The door should be left ajar for several minutes before trays are removed so that the bags and other materials have a chance to dry before they are stored. Even after a few minutes of cooling, however, the metal trays and their contents will still be hot and should be handled with care.

Monitoring sterilization. The effectiveness of any sterilization procedure cannot be guaranteed unless the clinician is certain that the desired conditions such as temperature, pressure, time, and/ or chemical exposure are consistently being met. Even the best gauges are not foolproof, and periodic tests should be made to ensure the effectiveness of all equipment.

All accepted methods of sterilization can be reg-ularly monitored for effectiveness. Special bacterial spore test strips or vials are available for monitoring autoclaves, dry heat ovens, ethylene oxide sterilizers, and chemical vapor sterilizers. These strips or vials provide the most reliable test of sterilization effectiveness. Autoclaves and chemical vapor sterilizers are tested using the organism *Bacillus stearothermophilus,* a bacterial spore that can withstand all but the most stringent sterilization conditions. The organism *B. subtilis var niger* is used to test dry heat ovens and ethylene oxide sterilizing equipment. The spore-impregnated strips or spore-containing test vials should be placed at the center of a normal load in the device to be tested and submitted to the usual sterilization cycle. After treatment, the strip or vial can be cultured and incubated in the dental office or sent to a sterilization monitoring service laboratory for analysis. Evidence of bacterial growth following incubation indicates that some of the bacterial spores survived the sterilization process and that equipment malfunction or other errors have been made during the sterilization procedure. The American Dental Association recommends that sterilization equipment be tested weekly by this method (ADA Council on Dental Materials, Instruments, and Equipment [ADA-CDM], 1981).

Both heat-sensitive labels on autoclave bags and special heat-sensitive tape used to seal bags change color after being heat processed. Chemical indicators housed in glass or plastic tubes can be inserted into packs of instruments or supplies to be sterilized. These indicators will undergo a change in color or physical state when subjected to sterilizing conditions. Although these indicators provide an easy means of identifying processed items from nonprocessed ones, the color change or physical change is only an indication of exposure to sterilization temperatures or chemicals. They can provide no assurance that the exact conditions required for sterilization have been met for an adequate amount of time. In instances where the actual results from spore test monitoring are not immediately available, however, these types of indicators can assist in the detection of improper sterilization procedures or gross equipment malfunction.

Dry heat. Dry heat may be used for materials that cannot withstand steam under pressure. Examples of these materials are oils, powders, greases, and some dental instruments and handpieces. Dry heat is the method of choice for fine endodontic instruments that need to be sterilized. The dry heat oven is much like a regular oven. The same considerations for loading the oven apply as for loading the autoclave to ensure that the internal temperature of all packages is high enough to kill the pathogens that might be present. Instruments should be packed in a manner that will allow the heated air to circulate freely around the contents of the oven.

Since some microorganisms are extremely resistant to dry heat, it is necessary to maintain high temperatures for a prolonged period of time until all spores have been killed. An internal temperature of 160° to 170° C (320° to 340° F) must be achieved and maintained for a minimum of 1 hour. The length of time required to achieve this internal temperature is dependent on the size of the load, the materials being heated, and the wrapping materials used. For example, a few unwrapped metal instruments could be heated to sterilization temperatures much faster than a large number of heavily wrapped bundles. Since a certain amount of time is required to heat the entire contents of the oven to this temperature, a total sterilization period of 2 hours is often recommended. The temperature should be checked by means of a thermometer that indicates the internal temperature of the oven. More specific instructions as to the recommended temperatures and times required for certain materials are given in Table 3-6. Test bacterial spores are recommended to monitor the effectiveness of this equipment in achieving sterilization.

Ethylene oxide gas. A third method of sterilization is ethylene oxide gas. This method is used mainly by hospitals when it is necessary to sterilize huge quantities of materials and instruments at one time. It is also used for sterilization of some commercial products. Recently, smaller sterilizing units that are more suitable in size and expense for the dental office have been made available. The main advantage of ethylene oxide gas sterilization is that it does not require the high temperatures of either the autoclave or the dry heat oven, so that heat-sensitive materials, including plastic items and all handpieces, can be safely sterilized. Generally, a sterilization cycle requires 4 to 5 hours, and equipment for the procedure is expensive. In addition, ethylene oxide gas does have some toxic properties that make it irritating to the eyes and nose. These toxic effects can be retained by plastics or rubber materials that are sterilized in this manner. Rubber and plastic materials that can absorb the gas should be aerated for 24 hours before they are used. Prolonged inhalation of the gas in even low concentrations should be avoided (ADA-CDT, 1982).

Chemical vapor. Chemical vapor sterilization is another method that is available for use in dental practices. The chemical vapor sterilizer is an autoclave-like device that uses a mixture of chemical vapors as its sterilizing system. These chemicals may be a mixture of alcohols, ketones, formaldehyde, and water heated to a temperature of 27° C under 20 to 25 psi for 20 to 30 minutes. This method has been found to be effective against both spore-forming and non-spore-forming organisms (Coughlin et al., 1967; Haberman, 1962; Lyon and Devine, 1974). The chemical vapor sterilizer should not be used for any material that cannot withstand the necessary temperatures or that is incompatible with the chemical agents. Wrapping materials or containers that are used must be permeable to the chemical vapors to ensure effective exposure to all surfaces. It is effective for materials that are heat sensitive and cannot withstand autoclaving or dry heat temperatures. The risk of damage by rust or corrosion is also diminished by this method of sterilization. Chemical vapor sterilization should be monitored with spore test organisms to ascertain that all conditions for sterilization are being met.

Chemical solutions. The only chemical solution that has been shown to achieve true sterilization is glutaraldehyde. A 2% concentration of this solution has been shown to destroy fungi, viruses, and bacteria including *Mycobacterium tuberculosis* (disinfection) after immersion for 10 minutes. It is capable of killing resistant bacterial spores after an immersion period of 6¾ to 10 hours. Exposure times vary depending on the product used and the amount of biocidal activity desired (ADA-CDT, 1982). The manufacturer's directions should be followed carefully to ensure optimal results. Because the etiologic agent for viral hepatitis cannot be cultured, there is no guarantee that a 2% concentration of glutaraldehyde will destroy this virus. Although its effectiveness against the hepatitis virus at the 10-hour exposure level is probable, it cannot be recommended as a substitute for sterilizing pro-

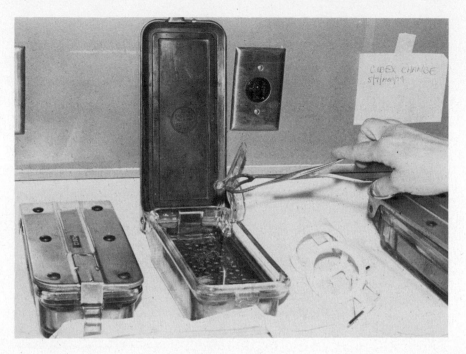

Fig. 3-3. Items that have been disinfected in a chemical solution should be removed from container with sterile forceps to avoid recontamination before use. Only items that cannot be sterilized are treated by chemical means. Note that the age of the chemical solution has been posted to prevent using it past the recommended time.

cedures such as the autoclave or dry heat oven. In spite of its potency, the 10 hours required for sterilization makes the use of this chemical somewhat impractical for routine treatment of instruments and other critical items between patients. It should be considered, however, for obtaining a high degree of disinfection or sterilization for any items that cannot be sterilized by heat, such as plastics or rubber items (Fig. 3-3).

Disposable supplies and instruments

The American Dental Association states that the proper handling and preparation of instruments in the dental office should provide the practitioner with instruments that are completely free of viable bacteria, viruses, and spores while maintaining their usefulness. This can be accomplished by sterilizing reusable instruments by one of the methods discussed previously or by using disposable items that are discarded after one use. Instruments and supplies that are used intraorally and cannot be sterilized should be avoided in dental practice.

Many dental supplies, such as tongue blades, cotton-tipped applicators, aspirator tips, saliva ejectors, radiograph holders, rubber polishing cups, fluoride trays, syringes, and needles, are disposable. These supplies are stored in sterile containers, used only once, and then discarded.

There are a number of advantages to using disposable supplies. The most important advantage is the prevention of cross-contamination, since these items are used only once and then discarded. The use of disposable needles is especially valuable in the prevention of serum hepatitis, since contaminated needles are known to be one of the chief causes of transmission of this serious disease. The use of disposable supplies saves considerable time and money that would otherwise be expended to clean and sterilize the supplies if they were to be reused. Disposable tray covers, patients' napkins, and headrest covers not only protect the patient and the working environment from contamination by bacterial aerosols and splatter, but also reduce significantly the time and effort needed to disinfect those surfaces between patients. Use of disposable hand towels is a necessity in the dental office. Cloth towels become contaminated after only one use and cannot be safely reused until they have been cleaned and sterilized (Eigener, 1977). The advantages of using disposable supplies should be weighed against the cost of purchasing them. Whenever possible, dental professionals should consider the use of disposable items for purposes of convenience and as a means of preventing cross-contamination.

Preparing instruments for sterilization

Cleaning instruments. Any instrument or other item that is to be sterilized or disinfected must be prepared by thorough cleaning, rinsing, and drying before it undergoes the chemical or heat process that will destroy the microorganisms it harbors. The presence of blood, saliva, soap films, and other organic debris not only increases the numbers of microorganisms that must be killed, but also protects them against the destructive agent. The more protected a microorganism is by insulating debris, soap residue, or other microorganisms, the longer it will take for it to be destroyed. Recommended sterilization and disinfection conditions (time, concentration, temperature) depend on the intimate contact of the chemical or heating agent with the microorganisms. This will only occur when thorough washing, rinsing, and drying of all instruments precedes the disinfecting or sterilization process.

Instruments should be cleaned as soon as possible after they have been used in order to expedite the removal of blood and debris before they dry. If immediate cleaning is not possible, instruments should be soaked in a cool detergent or disinfectant solution. Ultrasonic cleaning is preferred for instrument preparation over hand scrubbing because the ultrasonic cleaner can dislodge contaminated material from grooves, hinges, and other surfaces that are not easily reached with a brush. Ultrasonic cleaning is also safer because it reduces the need to handle contaminated instruments. Protective rubber gloves should always be worn when handling contaminated instruments to prevent accidental injury and infection of the handler.

When an ultrasonic cleaner is not available, it is necessary to scrub instruments with a brush. A sterilized brush should be reserved for scrubbing instruments. A detergent (not soap) is necessary for loosening blood and debris from the instrument surfaces and for reducing surface tension. During and after scrubbing, all loosened soil and blood should be rinsed off by running the instruments under cool water. All removable parts must be disassembled, and hinged instruments such as scissors must be opened to ensure that all surfaces have been cleaned. The final rinse should be in warm or hot water so that all residual detergent is completely removed. A NOTE OF CAUTION: Contaminated instruments used in the treatment of a known or suspected hepatitis carrier should not be scrubbed or ultrasonically cleaned prior to sterilization. After use, these instruments should be placed in a tray and sterilized before they are handled. Following sterilization, the instruments should be cleaned carefully and then resterilized.

Use of the ultrasonic cleaner. Gross debris may be rinsed from contaminated instruments prior to cleaning. They are then placed into the cleaning solution, which can be either a nonfoaming commercial detergent (see manufacturer's instructions) or a solution of one part iodine surgical scrub to 19 parts detergent (Crawford, 1978). The instruments should be treated for 5 minutes in the ultrasonic bath with the cover in place to avoid splattering of the solution onto adjacent surfaces. Following cleaning, the instruments should be removed with forceps or heavily gloved hands, rinsed, inspected for debris, and then either rinsed in alcohol to enhance drying or dried with paper towels. Instruments that will be sterilized by dry heat, chemical vapor, ethylene oxide gas, or glutaraldehyde solution must be dry prior to being sterilized. Carbon steel instruments or low-quality stainless steel instruments that are likely to rust as a result of autoclaving should be dipped in protective solutions such as 1% sodium nitrite (ADA-CDT, 1982) or amine compounds to prevent corrosion. The cleaned instruments can then be wrapped or placed in trays for sterilization. At the end of the day, the cleaning solution in the ultrasonic cleaner should be discarded, and the reservoir and tray should be disinfected with 0.5% sodium hypochlorite (Crawford, 1978; Parker, 1976).

Wrapping instruments. Unless an instrument or item will be used immediately after it is sterilized, it should be wrapped in a paper or plastic bag specifically made for storage of instruments during

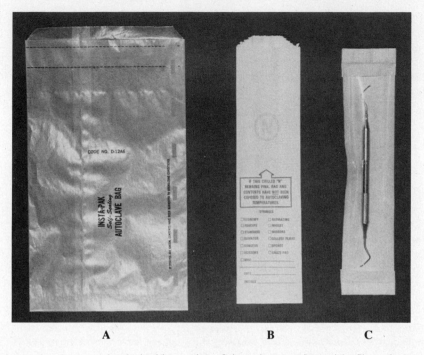

A   **B**   **C**

Fig. 3-4. Autoclave bags may be obtained in a variety of sizes, shapes, and materials. Shown here are three different types of bags. **A,** Autoclave bag that is large enough to facilitate items such as impression trays or cheek retractors, which are normally too wide for the smaller bags. **B,** Common type of opaque paper bag designed for easy labeling. Note faint heat-sensitive symbol at top portion of bag. **C,** Bag made of opaque paper on one side and clear plastic on the other so that the instrument can be easily identified without opening the bag.

and after heat sterilization (Fig. 3-4). These bags are constructed of materials that can withstand the conditions of sterilization without interfering with the sterilization of their contents. Sterilization bags are usually constructed so that once they are sealed, they maintain the sterility of their contents unless the bag is torn or punctured. Damage to sterilization bags can be prevented by wrapping sharp instruments in a paper towel or shielding sharp edges with cotton rolls or gauze sponges before inserting them into the bag. Prior to packaging, jointed instruments must be disassembled and hinged instruments must be opened. This procedure will ensure that all parts of the instruments that may be contaminated are subjected to the sterilizing agent. Instruments that can be damaged by contact with other instruments, such as the head of the mouth mirror, should be wrapped separately so that they are protected from damage.

The most common type of sterilization bag is made of paper and is disposable. These bags come in a variety of shapes and sizes, depending on the number and type of instruments that are being sterilized. To increase practice efficiency, it is advisable to wrap instruments together as a "tray" specific to a designated procedure. By wrapping instruments according to their intended use, only one or two sterile packages need to be opened to furnish the entire tray setup. This is important, since whenever a bag is opened, its entire contents are exposed to environmental contaminants and can no longer be considered sterile. By wrapping instruments with this in mind, bags need not be opened unless all instruments are to be used. Instruments that are used infrequently should be packaged individually. Each bag should be labeled so that instruments for any given tray setup can be easily identified. As an added convenience, some sterilization bags are made of transparent materials so that the contents can be identified without the need for labeling or opening the bag. These are especially useful for singly wrapped instruments. Following are examples of instruments that may be packaged together:

Treatment procedure	Tray setup (package together)
Initial examination	Mirror, explorer, probe, gauze sponge, tongue blade
Scaling	Assorted scalers and/or curettes
Root planing/curettage	Gracey curettes, explorer, mirror
Polishing	Mirror, prophylaxis angle, rubber cup, occlusal brush, dappen dish

Once the wrapped instruments and supplies are inserted into the labeled bag, the open end of the bag should be closed with a double fold and sealed with a piece of specially designed sterilization tape. The tape should be long enough to seal the entire fold and lap slightly around to the opposite side on both ends. Sealing and taping in this way will help ensure that the bag is properly sealed against recontamination during storage. Muslin or paper-wrapped packs should be resterilized if not used within 30 days. Sealed paper and plastic packs should be resterilized after 4 months, and sealed plastic packs can last up to 6 months before requiring resterilization (ADA-CDM, 1981).

Instrument transfer. In preparing the tray for treatment, sterile supplies should be transferred to the bracket table or from one container to another by means of sterile forceps rather than with the fingers. This will help ensure that pathogens that may be transmitted by the hands are not introduced into an otherwise aseptic environment. Sterile cotton pliers may be included on each tray setup for this purpose. If transfer forceps are used, they should be kept in a container that has been sterilized and contains a phenolic disinfectant solution. The solution should be changed according to the manufacturer's instructions, and the whole assembly should be autoclaved weekly (Rowe and Brooks, 1978). The transfer forceps should not contact the sides of the container during removal. They should be held in a vertical position with tips down at all times so that the disinfecting solution does not run over a contaminated part of the forceps and then back onto the disinfected part that touches the supplies. Since the objective is to keep the forceps as

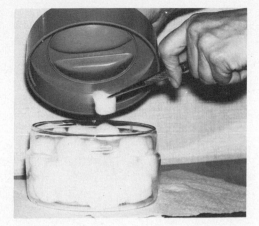

Fig. 3-5. Transfer of supplies from a sterile container should always be accomplished by means of sterile forceps and *not* by hand. Note that lid of container is held so that sterile inner surface is not exposed to dust and particles in air and is not laid down on counter top.

free from contamination as possible, they should be autoclaved regularly, and the container should be covered to prevent contamination from airborne bacteria and other sources of contamination.

When supplies are being transferred from a covered container, it is best to hold the lid top up with one hand while removing the supplies with the forceps in the other hand (Fig. 3-5). This prevents airborne bacteria from settling onto the inside of the lid, which is then replaced on the sterile container. If it is necessary to lay the lid down, however, it should be put down with the inside surface up so that the rims of the lid are not contaminated by the counter top.

Removing sterile instruments from an autoclave bag for positioning on the tray requires a special procedure also. Since the outside of the bag has contacted the storage drawer and has been handled since it left the autoclave, the outside is no longer sterile. Therefore placing the bag on the tray contaminates the whole tray. The proper procedure is to tear off the end of the bag and slide the wrapped instruments onto the tray without the outside of the bag contacting the tray. The bag should be discarded, and the clinician's hands should be washed before handling the sterile instruments. The tray setup should be covered with a disposable cover. The inside of the folded cover should be toward the instruments, since this surface is relatively free of microorganisms (because of its heat processing) and has not been in contact with the storage area and human hands, as has the outside of the cover.

Hand scrubbing and washing

One important point that has been stressed is that everything and anything that goes into a patient's mouth should be sterilized if possible, or disposable supplies should be used so that the chance of cross-contamination is minimized. The most obvious and unavoidable failure of this rule is the clinician's hands. There is no acceptable way to sterilize human hands. Certainly, there is less chance of cross-contamination if the clinician wears a new pair of disposable gloves for each patient, but there is always the possibility that the gloves will tear. It is imperative that dental care providers give close attention to the washing and care of the hands to prevent contamination. For the clinician's own protection, a close inspection of the hands should be conducted to ensure that there are no potential portals of entry for bacteria. Hangnails or small cuts or irritated areas are potential gates for infectious bacteria to enter the bloodstream. Any breaks in the skin should be protected by gloves or finger cots. Whether or not the clinician is planning on using disposable gloves, the hands should be carefully scrubbed to remove as many as possible of the microorganisms that are present.

There are two levels of bacterial residence on the hands. There is a superficial layer of microorganisms, or *transient bacteria*, on the outer layers of the skin, under the fingernails, and around the nails. These include all the microorganisms that are picked up in the environment. There is also a deeper level, called *resident bacteria*. These bacteria are part of the normal flora of the skin and lie deep in the crevices and folds of the skin. A quick, superficial washing will not dislodge these bacteria. This is significant, since many of these types are potential pathogens. Any technique of washing must be thorough enough to remove most transient bacteria and as many of the resident microorganisms as possible.

There are many different theories as to the best way to wash the hands so that disease transfer is minimized. Some methods depend on scrubbing the surfaces of the hands for a prescribed number of strokes. This is referred to as a *stroke-count method*. Other authorities advocate continual scrubbing of all surfaces for a minimum length of time. Studies have shown that the rate of reduction of normal skin flora or resident bacteria is roughly 50% for every 6 minutes of scrubbing (Perkins, 1978). One can assume from that statistic, then, that the initial scrub has probably removed most of the transient bacteria but has only begun to affect the bacterial counts of the resident flora of the skin. No matter what method is used, there seems to be general agreement that the desired goals include the following: the removal of all surface dirt and organic matter, which will destroy transient bacteria; dissolution of the normal greasy film that contains some of the more accessible resident bacteria of the skin; and a final "degerming" of the more resistant resident bacteria of the skin through the use of disinfecting soaps or solutions (Hooley, 1970).

An effective handwashing procedure should start with an initial scrub that includes a thorough lathering and scrubbing of all surfaces of the nails, fingers, hands, and lower arms. This is possible only if the hands and arms are bared of all jewelry and clothing, at least to the elbow. This initial scrub should be a series of three latherings, each followed by a thorough rinsing, and may last for 2 to 3 minutes (Crawford, 1978). During the entire scrubbing procedure it is important that there be copious amounts of running water to remove loosened microorganisms and flush them away. The initial scrub should be done with a soft, sterile brush or sponge. Overzealous use of stiff bristle brush can abrade and lacerate the skin, increasing the risk of infection by oral pathogens. Soap or detergent is helpful in loosening dirt, oils, and bacteria from the skin. The use of a liquid soap dispenser rather than a bar of soap will reduce cross-contamination during handwashing. A cake or bar of soap can serve as a nutrient source and reservoir for bacterial growth once it has been used (Parker, 1976). There is some benefit in using soaps that contain antiseptic materials, since they will enhance the destruction of bacteria in the deeper recesses of the skin. The professional should be aware of the claims made by whatever product is being used, since the bactericidal and bacteriostatic effects of these soaps differ. It is important that whatever product is chosen, it is nonirritating and gentle to the skin. Excessive drying and skin irritation can result from the constant use of a harsh product, reducing the ability of the skin to form an effective barrier against infection.

Scrubbing should start at the fingertips and nails. An orangewood stick can be used to clean thoroughly under the nails. The washing should continue to all sides of the fingers, hands, wrists, and lower arms. It is important that there be at least three latherings followed by thorough rinsing to achieve a satisfactory degree of cleanliness. The most important aspect of handwashing is the mechanical rubbing of all surfaces to remove soil and microorganisms, which are then rinsed away by the running water. When the hands are being rinsed, the water should flow from the fingertips down toward the elbow. The water should not be allowed to run back over an area that has been previously rinsed. Contaminated rinse water should not contact already clean areas.

After the hands have been scrubbed, washed, and rinsed, they should not touch anything that is not within the aseptic chain. The hands should be dried with a paper towel, starting with the fingers, then the hands, and finally the surfaces of the arms. A separate paper towel should be used for each hand. The faucet should be turned off either by means of foot controls or with a paper towel if hand controls are used. The paper towels should then be discarded. Care should be taken not to touch the sink, paper towel dispenser, or waste receptacle after the hands have been washed. Between patients, the hands should be washed for 1 to 2 minutes, with care taken to lather and rinse at least three times within that period (Crawford, 1978).

Wearing disposable gloves. The initial scrub should precede regular handwashing, both at the beginning of each treatment period (morning and afternoon) and prior to putting on disposable gloves. It is incorrect to assume that hands do not need to be scrubbed thoroughly if gloves are worn. Actually, the warm, moist environment of the skin beneath the gloves is especially conducive to bacterial growth. If microbes enter this environment through a tear in the gloves or from contaminated rinse water, they can multiply quickly and are protected by the gloves from subsequent handwashing. Once the gloves are removed, a potent reservoir of microorganisms may be present. Care should be

taken to inspect gloves routinely for rips or tears and to discard them if they are not intact. In addition, rinse water from handwashing should not be allowed to seep beneath the gloves (Mitchell et al., 1983).

The use of sterile gloves by dental clinicians will afford the highest degree of hand hygiene and protection against cross-contamination. Sterile, disposable gloves can permit the achievement and maintenance of a safer level of contamination control than can be achieved with bare hands alone. Gloves are sterile or clean when received and can be cleaned more effectively by handwashing procedures than can bare hands. The same handwashing routine of two to three latherings followed by a thorough rinsing should be followed. Gloves also protect the hands against the drying effect of continual washing before, during, and after patient treatment. Most important, they provide an effective barrier against the entry of serious pathogens, including those responsible for syphilis, hepatitis, and other diseases transmitted by the blood or saliva of infected patients. Since it is not always possible to detect which patients may be carriers of infectious diseases, *the dental professional is well-advised to wear gloves for all intraoral procedures* and especially for those procedures in which bleeding is likely to occur (Giangrego, 1980; Goebel, 1979).

Sources of contamination

The first step in preparing the clinical site is complete and frequent sanitization of all surfaces. This should be followed by appropriate use of surface disinfectants. Finally, all critical items should be sterilized or made of disposable materials. Following these initial cleaning and disinfecting procedures, the challenge remains to maintain this environment in a manner that will prevent cross-contamination from occurring between patient and clinician, between patient and environment, and between one patient and another. Each source of contamination should be examined for its potential role as a disease-transmitting agent, the number and type of microorganisms that are likely to be present, and the level to which contamination control is possible. With this information in hand, it should be possible to select the most effective methods of disease control for each component of the dental environment.

To increase the efficiency of contamination control procedures, members of the dental staff should compile a comprehensive list of each critical, semicritical, and noncritical surface or item in the dental office and identify the appropriate method of contamination control to be used. In addition, care must be taken during treatment of patients not to enlarge the list of critical surfaces by touching and contaminating additional surfaces. Once they have been contaminated by the patient's oral flora, the dental professional's hands should not touch any surface that is not routinely sterilized or disinfected until the hands have been washed. By making a conscious effort not to break the so-called contamination chain, the dental staff will be saved additional effort and time during the preparation of the operatory for the next patient.

The major sources of contamination include the patient, the general working environment, surfaces and equipment of the operating area, dental instruments and supplies, and dental personnel. Frequent sites of surface contamination appear as shaded areas in Fig. 3-6. As specific sites of contamination are considered, appropriate disinfection and sterilization methods are suggested, as well as additional guidelines for contamination control.

The *dental chair* is contacted by each patient and by the hands of the operating personnel. The patient's clothing and body contaminate the headrest and the armrest. Bacteria-laden dust, dirt, and dandruff can be shed from these hair-bearing areas onto the chair, where they may contact the next patient. The patient's hands and arms may be contaminated by any number of different pathogens, which are then transferred to the armrest. In addition to a thorough cleaning and dusting, use of a mild disinfectant that will not harm the chair material is suggested. Headrests should have a disposable cover placed for each patient. Armrests may be either disinfected after each patient or covered with a disposable paper cover. Chair control switches that are operated by the hands of the dental personnel

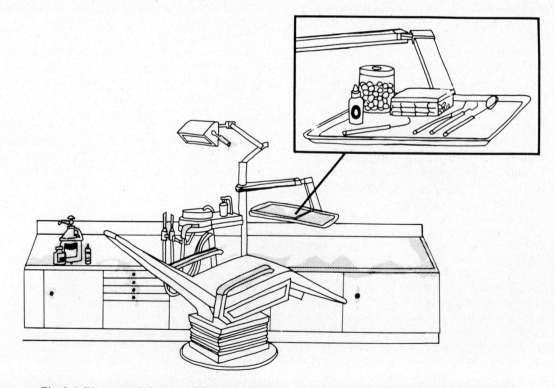

Fig. 3-6. Diagram depicting potential sources of contamination that exist in dental offices. Shading identifies objects and areas that must be sterilized or disinfected between patients to prevent cross-contamination.

should also be carefully disinfected after each patient with a recommended surface disinfectant or kept covered during treatment with a disposable material such as transparent film or foil to prevent their contamination by the clinician's hands.

All *unit controls,* including controls for power, air, water, and lights, should be carefully disinfected before each patient arrives. The bracket table and all operatory counter tops should be covered with a disposable patient napkin or other covering. All drawer and cabinet handles should be kept disinfected. To avoid unnecessary handling of these surfaces, all supplies and instruments should be dispensed and placed on the bracket table or adjacent counter top prior to each appointment by noncontaminated hands. Light handles and bracket table handles should be disinfected or covered with a disposable paper towel or foil to prevent cross-contamination. Dental personnel should avoid touching any surface that is not routinely disinfected between patients. The *high-speed suction* and *saliva ejector tubes* should be cleaned out daily to remove residual saliva, blood, and debris. To accomplish this, the entire system should be flushed with water and a disinfectant solution at the end of each operating day. Exact instructions as to how this should be accomplished should be obtained from the manufacturer of the equipment. In addition, the part of these items that will be handled during patient treatment should be carefully wiped with a 4 × 4 inch sponge that has been saturated with a recommended surface disinfectant such as a 1:20 iodophor and alcohol mixture or 2% glutaraldehyde. The suction tips that will enter the patient's mouth should be made of a material that can be sterilized or is disposable.

In many instances the *water supplies* within dental units can become contaminated with bacterial concentrations higher than those levels considered acceptable for public consumption. When water supplies are allowed to sit for long periods without being used, the effectiveness of chlorine to control bacterial growth begins to decrease. The subsequent growth of microorganisms provides a source of contamination when the water lines are again used and delivered directly into the patient's mouth by way of the drinking cup, the tri-syringe, the ultrasonic scaler, and the water-cooled handpiece. In addition, many modern handpieces and tri-syringes have been equipped with retraction devices that are designed to prevent water from dripping out of the ends of these items after they have been used. When this excess water is retracted back into the handpiece or syringe, it is often accompanied by contaminated water and saliva, which then contaminate the water line and the next patient treated with this equipment. The best way to prevent this contamination is to remove the retraction devices from tri-syringes and handpieces. In addition, all hoses that deliver water from the dental unit should be flushed for 3 to 5 minutes at the beginning of the day. Handpieces and syringes should be flushed for 1 minute between patients (Abel et al., 1971; Scheid et al., 1982).

The *tri-syringe* is another major source of contamination, since it is contaminated by both the clinician's hands and the mouth of the patient. Many modern syringes are now made with removable tips that can be autoclaved after patient treatment. If sterilization of the tip is not possible, it must be carefully disinfected along with the rest of the syringe with an effective surface disinfectant. Because of the high contamination potential of this item, it should be thoroughly scrubbed with a brush and a high- or intermediate-level disinfectant at the sink (if the hose length will allow), or scrubbed twice with two separate gauze sponges that are saturated with the disinfectant (Crawford, 1978).

Dental handpieces are also critical items. They are contaminated by the patient's oral bacteria, by aerosols created during their use, and by the hands of the clinician and those of the assistant. Until recently, most handpieces could not be sterilized in the autoclave, so disinfection was the only means of contamination control. There are now several manufacturers of dental instruments who produce handpieces and prophylaxis angles that can be sterilized. The use of sterilized handpieces is necessary to ensure optimal treatment safety (Sanger et al., 1978). Specific instructions regarding sterilization of dental handpieces and prophylaxis angles should be obtained from the manufacturer. Some dental handpieces can be sterilized by chemical vapor sterilizers, and all types of handpieces can be sterilized with ethylene oxide gas, but this requires expensive equipment and a sterilization cycle of several hours. If the operatory is equipped with a handpiece that cannot be safely sterilized in the autoclave and ethylene oxide sterilization is not available, then the handpiece must be treated with an ADA-recommended high- or intermediate-level disinfectant. It can be scrubbed at the sink with a brush or thoroughly scrubbed with two separate 4 × 4 inch gauze sponges.

The *nitrous oxide nosepiece* should be disinfected after each use to prevent transmission of viral and upper respiratory tract infections from one patient to another. This equipment cannot be routinely sterilized, because it is composed of rubber or plastic materials that cannot withstand the high temperatures of the autoclave or dry heat oven. Yagiela et al. (1979) compared the effectiveness of a number of different methods for disinfecting this equipment and concluded that the most effective procedure was to wash the nosepiece thoroughly after each use with soap and water and then immerse it in a 2% alkaline glutaraldehyde solution for 10 minutes to achieve disinfection, followed by thorough rinsing in tap water. Sterilization of this equipment should be accomplished nightly, when immersion for the full 10-hour period, followed by a 1-hour rinse, can be accomplished.

The *x-ray cone, head,* and *controls* must also be disinfected after each use. Since the clinician is constantly going back and forth between the intraoral placement of radiographic films and the x-ray equipment, these are prime sources of cross-contamination. Whenever possible, disposable paper towels should be used to handle the head and the cone to avoid excessive contamination. All radiographic film holders are critical surfaces and should be made of materials that are disposable or that can be sterilized between patients. Plastic film holders must be treated with high-level disinfectants, since they cannot be autoclaved.

The *pens and pencils* used for recording patient data and *patients' charts* are often overlooked as sources of contamination. Pens and pencils should be wiped thoroughly with a high-level disinfectant after each patient appointment. Another safeguard is to delegate all recording and chart handling to an assistant so that the clinician's contaminated hands never touch them. If an assistant is not available, the clinician's hands must be washed prior to handling these items and then washed again before resuming intraoral procedures. An alternative is to use one hand for intraoral examination and the other hand to record all data on the chart forms. Pens and pencils that are used in the treatment room

should remain there and not be carried to other areas where they could transfer pathogens to other patients or family members.

All operating *personnel*—the dentist, the hygienist, and the assistant—participate in patient treatment and are potential sources of contamination. Dental personnel, by means of their occupation, are exposed to more disease-producing microorganisms than are most other people (Micik et al., 1971; Miller et al., 1971. If a member of the dental team contracts any sort of contagious disease, all efforts should be made to avoid transmission to other people in the office and to patients. A responsible health care provider will not risk transmitting active disease. When known disease is present in either the clinician or the patient, elective procedures should be postponed if possible. Otherwise, the use of face masks, safety glasses, and gloves by dental personnel may be necessary to avoid cross-contamination.

Even a healthy individual, be it patient or professional, carries potentially harmful bacteria on clothing, skin, and hair and in the mouth and nose. Even though the carriers may be unaffected by these microbes, other, more susceptible individuals can contract disease if they encounter these pathogens. Health care providers can control contamination by wearing freshly laundered clothing while in the dental environment. Many persons prefer to wear uniforms because they are easily cleaned and are usually constructed of materials that do not readily give off bacteria-laden lint and threads. The uniformed professional also avoids carrying in the many germs that can be picked up by street clothes that are worn outside the dental environment. Many dental professionals find that wearing a clean lab coat or clinic coat over clean street clothes serves the same purpose. In any case, uniforms and clinic coats should be laundered thoroughly at the end of each day and should not be worn when the professional is with family members at home or with other persons outside the dental environment. Obviously, clinic attire should be removed before preparing food.

Since it is also known that bacteria are shed along with the skin cells, dandruff, and dust from the hair and body, it is necessary that all exposed skin and hair be as clean as possible. In addition, the longer the hair, the more likely it is that dandruff and bacteria may be shed because of its movement and contact with the shoulders and face. The clinician's head and face are kept close to the patient during treatment, so cross-contamination between oral pathogens and the clinician's hair (including a beard or mustache) can pose a health problem. Longer hair may also be a problem for the clinician in terms of maintaining a clear field of vision. For these reasons it is advisable that hair be kept short, pinned, or tied close to the head and out of the field of operation.

Jewelry may be another source of contamination and should be kept to a minimum, if worn at all. Since hands and wrists cannot be adequately cleaned unless they are bare, it is recommended that jewelry not be worn on the hands while treating patients. Not only will rings prevent adequate hand cleansing, but they are also difficult to clean and can become potent sources of cross-contamination between patients and the wearer. Contrary to a popularly held belief, wedding rings are no less hazardous as sources of contamination than are other rings.

Dental personnel must be careful not to touch any part of their clothing or body during patient treatment. If this occurs, the hands must be rewashed before returning to the patient's mouth or touching any other part of the operating environment.

Dental aerosols and splatter

Dental aerosols are tiny, invisible particles of contaminated water, blood, and saliva that are generated from the patient's mouth during dental procedures. Significantly large numbers of aerosols are produced during use of the high-speed handpiece, the tri-syringe, and the ultrasonic scaler, and during procedures such as polishing and toothbrushing. The small size of these particles permits them to enter the body through the nose, mouth, and eyes. Once they have entered the respiratory tract, they can penetrate deeply into the lungs. Aerosols remain suspended in the air for as long as 24 hours (Micik et al., 1969), where they continue to be sources of contamination long after the patient has left.

In addition to aerosols, the air can also be contaminated by larger droplets of saliva-borne microorganisms and debris known as *splatter*. Splatter droplets are usually large enough to be visible. Their larger diameter and weight cause these particles to fall out of the air more quickly than aerosols, so that they land on nearby surfaces and contaminate them with the patient's oral flora.

Miller et al. (1971) compared the aerosol and splatter production of specific dental procedures with those of common nasal-oral activities. They found that using the high-speed handpiece or washing the teeth with a combined air-water spray produced contamination equal to sneezing, hissing, or toothbrushing. A prophylaxis produced the same amount of aerosol contamination as gargling, and using the ultrasonic scaler produced the same amount of contamination as a cough. Certainly, anyone would dislike having another person sneeze, hiss, gargle, or cough directly at him/her within a close personal distance of only 8 to 12 inches, and yet most dental clinicians have to contend with these same levels of aerosol and splatter contamination continuously.

Both aerosols and splatter can contaminate the mucous membranes of the oral cavity, nose, or eyes and can lead to disease in a susceptible host. Aerosols can be the source of transmission for serious diseases, including hepatitis, tuberculosis, herpes simplex and other viral infections, and respiratory tract infections. Treatment of patients known to have these conditions should be postponed until they are no longer infectious. Cross-contamination due to aerosols and splatter should be controlled by using disposable paper covers on all counter tops; keeping all clean and sterile supplies in closed containers, drawers, or cabinets; and disinfecting all contaminated surfaces thoroughly between patients.

Reducing aerosol production. There are a number of ways in which the dental professional can control and reduce the amount of dental aerosols and splatter generated during treatment. The use of the rubber dam during operative procedures or at other times when this type of isolation would be practical will reduce aerosol production. High-speed evacuation during procedures involving the ultrasonic scaler or high-speed handpiece or when rinsing the mouth is also helpful. When the tri-syringe is used, the clinician should apply water to the area, followed by air, rather than dispensing both at the same time to produce a forced spray of water. Bristle brushes generate more splatter during polishing procedures than do rubber cups or polishing points, so use of brushes should be limited.

The direction of airflow within the dental operatory will also affect aerosols. Installation of a ceiling-to-floor laminar airflow system to direct the circulation of air in the operatory has been shown to reduce aerosols in the treatment area. The use of laminar airflow will also reduce the amount of surface contamination resulting from airborne particles (Pollock et al., 1970).

Use of mouthwashes. The numbers of microorganisms within the patient's mouth can be significantly reduced through the use of an antiseptic mouthwash prior to dental treatment (Litsky et al., 1976). Wyler et al. (1971) demonstrated that the use of a pretreatment rinse with a commercially available antiseptic mouthwash reduced bacterial counts by 10 to 100 times. Crawford (1978) suggested that although the main effect of mouth rinsing is one of mechanical removal, the antiseptic properties of some mouthwashes could enhance the overall reduction of microorganisms.

Use of face masks. A face mask is an effective means of protection in two ways. First, it may protect the patient from contamination by a clinician who has a cold or other condition that is transmittable by respiratory droplets. Since the clinician's face is in such proximity to the patient, this kind of transfer could easily occur. It may also be a source of protection for the clinician from bacteria-laden aerosols that may originate from the patient while breathing, talking, sneezing, or coughing during dental treatment. The use of a face mask is indicated for treatment of a patient with any disease that is transmittable by respiratory droplets, including hepatitis, tuberculosis, colds, and influenza (Coughlin et al., 1967; Micik et al., 1971).

An effective mask is one that will not only mechanically block larger particles of blood, saliva, and oral debris, but also will filter out aerosols with very small particles such as those generated by high-speed handpieces and ultrasonic scalers. Face masks should also be comfortable, fit well, and have minimal marginal leakage (Micik et al., 1971).

Face masks are available in a wide variety of styles and materials, including paper, cloth, foam, fiberglass, and other synthetic materials. Of these, the paper, cloth, and foam masks have shown the least effectiveness, whereas the masks made of glass or synthetic fiber have been most effective in filtering aerosols (Micik et al., 1971).

Most face masks available to dental personnel are disposable. Although disposable face masks have been shown to be effective in reducing contamination, they do not totally prevent the passage of potentially dangerous microorganisms. More effective control of dental aerosols depends on reducing the numbers of bacteria at the source and interrupting the process of transmission by using high-speed suction at the operating site as well as masks to protect those who may be affected.

Use of protective eyeglasses. Protective eyeglasses should be worn by all dental personnel involved in chairside treatment and by patients. This important safety measure can prevent damage caused by bacteria-laden aerosols, accidental trauma, or flying debris. The patient's eyes are extremely vulnerable to damage from oral debris and aerosols, and from falling or mishandled instruments and dental materials. This is especially true for patients in the supine position (Cooley et al., 1978). Incorrect instrument or supply transfer over the patient's face could result in trauma to the eye or impaction of a foreign body. The use of ultrasonic scalers and high-speed handpieces increases the presence of aerosols containing large numbers of infectious bacteria that pose a risk to clinician and patient alike. The herpes virus is one example of a pathogen that could be transmitted from saliva or an active lesion into the eye by means of aerosols or splatter droplets. The resultant infection, recurrent herpetic keratitis, leads to impaired vision and, in some cases, blindness (Brooks et al., 1981; Crawford, 1978).

The clinician is also at risk from flying debris from the mouth during dental treatment. Safety glasses prevent damage to the eyes that could result from a particle of calculus being snapped from the tooth and propelled out of the mouth or from a slurry of abrasive and saliva that might splatter against the clinician's face during polishing procedures. Those clinicians who wear glasses can see the evidence of splatter and debris on their safety lenses following patient treatment. Since both the patient's eyes and those of the dental team are in such close proximity to the working area, the risk of eye injury is high. In a survey of dental hygienists, 44% had suffered the following foreign bodies in their eyes as a result of treatment procedures: pumice/prophylaxis paste, calculus, dental materials, and contaminated water spray (Gravois and Stringer, 1980). Those professionals who decide not to protect themselves and their patients with safety glasses should carefully consider the economic and ethical implications of that choice.

Most eyeglasses fitted by prescription are now made of shatter-resistant materials. Patients who already wear glasses should be advised to wear them during dental treatment. Safety glasses should be provided for patients who do not normally wear glasses. These may be of a disposable design, or they should be sterilized or disinfected between patients. Most patients will appreciate this precaution if the dental professional explains that it is recommended out of concern for their health and safety. Tinted lenses in the glasses provided for patient use will also provide shielding from overhead lighting. The clinician's glasses can be treated with antifogging cloths or cleaners that are commercially available to prevent the problem of fogging.

CONCLUSION

It should be apparent that control of contamination when preparing the site for the patient is a very important step in patient care. It makes possible a comfortable, efficient, and safe environment for the patient and thus affords the dental personnel those same considerations.

Although the time needed for this preparatory phase may diminish with experience, its importance in providing quality care should remain a primary consideration in all phases of care.

ACTIVITIES

1. Purchase or prepare Petri dishes that contain an agar medium that will support the growth of several types of organisms. Using sterile cotton swabs, collect microbial samples from different parts of the clinic (such as counter tops, sinks, tri-syringes, dental chair) or from yourself (such as skin, clothing, shoes). Wipe the contaminated swab over the agar medium and incubate for 24 to 48 hours. Observe the growth on the plates for a visual representation of the organisms present in the clinical area. As an extension of the activity, compare culture samples from both before and after sterilization and disinfection procedures. Evaluate the success of contamination control practices in the clinic.
2. View the 16 mm film, *Oral Sepsis: The Unseen Problem.* (DTB-294, 20 minutes, produced by the American Dental Association, Bureau of Audio Visual Service. Available for rental.)

3. With a lab partner, role play performing an intraoral procedure. Identify the possible sources of contamination in the area. Demonstrate how direct and indirect transmission occur.
4. Observe and report on aseptic practices in other parts of the school or other clinics.
5. Observe asepsis control in a hospital operating room.
6. Review the literature for statistics relating to the incidence of hepatitis among dental professionals and patients.
7. Discuss the implications of contracting serum hepatitis for the career of a dental professional.
8. Discuss the legal ramifications of endangering safety of practice through ineffective contamination control. Determine if there have been any malpractice suits related to this issue brought against health professionals in your state or others. Consult a lawyer about the legalities of such an issue.
9. Make a specific list of each item in the student's instrument kit, and determine how it would best be sterilized/disinfected.
10. Ask students to inspect their safety glasses after a patient appointment for signs of splatter droplets of blood and saliva or other debris.
11. Compare the germicidal effects of all disinfectants, soaps, and antiseptics available in the clinic from manufacturers' descriptions and descriptions in *Accepted Dental Therapeutics.*
12. Wipe red tempora paint on a surface normally contaminated during dental treatment to simulate saliva contamination. Have students attempt to remove it with disinfectant-soaked gauze squares. Discuss how much scrubbing was necessary to remove all traces of the paint. Draw comparisons with the amount of wiping students may normally use.

REVIEW QUESTIONS

1. Discuss the susceptibility of the dental clinician to sources of infection.
2. State the bacterial or viral disease caused by the following organisms (give the mode of transmission for each):
   a. *Mycobacterium tuberculosis*
   b. *Treponema pallidum*
   c. *Clostridium tetani*
   d. Respiratory virus, e.g., adenovirus
   e. Hepatitis B virus
   f. Rubeola virus
3. True or false
   a. Hepatitis A usually has no residual effects after recovery.
   b. Jaundice occurs in all cases of hepatitis.
   c. Hepatitis B virus may be transmitted by means of the saliva.

d. *Mycobacterium tuberculosis* is routinely destroyed by surface disinfection.

e. Because of an increased opportunity for contracting tuberculosis, dental personnel should have periodic skin testing performed.

f. When the patient's saliva enters the clinician's blood by way of a break in the skin, direct transmission has occurred.

g. When the hygienist punctures his/her hand while cleaning instruments, indirect transmission has occurred.

h. Aerosol production is responsible for contaminating a major portion of the dental operatory.

i. Syphilis is only contagious in the primary stage.

j. A chancre is a primary stage syphilitic lesion.

4. Define the terms sanitation, disinfection, and sterilization.

5. Describe an effective handwashing procedure.

6. List five accepted methods for instrument sterilization.

7. Describe the conditions required for sterilization when using each of the methods listed in 6.

8. Describe the recommended procedure for decontaminating the tri-syringe and the handpiece between patients.

9. Under what conditions should the dental clinician wear a face mask?

REFERENCES

Abel, L.C., et al. 1971. Studies on dental aerobiology. IV. Bacterial contamination of water delivered by dental units. J. Dent. Res. **50**:1567.

ADA Council on Dental Materials, Instruments and Equipment. 1981. Current status of sterilization instruments, devices, and methods for the dental office. J. Am. Dent. Assoc. **102**:683.

ADA Council on Dental Therapeutics. 1976. Type B (serum) hepatitis and dental practice. J. Am. Dent. Assoc. **92**:153.

ADA Council on Dental Therapeutics. 1978. Quaternary ammonium compounds not acceptable for disinfection of instruments and environmental surfaces in dentistry. J. Am. Dent. Assoc. **97**:855.

ADA Council on Dental Therapeutics. 1982. Sterilization or disinfection of dental instruments. In Accepted dental therapeutics, ed. 39. Chicago: American Dental Association.

ADA Councils on Dental Materials and Devices and Dental Therapeutics. 1978. Infection control in the dental office. J. Am. Dent. Assoc. **97**:673.

Alexander, R.E. 1981. Hepatitis risk: a clinical perspective. J. Am. Dent. Assoc. **102**:182.

Allen, A.L., and Organ, R.J. 1982. Occult blood accumulation under the fingernails: a mechanism for the spread of bloodborne infection. J. Am. Dent. Assoc. **105**:455.

Auteo, K., et al. 1980. Studies on cross contamination in the dental clinic. J. Am. Dent. Assoc. **100**:358.

Bertolotti, R.L. 1978. Inhibition of corrosion during autoclave sterilization of carbon steel dental instruments. J. Am. Dent. Assoc. **97**:628.

Bond, W.W., et al. 1977. Viral hepatitis B: aspects of environmental control. Health Lab. Sci. **14**:235.

Brooks, S.L., et al. 1981. Prevalence of herpes simplex virus disease in a professional population. J. Am. Dent. Assoc. **102**:31.

Burnett, G.W., and Schuster, G.S. 1978. Oral microbiology and infectious disease. Baltimore: Williams & Wilkins.

Buyrak, E.B., et al. 1976. Vaccine against human hepatitis B. JAMA **235**:2832.

Cooley, R.L. 1983. AIDS: an occupational hazard. J. Am. Dent. Assoc. **107**:28.

Cooley, R.L., and Lubow, R.M. 1982. Hepatitis B vaccine: implications for dental personnel. J. Am. Dent. Assoc. **105**:47.

Cooley, R.L., et al. 1978. Ocular injuries sustained in the dental office: methods of detection, treatment, and prevention. J. Am. Dent. Assoc. **97**:985.

Coughlin, J.W., et al. 1967. Comparison of dry heat, autoclave and vapor sterilizers. J. Tenn. Dent. Assoc. **47**:350.

Crawford, J.J. 1978. Clinical asepsis in dentistry: advanced instruction, ed. 2. Dallas: R.A. Kolstad, Publisher.

Crawford, J.J. 1979. Office sterilization and asepsis procedures. Dent. Clin. North Am. **23**:717.

Crawford, J.J. 1982. Sterilization, disinfection and asepsis in dentistry. In McGhee, J.R., Michalek, S.M., and Cassell, G.H., editors. Dental microbiology. New York: Harper & Row, Publishers, Inc.

Dayoub, M.B., et al. 1978. A method of decontamination of ultrasonic scalers and high speed handpieces. J. Periodontol. **49**:261.

Eigener, U. 1977. Hand hygiene in dental practice. Quintessence Int. **8**:79.

Frances, D.P., et al. 1982. The prevention of hepatitis B with vaccine: report of Centers for Disease Control multicenter efficacy trial among homosexual men. Ann. Intern. Med. **97**:362.

Giangrego, E. Aug. 1980. HBV: the hidden killer. Horizons **1**:1.

Goebel, W.M. 1979. Reliability of the medical history in identifying patients likely to place dentists at an incresed hepatitis risk. J. Am. Dent. Assoc. **98**:907.

Gravois, S.L., and Stringer, R.B. 1980. Survey of occupational health hazards in dental hygiene. Dent. Hyg. **54**:518.

Gross, M.L. 1981. Herpes: an overview on diagnosis and treatment. J. Ky. Dent. Assoc. **33**(3):26.

Haberman, S. 1962. Some comparative studies between a chemical vapor sterilizer and a converted steam autoclave on various bacteria and viruses. J. South. Calif. Dent. Assoc. **30**:163.

Hartley, J.L. 1978. Eye and facial injuries resulting from dental procedures. Dent. Clin. North Am. **22**:505.

Hooley, J.R. 1970. Hospital dentistry. Philadephia: Lea & Febiger.

Johnson & Johnson. 1969. Handbook of dental practice asepsis. East Windsor, N.J.: Dental Products Co.

Ketterl, W. 1980. Disposable materials, II. Quintessence Int. **11**:79.

Kolstad, R.A., and Crawford, J.J. 1978. Sterilization, disinfection, and asepsis in dental practice, ed. 2. Dallas: R.A. Kolstad, Publisher.

Krugman, S., et al. 1981. Immunogenic effect of inactivated hepatitis B vaccine: comparison of 20 microgram and 40 microgram doses. J. Med Virol. **8**:119.

Litsky, B.Y., et al. 1976. Use of an antimicrobial mouthwash to minimize the bacterial aerosol contamination generated by a high speed drill. Oral Surg. **29**:25.

Lyon, T.C., and Devine, M.J. 1974. Evaluation of a new model vapor pressure sterilizer. J. Dent. Res. (Abstract 634, Special Issue) **53**.

MacFarlane, T.W. 1980. Sterilization in general dental practice. J. Dent. **8**:13.

MacQuarrie, M.B., et al. 1974. Hepaitis B transmission by human bite. JAMA **230**:723.

Mair, J.H., et al. 1982. The implications of viral hepatitis for the practice of dentistry. Can. Dent. Assoc. J. **48**:756.

Merchant, V.A. 1982. Herpes simplex virus infection: an occupational hazard in dental practice. J. Mich. Dent. Assoc. **64**:199.

Merck, Sharp & Dohme. 1982. Hepatitis B and the Dental Profession. West Point, Penn.: Division of Merck and Co., Inc.,

Micik, R.E., et al. 1969. Studies on dental aerobiology. I. Bacterial aerosols generated during dental procedures. J. Dent. Res. **48**:51.

Micik, R.E., et al. 1971. Studies on dental aerobiology. III. Efficiency of surgical mass in protecting dental personnel from airborne bacterial particles. J. Dent. Res. **50**:626.

Miller, R.L., and Micik, R.E. 1978. Air pollution and its control in the dental office. Dent. Clin. North Am. **22**:453.

Miller, R.L., et al. 1971. Studies on dental aerobiology. II. Microbial splatter discharges from the oral cavity of dental patients. J. Dent. Res. **50**:621.

Mitchell, R., et al. 1983. The use of operating gloves in dental practice. Br. Dent. J. **154**:372.

Nolte, W.A. 1982. Oral microbiology, ed. 4. St. Louis: The C.V. Mosby Co.

Palenik, C., and Miller, C. 1981. Monitoring the dental office sterilzer. Ind. Dent. Assoc. J. **60**:25.

Parker, R.B. 1976. Dental office procedures for breaking an infection chain. Am. Soc. Prevent. Dent. **6**:18.

Parker, R.B., and Kolstad, R.A. 1982. Effects of sterilization on periodontal instruments. J. Periodontol. **53**:434.

Pelleu, G.B., and Wachtel, L.W. 1970. Microbial contamination in dental unit warm water systems. IADR Program and Abstract No. 298.

Perkins, J.J. 1978. Principles and methods of sterilization in health sciences. Springfield, Ill.: Charles C Thomas, Publisher.

Pollock, N.L., et al. 1970. Laminar air purge of microorganisms in dental aerosols. J. Am. Dent. Assoc. **81**:1131.

Rimland, D., et al. 1977. Hepatitis B outbreak traced to an oral surgeon. N. Engl. J. Med. **296**:953.

Rothstein, S., and Goldman, H.S. 1980. Sterilizing and disinfecting for hepatitis B virus in the dental operatory. Clin. Prevent. Dent. **2**:9.

Rothstein, S., Goldman, H.S., and Arcomano, A.S. 1981. Hepatitis B virus: overview for dentists. J. Am. Dent. Assoc. **102**:173.

Rowe, N.H., and Brooks, S.L. 1978. Contagion in the dental office. Dent. Clin. North Am. **22**:491.

Rowe, N.H., et al. 1982. Herpetic whitlow: an occupational disease of practicing dentists. J. Am. Dent. Assoc. **105**:471.

Sach, H. 1981. Dentistry and hepatitis B: the legal risks. J. Am. Dent. Assoc. **102**:177.

Sanger, R.G., et al. 1978. An inquiry into the sterilization of dental handpieces relative to transmission of hepatitis B. J. Am. Dent. Assoc. **96**:621.

Scheid, R.C., et al. 1982. Reduction of microbes in handpieces by flushing before use. J. Am. Dent. Assoc. **105**:658.

Smith, A.L. 1982. Principles of microbiology, ed. 9. St. Louis: The C.V. Mosby Co.

Smith, J.L. 1976. Comparative risk of hepatitis B among physicians and dentists. J. Infect. Dis. **133**:705.

Smith, Q.T. 1976. Viral hepatitis: an occupational risk of dentists. Northwest Dent. **55**(4):20.

Smith, R.J. 1968. Clean working in conservative dentistry. Br. Dent. J. **124**:27.

Spaulding, E.H. 1972. Chemical disinfection and antisepsis in the hospital. J. Hosp. Res. **9**:5.

Stortebecker, T.P. 1967. Dental significance of pathways for dissemination from infectious foci. J. Can. Dent. Assoc. **33**:301.

Szmuness, W., et al. 1982. Hepatitis B vaccine in medical staff of hemodialysis units: efficacy and subtype cross-protection. N. Engl. J. Med. **307**:1481.

Tankersley, R.W. 1964. Amino acid requirements of herpes simplex virus in human cell. J. Bacteriol. **87**:609.

Terezhalmy, G.P., et al. 1978. The use of water-soluble bioflavonoid-ascorbic acid complex in the treatment of recurrent herpes labialis. Oral Surg. **45**:56.

Villarejos, V.M., et al. 1974. Role of saliva, urine, and feces in transmission of type B hepatitis. N. Engl. J. Med. **291**:1375.

Ward, R., et al. 1972. Hepatitis B antigen in saliva and mouth washings. Lancet **2**:726.

White, S.C., and Glaze, S. 1978. Interpatient microbiological cross-contamination after dental radiographic examination. J. Am. Dent. Assoc. **96**:801.

Williams, G.H., et al. 1970. Laminar air purge of microorganisms in dental aerosols: prophylactic procedures with the ultrasonic scaler. J. Dent. Res. **49**:1498.

Wyler, D., et al. 1971. Efficacy of self-administered preoperative oral hygiene procedures in reducing the concentration of bacteria in aerosols generated during dental procedures. J. Dent. Res. **50**:509.

Yagiela, J.A., et al. 1979. Disinfection of nitrous oxide inhalation equipment. J. Am. Dent. Assoc. **98**:191.

4 THE COMPLETE DENTAL RECORD

OBJECTIVES: *The reader will be able to*

1. Explain the purposes of a complete dental record.
2. List the components of a complete dental record and justify the inclusion of each component.
3. Describe and follow the guidelines for making chart entries, especially progress notes.
4. Compare and contrast treatment-oriented and problem-oriented approaches to records.
5. Define the phrase *chart audit* and explain the purposes of a chart audit.
6. Discuss the uses of computers for maintaining dental records.

In all likelihood, you, the reader, have at one time or another been treated by a physician, nurse practitioner, nurse, dentist, or dental hygienist. Think about your treatment and the records of your treatment that the health care providers have used to assist them. What would you expect to be in the record? What would you want to be excluded from the record? Have you ever read (or peeked at) the record? If so, what was your impression of its contents and of the health care providers who had written in the record?

Undoubtedly, you have come to expect that the health care provider will have an accurate, legible recording of each of your conditions or problems, visits, treatments, tests, and test results, as well as of the progress of your condition. In a nutshell, you expect that the provider will be able to glean from the record all the pertinent information needed to knowledgeably and adequately treat your present condition. In addition, you probably expect that entries will be written objectively and that the entire record will be treated with respect and confidentiality.

As a dental health care provider, patients will have these expectations of you regarding their dental record. Patients rightfully expect health care providers to maintain accurate, adequate records about their past and present conditions, treatments, and the progress of treatment. The purpose of this chapter is to familiarize you, the reader, with the functions of the dental record, its inclusions, and the approaches to maintaining a complete dental record. In addition, confidentiality, legal respon-

sibility, chart audits, and the use of computers are discussed.

A MEDICOLEGAL DOCUMENT

A complete dental record should include all of the information necessary to safely and knowledgeably treat a patient. The record must contain a data base that includes the patient's past and present medical and dental histories, present dental status, diagnosis of present conditions, treatment plan, treatment rendered, and financial records. The complete dental record and associated materials, such as study models, radiographs, laboratory test results, and photographs, are medicolegal documents. The records are related to medicine because they concern the general health of a patient and the ensuing treatment. They are related to the law because the records are admissible in a court of law as evidence either for or against the health care provider or the patient (Miller, 1979). As a legal document, the chart protects both the patient and the clinician, so the chart should be complete, thorough, accurate, and legible.

Miller (1979) states, "A cautious dentist (dental hygienist) will never rely on memory. He (she) will record *all* facts pertinent to a patient's history, examination, diagnosis, visits, treatments, fees, and observations, and will identify each fact by specific date. . . . Everything pertinent to a dentist's (dental hygienist's) treatment should be included in the record file. . . . " Any treatment, diagnostic aid, or diagnosis performed with the patient must be noted in the permanent record. It is important to document every interaction and treatment to ensure continuity of care for the patient and legal protection for the patient and dental personnel.

The dental record is important not only for the provision of quality care for the patient, but also as legal protection. The dental health care provider is legally responsible for protecting and respecting the personal and property rights of the patient, for providing only necessary and agreed-on care, for completing care within a reasonable amount of time, for achieving reasonably satisfactory results, for exercising "reasonable care" in performing services, and for charging reasonable fees (Miller, 1979; Morris, 1971; Woodall, 1983). In turn, the patient is responsible for paying the fee and cooperating in treatment (Miller, 1979; Morris, 1971; Woodall, 1983). If either the health care provider or the patient does not fulfill any of the responsibilities, the other party can take legal action. In most such legal cases the dental record would be used as evidence; therefore it is crucial that the record be accurate and legible. For a further discussion of patient and health care provider responsibilities, as well as malpractice, consult Woodall (1983).

Two elements of the health care provider's responsibility for protecting and respecting the personal and property rights of the patient—confidentiality and informed consent—must be emphasized. Protecting the patient's confidentiality involves respecting communications among the health care providers and the patient. It does not mean that everything between the patient and the health care provider is secret; if that were so, continuity of care would be impossible. Rather, protecting a patient's confidentiality involves ensuring that the records are not visible to other patients and that the patient's name or identifying information is removed from records being used in a professional presentation. Another example of protecting this confidentiality is not releasing a patient's records without his/her permission. Perhaps the most important way to respect a patient's confidentiality is by writing objective, truthful, and respectful chart entries. Such chart entries are discussed later in the chapter.

Informed consent, discussed in Chapter 18, means that the patient has enough information about his/her condition to be able to accept or reject the recommended treatment. The patient's informed consent should be recorded in the dental record.

NECESSARY INCLUSIONS AND RECORD ORGANIZATION

Considering the importance of the dental record, dentally and legally, it becomes apparent that a health care provider should know the inclusions of a complete dental record. The necessary inclusions for a dental record are the patient's name on all pages; the patient's residence and employment addresses and phone numbers; the patient's date of birth, sex, and occupation; the physician's name, address, and phone number; the name of the person to contact in an emergency; medical and dental histories; examination findings and diagnosis; treatment goals; the treatment plan; the treatment provided with dates and signatures; results of treatment, especially unexpected results; radiographs; fees charged and paid; and copies of all correspondence (Miller, 1979).

The chart should be logically organized so that it is easily read and understood. Records can be organized in many different ways. The most common format is to have a folder or envelope that contains all the forms and radiographs. It is helpful if chart folders have an envelope or pocket attached to hold the radiographs and intraoral photographs. Forms should be fastened in the sequence in which they will be prepared or reviewed at the time of the appointment.

The usual sequence of forms is basic demographic data, the patient's past and present medical and dental histories, examination findings and diagnosis, treatment goals, the treatment plan, the treatment provided with dates and signatures, results of treatment, and fees charged and paid. Radiographs, intraoral photographs, and copies of correspondence follow or are stored in the folder pocket (Miller, 1979).

Medical alerts notifying the clinician of patient conditions such as penicillin allergy, rheumatic heart disease, hepatitis, or a heart condition should be plainly visible on the front of the chart (Kilpatrick, 1974). Some charts have a symbol, colored tape, or the words "medical alert" in a prominent position on the front of the chart to alert the clinician to a medical condition that must be considered *before* treatment is begun. On seeing such an alert, the health care provider can then open the chart, refer to the medical history, and become familiar with the patient's condition. This system of symbols, tape, or "medical alert" is preferable to the system of writing the condition (e.g., "hepatitis") on the front of the chart, because it is more respectful of the patient's right to confidentiality.

The chart should also have an area for notation of special needs of the patient. Such needs may include special provisions to accommodate a wheelchair or referral to a specialist.

Some charts provide an area for notation of nicknames, hobbies, or special interests of the patient (Kilpatrick, 1974); these may provide the dental professional with information to put the patient at ease. It is also helpful to note emotional traumas a patient may mention to the provider, such as the death of a spouse or a recent separation; these emotional traumas may affect the patient's overall and dental health. The health care provider should remember to write these statements objectively and descriptively without violating the patient's privacy.

GUIDELINES FOR CHART ENTRIES

Considering the importance of the complete dental record, some general guidelines to help a student complete a chart are helpful. The following should be considered whenever making an entry in a patient's record.

All entries should be made *clearly, legibly,* and *in ink* or some other *permanent form* (Woodall, 1983). To be admissible as evidence in court, the data must be discernible, and it must be obvious that entries were made during the course of treatment and not after a suit was filed. Ink and computer entries can be evaluated for the length of time since they were made; thus they are valid as evidence if they reflect legitimate records of the progress of care. Pencil entries are easily changed and are difficult to evaluate concerning the time of entry; therefore pencil records in some instances may not be admissible as evidence. It should be obvious from these facts that entries should be made at each visit and that, in the face of a suit, *no attempt should be made to alter records* to try to prove a point. Such an attempt is foolish and is an obstruction of justice (Stetler, 1962; Woodall, 1983).

Records should be retained for at least 10 years past the time a file becomes inactive (Miller, 1979).

Depending on the state, a patient may file suit against a health care provider up to 6 to 10 years *after* the encounter that triggered the dissatisfaction (Stetler, 1962). The record may be the only evidence in support of the health care provider. Therefore, even if the only treatment rendered for that patient was an extraction, the record must be kept for the duration of the state's statute of limitations.

Documentation of all services rendered, data collection as well as procedures performed, should be entered in the record when they are performed. The progress notes should reflect the patient's needs identified during data collection, the diagnosis, and treatment planning. For example, a progress note stating that an amalgam was placed in tooth No. 30 should only be present if a carious lesion was charted for tooth No. 30 during data collection and subsequently included in the treatment plan.

The progress note should contain descriptive, objective statements dated and signed by the health care provider. It is always wise to compose the progress notes in a specific order so that the necessary information is always present. One such order is to report the patient's subjective findings, if any; the clinician's objective findings; any medication administered, such as a local anesthetic; the procedure performed; complications and/or results observed; the patient's reactions; whether the treatment is complete or incomplete; the treatment to be performed at the next appointment; and the amount of time required before the next appointment. Following is a sample progress note:

6/11/84: Patient reports bleeding gums whenever she brushes. Tissues are swollen, tender, and bleed on probing; moderate to heavy subgingival calculus. Plaque and bleeding indices recorded; demonstrated Bass brushing technique. Patient performed technique and agreed to brush twice daily. Flossing reviewed; patient was not carrying floss subgingivally and was corrected. Lidocaine 2% with 1:200,000 epinephrine (72 mg lidocaine/ 0.038 mg epinephrine) administered in upper right quadrant: posterior superior alveolar, middle superior alveolar, anterior superior alveolar, greater palatine, nasopalatine. Ultrasonic scaler and hand instruments used to scale, root plane, and perform soft tissue curettage. Area should be evaluated at next visit and upper left quadrant treated. No adverse reactions to local anesthetic or to treatment reported observed. Next appointment. 1 week.
LWF

By using commonly accepted abbreviations, this chart entry could be shortened as follows:

6/11/84: Pt. reports bleeding on brushing. Ging. edem., tender, BOP; mod. to heavy sub. calculus. PI & BI recorded. Bass brushing demon. & pt. performance acceptable. Pt. agreed to brush 2 X's daily. Flossing reviewed; not carrying sub., was corrected. Lido. 2% with Epi. 1:200,000 (72 mg lido.; 0.038 mg Epi.) admin. UR quad.: PSA, MSA, ASA, GP, NP. Scaled with ultra. & hand; RP & STC performed UR quad. Eval. next visit & scale, RP, STC UL quad. No adverse reactions to LA or tx. reported or observed. Next visit: 1 wk.

LWF

It is important to enter progress notes using accepted dental terminology or abbreviations and descriptive, objective sentences for two reasons. First, other health care providers must be able to understand the terminology used in the entry to continue care; second, the patient can gain access to the record, so no derogatory or subjective comments should be entered in the record (Howard, 1975). For example, it is highly inappropriate to enter, "Ms. Jones is a real complainer—ignore her for her own good." The following sample entry may be more appropriate: "Ms. Jones said that she hates the scraping noise of the instruments on her teeth and that she does not want me to make that noise. I explained why the noise was necessary and reassured her that the scaling was being done properly. At the end of the appointment, Ms. Jones said, 'I still don't like that sound, but my teeth feel smooth.'" The second entry describes the situation more completely, and if the patient ever read the entry, it is not likely that she would be offended or feel discredited. Abbreviations could be used to shorten the length of this entry.

An entry should be supported with data whenever possible so that the next health care provider can better understand the situation. If an entry stated, "Patient has poor home care procedures," the next health care provider would not have much concrete information to evaluate. However, the entry "Patient has consistently high plaque and bleeding indices; patient reports that she brushes once a day when she remembers to brush" gives the next health care provider more information about the patient's dental status without subjective judgments.

APPROACHES TO RECORD STYLE

The necessary inclusions in a dental record have been discussed, but the styles of record keeping have not. At the present time two approaches are popular. The first is the *treatment-oriented approach,* and the second is the *problem-oriented approach* (Sanger, 1973; Weed, 1969). The treatment-oriented approach has three major components: data base, treatment plan, and progress notes. The problem-oriented approach has four components: data base, problem list, treatment plan, and progress notes (Sanger, 1973; Weed, 1969). The major difference between the two approaches is the formulation of the problem list. Weed (1969) maintains that an essential element, the problem list, is missing in the traditional treatment-oriented approach.

In the treatment-oriented approach, after the data are collected, the dentist analyzes the data and formulates a treatment plan that should meet all the needs of the patient that were identified by the data collection. If the patient has complex needs, such as systemic problems as well as multiple carious lesions and areas of mobility, pocketing, and bleeding, the treatment plan may become complex and difficult to properly complete.

In the problem-oriented approach, the dentist compiles a problem list from all of the data collected. Each sign and/or symptom is identified as a problem, and each problem has an individual treatment plan with a priority number so that the most threatening problems are treated first (Weed, 1969). For example, if a patient being treated complained of bleeding gums, had gingivitis, and had one carious lesion, the problems, in order of priority, would be (1) bleeding gums, (2) gingivitis, and (3) carious lesion. In the problem-oriented approach, there is a specific step, formulating the problem list, for analysis of the data and then logical assignment of priorities. In the treatment-oriented approach, this step is not present; rather, the dentist analyzes the data as part of the treatment plan (Fig. 4-1).

After the problem list has been formulated, a treatment plan addressing each of the problems is designed. Since the problems have already been assigned priorities, the treatment plan for the above example would be (1) bleeding gums—take baseline indices; teach modified Bass brushing and

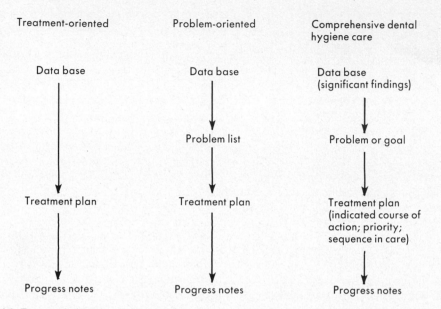

Comparison of record approaches

Fig. 4-1. Treatment-oriented and problem-oriented approaches are compared in the first and second columns: note that the treatment-oriented approach does not include a problem list. The approach presented in this book, a problem-oriented approach, is in the third column. Consult Chapter 18 for further explanation of terms in parentheses.

flossing; monitor patient's progress via indices; (2) gingivitis—scaling and prophylaxis; and (3) carious lesions—amalgam restoration No. 30. As can be seen, the treatment plan flows from the problem list. The problem-oriented approach is particularly helpful when a patient presents complex systemic and/or dental problems leading to an involved treatment plan. This approach is also helpful during the case presentation to the patient, since the treatments are geared to the patient's problems. Once the clinician has explained the problems to the patient in an organized fashion, the treatments are more likely to be understood by the patient.

Weed (1969) has an excellent description of the problem-oriented approach to records and a sample case, which can be studied to understand the problem-oriented approach in greater detail. The approach to records and treatment planning presented in this book (Fig. 4-1) is a problem-oriented one. The approach is described more fully in Chapter 18.

COMPUTERS IN DENTISTRY

The use of computers within dentistry is varied and continually expanding. Computers are used in research (Mahler et al., 1980), orthodontics (Sloan, 1980), oral medicine (Kramer, 1980), and office management (Council on Dental Practice, 1980; Crandell, 1980), to list some of the areas. Within the area of office management, computers are used for maintenance of data and for analysis concerning patients' records and accounts, clinician productivity and competency, practice productivity and costs, and recall systems and appointment planning (Crandell, 1980). Increasingly, clinicians will be exposed to computers and will use them in many facets of clinical practice, including patient record keeping.

RECORD AUDITS

With the increasing emphasis among health care providers on thorough, complete, and accurate records and with the increasing interest of third-party

Patient_____ Date_____

Chart number_____ Reviewer_____

Note in each box whether the item is Satisfactory (S), Unsatisfactory (U), or

Not Applicable (NA). Note the reason of each NA on the back of this form.

Place your initials and the date of the review in the appropriate boxes.

Initials

Date

1. Medical history complete, updated, signed

2. Physician's letter present, if needed

3. Oral exam complete, updated, signed

4. Chartings complete, updated, signed

5. Satisfactory radiographs taken/present

6. Satisfactory study models present, if taken

7. Satisfactory photographs present, if taken

8. Additional records present, if taken

9. Home care procedures assessed

10. Treatment plan recorded

11. Home care planned, implemented, evaluated

12. Treatment plan followed/revised

13. Progress notes complete, dated, signed

14. Recall date recorded

15. Financial records complete

16. Demographic data complete

Additional comments:

Fig. 4-2. Sample dental record audit form. See text for explanation of how to use this form.

carriers, such as insurance companies, in the prevention of fraud in filing claims, many health care practices have instituted record audits among the dental personnel to ensure that the charts are being completed accurately and that the necessary inclusions are present (Woodall, 1983). Fig. 4-2 is a sample chart audit form that has been used in a health care practice to audit dental records.

The audit form is completed at the conclusion of a patient's course of treatment by a clinician other than the one responsible for the patient's treatment. When performing an audit, the clinician checks the record to ensure that each of the items listed in the left column is present. If the item is present and satisfactory, an ''S'' is placed in the appropriate space; if the item is missing or unacceptable, a ''U'' is placed in the space. Once the audit is completed, the person doing the audit initials and dates the form at the top of the column. If any items are missing or unsatisfactory, the clinician responsible for the patient's care is asked to rectify the situation. Since there are several columns, the same audit form can be used after each course of a patient's treatment.

It is a wise practice to review all patient records regularly using an audit form to identify missing or inaccurate entries and to be certain that the care being delivered is appropriate for the patient's needs. By maintaining thorough, complete, and accurate charts, the health care provider will be better able to provide continuous high-quality care and provide protection for both the dental personnel and the patient.

ACTIVITIES

1. Secure sample charts from several dental care practices and:
   a. Review the charts for organization.
   b. Review the charts for the necessary inclusions.
   c. Review the progress notes for thoroughness and completeness.
   d. Rewrite some of the progress notes in a format that meets the criteria described in the chapter.
2. Invite a speaker from one of the companies that print dental records to explain the company's record forms.
3. Develop a chart audit system that could be used in a dental practice.
4. Read Chapter 19, ''Problem-oriented dental record system—an alternative'' and Chapter 20, ''Problem-oriented record system—case example,'' in *Treatment Planning: A Pragmatic Approach* (Wood, 1978).

REVIEW QUESTIONS

1. Explain the purposes of dental records.
2. List the inclusions that should be part of a dental record and justify each item.
3. Name one major difference between the treatment-oriented and the problem-oriented approaches to record keeping.
4. What is the purpose of a chart audit?
5. Describe a format for writing progress notes.

REFERENCES

Conger, S.X. Sept. 1983. The law and dental hygiene practice. Dent. Hyg. **57:**14.

Corby, C.S. 1978. Are you ready for a computer? Dent. Econ. **68:**35.

Council on Dental Practice. 1980. Computer technology in dental practice. J. Am. Dent. Assoc. **101:**938.

Crandell, C.E. 1980. Use of computers in dental office management. Int. Dent. J. **30:**226.

Ehrlich, A., et al. 1981. Selecting a computerized account receivable system. Dent. Clin. North Am. **25:**731.

Gairola, G., and Skaff, K. Feb. 1983. Ethical reasoning in dental hygiene practice. Dent. Hyg. **57:**16.

Granger, B. July 1980. Legal aspects of dental hygiene practice. Dent. Hyg. **54:**43.

Howard, W.W.: 1975. Dental practice planning. St. Louis: The C.V. Mosby Co.

Johnson, D. May-June 1979. Structured case presentations: cornerstone to informed patients. Gen. Dent. **27:**62.

Kilpatrick, H.C. 1974. Work simplification in dental practice: applied time and motion studies. Philadelphia: W.B. Saunders Co.

Kramer, I.R.H. 1980. Computers in clinical and laboratory diagnosis. Int. Dent. J. **30:**214.

Mahler, T.M., et al. 1980. Computers in preventive dentistry. Int. Dent. J. **30:**201.

Miller, S.L. 1979. Legal aspects of dentistry. New York: G.P. Putnam's Sons.

Morris, W.O. 1976. Some thoughts on dental malpractice. Int. Dent. J. **26:**175.

Sanger, R.G., and Boone, M.E. 1978. Problem-oriented dental record system—an alternative. In Wood, N.K., editor. Treatment planning: a pragmatic approach. St. Louis: The C.V. Mosby Co.

Sloan, R.F. 1980. Computer application in orthodontics. Int. Dent. J. **30:**189.

Stetler, C.J., and Moritz, A.R. 1962. Doctor and patient and the law. St. Louis: The C.V. Mosby Co.

Warner, R., and Segal, H. 1980. Ethical issues of informed consent in dentistry. Chicago: Quintessence Publishing Co., Inc.

Weed, L.L. 1969. Medical records, medical education, and patient care. Cleveland: Case Western Reserve University, Year Book Medical Publishers, Inc.

Wood, N.K., editor. 1978. Treatment planning: a pragmatic approach. St. Louis: The C.V. Mosby Co.

Woodall, I.R. 1983. Legal, ethical, and management aspects of the dental care system, ed. 2. St. Louis: The C.V. Mosby Co.

5 BASIC INSTRUMENTATION AND POSITIONING

OBJECTIVES: *The reader will be able to*

1. Describe the basic purposes of the following instruments in assessment phases of dental hygiene care:
   Mouth mirror
   Retractor
   Explorer
   Periodontal probe
2. Given an instrument, identify its handle, working end(s), shank, and terminal shank.
3. Given a variety of instruments, identify single-ended, double-ended, and paired instruments.
4. Give two reasons for the importance of being able to identify instruments by their shapes and recognize variations in shape and design.
5. Explain how proper positioning at the dental chair enhances proper instrumentation.
6. Describe the properly seated clinician, patient, and chairside assistant.
7. Adjust the positions of the clinician, patient, and chairside assistant for maximum access and visibility for any area in the dentition.
8. Given any tooth surface, adjust himself/herself to the proper position; adjust the patient's head position and the overhead light; use the mouth mirror to maximize access and vision; and establish a modified pen grasp, a fulcrum, and a wrist rock to generate vertical, overlapping strokes on a tooth.
9. Establish proper positioning, access, vision, grasp, fulcrum, wrist rock, and stroke for each area in the recommended sequence of positions.
10. Use proper positioning, grasp, wrist rock, instrument adaptation, and stroke for the:
    Periodontal probe
    Paired explorer (cowhorn, pigtail)
    Straight-shanked explorer (No. 17 or 20)
11. Use the shepherd's hook (No. 23) to explore for caries.

PURPOSE OF HAND INSTRUMENTS IN DENTAL HYGIENE CARE

The hand instruments used in dental hygiene care serve a variety of functions in the assessment, implementation, and evaluation phases of care. Before learning and performing any additional assessment procedures, it is important to develop some basic skills in handling instruments and in learning to work at the chairside.

Mouth mirrors

One of the most important instruments in dental hygiene care is the mouth mirror. It is an instrument used to *enhance vision* in the recesses of the oral cavity. Mirrors are available in a variety of sizes and may have a magnifying surface. The mouth mirror is used for retracting tissues such as the cheek and tongue, for reflecting light onto an area that otherwise would be in a shadow, for indirect vision of an area that cannot be seen directly (such as the distal aspect of the most posterior molar), and for transillumination (casting light through teeth to determine the presence of caries or calculus by detecting variations in translucency).

An essential prerequisite skill in learning to use dental instruments is the effective use of the mouth mirror to ensure comfortable, adequate vision of all areas of the mouth. An exercise at the end of this chapter outlines a method for developing this skill prior to the introduction of "working instruments." The goal should be careful, assertive placement of the mirror to obtain a clear view of the operative site and adequate space to locate a firm fulcrum or finger rest for the working hand. This should be done without clanking the mirror against the teeth, without pinching the lip against the teeth, without pressing the mirror head against the gingiva, and without impinging soft tissue against bone.

Retractors

Another example of a dental instrument that enhances vision is the cheek retractor, most often used to extend the cheeks and lips away from the mouth to assist in intraoral photography. Other intraoral retractors can be used to keep the tongue from

SINGLE END

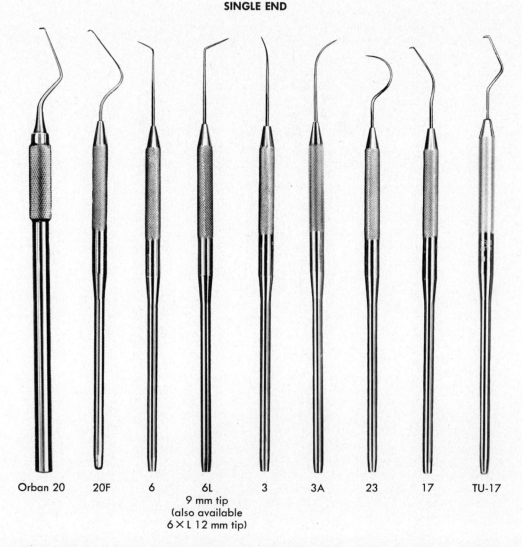

Orban 20   20F   6   6L   3   3A   23   17   TU-17

9 mm tip
(also available
6 × L 12 mm tip)

Fig. 5-1. Explorers used for detection of caries and for examining teeth for calculus and other irregularities are available in a variety of shapes and sizes. (Courtesy Hu-Friedy Co., Chicago.)

wandering toward the operative site, thus preventing accidental trauma.

Explorers and probes

Other instruments are used to *examine* teeth and tissues by exploring the teeth and by measuring the size and location of tissue entities. Explorers are instruments used primarily to examine the teeth for caries and for the presence of tooth irregularities such as calculus deposits, root roughness, anatomic defects, and margins of restorations. Explorers come in a variety of shapes and sizes—some best suited for exploring for caries and others for the detection of fine subgingival irregularities. (Figs. 5-1 and 5-2 show several common types of explorers.) Because the dental hygienist's role includes identifying tooth characteristics and monitoring a patient's oral health, it is important to master the use of explorers early in clinical practice.

The periodontal probe is used for examining oral tissues also. It is not used for caries detection, since

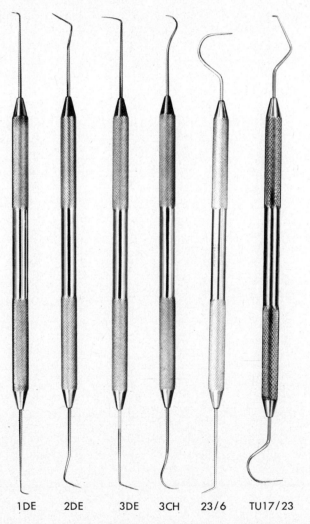

1DE   2DE   3DE   3CH   23/6   TU17/23

Fig. 5-2. Explorers are available in pairs to gain access to a tooth from facial aspect with one end from the lingual aspect with the other end. Double-ended instruments may have two entirely different styles of working designs, such as the 23/6. (Courtesy Hu-Friedy Co., Chicago.)

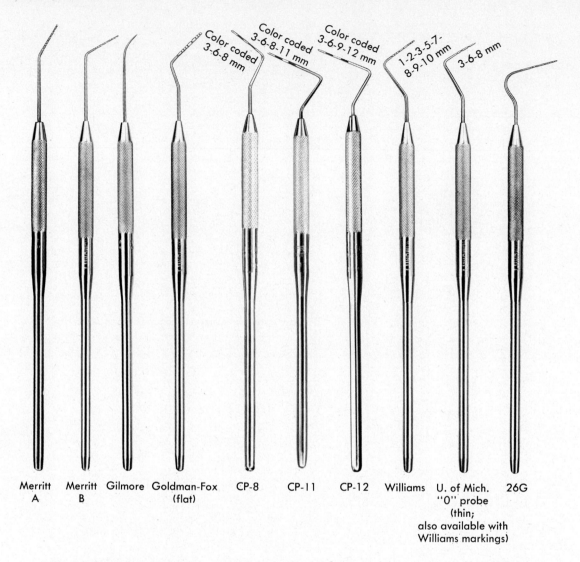

Fig. 5-3. Periodontal probes, used primarily for examining sulcus and measuring its depths, are calibrated in millimeters. Some are color coded to improve readability. Shank length, angle, and working tip shape vary. (Courtesy Hu-Friedy Co., Chicago.)

it does not have a sharp point for retention in carious areas. Probes that are noted for their delicate design can be used for detection of root irregularities and hard deposits. However, the probe's primary use is for measuring the depth of the gingival sulcus or periodontal pocket (Pattison and Behrens, 1973; Ward and Simring, 1978). The periodontal probe's unique characteristic is its calibrations, marked in millimeters. How far the probe slides into the sulcus or a pocket indicates the level of the attachment of the gingiva to the tooth. The probe can trace the topography of the attachment around the tooth, providing the hygienist with an idea of the extent of disease and the health status of the periodontium.

The calibrated probe also can be used to measure recession of the free gingiva, the amount of attached masticatory mucosa, or the size of a lesion.

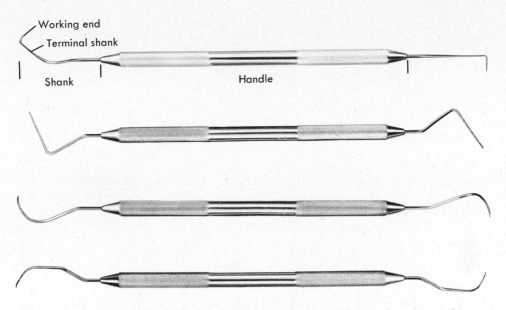

Working end
Terminal shank
Shank
Handle

Fig. 5-4. Handle of instrument is connected to a thinner shank that is angled to permit access to various areas of the dentition. Working end is at tip of instrument. Part of shank closest to working end is called the *terminal shank*. All instruments shown are double ended. Bottom two instruments are paired. (Courtesy Hu-Friedy Co., Chicago.)

It is critical to know how the probe is calibrated, since some are marked in 3 mm increments and others are marked at 1, 2, 3, 5, and 7 mm and other variations (Fig. 5-3).

Exercises described in this chapter provide opportunities for using the mouth mirror for vision and the periodontal probe for exploring and measuring subgingival areas. A subsequent exercise advances the student to the use of a cowhorn explorer and a No. 17 explorer.

Once the mouth mirror, probe, and explorers can be used competently, the clinician is prepared to assess the intraoral dental findings for a patient.

Other instruments

Instruments used in the implementation of care are those used to *remove deposits* from teeth such as scalers and curettes and those used to *recontour or excise tissue*. Other working instruments, particularly those used in restorative dentistry, are used to *place materials on or in the teeth and the surrounding tissues*. As each phase of implementation of dental hygiene care is addressed in later chapters, the design and use of each instrument are also discussed.

BASIC INSTRUMENT DESIGN

The basic terminology used to describe most dental instruments makes it easier for the student and faculty member or for the clinician and assistant to understand each other when discussing instrument selection and use. Refer to Fig. 5-4 as the parts of the instruments are described.

The *handle* is the part grasped by the clinician or assistant. Handles come in various shapes and sizes, including variations of hexagonal, round, and tapered. They can be smooth or have knurls or a grooved pattern to prevent the handle from slipping in the user's hand (Pattison and Behrens, 1973; Ward and Simring, 1978).

The *working end* of the instrument refers to the end of the instrument that contacts the tooth and performs the intended task. The working end can have a point, a blade, a blunt nib, pincers for grasping an object, or some other useful configuration (Pattison and Behrens, 1973; Ward and Simring, 1978).

Joining the working end and the handle is the *shank*, which determines the accessibility of the instrument to various places in the mouth and the flex and strength of the instrument. The angles and convolutions in the shank permit access to posterior areas and proximal surfaces while allowing the clinician's hand to enter from the front of the mouth. The thickness and tensile strength of the shank dictate the amount of stress that the shank can endure in intraoral procedures requiring considerable pressure. Shank shape and strength are therefore particularly important considerations when selecting instruments for removing particularly heavy, tenacious deposits from the teeth (Pattison and Behrens, 1973; Ward and Simring, 1978).

The *terminal shank* is the part of the shank that is closest to the working end. It is important to be able to locate the terminal shank on instruments with simple and complex shanks, since the terminal shank is one important cue in adapting the instrument to the tooth. This term is used frequently in this chapter in describing the procedure for selecting the correct end of the instrument and for ensuring that it is being used safely and correctly.

Instruments are available with two working ends, one at each end of the handle. These are referred to as *double-ended* instruments. Using double-ended instruments necessitates fewer instrument changes and minimizes the number of individual instruments on the tray, reducing clutter. However, when changing ends of an instrument, one must take care to prevent contacting the patient with the instrument. Instrument changes should occur away from the patient's face, usually over the patient's chest, as is the practice in four-handed dentistry. All the instruments in Fig. 5-4 are double ended.

Two of the double-ended instruments in Fig. 5-4 are also examples of *paired instruments*. The ends of a paired instrument are mirror images of each other. One end is intended for use on a proximal surface of a tooth from the facial aspect. Its pair is intended for entry from the lingual aspect. Thus the bends in the shank allow access to a given proximal surface from both aspects.

A more complete discussion of where instruments may be used and how pairs are identified is presented in later chapters. At this point in developing an awareness of instruments and their use, it may be helpful to remember that many instruments are used in pairs, permitting universal access to tooth surfaces.

As each instrument is introduced and used in assessing patient needs and implementing care, it may be helpful for the clinician to identify the parts of the instrument and to project what function it might serve and where it could be adapted. Such an approach to instruments will make it possible for the clinician to identify instruments on the basis of their shapes and sizes rather than by the numbers engraved in the handle. It also will help the clinician develop a working familiarity with instruments that will enable experimentation with a variety of designs as skill and experience grow.

Another important reason for knowing and analyzing instrument design is that the original shape must be preserved as instruments are sharpened. Strokes with a sharpening stone are more likely to sharpen without damaging the working end if the clinician has a clear concept of the proper shape.

HOLDING AND USING INSTRUMENTS: THE GRASP, FINGER REST, AND WRIST ROCK

Holding an instrument is different from the way most people hold writing implements. Fig. 5-5 shows a typical pen grasp with the thumb and first finger grasping the handle, supported by the middle finger under the handle. Fig. 5-6 shows the modified pen grasp, in which the first and second fingers are placed on the instrument, opposed by the thumb. Fig. 5-7 shows a common error made in grasping a dental instrument. The first two knuckles of the first finger should be flat on the instrument to improve stability and to ensure tactile sense. The third finger should serve as a *fulcrum,* or pivot point, often called a *finger rest.* With this grasp and fulcrum, it should be possible to see the palm of the hand when looking past the instrument from the thumb, as evident in Fig. 5-6. The wrist rock begins in this position and moves on the fulcrum point as a unified movement of arm, wrist, and hand in a side-to-side, rock-and-return oscillation (Fig. 5-8). With the wrist rock, the instrument should be moved up and down the tooth without changing the angle of the shank to the tooth with each stroke. A heavily accentuated wrist rock that starts with the palm cupped downward can cause the shank to move in and out from the tooth, and this is undesirable.

Another motion that can be useful in areas where lateral rocking is difficult is the vertical, or forward-and-back, wrist rock (Fig. 5-9). The instrument is moved up and down the tooth in the same stroking pattern, but the hand movement is done by lowering the wrist while maintaining a fulcrum.

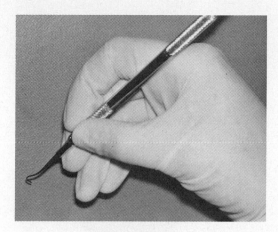

Fig. 5-5. Typical pen grasp with thumb and first finger grasping handle. Middle finger supports instrument from underneath.

Fig. 5-6. *Modified pen grasp* with both first and second fingers holding handle, opposed by thumb. Third finger is in position to rest on tooth structure to create stability and to create a fulcrum point for moving the instrument.

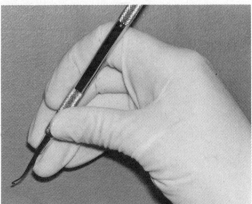

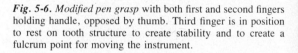

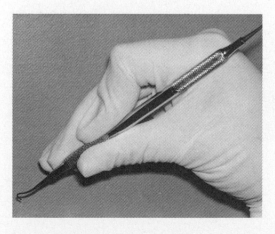

Fig. 5-7. *Incorrect* modified pen grasp because knuckle of first finger is buckled. Handle should lie flat against first two sections of first finger as shown in Fig. 5-6.

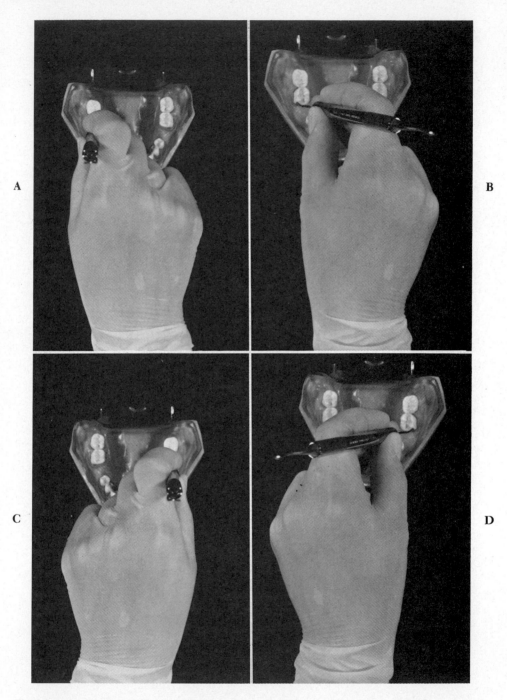

Fig. 5-8. A, Beginning position for lateral wrist rock, with pen grasp and solid fulcrum **B,** Hand rocks laterally to the right, moving working end of instrument in coronal direction. Rocking back to position in **A** moves working end of instrument apically. Thus instrument strokes are accomplished by rocking the hand back and forth. **C,** Beginning position for left-handed clinician. **D,** Hand rocked laterally to the left.

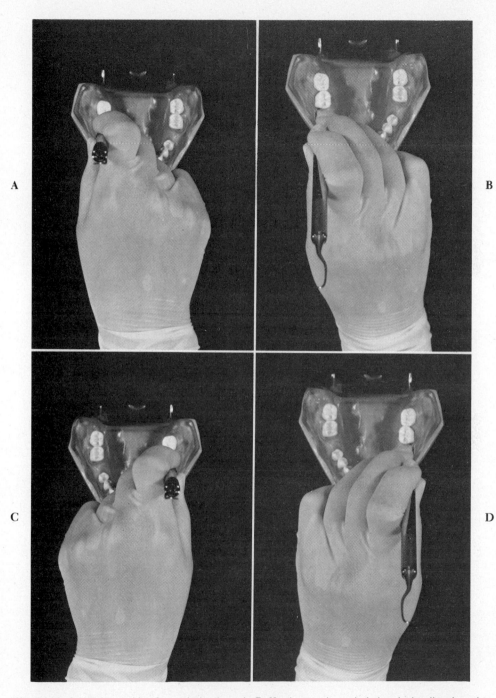

Fig. 5-9. **A,** Beginning position for vertical wrist rock. **B,** Hand moves in vertical plane by bending the wrist. Bending the wrist moves instrument tip coronally, and returning to position in **A** moves instrument tip apically. **C,** Beginning position for left-handed clinician. **D,** Hand moved by lowering the wrist while maintaining a fulcrum.

EFFICIENCY AND MOTION ECONOMY IN INSTRUMENTATION

When any instrument is used in performing intraoral procedures, effectiveness is improved and fatigue can be reduced if a few simple guidelines are followed. Proper positioning of the clinician, the patient, and the dental assistant during the very first efforts at instrumentation can help the dental hygienist develop safe practice habits that will enhance efficiency and aid in mastery of instrumentation skills.

Proper positioning at the chair makes it easier to see the operative site, to maintain a stable fulcrum or finger rest, and to adapt the instrument. Finally, good positioning reduces muscle strain and fatigue for the entire dental team, including the patient.

Therefore, as the basic principles of instrumentation are introduced and practiced, principles of motion economy, including proper positioning, will be implemented as well. The basic premises underlying this approach are that good instrumentation learned from detrimental or impossible clinician and patient positions does not transfer readily to a useful pattern of clinical practice, and instrumentation learned from ideal positions at the chair makes mastery of basic manipulation much easier, since it is enhanced by good vision, fulcrum placement, and access.

BASIC POSITIONS OF THE DENTAL TEAM

To begin instrumentation, the patient should be placed in a supine position. As described in Chapter 2, this is best accomplished by tilting the entire chair back to ensure seating the patient's hips in the angle of the chair. The back of the chair is then lowered to just above the lap of the seated clinician. The headrest should be adjusted, and a protective napkin or bib placed on the patient. The patient's feet should be at approximately the same height as the patient's head.

The clinician should be seated so that the thighs are parallel to the floor and the feet are flat on the floor. If the clinician's stool has an abdominal rest, the rest should be located just below the clinician's ribs to provide support as he/she inclines the upper body forward from the waist.

The chairside assistant should be seated so that his/her eye level is 4 to 6 inches above the clini-

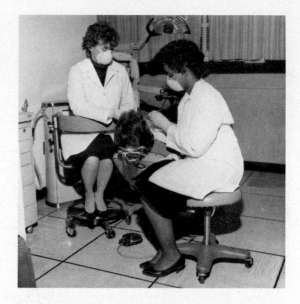

Fig. 5-10. Properly positioned patient, right-handed clinician, and assistant.

cian's eye level. Depending on the assistant's height, this may necessitate a foot support on the stool to enable the thighs to be parallel to the floor.

With the three members of the team in this basic seating arrangement, the clinician may move from a front to a rear position at the chair with the assistant making appropriate minor adjustments to ensure proper instrument transfers and visibility. The right-handed clinician's position is at approximately 8:30 to 10 o'clock at the chair for the front position and at 10:30 to 12 o'clock for the rear position. Left-handed clinicians occupy 3:30 to 2 o'clock and 2:30 to 12 o'clock positions for front and rear positions, respectively (Figs. 5-10 and 5-11).

In addition to the flexibility of moving from front to rear, there is additional flexibility and access as the patient turns his/her head toward or away from the clinician. Additionally, the patient can raise or lower the chin. The back of the chair can be raised or lowered 1 to 2 inches for access to specific areas.

The combination of clinician position, patient head movement, and the wisely used mouth mirror eliminates the need for contorted positions for adequate vision. It is possible to gain access to all areas of the mouth while maintaining a healthful posture.

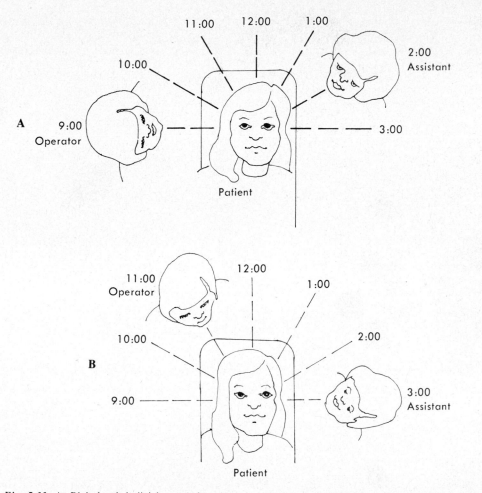

Fig. 5-11. **A,** Right-handed clinician seated at approximately 9 o'clock position with assistant at 2 o'clock position. **B,** Right-handed clinician seated at 11 o'clock position with assistant at 3 o'clock position. Left-handed clinician sits at 3 o'clock and 1 o'clock positions for front and rear positions, respectively.

POSITIONING EXERCISES

To develop skill in gaining access to all areas of the mouth, students should divide into groups of three to practice the basic positions, each serving once as patient, clinician, and assistant. As each student serves as chairside assistant, he/she should prepare the dental unit by disinfecting equipment and placing sterile instruments on the tray (including a mouth mirror and a cotton-tipped applicator), seat the patient in a supine position, and place the bib. The assistant should adjust his/her stool to the proper height in relation to the clinician and ensure

that he/she has an adequate view of each operative site by making minor adjustments in position.

The dental assistant should ensure proper adjustment of the overhead light by observing the target of the primary beam of light and adjusting the overall position and angle of the lamp so that the beam is on the operative site and is not blocked by a hand, the clinician's head, or some other obstacle. A general rule is to bring the lamp up over the patient's face and angle it downward (nearly perpendicular to the floor) for mandibular sites and to bring the lamp back over the patient's lap and

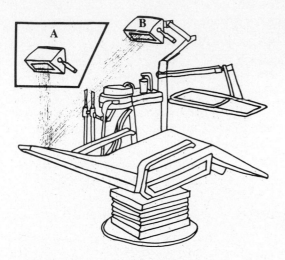

Fig. 5-12. A general rule in obtaining optimal intraoral illumination is to angle beam of overhead lamp nearly perpendicular to floor, **A**, for mandible and more parallel to floor, **B**, for maxilla. Range of angulation for maxilla is usually between 45 and 10 degrees to floor.

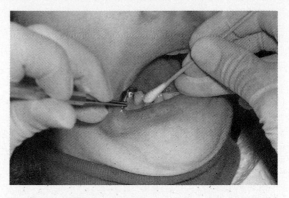

Fig. 5-13. Modified pen grasp for *right-handed* clinician, showing cheek retraction and stable third-finger fulcrum on teeth for access to mandibular right buccal area.

angle it toward the mouth so that the primary beam is nearly parallel to the floor for maxillary sites (Fig. 5-12). From these two basic positions it is possible to angle the lamp from one side or the other to eliminate shadows created by the hands.

The clinician should adjust his/her stool to the proper height and use the mouth mirror for retraction, indirect vision, and/or light reflection as appropriate for each area of the mouth. The mouth mirror should be held in the nonworking hand. The cotton-tipped applicator should be held in the working hand (right-handed people use the right hand; left-handed people use the left hand).

Moving sequentially from area to area of the dentition, the clinician should use the mouth mirror as indicated in Table 5-1 or 5-2. The clinician should establish a solid modified pen grasp with the working hand as shown in Figs. 5-13 and 5-14 for right- and left-handed clinicians, respectively, establish a fulcrum or finger rest on the teeth, and use the wrist rock so that the cotton tip rides up and down the tooth in a vertical pattern of overlapping strokes. Two or three teeth in each area should be traced to provide practice in maintaining retraction and in using a stable grasp, fulcrum, and wrist rock.

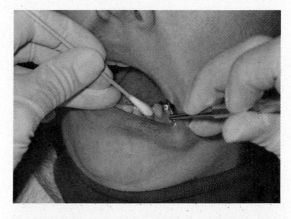

Fig. 5-14. Modified pen grasp for *left-handed* clinician, showing cheek retraction and stable third-finger fulcrum on teeth for access to mandibular left buccal area.

Figs. 5-15 to 5-26 show sample hand positions for right-handed clinicians; left-handed clinicians should follow Figs. 5-27 to 5-38. These hand positions should be referred to for this exercise. The student may progress to the probe and then to the cowhorn (as shown in these illustrations) after basic skill is achieved with the cotton-tipped applicator.

Text continued on p. 84.

Table 5-1. Positioning for right-handed clinicians

Area of operation	Patient's head position*	Clinician position	Finger rest	Vision	Use of mirror
Mandible					
Right buccal	Left	9 o'clock	Bicuspid/cuspid	Direct	Retract cheek
Left lingual	Left	9 o'clock	Bicuspid/cuspid	Direct	Retract tongue
Right lingual	Right	9 o'clock	Bicuspid/cuspid	Indirect	Retract cheek; indirect vision and illumination
Left buccal	Right	11 o'clock	Bicuspid/cuspid	Direct	Retract cheek
Anterior lingual	Straight†	11 o'clock	Cuspid	Direct	Reflect light; retract tongue
Anterior labial	Straight†	11 o'clock	Cuspid	Direct or indirect	Indirect vision; retract lip
Maxilla					
Right buccal	Left	9 o'clock	Occlusal surface of tooth posterior to area of operation	Direct	Retract cheek
Left lingual	Left	9 o'clock		Direct	Reflect light
Right lingual	Right	11 o'clock		Indirect	Indirect vision; reflect light
Left buccal	Right	11 o'clock		Direct	Retract cheek
Anterior lingual	Straight†	11 o'clock	Incisal edge	Indirect	Indirect vision; reflect light
Anterior labial	Straight†	11 o'clock	Incisal edge	Direct	None

*Patient is in the supine position.
†Patient is asked to turn his/her head slightly as clinician moves from cuspid to cuspid in the anterior areas.

Table 5-2. Positioning for left-handed clinicians

Area of operation	Patient's head position*	Clinician position	Finger rest	Vision	Use of mirror
Mandible					
Left buccal	Right	3 o'clock	Bicuspid/cuspid	Direct	Retract cheek
Right lingual	Right	3 o'clock	Bicuspid/cuspid	Direct	Retract tongue
Left lingual	Left	3 o'clock	Bicuspid/cuspid	Indirect	Retract cheek; indirect vision and illumination
Right buccal	Left	1 o'clock	Bicuspid/cuspid	Direct	Retract cheek
Anterior lingual	Straight†	1 o'clock	Cuspid	Direct	Reflect light; retract tongue
Anterior labial	Straight†	1 o'clock	Cuspid	Direct or indirect	Indirect vision; retract lip
Maxilla					
Left buccal	Right	3 o'clock	Occlusal surface of tooth posterior to area of operation	Direct	Retract cheek
Right lingual	Right	3 o'clock		Direct	Reflect light
Left lingual	Left	1 o'clock		Indirect	Indirect vision; reflect light
Right buccal	Left	1 o'clock		Direct	Retract cheek
Anterior lingual	Straight†	1 o'clock	Incisal edge	Indirect	Indirect vision; reflect light
Anterior labial	Straight†	1 o'clock	Incisal edge	Direct	None

*Patient is in the supine position.
†Patient is asked to turn his/her head slightly as clinician moves from cuspid to cuspid in the anterior areas.

Right-handed clinician

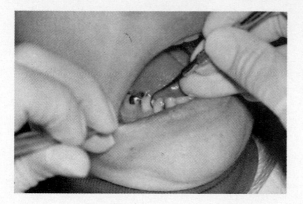

Fig. 5-15. *Right-handed clinician:* Hand position for instrumentation on mandibular right buccal aspect. Once cotton-tipped applicator has been used in each area, student may progress to periodontal probe to learn subgingival insertion and to explorer to learn adaptation. Mirror retracts cheek; fulcrum is anterior to operative site, resting on occlusal surfaces.

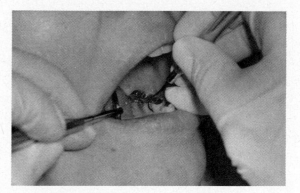

Fig. 5-16. *Right-handed clinician:* Hand position for instrumentation on mandibular left lingual aspect. Mirror retracts tongue. Fulcrum is on facial-occlusal aspect of teeth in that sextant.

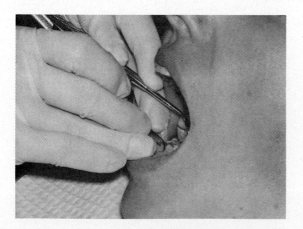

Fig. 5-17. *Right-handed clinician:* Hand position for instrumentation on mandibular right lingual aspect. Mirror retracts tongue but faces teeth, directing light onto area and providing indirect vision. Some clinicians prefer to approach this area from a rear position, with patient's head turned well toward clinician to enable direct vision.

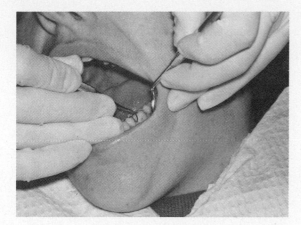

Fig. 5-18. *Right-handed clinician:* Hand position for instrumentation on mandibular left buccal aspect. With patient's head turned toward clinician, mirror retracts cheek, enabling direct vision. Clinician is seated in rear position.

Fig. 5-19. *Right-handed clinician:* Hand position for instrumentation on mandibular anterior lingual aspect. Seated in rear position, clinician uses mirror to retract tongue and reflect light on area for direct vision.

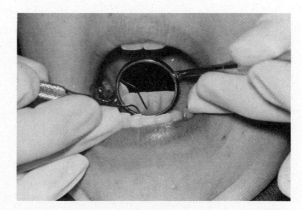

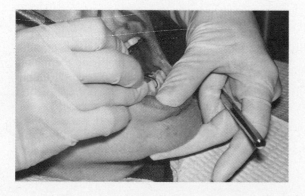

Fig. 5-20. *Right-handed clinician:* Hand position for instrumentation on mandibular anterior facial aspect. Clinician is seated in rear position. Lower lip is retracted by thumb, forefinger, or mouth mirror, Direct vision is used. When direct vision is difficult to achieve, mouth mirror can retract lip and provide indirect vision.

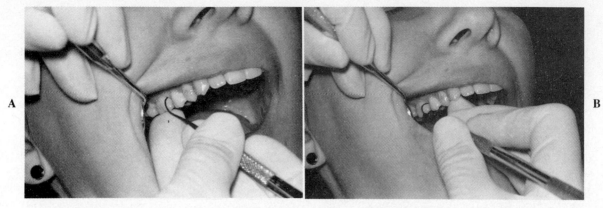

Fig. 5-21. *Right-handed clinician:* Two approaches to maxillary right buccal aspect. **A,** Palm up, fulcrum on or posterior to operative site, giving stability and greater leverage for deposit removal during scaling. Clinician is seated at approximately 9:30 position. **B,** Palm down, fulcrum anterior to area being explored. Clinician is seated in front position. While this technique is easier to learn and is adequate for exploring, it provides less control and leverage during scaling. A vertical wrist rock (see Fig. 5-9) is used for this approach.

Fig. 5-22. *Right-handed clinician:* Hand position for instrumentation on maxillary left lingual aspect. Fulcrum is placed on occlusal surface of tooth or slightly on buccal aspect. All fingers are kept together as single unit to ensure a solid wrist rock and stroke. Mirror reflects light onto area. Direct vision is used, with patient's head tilted away. Clinician is seated in front position.

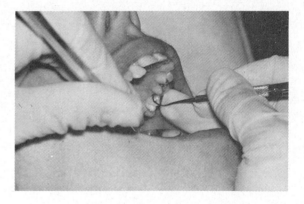

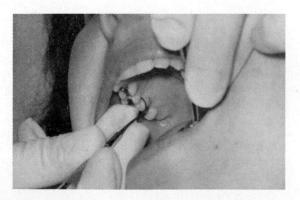

Fig. 5-23. *Right-handed clinician:* Hand position for instrumentation on maxillary right lingual aspect. Clinician is in rear position. Mirror reflects light and provides indirect vision. Fulcrum is on occlusal aspect of sextant. Maintaining good posture, clinician holds mirror so it is visible, then angles mirror until light is cast on area to be explored and image is visible in mirror.

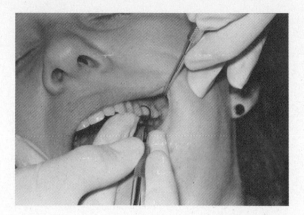

Fig. 5-24. *Right-handed clinician:* Hand position for instrumentation on maxillary left buccal aspect. Clinician is in rear position. Mirror retracts cheek, and fulcrum is on occlusal aspect of teeth, with patient's head turned toward clinician for direct vision.

Fig. 5-25. *Right-handed clinician:* Hand position for instrumentation on maxillary anterior lingual aspect. Clinician remains in rear position and uses mirror to reflect light and provide indirect vision. Maintaining good posture, clinician holds mirror so it is visible, then angles mirror until area is illuminated and visible in mirror. Fulcrum is on incisal edge, with palm up for efficient wrist rock.

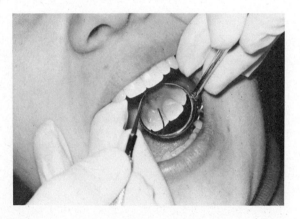

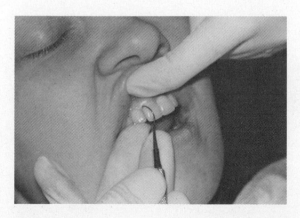

Fig. 5-26. *Right-handed clinician:* Hand position for instrumentation on maxillary anterior labial aspect. To ensure a stable fulcrum, rear position is preferred. Hand remains a solid unit, with all fingers resting on fulcrum, palm up. Direct vision is used, with forefinger retracting lip.

Left-handed clinician

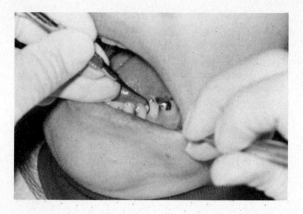

Fig. 5-27. *Left-handed clinician:* Hand position for instrumentation on mandibular left buccal aspect. Once cotton-tipped applicator has been used in each area, student may progress to periodontal probe to learn subgingival insertion and to explorer to learn adaptation. Mirror retracts cheek; fulcrum is anterior to operative site, resting on occlusal surfaces.

Fig. 5-28. *Left-handed clinician:* Hand position for instrumentation on mandibular right lingual aspect. Mirror retracts tongue. Fulcrum is on facial-occlusal aspect of teeth in that sextant.

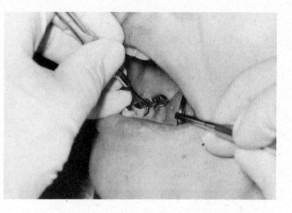

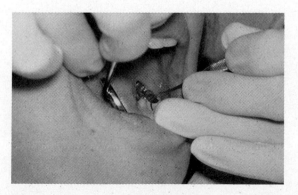

Fig. 5-29. *Left-handed clinician:* Hand position for instrumentation on mandibular left lingual aspect. Mirror retracts tongue but faces teeth, directing light onto area and providing indirect vision. Some clinicians prefer to approach this area from a rear position, with patient's head turned well toward clinician to enable direct vision.

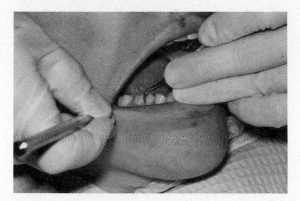

Fig. 5-30. *Left-handed clinician:* Hand position for instrumentation on mandibular right buccal aspect. With patient's head turned toward clinician, mirror retracts cheek, enabling direct vision. Clinician is seated in rear position.

Fig. 5-31. *Left-handed clinician:* Hand position for instrumentation on mandibular anterior lingual aspect. Seated in rear position, clinician uses mirror to retract tongue and reflect light on area for direct vision.

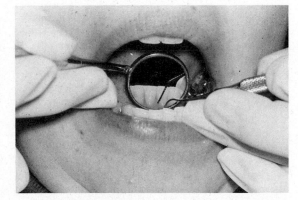

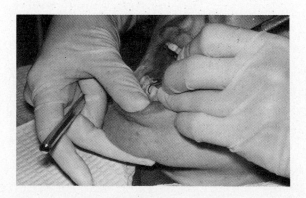

Fig. 5-32. *Left-handed clinician:* Hand position for instrumentation on mandibular anterior facial aspect. Clinician is seated in rear position. Lower lip is retracted by thumb, forefinger, or mouth mirror. Direct vision is used. When direct vision is difficult to achieve, mouth mirror can retract lip and provide indirect vision.

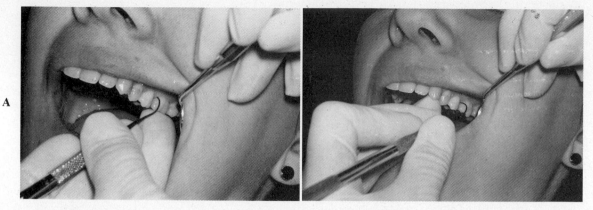

Fig. 5-33. *Left-handed clinician:* Two approaches to maxillary left buccal aspect. **A,** Palm up, fulcrum on or posterior to operative site, giving stability and greater leverage for deposit removal during scaling. Clinician is seated at approximately 2:30 position. **B,** Palm down, fulcrum anterior to area being explored. Clinician is seated in front position. While this technique is easier to learn and is adequate for exploring, it provides less control and leverage during scaling. A vertical wrist rock (see Fig. 5-9) is used for this approach.

Fig. 5-34. *Left-handed clinician:* Hand position for instrumentation on maxillary right lingual aspect. Fulcrum is placed on occlusal surface of tooth or slightly on buccal aspect. All fingers are kept together as single unit to ensure a solid wrist rock and stroke. Mirror reflects light onto area. Direct vision is used, with patient's head tilted away. Clinician is seated in front position.

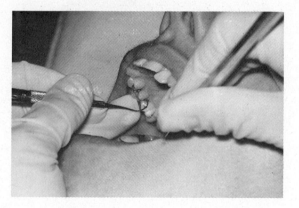

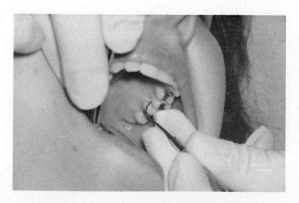

Fig. 5-35. *Left-handed clinician:* Hand position for instrumentation on maxillary left lingual aspect. Clinician is in rear position. Mirror reflects light and provides indirect vision. Fulcrum is on occlusal aspect of sextant. Maintaining good posture, clinician holds mirror so it is visible, then angles mirror until light is cast on area to be explored and image is visible in mirror.

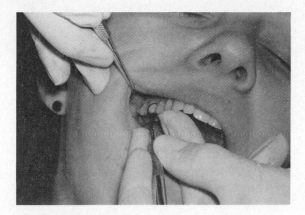

Fig. 5-36. *Left-handed clinician:* Hand position for instrumentation on maxillary right buccal aspect. Clinician is in rear position. Mirror retracts cheek, and fulcrum is on occlusal aspect of teeth, with patient's head turned toward clinician for direct vision.

Fig. 5-37. *Left-handed clinician:* Hand position for instrumentation on maxillary anterior lingual aspect. Clinician remains in rear position and uses mirror to reflect light and provide indirect vision. Maintaining good posture, clinician holds mirror so it is visible, then angles mirror until area is illuminated and visible in mirror. Fulcrum is on incisal edge, with palm up for efficient wrist rock.

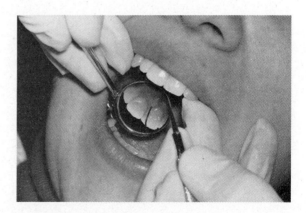

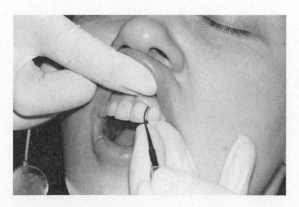

Fig. 5-38. *Left-handed clinician:* Hand position for instrumentation on maxillary anterior labial aspect. To ensure a stable fulcrum, rear position is preferred. Hand remains a solid unit, with all fingers resting on fulcrum, palm up. Direct vision is used, with forefinger retracting lip.

The student playing the role of patient should comply with requests to turn the head to the right or to the left or to tilt the head up or down to facilitate access. It is also appropriate for this student to provide feedback about the careful use of the mouth mirror (reporting pain or discomfort) and to comment on the sense of confidence inspired by the stability of the fulcrum and the clinician's caring approach to the ''patient.'' From the beginning, the clinician should treat the patient as a person rather than as a mannequin or ''object of care.'' The student playing the role of the patient may also hold the table of positions, areas and approaches for the clinician's reference as the sequence is learned. As the sequence is learned and approaches become more comfortable, the student-patient may wish to observe the student-clinician in a hand mirror.

All three students should feel free to discuss comfortable ways of implementing each position. The instructor should circulate among the groups of students to check mirror use, pen grasp, fulcrum placement, and wrist rock as well as basic positions and the location of the overhead lamp.

In order to see how the mirror can be used to *reflect light through tissue (transillumination),* the clinician should place the mirror behind the teeth and angle it until the teeth brighten from the light being reflected through them. The clinician should look at the teeth rather than the image in the mirror. The shadow of restorations should be visible, as well as caries and interproximal or lingual calculus. The light passing through substances other than healthy tooth structure is not as easily transmitted. These substances or defects are thus usually visible as dark shadows.

As each clinician practices and completes the sequence of positions, the team should rotate to ensure each student an experience as clinician, assistant, and patient. All the basic principles of contamination control, including unit preparation, instrument sterilization, hand scrub, and aseptic chain should be practiced to reinforce previously learned skills.

After one or two practice sessions and study of the table of positions, students should be prepared to assume the proper position for any given area of the mouth and, also, to assume each position in sequence. Skill with the mouth mirror should be considerable, and beginning skills for instruments used with the working hand should be apparent.

As the positioning exercise is implemented, the skills of the modified pen grasp, fulcrum, and wrist rock should improve.

Following the arbitrary sequence of positions found in Tables 5-1 and 5-2 allows integration of time and motion economy with mastery of most dental hygiene instruments as each instrument is learned. The sequence is designed to minimize position and instrument changes and to provide a systematic approach to completing each arch or quadrant. Experienced clinicians may have variations in approach to specific areas that complement or replace some of the suggested positions and sequence.

Typically difficult areas to master are (1) the lingual surfaces of the mandibular quadrant closest to the clinician (Fig. 5-17 or 5-29), (2) the buccal surfaces of the maxillary quadrant closest to the clinician (Fig. 5-21 or 5-33), and (3) the lingual surfaces of that quadrant as well (Fig. 5-23 or 5-35).

Problems with the positions shown in Figs. 5-17 and 5-29 usually arise from the dual role of the mouth mirror. It is both retracting the tongue and cheek and serving as a source of indirect vision. Many times it also acts to reflect light on an otherwise dark area. Therefore the beginning clinician needs to acquire a high degree of control with the mirror. The shank retracts the cheek, the back of the mirror head retracts the tongue, and the face of the mirror serves as the primary source of vision and illumination. The patient's head position is critical in enabling all this to happen. Many clinicians prefer to approach this area from a rear position, with the patient's head turned well toward them.

The maxillary right buccal (for right-handed clinicians) and the maxillary left buccal (for left-handed clinicians) are controversial as well as difficult areas. Most people agree that the mirror retracts the cheek. The controversy centers around fulcrum placement and hand position. The easiest approach to learn is to place the fulcrum anterior to the area to be examined with the palm down. The wrist rock then becomes a back-and-forth vertical rock rather than a rock to the side (Figs. 5-21, *B,* and 5-33, *B*).

The more difficult position to learn is the placement of the fulcrum finger on the occlusal surface of the tooth posterior to the tooth being examined, with the palm up. Although the clinician is in a front position, it usually is at 9:30 o'clock, (or 2:30 o'clock for left-handed clinicians) with the body turned toward the patient. For beginners it is best to practice this position on the premolars, moving posteriorly tooth by tooth. As the clinician's hand moves back toward the last molar, the actual fulcrum is less on the fingertip on the tooth and more on the side of the finger on the muscular resistance of the obicularis oris (Figs. 5-21, *A*, and 5-33, *A*).

This palm-up position may be more difficult to master, but according to the laws of physics, it increases control of the instruments, makes it possible to maintain proper terminal shank relation to the tooth, and allows for more efficient use of strength in engaging and removing hard deposits from the teeth and in root planing.

The difficulties encountered with the lingual side of that quadrant are simpler to identify and overcome. Usually, at first the student has difficulty working with a mirror image. This area relies heavily on indirect vision by means of the mirror. Ways to overcome this are to bring the mirror to the front of the mouth and to maintain good posture. With the mirror located in the anterior area, the reflective surface can be seen clearly by the seated clinician. The mirror is then angled until the area to be examined is visible in the mirror. Skill in moving the working hand in the intended direction while looking at a mirror image will develop with practice. This is one reason why rubbing the cotton-tipped applicator up and down the tooth structure is good practice. It is a "safe" instrument with which to learn indirect vision and instrument control.

Exercises with the periodontal probe

Once the student can move quickly and easily from area to area using the proper positioning, mirror function, grasp, fulcrum, and wrist rock, he/she is ready to learn to use the periodontal probe.

Since the periodontal probe can be used on all surfaces (universally) and has no cutting edge or sharpened point, it is a relatively safe beginner's instrument. In addition, it is a key instrument in assessing oral health. Sliding it into the gingival sulcus reveals the depth of the sulcus and the presence of root irregularities and hard deposits. Gently

bobbing the instrument up and down in the sulcus (using an overlapping *stroke* pattern) as it travels around the tooth helps the clinician trace the topography of the attachment. Thus, even in the first phases of learning instrumentation, the clinician can learn about his/her partner's oral conditions.

Guidelines for using the probe include the following:

1. Using the same positioning, grasp, fulcrum, and wrist rock as was practiced in the previous exercise
2. Sliding the probe into the sulcus until it meets the elastic resistance of the epithelial attachment
3. Using approximately 1 mm of the tip of the calibrated portion of the instrument to feel the side of the tooth as it slides in and out of the sulcus and around the tooth
4. Keeping the calibrated portion of the instrument parallel to the long axis of the tooth, except for modifications necessary to accommodate the flare of the crown of the tooth
5. Using the wrist rock to move the instrument coronally for each stroke
6. Pivoting on the fulcrum finger and rolling the instrument slightly in the fingers to move the bobbing instrument around the tooth

The probe should slide in gently so as to avoid causing pain; yet it must travel the full depth of the sulcus or pocket to yield valuable, accurate information. One frequent error is failure to "instrumentate" far enough across the proximal surfaces (Ward and Simring, 1978). If the probe is not placed to the base of the sulcus at the middle portion of the proximal surface, the most frequent site of early periodontal disease will remain unexamined. Examining this area, particularly below contact areas, may necessitate a *slightly* angled approach with the probe.

One way to begin probing a tooth is to *insert* the probe into the sulcus at the distofacial line angle and *bob* or *walk* the instrument across the distal surface (at least slightly more than halfway); *retrace* the probing to the distofacial line angle and *across the facial* surface, past the facial line angle at least slightly more than halfway *across the mesial;* and *back out* to the mesial line angle. The probe should not emerge completely from the sulcus with each stroke. Rather, the probe should remain subgingival as it travels around the tooth (Fig. 5-39).

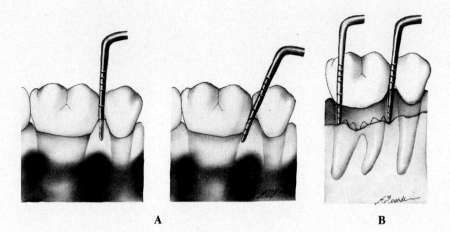

A   B

Fig. 5-39. A, Incorrect *(left)* and correct *(right)* adaptations of probe to tooth. Correct adaptation ensures that tip is adapted and is not free to engage soft tissue in sulcular wall. Walking, or bobbing, motion of probe in sulcus is shown in **B.** Note that probe follows topography of attachment.

If there is a student serving as the assistant, he/she should record millimeter readings for the distal, facial, and mesial surfaces and then for the distal, lingual, and mesial surfaces for each tooth as it is probed in sequence. Otherwise, the clinician should record findings for at least two teeth in each sextant. The faculty member should circulate to help students improve their grasp, fulcrum position, wrist rock, stroke (in and out of the sulcus), adaptation of the tip to the tooth, and pivot motion around the tooth.

By the end of the exercise, the student should have probed all areas of the mouth and measured two teeth for sulcus depth in each sextant of teeth. The student should have acquired entry-level competence in at least six of the following skills:

Proper positioning
Grasp of instrument
Fulcrum placement and use
Wrist rock
Adaptation of tip to tooth
Smooth sulcular bobbing and walking strokes around tooth
Maintenance of calibrated portion in parallel relation to long axis of tooth
Guidance of instrument at least slightly more than halfway across proximal surfaces
Measurements of sulcus accurate within 1 mm
Further practice sessions should allow students to concentrate on those areas in which they are not yet skilled.

Exercises with the paired explorer

Many of the basics of instrumentation given in the previous two exercises will prove helpful in learning to use the paired explorer (such as the cowhorn or pigtail). As the student learns to use this instrument, he/she will learn to (1) select the appropriate end of the explorer for adaptation in each area of the dentition, (2) adapt the side of a sharp tip against the tooth to minimize discomfort, and (3) change (pivot) the direction of a tip moving out from the distal surface so that it can be guided in an anterior direction across a facial or lingual surface, around the mesial line angle, and across the mesial surface.

For this exercise the same positioning, use of the mouth mirror, pen grasp, fulcrum, and wrist rock are used. The stroke with the instrument is an overlapping pattern of vertical strokes around the tooth. The purpose for using the instrument subgingivally is to detect the presence of calculus, root irregularities, normal anatomic landmarks such as the cementoenamel junction (CEJ), and root furrows and contours. The thin shank and working end facilitate the transmission of vibrations to the clinician's fingers and thumb holding the shank and handle. It can be used supragingivally to examine

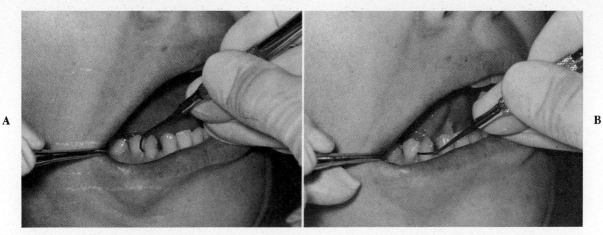

A   B

Fig. 5-40. **A,** Adaptation of one end of cowhorn explorer to mesial surface of tooth with point directed across mesial surface. Terminal shank is parallel to long axis of tooth; point is curved in toward tooth. **B,** Opposite end of explorer, which, although adapted in same area, has terminal shank in horizontal relationship with point curved toward gingiva. These cues help in selecting correct end of paired cowhorn explorer.

the tooth for roughness and contours to confirm what is visible.

In selecting which end to use, it is helpful to (1) select either end of the paired explorer, (2) assume the proper position for the first sextant (mandibular facial area closest to the clinician), (3) establish a proper pen grasp and fulcrum, and (4) place the randomly selected end so that the tip is aimed across the mesial surface from the facial aspect in one of the teeth in the sextant. One of the two views in Fig. 5-40 should resemble this first effort.

The next step is to assess whether the instrument point is curling out toward the tissue as if ready to penetrate it if it were moved subgingivally. Depending on the selected end, the point will be directed either toward the soft tissue or toward the tooth. The latter, for obvious reasons, is preferable.

Another cue is whether the terminal shank (which is contiguous with the working tip) is horizontal or vertical. The point is curved toward the tooth when the terminal shank is vertical. Thus a handy guide for determining which end to use is to look at the direction of the point and the terminal shank's relation to the long axis of the tooth. The end that aligns the terminal shank with the long axis of the tooth will provide correct adaptation for distal, facial, and mesial surfaces on the first sextant of teeth. Fig. 5-40, *A,* meets these criteria.

Once the proper end is selected, the side of the

tip (1 to 2 mm) should be placed on the distobuccal line angle. A wrist rock should be activated to move the instrument up and down. A pivot on the fulcrum finger and a slight rolling of the instrument in the fingers should guide the tip around the line angle and across the distal surface at least slightly more than halfway (Pattison and Behrens, 1973). The clinician should concentrate on what he/she feels with 1 mm of the side of the tip. He/she should explore for calculus, the CEJ, rough margins of restorations, and the root shape.

Then the side of the tip should be bobbed back out to the distobuccal line angle. The tip should be pivoted so that it is aimed toward the anterior of the mouth, and the side of the tip should contact the facial aspect of the tooth. Again, a pivot of the hand on the fulcrum finger and a slight rolling of the instrument in the fingers should allow the side of the tip to move past the mesiobuccal line angle onto and across the mesial surface. The tip is then backed out to the mesiobuccal line angle and removed from the tooth (Figs. 5-41 to 5-46). It is critical to keep 1 to 2 mm of the tip in contact with the tooth. No more and no less should be used; otherwise (1) the tip may wander into the tissue, (2) it is less possible to determine exact locations of deposits, and/or (3) the point will merely scratch over the tooth, sending misleading vibrations to the clinician's hand (Pattison and Behrens, 1973).

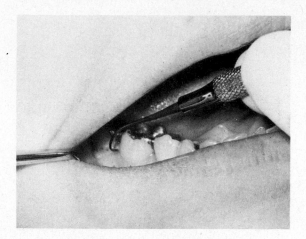

Fig. 5-41. Explorer is inserted on tooth's distobuccal line angle and is moved with vertical strokes around line angle into proximal area to fully explore distal surface.

Fig. 5-42. Once explorer is more than halfway across distal surface and has explored from attachment to margin of gingiva, it should be backed out to distobuccal line angle with overlapping strokes.

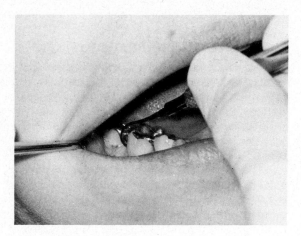

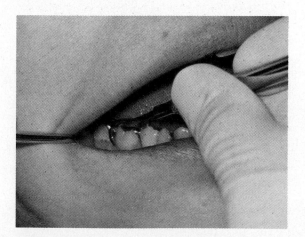

Fig. 5-43. At distolingual line angle the point is pivoted so that it is directed toward mesial aspect of tooth and stroked in overlapping pattern across facial surface.

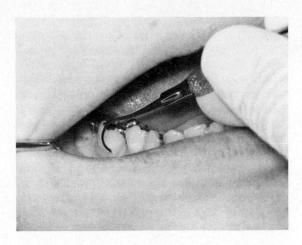

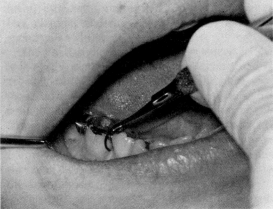

Fig. 5-44. When explorer reaches mesiobuccal line angle, tip is pivoted so that it stays in adaptation with tooth and does not wander into soft tissue. Stroking pattern continues around line angle and into mesial aspect to fully explore proximal surface.

Fig. 5-45. Thorough exploration of mesial surface includes moving explorer in vertical and oblique pattern over all subgingival tooth surface, ensuring that area is fully explored to base of sulcus more than halfway across tooth.

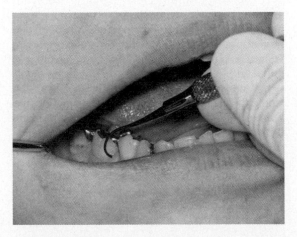

Fig. 5-46. After fully exploring mesial aspect of tooth, explorer is backed out to mesiobuccal line angle, where it is removed from sulcus. Tip of explorer should remain in subgingival position throughout its course around tooth to minimize trauma of reentering sulcus with each stroke.

It is also important to use overlapping strokes that cover the area. A few long sweeping strokes do not thoroughly evaluate a tooth surface for the presence of miniscule deposits and root roughness (Pattison and Behrens, 1973).

As with probing, exploring must drop to the attachment with each stroke to complete a thorough evaluation of subgingival areas (Pattison and Behrens, 1973). Gentle subgingival exploring does not allow the explorer to exit completely from the sulcus with each stroke. Reentry to the sulcus for each downward motion is unnecessary and may cause trauma to the margin of the gingiva.

As each student explores a partner's teeth, he/she should identify calculus, root irregularities, and margins of restorations while focusing on stroke and adaptation. The faculty member should circulate to help students improve form and approach. Each student should be able to identify all areas in the dentition where each end of the explorer can be adapted simply by testing the direction of the point and the relationship of the terminal shank to the tooth's long axis. If one end can be adapted on the facial aspect of teeth No. 28 to No. 32, where else in the dentition can the *same end* be used?

At the completion of the exercise the student should have improved his/her performance in the following basic skills:

Positioning and maintenance of vision
Grasp
Fulcrum location and maintenance
Wrist rock
Exploratory stroke

The student should have learned how to select the correct end of a paired explorer for any sextant in the dentition and be able to adapt the tip safely and effectively. Safety and effectiveness should improve with practice.

Exercises with the "anterior" explorer

Once adaptation of the tip to the tooth has been added to the student's repertoire of entry-level skills, it is possible to move from the paired contra-angled explorer to the more simply designed "straight shanked" explorer such as the No. 17 or No. 20. The shanks for these explorers do have bends and angles, but they do not have the contra-angles that necessitate their use in pairs. The No. 20 explorer is shaped similarly to the No. 17; however, it is much finer and has a longer shank and thus more flex.

The No. 17 or No. 20 can be used almost universally; accessibility is limited to the relatively straight shank that makes it difficult to obtain a solid fulcrum and adaptation in posterior areas. For purposes of simplicity (and with the full acknowledgment that the instrument *can be* and *is* used in posterior areas), the instrument is referred to here as an *anterior* instrument. The maxim "the simpler the shank, the more anterior the intended use of the instrument," is applied here for explorers and later in those chapters in which scalers and curettes are discussed. Variations in areas of use can be added as the student gains experience and confidence.

One of the reasons for calling the No. 17 or No. 20 explorer an *anterior* instrument is that it allows the student to learn some basic principles associated with adapting instruments in anterior teeth prior to learning about cutting edges and angulation.

When an anterior instrument is being used, the terminal shank is kept parallel to the long axis of the tooth. To do this, the fulcrum must be on the same tooth or on the immediately adjacent one (Fig. 5-47). Allowing the fulcrum to rest two or three teeth away causes the terminal shank to angle in the direction of the fulcrum rather than remaining parallel to the tooth's long axis.

Many straight-shanked instruments can be used with a circumferential or horizontal stroke (as opposed to a vertical stroke) on the facial and lingual

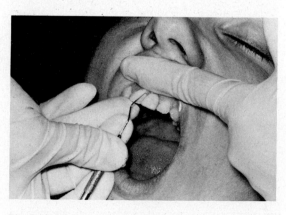

Fig. 5-47. When an anterior-design instrument is used, fulcrum must be on same tooth or nearby tooth to ensure that shank is parallel to long axis of tooth.

surfaces of teeth, including posterior teeth. The tip is angled more apically, the shank is *not* parallel to the long axis of the tooth, and the tip moves in short overlapping oblique strokes from line angle to line angle (Fig. 5-48).

Another key factor is the need to accommodate the sharp line angles of the anterior teeth. If the tip is not carefully adapted to the tooth as the surface changes from facial to proximal, the sharp point will catch the gingiva, causing an iatrogenic hemorrhage point and its accompanying discomfort.

Therefore practice in adapting the instrument is the focus in learning anterior instruments. The exercise also allows the student to improve skills in the following:

Positioning and maintenance of vision
Grasp
Fulcrum location and maintenance
Wrist rock
Exploratory stroke
Detection of irregularities, landmarks, and calculus

At the completion of exploring the anterior teeth, the student should have achieved entry-level competence in all of the aforementioned skills and be able to explore anterior teeth and the direct facial and lingual surfaces of any tooth in the dentition without creating hemorrhage points or pain.

Another straight-shanked explorer is the shepherd's hook (No. 23). It can be used for calculus detection, but its use is frequently limited to caries detection because of the thickness of its tip and shank (Pattison and Behrens, 1973).

Fig. 5-49 shows the No. 23 explorer adapted for caries detection in the distal pit of tooth No. 28. The sharp point of the explorer is pressed into the pit to see if it sticks in soft tooth structure (caries). If resistance is felt as the explorer is removed from the tooth structure, the area is usually considered carious and worthy of further evaluation for restoration.

In addition to exploring pits for caries, the explorer can be used to check grooves, margins of restorations, and other caries-prone areas of the teeth, such as the gingival third of the facial and lingual surfaces and the proximal surfaces. While it is usually necessary to examine a patient radiographically in order to rule out proximal caries, large lesions can often be found with an explorer.

The student should explore a partner's teeth for caries and for defective margins of restorations by placing the point into the pits and grooves, applying pressure, and detecting *retention* of the point in a *soft area*. Similarly, tracing the margins allows the detection of caries and other defects around restorations.

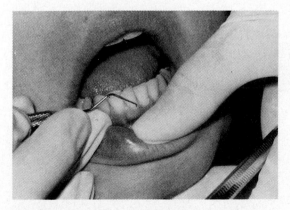

Fig. 5-48. Instruments may be used with a circumferential or horizontal stroke around tooth. Tip is placed so that it is inclined apically and with terminal shank at 45-degree angle to long axis of teeth. Care must be taken to adapt carefully at line angles when using this stroke on facial and lingual aspects.

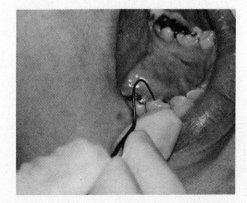

Fig. 5-49. Shepherd's hook (No. 23) explorer is usually reserved for caries detection because of its thick, resilient shank. Its sharp point is pressed into pits and grooves and suspicious margins of restorations to see if it sticks in soft tooth structure (caries).

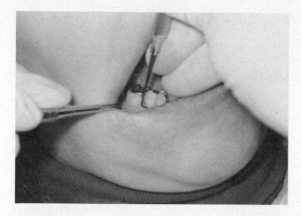

Fig. 5-50. Exploring for calculus with No. 6 explorer, a simply designed instrument with universal use.

ADJUNCT EXPLORERS

Refer again to Figs. 5-1 and 5-2 and note the variety of explorers available for calculus and caries detection. With greater experience a clinician can experiment with the variety that is available.

Fig. 5-50 shows the No. 6 explorer being adapted in the posterior teeth. It has a simple design with only one angle in the shank. The terminal shank is the portion that is in the same plane with the handle, and it is maintained in a nearly parallel relationship to the long axis of the tooth. The tip is angled slightly downward into the sulcus, but not so that it is pointed directly apically. This instrument can be used universally; its versatility makes it a popular choice.

SUMMARY

The probe and explorers are valuable tools for assessing dental health. They also provide a framework for learning basic positioning and instrumentation skills, which can be generalized to apply to the use of other instruments.

Once the student is familiar with the probe, a paired contra-angled explorer, and a straight-shanked explorer, other instruments used for exploring can be learned. Students should then use the instruments to prepare assessment data for partners or for the patients of more advanced students.

ACTIVITIES

1. Compare a variety of instruments to determine the parts of the instruments, to distinguish between double-ended and paired instruments, and to examine shank shape and strength and the location of the terminal shank.

2. Ask a partner to grasp the handle of an instrument you are holding and try to move it while you are using each of the following grasps. Which grasp provides the most stability against movement? How would this grasp ensure best control of the instrument?
   a. A typical pen grasp used in holding a pencil
   b. The modified pen grasp, but with the knuckle buckled as shown in Fig. 5-6, *B*
   c. The modified pen grasp as shown in Fig. 5-6, *A*
3. *Exercises in positioning.* In groups of three, rotate from clinician to assistant to patient roles in completing the following procedures:
   a. As chairside assistant
      (1) Disinfect unit.
      (2) Place sterile mirror and cotton-tipped applicator on covered tray.
      (3) Clear pathway for patient entry to chair.
      (4) Position patient:
         (a) Tilt chair back.
         (b) Lower back of chair.
         (c) Adjust headrest.
         (d) Place bib.
      (5) Adjust assistant's stool to proper height and location.
      (6) Adjust overhead light to ensure illumination of each area.
   b. As patient
      (1) Comment on seating comfort.
      (2) Comment on comfortable use of mouth mirror and cotton-tipped applicator.
      (3) Turn head as requested by clinician.
      (4) Hold table of positions for clinician and assistant reference.
   c. As clinician
      (1) Adjust stool properly (thighs parallel to floor; feet flat on floor; abdominal rest below rib cage).

(2) Seat self at chairside at 9 o'clock position (for right-handed clinician) or at 3 o'clock position (for left-handed clinician).

(3) Use Table 5-1 or 5-2 to guide position, mouth mirror use, and fulcrum placement for each of the following areas of the mouth:

Right-handed clinician	Left-handed clinician
Mandibular	Mandibular
Right buccal	Left buccal
Left lingual	Right lingual
Right lingual	Left lingual
Left buccal	Right buccal
Anterior lingual	Anterior lingual
Anterior labial	Anterior labial
Maxillary	Maxillary
Right buccal	Left buccal
Left lingual	Right lingual
Right lingual	Left lingual
Left buccal	Right buccal
Anterior lingual	Anterior lingual
Anterior labial	Anterior labial

(4) Use mouth mirror as indicated for each area.

(5) Use cotton-tipped applicator as dental instrument to explore two teeth in each area, using
 (a) Modified pen grasp
 (b) Fulcrum
 (c) Wrist rock
 (d) Stroking pattern

(6) Reflect light through anterior teeth with mirror and observe the presence of caries, restorations, or calculus.

4. *Exercises with periodontal probe.* In dyads, serve as patient and as clinician in completing the following procedures:
 a. As patient
 (1) Comment on seating comfort.
 (2) Comment on comfortable use of mouth mirror and probe.
 (3) Monitor proper positioning of clinician.
 b. As clinician
 (1) Use proper seating and positioning of self, patient's head, and mouth mirror for each area as described in Tables 5-1 and 5-2.
 (2) With periodontal probe in working hand
  (a) Maintain modified pen grasp.
  (b) Maintain firm fulcrum.
  (c) Gently insert probe in sulcus.
  (d) Explore first area with probe
   From distobuccal line angle to direct distal
   From distal to distobuccal line angle and across facial aspect
   Past mesiobuccal line angle to direct mesial and back to mesiobuccal line angle
  (e) Explore with 1 mm of tip adapted to tooth.

 (f) Maintain calibrated working end parallel to long axis.
 (g) Bob or walk instrument from base of sulcus to free margin of gingiva while traveling around tooth.
 (h) Measure depth of sulcus in millimeters.
 (3) Record measurements of sulcus depth for at least two teeth in each sextant.

5. *Exercises with paired explorer.* In dyads, serve as patient and as clinician in completing the following procedures:
 a. As patient
 (1) Comment on seating comfort.
 (2) Comment on comfortable use of mouth mirror and paired explorer.
 (3) Monitor proper positioning of operator.
 b. As clinician
 (1) Use proper seating and positioning of self, patient's head, and mouth mirror for each area as described in Table 5-1 or 5-2.
 (2) With paired explorer in working hand
  (a) Maintain modified pen grasp.
  (b) Maintain firm fulcrum.
  (c) Select proper end of explorer.
  (d) Adapt side of point (1 mm) to tooth at distobuccal line angle in first area.
  (e) Activate wrist rock to stroke instrument in overlapping vertical pattern around distal surface and back out to line angle.
  (f) Pivot point at line angle so that it is aimed anteriorly, stroking vertically across facial surface.
  (g) Continue stroking past mesiobuccal line angle and across mesial surface, using pivot on fulcrum finger and rolling instrument slightly with fingers.
  (h) Back instrument out to mesiobuccal line angle using vertical stroking pattern.
  (i) Remove instrument from sulcus.
 (3) Explore root anatomy, margins of restorations, and calculus deposits.
 (4) Watch for iatrogenic hemorrhage points, and correct adaptation to ensure that side of point is in contact with tooth.

6. *Exercises with anterior explorer.* In dyads, serve as patient and as clinician in completing the following procedures:
 a. As patient
 (1) Comment on seating comfort.
 (2) Comment on comfortable use of mouth mirror and anterior explorer.
 (3) Monitor proper positioning of clinician.
 b. As clinician
 (1) Use proper seating and positioning of self, patient's head, and mouth mirror for each area as described in Table 5-1 or 5-2.

(2) With straight-shanked explorer in working hand
  (a) Maintain modified pen grasp.
  (b) Establish fulcrum close to site of operation in anterior teeth.
  (c) Maintain terminal shank parallel to long axis of tooth.
  (d) Adapt 1 mm of tip at line angles and activate vertical overlapping strokes with wrist rock to move instrument across proximal surfaces.
  (e) Use horizontal or oblique stroke with terminal shank horizontal to long axis of tooth to explore direct facial and lingual surfaces of anterior and posterior teeth (tip toward base of sulcus).
  (f) Explore tooth for normal anatomy, margins of restorations, calculus, and irregularities.
(3) Using shepherd's hook explorer, explore for caries. Direct point into pits, grooves, and around restorations with pressure to find areas of retention that feel soft.

REVIEW QUESTIONS

1. What are four functions of a mouth mirror?
2. What are the functions (at least four) of a periodontal probe?
3. What are the functions (at least two) of explorers?
4. True or false
   a. The terminal shank is that part of the shank closest to the working end.
   b. In exploring, the full length of the working end should contact the tooth.
   c. Generally, the simpler the shank, the more anterior the use intended for the instrument.
   d. In selecting one end of a paired instrument for a given area, one cue in selecting the right end is that the terminal shank is perpendicular to the long axis of the tooth.
5. Identify the proper clinician and patient's head position for each of the following areas. For each area designate whether the positions are for a right-handed or a left-handed clinician.
   a. Labial No. 8
   b. Lingual No. 18
   c. Buccal No. 3
   d. Buccal No. 12
   e. Lingual No. 5
   f. Lingual No. 14
   g. Buccal No. 31

REFERENCES

Carter, L.M., and Yaman, P. 1981. Dental instruments. St. Louis: The C.V. Mosby Co.

Nield, J.S., and O'Connor, G.H. 1983. Fundamentals of dental hygiene instrumentation. Philadelphia: W.B. Saunders Co.

Pattison, A.M., and Behrens, J. 1973. Dental hygiene: the detection and removal of calculus. Reston, Va.: Reston Publishing Co., Inc.

Pattison, G.L., and Pattison, A.M. 1979. Periodontal instrumentation. Reston, Va.: Reston Publishing Co., Inc.

Ward, H.L., and Simring, M.R. 1978. Manual of clinical periodontics, ed. 2. St. Louis: The C.V. Mosby Co.

6 INSTRUMENT SHARPENING

OBJECTIVES: *The reader will be able to:*

1. State the advantages of using sharp periodontal instruments.
2. Discuss three methods used to identify sharp versus dull cutting edges.
3. Describe the design features of universal curettes, Gracey curettes, and sickle scalers that must be maintained during the sharpening procedure.
4. State three different techniques of instrument sharpening.
5. State the rationale for sharpening the lateral surfaces of curettes and sickle scalers.
6. Discuss the care of an Arkansas sharpening stone.
7. Describe two techniques of sharpening curettes and sickle scalers using a hand-held sharpening stone.

A clinician's success during all instrumentation procedures is directly related to the quality of the instruments being used. Effective scaling, root planing, and soft tissue curettage depend on the use of sharp instruments for their success. There are a number of advantages to using sharp instruments. First, a sharp cutting edge is more effective in removing calculus and cementum from tooth surfaces. Dull instruments are more likely to simply rub over or burnish calculus deposits rather than remove them cleanly from the tooth surface. A sharp cutting edge, however, can shear off deposits and plane root surfaces with less effort and fewer strokes. A sharp cutting edge will also deliver finer tactile sensations to the clinician during the scaling and root planing procedures so that more effective exploring strokes are possible. Soft tissue curettage requires a cutting edge that is supremely sharp so that inflamed tissues are sliced away from the healthy gingiva, rather than being torn or ripped away. Using a dull instrument for soft tissue curettage would be about as effective as trying to peel an apple with a plastic spoon. It could be done, but would there be any apple left when it was over?

Sharp instruments are more efficient than dull instruments. They can accomplish the same procedures in a much shorter period of time. Fewer strokes are needed to remove deposits or cementum from the tooth. Better tactile sensitivity with the scaling or root planing instrument allows the clinician to do more exploring with that instrument rather than having to constantly switch back and forth between an explorer and the scaling instrument.

The use of a sharp instrument produces a more pleasant experience for both the clinician and the patient. The clinician will not have to exert as much energy behind working strokes in order for them to be effective. The patient will appreciate a light and gentle approach to scaling and root planing that is more likely if sharp instruments are used. The clinician is also more likely to cause unnecessary pain and trauma when using dull instruments because working strokes must be repeated again and again in the same areas until the deposits are finally removed. Both patient and clinician will benefit from the time saved during the appointment by using sharp instruments. It is easy to understand that the short amount of time it takes to effectively sharpen the instruments used during periodontal treatment is certainly justified by the benefits that are gained.

IDENTIFICATION OF SHARP VERSUS DULL INSTRUMENTS

The first step in learning how to sharpen instruments is to develop the ability to determine whether or not an instrument is optimally sharp. There are a number of ways to evaluate instrument sharpness. Experienced clinicians can determine when their instruments are getting dull by the ease with which they can remove calculus deposits and cementum.

A beginning clinician, however, has not had the opportunity to develop a sense for what a sharp instrument can be expected to accomplish. Several other ways to detect a dull instrument are available that may be easier to use at first.

One of the best ways to test instrument sharpness is by applying the cutting edge to be tested against an acrylic or plastic rod. Special testing sticks have been designed specifically for this purpose and are available from instrument manufacturers (Fig. 6-1). The instrument's cutting edge is applied to the surface of the testing stick at the same angle that

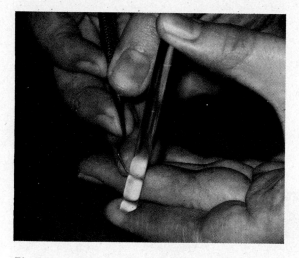

Fig. 6-1. Acrylic testing stick is used by applying light pressure against stick at a working angulation.

would be used to implement a working stroke against the tooth surface. If the edge is sharp, it will "bite" into the plastic surface when only light pressure is applied. If the instrument tends to drag or grate across the surface, it is not sharp. The entire length of the cutting edge should be evaluated for dullness. If a commercial testing stick is not available, a plastic disposable cotton-tipped applicator can serve the same purpose. Commercially designed testing sticks are made of materials that can be autoclaved so that they can be included on each tray setup to ensure sharp instruments during treatment procedures.

Another method of detecting a dull cutting edge is to examine it under a microscope or a magnifying lens. The instrument is held so that the cutting edge faces a strong light source. A dull surface will reflect light, so that a white area or a bright line will be visible where the cutting edge should be (Fig. 6-2, *B*). If the cutting edge is truly sharp, there should not be a flat surface at the junction of the facial and lateral surfaces. Only a dark line will be visible where these two surfaces meet when the instrument is correctly sharpened (Fig. 6-2, *A*). This evaluation method is particularly useful when time has been set aside specifically to sharpen instruments and a special working area is available that has a good light source and a microscope or magnifying lens. This technique would take too much time to use during a patient appointment.

One method that should not be used to test instrument sharpness is to apply the edge to a fin-

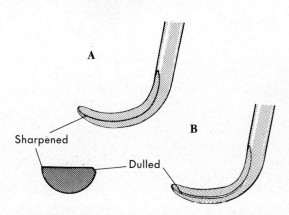

Fig. 6-2. A, A sharp cutting edge will not reflect light. **B,** A dull cutting edge will appear as a bright area at junction of face and lateral surface.

gernail. Not only is this hard on the clinician's fingernail, but it is also a violation of aseptic technique. Instrument sharpening is often performed at the chairside during a patient appointment. If the clinician used this method to test the sharpness of scaling instruments, the instruments would be contaminated and no longer acceptable for patient treatment. All clinicians who perform intraoral procedures should wear disposable gloves to protect themselves and the patient from cross-contamination. It would be very time consuming and inconvenient to have to remove the gloves, wash the hands, test the instruments, sharpen them, wash the hands, and put the gloves back on each time instrument sharpening was necessary. It is much easier to use a testing stick or other method to evaluate instrument sharpness.

APPLICATION OF INSTRUMENT DESIGN TO SHARPENING TECHNIQUES

Each type of periodontal instrument has specific design characteristics that must be preserved during sharpening. The clinician must understand exactly how these design principles affect the use of each type of instrument so that sharpening techniques can be implemented effectively. The two types of instruments that are used most frequently for scaling and root planing procedures are the sickle scaler and the curette. Design characteristics of both of these instrument types are discussed.

Sickle scalers

Design features of sickle scalers are shown in Figs. 6-3 and 6-4. There are actually two different blade designs for sickle scalers. The straight blade design is shown in Fig. 6-3. The side view shows that the two cutting edges of this sickle form a gentle arc that converges in a sharp tip. Both cutting edges are used, so both must be sharpened. The pointed tip of the sickle scaler provides access beneath tight supramarginal contact areas. A significant design feature of the straight sickle blade is the squared-off design of the back of the blade, which can be seen in the cross-sectional view in Fig. 6-3.

Fig. 6-4 shows the design characteristics of a curved sickle blade. The facial surface of this instrument forms a slight curve as it extends from the shank of the instrument to the pointed tip. The lateral surfaces of this sickle are flat and converge at the pointed back. Differences in the back design can be seen by comparing the two cross-sectional views of these sickle scalers.

In both of these instruments, the internal angle formed by the lateral surfaces and the facial surface is approximately 70 to 80 degrees. This angle determines the angle at which the sharpening stone must be applied in order to preserve the original cross-sectional design. When properly applied, the sharpening stone will form a complementary angle of 100 to 110 degrees with the face of the sickle blade.

Curettes

Design characteristics of the universal curette are shown in Fig. 6-5. The side view of the universal curette blade shows two parallel cutting edges, both of which are used during scaling and root planing. The two cutting edges converge in a rounded toe. It is important to maintain a rounded toe during the sharpening procedure, since this is one of the

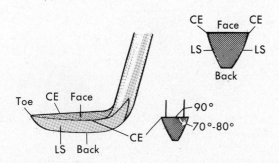

Fig. 6-3. Straight sickle. Face is basically flat; back surface is also flat.

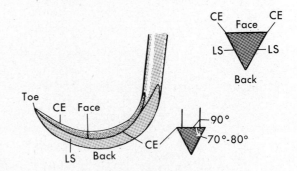

Fig. 6-4. Curved sickle. Note pointed back.

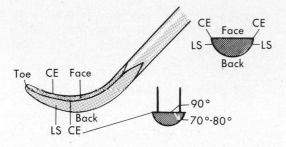

Fig. 6-5. Universal curette. Note that the two cutting edges are parallel. Rounded back and toe are important design features.

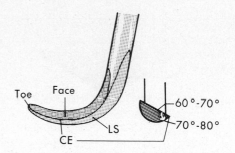

Fig. 6-6. Gracey curette. Note offset relationship of cutting edges so that one blade appears lower than the other.

design features that allows this instrument to be used safely in subgingival areas. Failure to maintain this design could result in trauma to the soft tissues when the curette is inserted below the gingival margin. Another important characteristic of the curette is that the lateral surfaces are curved, rather than flat, and they form a rounded back surface. A cross-sectional view of the universal curette looks like a half circle. This is the second design feature that allows this instrument to navigate in tight pockets without damaging the adjacent soft tissues. The rounded back must be preserved during sharpening. The cross-sectional view of the universal curette shows that the facial surface of the blade forms a 90-degree angle with the shank of the instrument. The internal angle of the curette blade is the same as that of the sickle scaler: 70 to 80 degrees.

The design features of the Gracey curette (Fig. 6-6) are the same as those of the universal curette with two notable exceptions. The blade is slightly offset at an angle of about 60 to 70 degrees from the shank of the instrument, so that the two cutting edges are not parallel to each other. Instead, one of the cutting edges appears to be lower than the other when the instrument is held so that the last bend in the shank (terminal shank) is perpendicular to the floor, as pictured in Fig. 6-6. Only this "lower" cutting edge is used during periodontal procedures, so only one of the cutting edges will be sharpened on a Gracey curette blade. Other design characteristics of a curette blade described earlier for the universal curette (e.g., rounded back, rounded toe, internal angle of 70 to 80 degrees) are also present on a Gracey curette blade.

SHARPENING TECHNIQUES

There are a number of different techniques for sharpening periodontal instruments. Probably the most common technique is performed with a hand-held sharpening stone. An advantage of this technique is that it can be performed anywhere in the dental office where there is adequate light and a good working surface. The use of a hand-held stone also allows the clinician to control the exact speed and pressure with which the instrument is being sharpened so that there is no unnecessary loss of the instrument surface due to oversharpening. This technique is recommended for routine sharpening of instruments. There are two ways in which a hand-held stone can be used for sharpening. One method is to hold the instrument stationary while moving the stone against it. The second method is to stabilize the stone and draw the instrument blade across the surface of the stone. Both techniques are discussed and shown in this chapter so that the clinician can decide which approach is preferable.

Sharpening or honing machines are also available for sharpening periodontal instruments. The use of these machines involves the same principles applied in the hand-sharpening methods, except that the sharpening stone is mechanically rotated or moved while the instrument blade is applied to it. The amount of metal that is removed with this method of sharpening is dependent on the amount of pressure applied to the instrument. These machines can be time-savers if the clinician is skilled in placement of the blade against the stone at the correct angle and if the instrument requires a great deal of contouring. Inexperienced clinicians or those unfamiliar with instrument design can ruin instruments much more quickly with this technique than with a manual technique. In addition, the need for special equipment limits the clinician's access to this method of sharpening during patient treatment, so that it is more useful when a special time has been allotted for instrument sharpening. For routine instrument sharpening and sharpening that must occur during patient treatment, a manual technique is more useful.

A third approach to instrument sharpening is through the use of small cylindrical or conical stones that can be mounted on a handpiece. This method has the same advantages and disadvantages as a honing machine. The clinician has less control over the speed of metal removal with this method than with hand methods. If used properly and with concern for preserving the original instrument design, it can be a timesaving device and is useful for sharpening instruments that require a great deal of sharpening or recontouring. An added advantage of this method is that the sharpening stones can be available at the dental unit and readily mounted on a slow-speed handpiece for sharpening instruments during patient treatment. These mounted stones can be sterilized after use.

Approach to sharpening

There are two approaches to creating a sharp cutting edge. One approach is to remove the facial surface of the instrument to create the sharp cutting edges. The other approach is to remove part of the lateral surfaces. Many clinicians have tried the former approach because it appears to be easier and less time consuming. The disadvantage of this approach, however, is a major one. The thickness of the instrument from back to facial surface is a critical factor in maintaining the strength of the blade. If the facial surface of the blade is removed during sharpening (Fig. 6-7, *A*), this strength factor is gradually reduced. This loss of strength would soon affect the ability of the instrument blade to withstand the stress of removing large or tenacious calculus deposits. This approach to sharpening creates the potential danger of breaking an instrument tip within a pocket area—a situation that is unpleasant for both the patient and the clinician.

The blade strength necessary for calculus removal can be maintained in an instrument longer if the lateral surfaces of the blade are removed during sharpening. This is shown in Fig. 6-7, *B*.

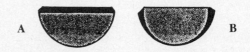

A   **B**

Fig. 6-7. A, Sharpening facial surface weakens blade strength. **B,** Sharpening lateral surfaces preserves strength and design.

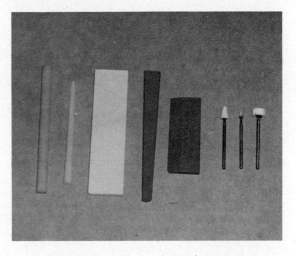

Fig. 6-8. Stones used to sharpen instruments.

Although the instrument gradually becomes thinner from side to side, this design change will not stress the instrument blade as quickly as the facial-sharpening approach. In fact, many clinicians prefer the thinner blades because they offer access to areas that new, thicker instruments have difficulty reaching. The clinician will also save money by not having to replace instruments as often.

Selecting a sharpening stone

Sharpening stones come in a variety of materials and designs (Fig. 6-8). The most popular stone for sharpening periodontal instruments is a natural stone known as the Arkansas oilstone. This stone is composed of extremely fine abrasive crystals as compared with man-made, or artificial, stones. The quality of a cutting edge is determined by the fineness of the sharpening stone with which it is sharpened. The Arkansas oilstone is capable of producing a high-quality cutting edge and at the same time does not grind away the metal surface of the instrument at the same rate as a coarser stone.

Therefore it meets the objectives of sharpening better than other sharpening stones.

Several man-made stones are also available for use in dentistry. These include the ruby stone, the Carborundum stone, and the diamond hone. These stones are impregnated with abrasive crystals such as aluminum oxide, silicon carbide, or diamond particles, all of which are coarser than the particle size of the Arkansas stone. These stones may be useful, however, if a great deal of recontouring is needed, since they will grind the surface more quickly than the Arkansas stone.

Sharpening stones are available in rectangular, wedge-shaped, or cylindrical shapes. The choice of shape and size is dependent on clinician preference and on how the stone will be used. Small cylindrical stones can be mounted for use in a slow-speed handpiece. Larger or tapered cylinders are used to sharpen the facial surfaces of instruments. Rectangular stones are used to sharpen the lateral surfaces of instruments.

Preparation for sharpening

The most convenient way to sharpen instruments is to have a workbench or counter top that is reserved for that purpose, so that all necessary supplies are within easy access, including an effective light source, a magnifying lense, sharpening oil, applicators, and alcohol-soaked gauze. If space is not available for this purpose, the methods of sharpening discussed in this chapter can be accomplished wherever an adequate light source and working surface are available.

The supplies needed for instrument sharpening are shown in Fig. 6-9. They include a sterile cylindrical stone (optional), a sterile rectangular or wedge-shaped Arkansas stone, alcohol-soaked gauze, a testing stick or other means of evaluation, light-grade oil, and a cotton-tipped applicator. Only sterile stones should be used to sharpen instruments, and these must be resterilized following their use on contaminated instruments. A light coating of oil should be applied to the stone with the cotton-tipped applicator. The purpose of the oil is to prevent metal filings from the sharpening procedure from becoming embedded in the surface of the stone. The oil also has a lubricating effect and enhances the ability of the clinician to implement smooth, even strokes over the stone's surface. Oil is also used to lubricate the India stone. Most man-

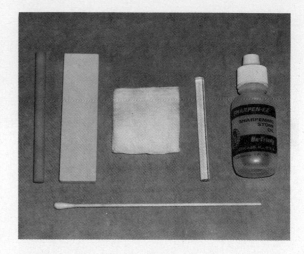

Fig. 6-9. Supplies used for instrument sharpening. *Left to right:* Cylindrical sharpening stone, rectangular Arkansas stone, alcohol gauze, testing stick, lubricating oil, and cotton-tipped applicator.

made stones can be lubricated with water if needed. The manufacturer's directions regarding the need for lubrication should be followed. The alcohol-soaked gauze sponge is useful for removing the oil and metal sludge from the sharpening stone and the instruments. The testing stick should also be sterilized prior to its use on sterile instruments.

Sharpening with a stationary stone and a moving instrument

When sharpening with a stationary stone, the Arkansas stone should be placed on a flat surface. The instrument should be held with a modified pen grasp, as shown in Fig. 6-10, with the third and fourth fingers providing support for the hand on the surface of the table. The fingers of the other hand should grasp and stabilize the stone, as shown. The instrument, in this case a universal curette, should be placed near the top of the stone so that the face forms a 90-degree angle with the stone's surface. The instrument handle can then be rotated slightly away from the clinician until the angle between the face and the stone is 100 to 110 degrees. This is the correct angle for sharpening all curettes and sickle scalers. This angle complements the internal angle of the instrument (70 to 80 degrees), so that the original design of the blade

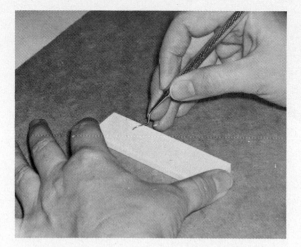

Fig. 6-10. Positioning of stone and instrument for stationary stone approach to sharpening.

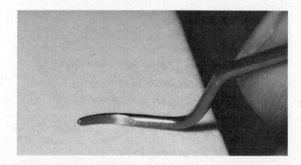

Fig. 6-11. Close-up view of facial surface of curette at 90-degree angle to stationary stone.

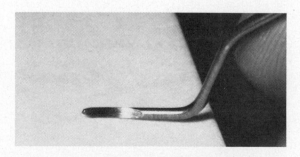

Fig. 6-12. Angle has been opened to 110 degrees prior to beginning sharpening stroke.

is maintained during sharpening. It is important that the clinician maintain this same angle for the entire length of the sharpening stroke. Until the clinician becomes experienced at identifying the correct angulation, it may be helpful to continue to place the instrument first so that the 90-degree angle is formed and then open it up slightly another 10 to 20 degrees. Figs. 6-11 and 6-12 show close-up views of the placement of the curette blade at both 90 and 110 degrees.

After the correct angulation has been established, the stroke should begin with the heel of the blade adapted to the stone. As the instrument is pulled toward the clinician, the instrument blade should be rotated toward the toe of the blade, so that the entire blade is sharpened during each complete stroke. The stroke is produced by moving the entire hand and arm as a single unit toward the clinician while rotating the wrist. At the end of the stroke, the toe should be rounded to preserve that curette design characteristic. The steps involved in implementing a single stroke are shown in Figs. 6-13 to 6-17. Several light strokes may be necessary to completely sharpen the entire cutting edge. After one cutting edge of the curette has been completed, the other edge should be sharpened in the same manner. The stone may need to be repositioned at the edge of the table to facilitate the placement of the opposite cutting edge. It is important when sharpening curettes to remember to round the toe each time the blade is sharpened so that a point is not created that would traumatize soft tissues.

Gracey curettes are sharpened in the same way, with only a few exceptions. Only one cutting edge of the Gracey curette should be sharpened. The clinician must first identify this lower cutting edge. Since the face of the Gracey curette is not perpendicular to the shank, care should be taken to first align the facial surface at a 90-degree angle to the stone and then open the angle to the proper sharpening angle of 100 to 110 degrees.

Sickle scalers can be easily sharpened by this method. The same principles of instrument placement and angulation apply. The only major difference is that the lateral surfaces of this instrument are flatter and straighter than those of the curette, so there is not as much rotation of the blade from heel to toe during each stroke. The stroke should stop at the tip of the instrument, since its point should be maintained. The sharpening strokes are

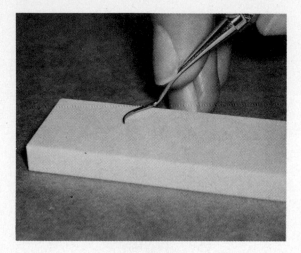

Fig. 6-13. Initial placement of curette against stone at 90-degree angle.

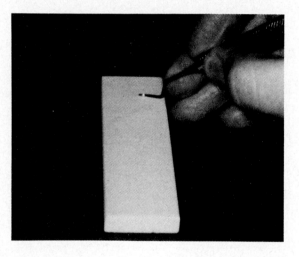

Fig. 6-14. Stationary stone and moving instrument: stroke begins at top of stone where heel of blade is in contact with stone at 100- to 110-degree angle.

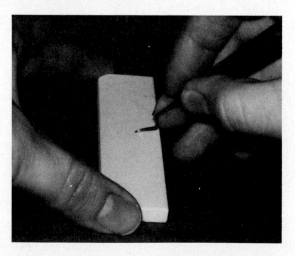

Fig. 6-15. As instrument is pulled forward across stone, blade is slowly rotated toward middle of cutting edge.

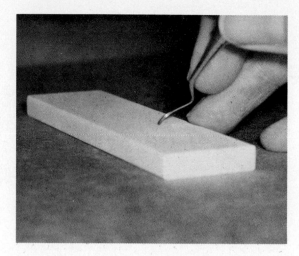

Fig. 6-16. As end of stroke approaches, back of cutting edge is lifted so that toe is in contact with stone.

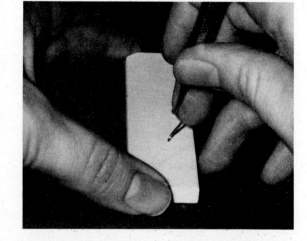

Fig. 6-17. Entire toe should be rounded off at end of stroke so that a sharp point is not created. Less pressure can be used at toe, since it is not a cutting surface.

repeated until the cutting edge is sharp, and the instrument is then repositioned to sharpen the opposite cutting edge.

Sharpening with a stationary instrument and a moving stone

A second method of sharpening curettes and sickles with a hand-held stone is to stabilize the instrument in one hand and move the stone across the lateral surfaces with the other hand. The first step is to grasp the instrument to be sharpened firmly in the left hand and brace the hand against the edge of a counter or table so that the instrument blade extends over the edge of the table with the toe pointing toward the clinician (Fig. 6-18). The sharpening stone should be grasped with the fingers of the other hand as shown in Fig. 6-18. The instrument should be oriented so that its facial surface is parallel to the floor. Fig. 6-18 shows the adaptation of the stone to the cutting edge of the straight sickle scaler at a 90-degree angle. The top of the stone is then rotated slightly away from the instrument until the correct angle of 100 to 110 degrees is formed between the stone and the facial surface (Fig. 6-19). With care being taken to maintain the stone at exactly the same angle, short up-and-down strokes (½ to 1 inch) are applied to the cutting edge of the blade. Pressure should be applied only to downstrokes to avoid the formation of a wire edge. A wire edge is a projection of metal that can form at the junction of the face and the lateral surfaces when the direction of the sharpening stroke moves

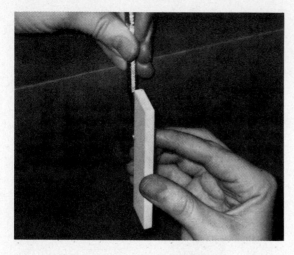

Fig. 6-18. Stationary instrument and moving stone technique. Note position of left hand, which is braced against tabletop. Facial surface of sickle is parallel to floor. Stone is placed at 90-degree angle.

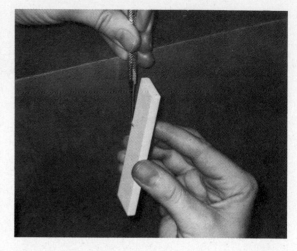

Fig. 6-19. Stone is correctly oriented at 100- to 110-degree angle to facial surface. This exact angle must be maintained for all strokes.

away from the cutting edge. If pressure is applied to both the upstroke and the downstroke using this technique, it may be necessary to smooth the facial surface with a cylindrical stone to remove any wire edges that have been created. Sharpening strokes should be applied first to the heel of the instrument, and then the stone should be rotated slightly until the entire cutting edge has been sharpened.

The same technique can be used to sharpen universal and Gracey curettes. Strokes should begin at the heel of the curette and move gradually toward the toe. Fig. 6-20 shows that approximately four adjustments of the stone position may be necessary to ensure that all parts of the blade have been equally sharpened. After the entire length of the blade has been sharpened, the cutting edge should be evaluated. If it is satisfactory, then the opposite cutting edge of the universal curette should be sharpened by repositioning the stone as shown in Fig. 6-21. Again, the clinician is reminded that only the lower cutting edge of a Gracey curette should be sharpened and that care should be taken to position the instrument so that the facial surface is parallel to the floor before positioning the stone to begin the sharpening stroke.

A separate stroke is needed to maintain the rounded toe of the curette. The stone should be adapted so that a 45-degree angle is formed between the bottom half of the stone and the facial surface of the curette. Short downstrokes should be applied around the curvature of the toe.

Occasionally a wire edge may be created using this technique. It can be easily removed by applying a cylindrical Arkansas stone to the facial surface (Fig. 6-22). The curvature of the instrument is matched to the diameter of the stone, and even pressure is applied to the facial surface while the stone is rotated in a counterclockwise direction. This grinding of the facial surface should only be necessary if wire edges are detected, since excessive grinding here could weaken the instrument design.

Sharpening explorers. Explorers used for detection of decay (No. 23) should be kept sharp. The points can be sharpened easily by applying the stone to the tip of the explorer at an angle of about 15 to 20 degrees. Short strokes should then be implemented around the entire point so that it becomes sharpened. Explorers that are used primarily for submarginal detection do not need to be sharpened as regularly as those used to explore for decay.

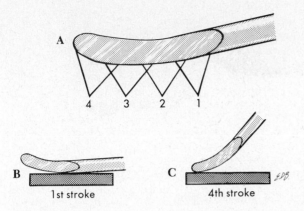

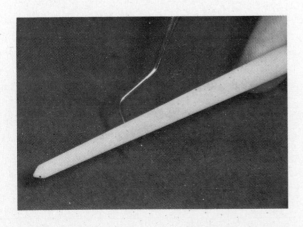

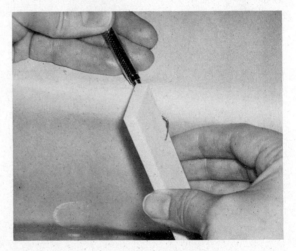

Fig. 6-20. **A,** Four different adaptations of stone are necessary to sharpen entire surface. **B,** First stroke should start at heel of blade. **C,** Last stroke should end at toe.

Fig. 6-21. Stone is adapted at 110-degree angle to sharpen opposite cutting edge of universal curette.

Fig. 6-22. Tapered cylindrical stone is applied to facial surface of curette to assist in removal of wire edges.

CONCLUSION

Following the sharpening procedure, all excess oil and debris should be wiped from the instruments, and they should be prepared for sterilization. Autoclaving will not dull the edges of instruments made of a fine-quality stainless steel, but this method of sterilization can dull carbon steel instruments (Parkes and Kolstad, 1981). Dry heat is preferred to protect the sharp cutting edges of carbon steel instruments.

A sterile sharpening stone and testing stick should be part of the tray setup for every periodontal procedure. Instruments should be sharpened at the first signs of dullness to increase the effectiveness of the treatment and so that unnecessary grinding and loss of metal will not be required to restore the original design and an optimal cutting edge. Frequent sharpening can extend the life of an instrument, since less metal will need to be removed to restore the instrument's form and function.

ACTIVITIES

1. Examine and compare the designs of the following types of instruments under a microscope:
   a. A new instrument
   b. A well-sharpened instrument
   c. A missharpened instrument
   d. A dull instrument
2. Compare the ease of scaling and root planing on extracted teeth when using an instrument that has been optimally sharpened versus using a dull instrument.
3. Inoculate a bacterial culture medium with shavings taken from a fingernail while testing instrument sharpness; incubate the test sample, and examine for bacterial growth.
4. Observe a demonstration of instrument sharpening using a handpiece-mounted stone or a honing machine and discuss the use of these techniques for routine instrument sharpening in terms of amount of metal removed, ability to control the application of the stone to the instrument, heat generated, contamination control, and access to equipment during patient treatment.

REVIEW QUESTIONS

1. Which of the following methods is *not* an acceptable way to determine instrument sharpness?
   a. Evaluation of the cutting edge during scaling procedures
   b. Evaluation of light reflection from the cutting edge when observed under magnification
   c. Evaluation of the cutting edge against a plastic testing stick
   d. Evaluation of the cutting edge against the clinician's fingernail
2. True or false
   a. The Arkansas stone is a man-made, or artificial, sharpening stone.
   b. Sterilization by autoclaving will not dull the cutting edges of stainless steel instruments.
   c. Both cutting edges of a Gracey curette should be sharpened.
3. What is the internal angle formed by the facial and lateral surfaces of curettes and sickle scalers?
   a. 45 degrees
   b. 70 to 80 degrees
   c. 90 degrees
   d. 100 to 110 degrees
4. Identify two design characteristics of curettes that must be preserved during sharpening.
5. Routine sharpening of the ＿＿＿ of a curette or sickle scaler will weaken the blade strength of the instrument and shorten its working life.
   a. Facial surface
   b. Lateral surfaces
   c. Back
   d. Toe
6. When a stationary instrument is being sharpened with a moving stone, pressure should be applied on the ＿＿＿ .
   a. Upstroke only
   b. Downstroke only
   c. Upstroke and downstroke

REFERENCES

Green, E., and Seyer, P.C. 1972. Sharpening curets and sickle scalers, ed. 2. Berkeley, Calif.: Praxis Publishing Co.

HuFriedy Dept. of Professional Education. 1982. Smarten up, sharpen up: a practical work-book on sharpening dental curets and scalers. Chicago: Hu-Friedy, Inc.

Paquette, O.E., and Levin, M.P. 1977. The sharpening of scaling instruments. I. An examination of principles. J. Periodontol. **48**:163.

Parkes, R.B., and Kolstad, R.A. 1981. Effects of sterilization on periodontal instruments. J. Periodontol. **53**:434.

Pattison, G., and Pattison, A.M. 1979. Periodontal instrumentation: a clinical manual. Reston, Va.: Reston Publishing Co., Inc.

U.S. Department of Health, Education, and Welfare, Project Acorde. 1976. Instrument sharpening. Castro Valley, Calif.: Quercus Corp.

Wilkins, E.M. 1983. Clinical practice of the dental hygienist, ed. 5. Philadelphia: Lea & Febiger.

PART TWO

ASSESSMENT

In the development of any program or project, it is wise to take time to *assess* the situation. Moving directly to implementation without taking time to determine the reasons for the project or the unique needs of the persons for whom the project is being developed can cause considerable difficulty, delay progress, or cause ultimate failure of the project. Even the best efforts in implementation can be fraught with difficulty if these efforts are aimed at nonexistent needs or at needs that the subjects of the project do not wish to have modified. A more scientific approach to project development is to set aside assumptions and personal beliefs about needs and reasons for a project and investigate objective data from which reasons can be inferred.

Assessment includes not only objective data, but also the more subjective responses and feelings of the people for whom or with whom the project will be carried out. Even though objective signs are clear indicators of the need for change, subjective responses may override those indicators. People may not want change, or they may want change to be gradual.

In providing clinical care for patients, the principle of assessment is particularly important. Assessment data provide the baseline information for determining the general and oral health status of each patient and provide the dental professional with the opportunity to evaluate the patient's perceptions of the need or desire for change. Assessment can prevent, or help the provider anticipate, emergency situations; it can allow for the individualization of care; it provides baseline data for comparing progress and outcomes with the entering status of the patient; and it allows for rational planning.

The following 10 chapters prepare clinicians to practice assessment skills with patients.

7 THE PATIENT'S PERCEPTIONS

OBJECTIVES: *The reader will be able to*

1. Describe briefly at least three possible motives for choosing a career as a health care provider that may influence the degree to which the patient is viewed as a partner in care.
2. Identify language patterns that may indicate to the patient the role he/she has in treatment.
3. Given case descriptions of two views of proposed treatment (the patient's and the hygienist's), identify discrepancies in wants, needs, and expectations.
4. Explain the probable impact of discrepancies in wants, needs, and expectations on the success of treatment.
5. Given case presentations, identify ways in which the dental hygienist can gather information regarding the patient's perspectives (wants, needs, and expectations).
6. Describe the helping relationship.
7. Differentiate between the helping relationship and a dependency relationship.
8. Differentiate between professional closeness and excessive familiarity.
9. Identify ways to blend responsiveness to patients' needs with professional responsibility to provide the "best" care.
10. Explain preliminary plans for assessment phases of care to a series of hypothetical patients who have a variety of wants, needs, and expectations regarding dental hygiene care.

As described in Chapter 1, there are many reasons for a person deciding to become a dental hygienist. The motivations related to self-esteem, a flexible working schedule, and a comfortable income and working environment form one basic group related mostly to "self" needs. A second group of motivations is based largely on the desire to perform technical kinds of procedures with one's hands and to work with fascinating equipment and instruments that can improve the function and appearance of teeth and their surrounding tissues. Although this second group is "other" oriented, it focuses largely on the procedural aspects of practice. A third kind of basic motivation is that of helping persons experience positive health changes or of helping them maintain health. In most instances health care providers have traces of all three motivations that, in balance, can provide satisfaction with the profession as well as favorable outcomes for patients.

According to communication theory regarding the building of interpersonal relationships, the person with a major interest in helping people maintain and achieve health is most likely able to encourage and develop the patient's role as a cotherapist or as a partner in care. If the health care provider's major interests are self-oriented or procedure oriented, the patient is more likely to be viewed as an object of care or as a means to an end.

THE PATIENT AS A PARTNER IN CARE

The health care provider who views the patient as a partner in care is more likely to be interested in finding out what the patient's wants, needs, and expectations are with regard to care rather than in creating an independent set of needs for the patient based solely on clinical data. The partner-in-care concept includes opportunities for the patient to self-assess personal needs, as well as oral conditions, under the guidance of the dental hygienist (Chapters 19 and 20). Partners in care arrive at mutually satisfying treatment plan configurations and appointment sequences that will best enable both members of the partnership to complete preventive and therapeutic phases of care (Clark and Morton, 1977).

Basic communications theory explains that people are more likely to feel a commitment to a project or a goal if they share in its development and if its development clearly meets their individual needs (Collins, 1977; Keltner, 1973). While sharing in the design of the plan, participants learn about needs they had not identified on their own and begin to feel some ownership of the entire proposal. Thus, in a partnership between the dental hygienist and the patient, the dental hygienist learns about the specific needs and limitations of the patient, and the patient learns about the needs and limitations of the hygienist (Cohen, 1975; Dworkin, Ference, and Giddon, 1978). Mutual respect for wants and needs can emerge, and a clear set of reasonable expectations can be defined, which both persons will be more likely to fulfill. Unshared expectations are difficult to meet. Unilateral treatment planning can often be unrealistic, because it is focused on what may be low priorities in the patient's view (Dworkin, Ference, and Giddon, 1978). The classic example is the treatment plan that is based on carefully gathered clinical, radiographic, and laboratory findings prepared by the brightest, most incisive diagnostician, scheduled into logical, perfectly spaced appointments, and presented to the patient with beautiful slides and a well-ordered outline of objective findings and related plans, but for which the patient never appears. Regardless of how well prepared the health care provider's procedures are, if the patient does not believe his/her needs are addressed and being met, the likelihood of compliance in care is remote. The patient has the final say in whether care will be delivered. If it is not in the form of a "no" at the time of the case presentation, it may be a cancelled or "forgotten" appointment.

The patient is usually able to detect whether he/she is an object or a partner in care. The language that health care providers use is an indicator. Do health care providers perform a procedure *for* someone or *with* someone, or do they do it *to* someone? Which expression connotes partnership and which connotes object? Is the person scheduled for an appointment at 3:00 PM referred to as the "Class III prophylaxis" or as the "Class II amalgam," or is that person referred to by name, with a diagnosis or planned treatment described as his/her condition? Compare the following two statements: "The upper denture case is in operatory 3." "Ms. Wolfe

is in operatory 3, waiting for a try-in of the upper denture." While the second phrasing may be a few words longer, it does connote a different image of just what is residing in operatory 3. Patients often hear our descriptions of them; if they are viewed as partners in care, they are likely to be referred to as people and not as conditions (Collins, 1977).

PATIENT INVOLVEMENT IN PLANNING CARE

Involving the patient in the preparation of a treatment plan and in designing appointment sequences is a difficult concept for many health care providers to accept. The most frequent response to such an idea is that the patient does not really know what he/she needs; that is why he/she has come to the health care provider—to find out what is wrong and to have it fixed. Although it is certainly true that the health care provider has far greater knowledge of the objective, observable needs of the patient's conditions, the patient may have some important information or notions regarding his/her health status or particular needs that can greatly influence the outcome of care. Such information may not emerge unless it is during a discussion of wants, needs, and expectations. Even if the patient has little to contribute to modify suggested care, inclusion in the decision-making process may improve the likelihood of the patient feeling a sense of commitment to the process and may help ensure that the disease state is avoided in the future (Clark and Morton, 1977; Collins, 1977; Keltner, 1973; Purtilo, 1978).

Evaluate the following two case presentations for the extent to which they include the patient in the decision-making process:

Presentation 1: Well, Mr. Brennan, I've taken a careful look at your examination findings and have decided that you need three appointments to completely clean your teeth and to complete four areas of soft tissue curettage. You have some problems with your gums, and the dentist and I concur that the best way to reverse that problem is to remove all the hard calculus from your teeth and to remove some of the necrotic lining of the gum tissue pockets around your teeth. Now, I know you are interested in having those front teeth turned so they are better looking, but I think your highest priority should lie with getting these gum problems under control. So, we have decided to delay discussing orthodontic treatment until these appointments are complete. If you'll see the receptionist, you can schedule those appointments some time in the next 2 weeks.

Presentation 2: As I remember our initial conversation, Mr. Brennan, your primary interest in dental care was to have those front teeth straightened. Is that still a primary concern for you? (Discuss with patient.) You may recall that during the guided self-assessment we did of your teeth and gums, we found a lot of red, swollen tissue and quite a bit of hard accumulations of calculus on your teeth. Well, the x-ray films confirm that you do have gum or gingival problems. Take a look at these films; I think if you compare the bone around the molars with the bone around your lower front teeth, you will see a difference in appearance and in height around the teeth. The bone around the molars appears to be in an active state of destruction. I consulted the dentist, and we agree that you may want to postpone the movement of the teeth until we modify the state of the supporting tissues for all your teeth. The bone and the gingiva should be made healthy before we put any additional stress on them. And even after their health has improved, we will have to decide whether tooth movement is advisable. The dentist has agreed that an orthodontist should completely review your case after the initial preparation is complete. We are suggesting that the efforts to move your teeth now might cause harm to the rest of your teeth if we don't attend to these other problems first. Is this advised set of priorities acceptable to you? Would you agree that we should proceed with the removal of these hard deposits? (Discuss with patient.) Once we have the irritants off your teeth, we'll show you a way to prevent their recurrence, since these gingival and bone problems will recur if plaque builds up on your teeth and if hard deposits form again. (Pause for response; check nonverbal response.) And, after the plaque is under control, we'll assess the gingiva to decide whether a soft tissue curettage is indicated to remove some of the lining of the gingival pockets around your teeth. Sometimes the gingiva are unable to heal completely unless necrotic tissue from those areas is removed and the root surfaces are hard and smooth. This will require three appointments, spaced over the next few weeks to allow time between each appointment for healing. Then, when all this is accomplished, we'll reevaluate orthodontic care. Does this sound reasonable to you? Do you have suggestions that could make it easier for us to accomplish our goal together? Are you as interested in having your supporting tissues heal and remain solid as you are in having those front teeth moved? (Discuss after each sample question.)

Which case presentation is more patient centered? Pick out the phrases that tell you the patient is viewed as a partner rather than a person expected to agree. In which case can you imagine the hygienist making eye contact frequently with the patient? What other differences in nonverbal behavior can you imagine would be evident between these two case descriptions? The differences intended between the two styles of case presentation are in the degree of opportunity the patient has to react to the suggested treatment plan and the extent to which the patient's need (tooth movement for esthetics) is kept in mind as a serious priority worthy of consideration. Patients may not necessarily value certain elements of dental health (or general health, for that matter) as much as health care providers do (Collins, 1977; Purtilo, 1978). Certainly, explanation regarding the rationale for an altered treatment plan and for including more in the plan than the patient expected is essential and valid. This explanation is given in patient-centered care with the underlying premise that the patient's wants and needs are equally important in designing the total plan and that the patient has the right to be involved in the discussion and in the decision making (Collins, 1977; Dworkin, Ference, and Giddon, 1978). The patient should always be asked if he/she is satisfied with the proposed treatment plan (Clark and Morton, 1977).

While this chapter focuses on the interpersonal responsibility and wisdom of keeping a patient fully informed and of seeking the patient's verbal consent, this responsibility is also a legal one. It is not enough to be "right" about what a patient needs. Thus the attitude of engaging a patient as a partner in decision making is supported by the law as well as by the need for harmony and cooperation (Rosoff, 1981).

An obvious outcome of sharing plans, discussing priorities, and asking opinions is that the patient may disagree with what the provider believes is right. There are times when the patient may not wish to compromise his/her desires for care, despite the careful discussion of rationale to include other phases of care or to delay or eliminate the phases of care the patient believes are needed to improve appearance or health. A case in point may be the person who appears with perfectly healthy teeth and periodontium but who insists that he/she will have all the teeth extracted and dentures made. A patient who is convinced that this course of treatment is best certainly deserves discussion of some alternatives and a careful analysis of why and how the patient came to this conclusion. In some cases it may not be possible to convince the patient sufficiently that other approaches should be followed. The health care provider then has to decide whether to provide the procedures the patient wants or refuse care. Generally speaking, if a patient requests care that, in the opinion of the dentist or hygienist, is totally inappropriate or dangerous, the health care provider is probably wise to refuse care. The only alternative is to write out all the adverse possible outcomes of such care and have the patient sign the statement. Such a statement should relieve the health care providers from responsibility for the negative outcomes of such treatment and place full responsibility on the patient. Because of the critical nature of such a disclaimer, it is absolutely essential that an attorney draw up such a document.

The patient who demands unreasonable care is certainly a challenge to health care providers, since the only realistic decision may be to refuse care. The professional must then allow the patient to leave with untended real problems as he/she seeks another professional to solve his/her imagined problems. For the patient, however, the labels for those problems are just the opposite, and efforts to solve what the patient sees as imaginary problems and the health professional sees as real will probably result in further patient dissatisfaction.

Another challenge is the patient who says he/she is satisfied but who does not act that way. The patient may act resentful or miss appointments. If there is a discrepancy between what is said and what is done, the patient should be asked about it (Purtilo, 1978).

LISTENING

The first step in developing an attitude that will "let the patient in" as a partner is to practice good listening skills. Many new clinicians are concerned about what to say to a patient. A clinician's first priority is to *listen* to what the patient says and to let the patient know the clinician understands. This is *not* accomplished by saying, "I understand." Even though these words of assurance are spoken, the patient is left wondering what it is the clinician thinks he/she understands.

Listening involves rephrasing (1) the *content* of the message the patient has sent and (2) the patient's *affect* or emotion behind it.

For instance, a new patient arriving for dental hygiene care says, "I sure hate coming to a dental office." Listening would involve reflecting back the content and affect by saying, "It sounds like you don't enjoy these visits very much and you'd rather be elsewhere right now." The patient responds to correct an inaccuracy, such as:

Well, no. I don't look forward to being here. But I know I should have this done. So here's the place to be.

Or the patient may confirm the hygienist's reflection and elaborate:

You bet. My mouth must be very sensitive, because I feel *everything*. Having my teeth cleaned really hurts.

Further listening would be:

So you've had your teeth cleaned many times before, and it always hurts.

The patient:

Yes, it does. Every time an instrument touches my teeth, I feel like a needle is touching the nerve.

The hygienist:

So what hurts is a metal instrument touching the tooth rather than your gums feeling sore.

The patient:

Yes. My gums don't bother me at all. It's the teeth. I just have to hang on for fear of crying. I wish someone could do something so I wouldn't feel the pain.

The hygienist:

It sounds like having your teeth cleaned must be awful for you—like you're 'white knuckling' it through the appointment. Anesthesia hasn't worked for you.

The patient:

Well, no one has given me anesthesia. I just put up with it and keep quiet.

After all that *listening* it may now be time for the hygienist to begin *talking*. It appears that the patient could benefit from anesthesia, and it could be suggested. But imagine that the hygienist had not used active listening. Typical responses to a patient's complaint about being in a dental office could be:

- Don't worry. I'll be gentle.
- Everyone hates to be in a dental chair—even I don't like it.
- Dentistry is an evil necessity, isn't it?

- Do you come to the dentist regularly?
- You should try relaxation exercises.
- Well, we're just cleaning your teeth today. It won't be bad.

Any one of those typical comments shuts off the communication. The patient either gives up and suffers again or has to start up with another entry to get the hygienist to listen. Even the question response shuts off communication because it redirects the patient to talk about what the hygienist suspects is behind the problem. The patient's message is lost, and thus a critical insight to the patient's needs and expectations is missed.

Practice in using active listening is essential in developing a partnership and helping relationship with a patient.

THE HELPING RELATIONSHIP

A basic element of the helping relationship in which the patient is a partner in care is the patient *wanting* to be helped (Purtilo, 1978). Patients must have the freedom to refuse help (even if help is *good* for them). If help is requested as a result of discussions with the patient, the relationship can grow.

The second basic element is that the helping relationship should build toward patient self-reliance (Purtilo, 1978). A sound helping relationship enables the patient to accept responsibility for self-care, for preventing disease, and for seeking professional help to maintain health. The alternative is a dependency relationship in which the patient sees the health care provider as the one responsible for the patient's dental health.

In the practice of dental hygiene, it is common to encounter patients who believe that as long as they have their teeth checked and cleaned every 6 months, their responsibility toward good dental health is fulfilled; the rest is up to the dentist and hygienist. Having clean teeth 2 days out of the year (every 6 months) and having restorations placed year after year result in detrimental long-term effects. Periodontists who treat patients who have "graduated" to their care from years of such a routine refer to this kind of care as supervised neglect. The patient has become dependent on the professionals for something they cannot possibly provide. Daily self-care in removing plaque and debris and in monitoring diet are critical components in dental health that cannot be assigned to the dental hygienist or dentist.

Certainly, there is a degree of dependence on the health care provider in some early stages of care when considerable therapeutic time and skill are required to correct disease status. The goal throughout these early stages, however, should be to shift primary responsibility from the health care provider to the patient (Purtilo, 1978), beginning with (1) involving the patient in the diagnostic phases of care by means of a guided self-assessment of oral conditions, (2) including the patient in decision making regarding treatment, and (3) facilitating the shift of responsibility for maintaining health by dental health education, nutritional guidance, and mechanisms for self-evaluation of oral status between appointments. Thus "constructive dependence" grows toward the interdependence of a partnership (Purtilo, 1978).

This relationship may be difficult to achieve for professionals whose major motives are self-oriented or technically oriented. Likewise, this may be a difficult relationship for the patient who would rather not be bothered with responsibility for health and who would rather say, "You're the doctor! Do what you need to." Usually the partnership relationship develops at different rates, depending on the perceptions and needs of the health care provider and the patient. In most cases it is the health care provider who leads the way in developing the partnership; in the era of consumer awareness, however, it may be the patient who leads the way by seeking information, input, and shared responsibility.

Values are changing among patients in tandem with the emphasis on consumer rights that has grown over the last 10 years. Such values include a greater sense of independence (less reliance on a health care provider's words), self-determination, and egalitarianism. Patients look past the status-claiming medical or dental degree and seek second opinions, inquire about alternatives, and question the conclusions presented (Gallagher, 1976). Thus the patients a hygienist or dentist encounters may expect to be involved more than the health care provider expects they will be.

PROFESSIONAL CLOSENESS

Since relationships with dental patients in particular may last many years and involve families of patients as well as individuals, there is considerable opportunity for developing trust and refining ways to move in and out of a dependency relationship with each person, depending on the patient's social and economic needs and growth as well as on overall health status (Purtilo, 1978). This may well be among the most satisfying aspects of the practice of dental hygiene.

This high degree of trust with a patient is professional closeness. During a series of appointments, and especially over a period of years, the patient and dental hygienist may be able to share personal ideas and judgments and perhaps feelings and emotions (Purtilo, 1978). They may be able to share laughter, grief, solutions to the world's problems, and a new recipe or an easy method for adjusting the carburetor. In any case, they will have passed the stage of limiting conversation to cliches about the weather and facts about plaque levels and gingival conditions (Purtilo, 1978). The critical balance (professional closeness) is between aloofness and excessive familiarity (Purtilo, 1978). Both verbal and nonverbal expressions declare which side of the balance the hygienist has found. Aloofness is cold, factual, precise, and uncomplicated with human feeling. Excessive familiarity is inappropriately casual or chummy, filled with expressions of feelings that are seen as overreactions, but still uncomplicated with much true understanding of human feelings. It is the lack of awareness of the other person's boundaries and freedom to move toward an open relationship or to reserve such a response for somewhere other than the dental environment. Professional closeness, in contrast to both extremes, is largely in response to the patient's expressed needs and is, above all, a genuine expression of caring for a fellow human being (Collins, 1977). It includes an interest in the patient as a person with values, needs, and beliefs that deserve respect (Collins, 1977; Goldberg, Plume, and Nacman, 1973; Murray and Weise, 1975; Purtilo, 1978), and it recognizes that efficiency and formality can express caring when they do not impose rigid limits on interaction (Purtilo, 1978). Issues regarding the use of white uniforms and the use of first names or last names with patients are regarded as moot points that require individual judgment of outcomes based on the *expressed* preferences of the patients and a careful analysis of personal preference (Purtilo, 1978).

One useful guideline in developing a professional relationship with a patient is to ask what the patient prefers: "What would you prefer I call you?" or "Do you prefer to have me talk to you during the appointment, or do you like it better if I work quietly?" After a while, experience seems to help the health care provider know when to talk, when to remain silent, when to work efficiently with minimal verbal exchange, and when to set aside instruments and discuss an issue. In some ways, developing a professional relationship is much like establishing a friendship, but with the complicating factors of specifying wants and needs, which hopefully will be considered appropriate by the patient for inclusion in a plan of care.

INTRODUCING THE PATIENT TO INITIAL PHASES OF CARE

Often the dental hygienist's initial encounters with the patient center on the critical issue of what shall or shall not be included in care. This issue can be a major one if the patient thinks that one or two specific procedures will be completed to meet his/her needs. For instance, if the patient has been accustomed to having his/her teeth cleaned on request, the patient may not expect to have a complete medical history, a complete series of radiographs, and plaque and gingival indices recorded. The patient may be even more aghast at having a facial massage (actually an extraoral examination) and blood pressure taken.

For this reason, it is wise to describe for the patient exactly what is routinely included in the first visit, how long it will take, and how much it will cost. The "laundry list" of procedures should be prefaced by a few introductory comments regarding the need at the first appointment to gather some baseline information on the basis of which decisions regarding treatment can be made. As each procedure is begun, the patient should be told what the procedure is, why it is important to perform the procedure, how it is done, and how the patient can cooperate in the effort. A simple request to proceed should precede performance of the procedure.

Some patients may be put at ease if the health care provider describes aloud what he/she is doing as each phase is performed. The patient may wish to observe in a hand mirror. Significant findings can be shared with the patient as long as no definitive diagnostic conclusions are given until after the dentist has completely reviewed the data. For instance, the hygienist may say, "I can feel the muscles in the floor of your mouth, and I see the normal structures that carry saliva to your mouth and that attach your tongue to the floor of the mouth. There is some normal tonsillar tissue on the side of your tongue." The hygienist probably should *not* say, "Everything looks and feels normal in the floor of your mouth. Nothing wrong there!" The first description is a report of findings. The second statement includes a diagnostic judgment, which should be confirmed with the dentist under current law.

Diagnosis of oral health over which the dentist has purview is best left unsaid. Comments about the healthy state of gingival tissue, which clearly relates to dental hygiene judgment, is less risky to divulge. For instance, an acceptable and helpful comment could be, "The firm, pink gum or gingival tissue you see here looks healthy."

Once the assessment data have been gathered and a diagnosis has been confirmed by the dentist, the hygienist may discuss in greater detail the significance of the findings with the patient. Most patients would like to know more about themselves, including their oral health, as long as the technical language is kept to a minimum and the descriptions are clear and relevant.

At the conclusion of the first appointment, the dental hygienist should tell the patient what will occur at the next appointment and approximately how long it will take (Clark and Morton, 1977). If an additional charge will be made, an estimate of cost should be provided. Usually all subsequent needs are addressed in a treatment plan as discussed in Chapter 18.

What if the patient refuses a phase of care? As mentioned earlier, the patient does have the right to refuse. For preliminary procedures, it may be helpful to explain how the missing data will affect the accuracy of the diagnosis. If the patient still elects to refuse a specific phase of care, the health care provider can elect to terminate care, can have his/her attorney draw up a disclaimer similar to that suggested for patients who request care that is not in their best interests, or can postpone that phase of care until other aspects not reliant on the rejected procedure can be completed. Sometimes, after a few appointments and some low-pressure discussion, the patient will reconsider and decide to include the procedure, especially if the undesir-

able result of its exclusion becomes increasingly apparent to the patient.

If the patient has the opportunity to see the health care provider as a trustworthy person who accepts the patient as an individual with unique needs rather than as one who views the patient as an object for demonstrating technical prowess or as a means to a lucrative end, it may be possible for him/her to lower defenses and see the dentist and hygienist as partners in care rather than as necessary evils. The patient may ask to have the omitted procedure performed.

In some instances this relationship depends on an initial lowering of apparent "control" over the environment. Sharing a bit of the control may yield more freedom in the long run to suggest and implement care. Insisting on immediate, total control may send many patients away or may unintentionally foster a dependency relationship in which the patient hears the message, "Doctor knows best. Hygienist heals all."

ACTIVITIES

1. Tape record interactions between a health care provider and a patient, and listen to the recording to determine signs of:
   a. Listening
   b. Dependence/partnership
   c. Aloofness, closeness, familiarity
   d. Conflicts of wants, needs, and expectations
2. Role play vignettes to demonstrate:
   a. A helping relationship
   b. A dependency relationship
3. Role play the explanation of preliminary assessment procedures to a patient who is:
   a. Interested only in restorative care
   b. Concerned about excess exposure to radiation from x rays
   c. Convinced he/she will need dentures in another 10 years
   d. Accustomed to *no* preliminary procedures in a dental office other than two x-ray films and a caries charting
   e. Afraid he/she has oral cancer

REVIEW QUESTIONS

1. The patient wants her front teeth polished so she will look nice for her son's wedding. The hygienist wants to do something about those inflamed gingivae and the heavy calculus on the molars. How might this discrepancy affect the outcome of care?
2. The patient wants his cavities filled. He does not want to hear the hygienist's eighteenth rendition of how to

floss and the need to eat fewer sweets. The hygienist wants to end this string of recurrent caries that is evident from the patient's record. How might this discrepancy affect the outcome of care?

3. A hygienist's patient looks up and says contentedly, "I know that as long as you take care of me, I'll never lose my teeth." What might that statement imply?

4. Identify whether each of the following vignettes reflects professional aloofness, professional closeness, or excessive familiarity:

   a. Hygienist slaps new patient on the back and says, "Well Joe, how's tricks?"

   b. Hygienist decides she prefers to wear a clinic jacket over street clothes. To verify this decision, she asks several patients what they think of the new garb.

   c. A long-term patient complains that she has been under considerable tension lately and that she knows she has not taken proper care of her teeth. The hygienist elects not to discuss the unusually bad state of the gingivae other than to show the plaque index and a few selected papillae (by means of the mirror) to the patient. Later during the appointment, the hygienist gently asks whether the patient has been able to get some help for her tension.

   d. The dental hygienist checks a plaque index and sees that it is actually worse than that from the previous visit. The hygienist launches into her "plan B" speech on the merits of brushing and flossing and states that care will fail if the patient does not comply with these directives.

5. What measures can a health care provider take if a patient refuses a phase of care that is essential for diagnostic or therapeutic purposes?

6. Give a listening response to each of these patient comments:

   a. "I don't think you are going to like the way my teeth look!"

   b. "I never have liked these dental chairs where I have to lie flat."

   c. "You really dig a lot deeper than other hygienists I've had."

   d. "I want the dentist to clean my teeth, not some girl."

7. How does each of these nonlistening replies to the statements in 6 cut off further communication and understanding?

   a. "Don't worry. I *always* like the way your teeth look!"

   b. "Well, these new ones are much better for posture than those old clunkers."

   c. "I could give you some anesthesia."

   d. "I'm not 'some girl.' I'm a licensed hygienist who is highly skilled at cleaning teeth and many other procedures."

REFERENCES

Clark, J.D., and Morton, J.C. 1977. Behavioral assessment: an appraisal of beliefs and behaviors relating to treatment. Dent. Clin. North Am. 21:515.

Cohen, D.W. 1975. Preventive periodontics. J. Indian. Dent. Assoc. (Special Issue), p. 273.

Cohen, L.C., et al. 1980. Caring and controlling dimensions in patient relations: the dental student perspective. J. Am. Coll. Dent. 47:180.

Collins, M. 1977. Communication in health care: understanding and implementing effective human relationships. St. Louis: The C.V. Mosby Co.

Dworkin, S.F., Ference, T.P., and Giddon, D.B. 1978. Behavioral science and dental practice. St. Louis: The C.V. Mosby Co.

Gallagher, E.B. 1976. The doctor-patient relationship in the changing health scene. Washington, D.C.: U.S. Department of Health, Education, and Welfare.

Goldberg, H.J., Plume, M., and Nacman, M. 1973. The importance of attitude in the delivery of health services. J. Public Health Dent. 33:35.

Keltner, J.W. 1973. Elements of interpersonal communication. Belmont, Calif.: Wadsworth Publishing Co., Inc.

Murray, B.P., and Weise, H.J. 1975. Satisfaction with care and the utilization of dental services at a neighborhood health center. J. Public Health Dent. 35:170.

Purtilo, R. 1978. Health professional/patient interaction. Philadelphia: W.B. Saunders Co.

Rosoff, A.J. 1981. Informed consent. Rockville, M.D.: Aspen Systems Corp.

Weinstein, P., et al. 1983. Oral self-care: a promising alternative behavior model. J. Am. Dent. Assoc. 107:67.

8 THE COMPREHENSIVE HEALTH HISTORY

OBJECTIVES: *The reader will be able to*

1. Explain the reasons for a comprehensive health history to a skeptical patient.
2. State the rationale for combining questionnaire and interview techniques to obtain the necessary patient information.
3. Identify and use the communication skills that help ensure a thorough health history.
4. List the components of a comprehensive health history and explain the relevance of each.
5. Identify responses that necessitate consultation with the dentist and/or physician.
6. Identify specific conditions and/or responses that indicate the need for antibiotic premedication, sedation, alteration of medication, special appointment planning, additional laboratory studies, and special precautions to prevent disease transmission and allergic reactions.
7. List history update questions to be asked at recall appointments.
8. Given various responses to questions, identify appropriate follow-up questions or procedures to ensure gathering of complete data.
9. Given a patient with a variety of medical problems, conduct a complete health history and prepare a review of systems.
10. Explain the rationale for a medical classification system.
11. Explain the rationale for a medical release letter.
12. Explain the need for use of the *Physicians' Desk Reference*.

Observing necessary precautions that may relate to specific medical problems or medications is a professional responsibility. Before dental services are offered to any patient, an assessment of the overall health status is necessary. Providing safe treatment is the prime objective in planning dental care consistent with a patient's health status. Advances in medical diagnosis and therapeutic agents enable many people with serious medical conditions to function at a near normal level of activity. For this reason, completing a comprehensive health history is essential to familiarize the health care provider with each patient's unique health profile.

RATIONALE FOR COMPLETING A HEALTH HISTORY

There are a number of reasons for completing a health history.

First, the information *provides continuity between medical and dental care*. Establishing communication and cooperation between the patient's physician and dentist helps ensure that all aspects of the patient's health needs can be addressed. Oral conditions and other physical conditions are often closely related. Measles, for instance, may be diagnosed by the recognition of Koplik's spots (white or bluish spots surrounded by an inflamed red zone) found on the buccal mucosa 24 hours before the general skin rash appears (Kerr and Ash, 1978). Conditions such as a red, swollen tongue and cracking skin at the corners of the mouth may be observed, which may indicate a nutritional deficiency in riboflavin. In chronic medical conditions such as diabetes mellitus, the patient's resistance to infection may be lowered, making him/her prone to periodontal disease.

Informing the patient about areas where medicine and dentistry are related is important in providing total patient care. For example, medications prescribed by the physician may affect oral conditions. Phenytoin (Dilantin) is an anticonvulsant medication often prescribed for the treatment of epilepsy. This medication has the potential to increase the gingiva's response to irritation (plaque, calculus) (Angelopoulous, 1975; Braham, 1977; Israel, 1974). For many patients the result of taking this medication is gingival enlargement, or hyperplasia.

A number of patients still find routine visits to a dentist anxiety producing. Patients with medical conditions such as angina pectoris or hypertension may be adversely affected by stress. Identifying patients who have medical or emotional conditions that may be aggravated by the stress of a visit to the dentist can be crucial for providing appropriate and successful treatment.

A complete health history may help the dental care provider *avoid medical emergencies and identify precautions the clinician and patient should observe*. It is not difficult to imagine what could happen if a medically compromised patient were treated without proper assessment of health status. Administering a local anesthetic agent to a patient who is sensitized or allergic to one of its constituents could produce a severe and possibly fatal anaphylactic reaction.

Patients who have heart valve disease due to rheumatic fever or congenital heart defects and patients with heart valves that have been surgically replaced with artificial prostheses must be medicated with an antibiotic prior to and following dental treatment. Patients with a history of surgical procedures in which foreign matter or prostheses have been implanted may require antibiotic protection, which should be determined by consultation with their physician. Examples of such implants are cardiac pacemaker implants and Dacron patches used to repair congenital heart defects. Patients with kidney disease who have hemodialysis shunts require antibiotic protection to prevent infection at the site of the prosthesis. Patients who have received prosthetic joints, and those who have organ transplants (e.g., kidney) also require antibiotic premedication. These patients are susceptible to subacute bacterial endocarditis following the inevitable bacteremia that occurs during procedures such as prophylaxis, curettage, endodontic therapy, tooth extraction, or more extensive periodontal surgery (''Reports of Councils,'' 1977, Weinstein and Schlesinger, 1974; Wintroke et al., 1970). Bacteremia refers to the presence of viable bacteria in the circulating blood. Antibiotic protection is rec-

ommended with all dental procedures that are likely to cause trauma to the tissue and allow oral bacteria to enter the bloodstream in these susceptible individuals.

A study by Baltch et al. (1982) describes 56 patients with moderate to severe periodontal disease. Twenty-eight with valvular heart disease received intravenous penicillin before a dental cleaning procedure was performed, and 28 without known disease did not receive the drug. None of the subjects had bacteremia before cleaning, but 5 minutes after the procedure, 61% of the group that had not received penicillin were bacteremic versus 11% of the treated group. From these patients 71 microorganisms were isolated, including 53 anaerobes and 18 aerobes. Only 11 of the isolates were found in the patients receiving prophylaxis with the antibiotic.

Since subacute bacterial endocarditis is of particular concern in dental care, the disease process is described in some detail. Following the bacteremia caused by a gingival procedure, the bacteria attaches to the susceptible person's affected cardiac valve endothelium or artificial prosthesis. *Streptococcus viridans* is the bacteria most commonly found as the cause of subacute bacterial endocarditis, although other bacteria, including *Staphylococcus aureus,* have been implicated as the cause of the infection (Durack, Kaplan, and Bisno, 1983; Wintroke et al., 1970). The organisms proliferate, forming bacterial masses and clumps. With the growth of these bacteria and the consequent infection and destruction of the cardiac tissue, the valve is unable to maintain its function. In other patients the surgical graft becomes infected and incompetent. Clinically, the patient exhibits a low-grade fever, slowly developing anemia, loss of appetite, and fatigue. With undiagnosed and untreated subacute bacterial endocarditis, the patient's life expectancy seldom exceeds 3 to 6 months. Sudden death may occur when a bacterial clump breaks off and causes a fatal embolism. The most common cause of death results from congestive heart failure attributed to valve destruction or myocardial damage (Weinstein and Schlesinger, 1974; Wintroke et al., 1970). The heart fails when the infected valve becomes incompetent, preventing the proper emptying of the heart chamber. The blood literally backs up because the valve is no longer able to close and permit the proper blood flow out of the heart to the rest of the body.

With early diagnosis and appropriate antibiotic treatment, 90% of patients survive subacute bacterial endocarditis (Durack, Kaplan, and Bisno, 1983). The clinician's role is to prevent the disease from occurring by screening susceptible patients with the comprehensive health history and providing the proper antibiotic protection prior to treatment.

In a recent study, 52 cases of endocarditis prophylaxis failure were reported to a national registry established by the American Heart Association (Durack, Kaplan, and Bisno, 1983). Forty-eight cases (92%) occurred after dental treatment. Only six patients (12%) had received the antibiotic treatment currently recommended by the American Heart Association. These data indicate that endocarditis prophylaxis failures may be more common than was previously believed, and most regimens used in patients with prophylaxis failure did not conform to current recommendations.

The American Heart Association's recommended prophylactic regimen (antibiotic premedication) for dental procedures is:

Penicillin V—2 g administered orally 30 minutes to 1 hour before the procedure, then 500 mg administered orally every 6 hours for 48 hours (8 doses)

For penicillin-allergic patients:
Erythromycin—1 g administered orally 1½ to 2 hours before the procedure, then 500 mg administered orally every 6 hours for 48 hours (8 doses)

For children under 60 pounds:
Penicillin V—1 g administered orally 30 minutes to 1 hour before the procedure, then 250 mg administered orally every 6 hours for 48 hours (8 doses)
Erythromycin—20 mg/kg administered orally 1½ to 2 hours before the procedure, then 10 mg/kg administered orally every 6 hours for 48 hours (8 doses)

Patients with a history of rheumatic fever without a residual organic heart murmur need not be premedicated. Patients classified as having "functional" heart murmurs or heart sounds not associated with structural defects do not need antibiotic protection. However, consulting the patient's physician for the exact nature of a cardiac condition is advisable. This can be accomplished by using a form of the medical release letter described later in this chapter.

Information gained through the comprehensive health history *aids in identifying the need for precautionary measures*. As mentioned in Chapter 3, disease transmission from patient to patient or patient to clinician can occur with some medical conditions. Hepatitis, venereal disease, and the common viral "cold" are examples. To prevent the transmission of such diseases the clinician is advised to wear a protective mask, gloves, and glasses; observe strict disinfection of the patient environment; and ensure proper sterilization of all instruments contacting the patient.

Undiagnosed conditions can also be detected as a result of the complete health history. A dental problem may be the one reason why a healthy person seeks any professional care over a period of years. A complete health history provides a unique opportunity to review the general health status of such a person. Perhaps, being unaware of its significance, the patient will discuss a symptom that could necessitate a medical consultation. Taking the blood pressure at each recall visit may reveal a jump in blood pressure levels or indicate a pattern worthy of medical advice. Additionally, taking the pulse and noting the ease and rate of respiration may help in assessing the patient's need to consult a physician. A discussion of vital signs, hypertension, and the role of the dental team in screening for these patients is contained in Chapter 9.

The health history *aids in diagnosis and treatment planning.* Questions related to dental status reveal the nature of the patient's chief complaint. For example, the patient may be aware of carious lesions in the posterior teeth but be most concerned about the appearance of a discolored front tooth. A patient may report sensitivity to hot or cold liquids in a particular area but be unable to locate the exact tooth that seems to be affected. Information such as this is helpful in guiding the dental team in performing diagnostic services (i.e., radiographs, vitality testing) and in directing care to satisfy patient concerns.

The overall physical and psychologic state of the patient can be assessed in general through the health history. The opportunity to talk candidly with the patient in discussing personal physical health allows the clinician to appreciate how the patient feels about himself/herself. Is the patient generally optimistic or pessimistic? Is the patient relaxed or anxious? The sensitive interviewer may be able to identify other significant tendencies. Is the patient cooperative or defensive? Compulsive or indifferent? In addition, the patient's ability and comfort in expressing himself/herself can be noted. Also, the patient's attitudes about dentistry are usually revealed during the interview. Evaluation of both the physical and psychologic factors will be helpful in providing individualized care.

Gathering the health history data is often the *first opportunity to establish professional interest*. Each patient desires to feel valued as an individual with special needs that the dental team will focus on. With an understanding of the patient's past and current health status and an appreciation of the patient's wants and needs, the dental care provider has guidelines on which to establish rapport and build a professional helping relationship. Within the framework of such a relationship, dental treatment issues become easier to address and trust in care increases.

Collecting detailed health information and updating the history at regular intervals provide a legal record as well as an important source of information about the patient when treatment is planned and delivered. The patient signs the health history to indicate that the information is accurate to the best of his/her knowledge. This record becomes an important reference when treating the patient over a period of time.

Occasionally, a patient may feel skeptical about the need for a comprehensive health history. Often this stems from feelings of privacy being invaded, defensiveness about medical problems, or a desire to simply get the dental visit over with as quickly as possible. Regardless of the reason for skepticism, it is important to dispel the patient's anxiety. The patient should be informed of the dental professional's responsibility to keep information confidential. The patient should be assured that the information she/he is asked for is necessary to provide safe treatment, and examples may be given of the way health information can affect dental treatment. One can agree that gathering information is time consuming, but it can be explained that this time means consideration for the patient's benefit. On occasion, some practitioners may choose not to provide elective treatment if the patient refuses to cooperate with the health history. Generally, most patients are agreeable and extremely helpful once the professional's sincere desire to provide the best possible care has been demonstrated.

COMMUNICATION: THE QUESTIONNAIRE/INTERVIEW

For gathering information, a questionnaire provides a thorough and timesaving tool for the professional. Fig. 8-1 is an example of one of the health questionnaires copyrighted by the American Dental Association. An interview provides a flexible and personal approach to obtaining and clarifying information. The combined questionnaire/interview technique is a practical and sensitive method for assessing the patient's health (Froelich and Bishop, 1977).

Although a lengthy interview or written health summary may not be necessary for every patient, the completed questionnaire should be closely examined prior to treatment. The patient may have missed an important question or misunderstood an item. Perhaps a medical condition was indicated that needs important follow-up information before dental care can begin. The following communication/interviewing principles will be helpful in conducting the review of the questionnaire with the patient.

The outcome of the comprehensive health history, using a questionnaire/interview technique, is determined to a great extent by the professional's ability to communicate. Conducting an interview demands a high level of communication skill. The interviewer must respond to both the attitudes and the behaviors of the patient. A good interviewer is nurturant, supportive, and helpful (Froelich and Bishop, 1977). It is not always easy for the patient to share highly private information about his/her personal or family history. The interviewer must listen and accept the patient's attitudes and perceptions without judging. As the interviewer responds to the patient by listening and clarifying statements, the patient begins to have a feeling that his/her problem is well understood. At this point, information may be shared with the patient to allay fears or anxiety related to his/her condition. In this way, the good interviewer may be able to convey to the patient a conceptual model by which the patient can better understand his/her illness, problem, or disease (Froelich and Bishop, 1977). When acquiring the comprehensive health history using a questionnaire/interview format, the health professional not only gathers information and builds rapport, but creates the environment and opportunity to educate and counsel the patient.

HEALTH QUESTIONNAIRE

Date _____

Name _____   Address _____
    Last   First   Middle   Number & Street

City   State   Zip Code   Home & Business Phone

Date of Birth _____ Sex _____ Height _____ Weight _____ Occupation _____

Married   Spouse _____   Single _____

Closest Relative _____   Phone _____

If you are completing this form for another person, what is your relationship to that person?

_____

In the following questions, circle yes or no, whichever applies. Your answers are for our records only and will be considered confidential.

1. Has there been any change in your general health within the past year .... YES   NO

2. My last physical examination was on _____

3. Are you now under the care of a physician... YES   NO
   a. If so, what is the condition being treated _____

4. The name and address of my physician is _____
   _____
   _____

5. Have you had any serious illness or operation .... YES   NO
   a. If so, what was the illness or operation _____

6. Have you been hospitalized or had a serious illness within the past five (5) years .... YES   NO
   a. If so, what was the problem _____

7. Do you have or have you had any of the following diseases or problems.
   a. Rheumatic fever or rheumatic heart disease.. YES   NO
   b. Congenital heart lesions.. YES   NO
   c. Cardiovascular disease (heart trouble, heart attack, coronary insufficiency, coronary occlusion,
      high blood pressure, arteriosclerosis, stroke).. YES   NO
      1) Do you have pain in chest upon exertion... YES   NO
      2) Are you ever short of breath after mild exercise...................................... YES   NO
      3) Do your ankles swell... YES   NO
      4) Do you get short of breath when you lie down, or do you require extra pillows when you sleep... YES   NO
   d. Allergy... YES   NO
   e. Sinus trouble.. YES   NO
   f. Asthma or hay fever.. YES   NO
   g. Hives or a skin rash .... YES   NO
   h. Fainting spells or seizures... YES   NO
   i. Diabetes... YES   NO
      1) Do you have to urinate (pass water) more than six times a day .... YES   NO
      2) Are you thirsty much of the time .... YES   NO
      3) Does your mouth frequently become dry .... YES   NO
   j. Hepatitis, jaundice or liver disease .... YES   NO
   k. Arthritis.. YES   NO
   l. Inflammatory rheumatism (painful swollen joints).. YES   NO
   m. Stomach ulcers .... YES   NO
   n. Kidney trouble .... YES   NO
   o. Tuberculosis .... YES   NO
   p. Do you have a persistent cough or cough up blood....................................... YES   NO
   q. Low blood pressure... YES   NO
   r. Venereal disease .... YES   NO
   s. Other _____

(over)

Fig. 8-1. American Dental Association health questionnaire. (Copyright by the American Dental Association. Reprinted by permission.)

8. Have you had abnormal bleeding associated with previous extractions, surgery, or trauma .... YES   NO
    a. Do you bruise easily .... YES   NO
    b. Have you ever required a blood transfusion.. YES   NO
       If so, explain the circumstances _____

9. Do you have any blood disorder such as anemia... YES   NO
10. Have you had surgery or x-ray treatment for a tumor, growth, or other condition of your mouth or lips .. YES   NO
11. Are you taking any drug or medicine.. YES   NO
    If so, what _____

12. Are you taking any of the following:
    a. Antibiotics or sulfa drugs...
    b. Anticoagulants (blood thinners)... YES   NO
    c. Medicine for high blood pressure.. YES   NO
    d. Cortisone (steroids).. YES   NO
    e. Tranquilizers... YES   NO
    f. Antihistamines .... YES   NO
    g. Aspirin.. YES   NO
    h. Insulin, tolbutamide (Orinase) or similar drug... YES   NO
    i. Digitalis or drugs for heart trouble .... YES   NO
    j. Nitroglycerin... YES   NO
    k. Other _____

13. Are you allergic or have you reacted adversely to:
    a. Local anesthetics..
    b. Penicillin or other antibiotics .... YES   NO
    c. Sulfa drugs... YES   NO
    d. Barbiturates, sedatives, or sleeping pills .... YES   NO
    e. Aspirin... YES   NO
    f. Iodine .... YES   NO
    g. Codeine or other narcotics... YES   NO
    h. Other _____

14. Have you had any serious trouble associated with any previous dental treatment .... YES   NO
    If so, explain _____

15. Do you have any disease, condition, or problem not listed above that you think I should know about... YES   NO
    If so, explain_____

16. Are you employed in any situation which exposes you regularly to x-rays or other ionizing radiation... YES   NO
17. Are you wearing contact lenses.. YES   NO

WOMEN

18. Are you pregnant .... YES   NO
19. Do you have any problems associated with your menstrual period............................... YES   NO

Remarks:

                 SIGNATURE OF PATIENT _____

                 SIGNATURE OF DENTIST _____

P1-HQ

Fig. 8-1, cont'd. American Dental Association health questionnaire.

Interviewing skills

Awareness of and sensitivity to the kinds of messages communicated are important to counseling and interviewing.

Communication involves words, facial expressions, gestures, body movements, tone of voice, rate of speech, and silence. The interviewer must become an active listener. This occurs through the interviewer's being aware of the patient's total communication effort and being able to respond in a way that the patient will interpret as attentive and concerned (Froelich and Bishop, 1977).

Body communication signifies to the patient that the interviewer is listening. The interviewer should find a comfortable and relaxed position for herself/ himself. The interviewer and patient should be at approximately the same eye level. Eye contact should be made with the patient when he/she is talking. Affirmative head nods also are used to indicate listening. Facial expressions should agree with the feelings being expressed by the patient.

The verbal communication and attitude of the interviewer can strongly influence the atmosphere of the interview. The following are techniques for verbal communication. Use a vocal tone that reassures the patient. Help the patient develop and pursue the topic using affirmative words to indicate understanding. Do not interrupt the patient if possible. Fit comments into the context of the topic. Use silence to aid the interview communication. For most inexperienced interviewers, silence is uncomfortable. Often, a question is hastily asked and may not be helpful. Interviewer-initiated silence can be used to communicate the desire for the patient to continue to provide information or to choose the topic. Silence allows the patient time to think about the response to the questions. Silence can be supportive and signify interest. Patient-initiated silence may mean that the patient needs time to think, is examining himself/herself, or wishes to avoid the topic. Each function of silence is important to the communication effort.

Interviewing suggestions (Froelich and Bishop, 1977)

1. Introduce yourself. Ask a direct, open question, such as "What situation brings you here today?"
2. Have a plan or order for obtaining information.
3. Guide the interview; do not dominate it.
4. Respond by showing support and empathy.
5. Restate or reflect a patient's response to clarify meaning.
6. Avoid questions that can be answered "Yes" or "No." Such questions permit the patient to avoid discussing a topic, or allow the patient to give a response he/she thinks the interviewer is looking for. An appropriately phrased question is "When does this pain bother you?" versus "Does it hurt when you eat something cold?"
7. Avoid antagonistic "why" questions that make the patient account for his/her behavior, such as "Why didn't you seek care sooner?"
8. Direct the patient to information closely related with current thoughts. Do not jump from one topic to another.
9. Use verbal and nonverbal signals to encourage the patient to say more.
10. Complete the interview with a summary to clarify what has occurred and affirm mutual understanding.

COMPONENTS OF THE COMPREHENSIVE HEALTH HISTORY

Three areas of information are explored in the comprehensive health history: the patient profile, the patient's current health status, and the patient's historical health data.

The *patient profile* includes the patient's name, address, telephone number, date of birth, and physician's name and office telephone number. Each practitioner may develop his/her own version of the patient profile section of the chart. Items that may be included are the patient's occupation, business telephone number, marital status, number of children, and dental insurance or preferred billing plan; the name of the person who referred the patient; and weekdays/times preferred for appointments. The patient completes this information on the questionnaire. The interviewer should be familiar with this basic information before greeting the patient. Follow-up on this information is usually indicated only when a response needs clarification.

The patient's *current health status* and *historical health data* require more attention. The interviewer should take a few minutes to review the patient's questionnaire responses and note the questions to

Comprehensive health history

Patient profile

NAME: Ms. Sample Case
ADDRESS: R.R. 10, Paradise, Pa.
TELEPHONE: 222-1234
OCCUPATION: Supermarket cashier and homemaker

PHYSICIAN: Dr. John D. Smith
PHYSICIAN TELEPHONE: 222-5678
REFERRAL: Neighbor, Ms. Mary Jones
DATE: May 1, 1984

Current status

CC: Patient is a 58-year-old woman who has come for treatment because of "bleeding gums for the past 3 months."

HPI: During the past 3 months patient noticed she expectorated blood each time she brushed her teeth. The bleeding would stop within 1 minute. Within the past 2 weeks her gingivae bled spontaneously 2 or 3 times.

MEDS: **Allergic to penicillin.** Reaction: immediate generalized body rash, and "My throat closed off."

1. Digoxin, 0.25 mg daily, for congestive heart failure
2. Hydrochlorothiazide (Hydrodiuril), 50 mg two times a day, for congestive heart failure
3. Chlordiazepoxide (Librium), 10 mg one to two times a week when she feels "nervous or upset"
4. Takes vitamin C and vitamin B_{12} supplement daily
5. Prefers acetaminophen (Tylenol) for headache, one to two times a week
6. Smokes cigarettes: one-half pack a day
7. Averages one to two alcoholic drinks a week

ROS:

Gen: Denies recent weight gain or loss, weakness, fever, insomnia, or change in general health
HEENT: Denies headache, dizziness, disturbance in vision, tinnitus, vertigo, nasal obstruction, difficulty in swallowing
Resp: Denies coughing blood or sputum; reports difficulty in breathing when walking one flight of stairs
CV: Reports difficulty in breathing when walking one flight of stairs and when lying flat; uses two pillows for sleeping at night; denies murmur
GI: Denies food intolerance, abdominal pain, change in bowel habits
GU: Denies pain or blood when passing urine, has nocturia due to diuretic (1 time); current menopause transition; experiences labile emotions; reports "hot flashes"
MBJ: Denies limitation of movement, back problems; reports "seasonal" stiffness and swelling of finger joints
CNS: Denies fainting, seizure, loss of feeling, stroke
Endo: Denies weakness, change in appetite, change in weight; reports occasional heat intolerance due to menopause
Hemo: Denies tendency to bruise or bleed, no recent blood transfusion or radiation exposure

Historical data

PMH: Patient denies history of rheumatic fever, diabetes, hepatitis, glaucoma, VD, TB, or bleeding disorders, Generally healthy childhood: measles, mumps, and chickenpox with no residual effects, all before age 10. Broken leg in car accident 1952. Hospitalized for normal childbirth, University of Pennsylvania, 1943, 1946, 1948. Myocardial infarction 3 years ago (see physician's letter); hospitalized for 3 weeks. Takes digoxin and Hydrodiuril for congestive heart failure. Sees physician every 3 months. Patient allergic to penicillin. Reports reaction of total body rash and swelling of mucosa after injection 10 years ago. Tolerates erythromycin well.

FH: Father: died age 74, myocardial infarction after history of hypertension 15 years. Mother: died age 79, cerebral vascular accident. Two brothers alive and well. Three children alive and well. Denies family history of diabetes, cancer, mental illness.

PDH: Had several restorations placed in childhood by private dentist; for past 30 years has been treated sporadically by several dental clinics, mostly for toothache or extraction. Tolerates local anesthesia well; brushes teeth one time a day; does not use floss or other home care aid; satisfied with dental care in past.

which an affirmative response has been indicated. These areas need specific follow-up during the patient interview. The following format with the accompanying descriptions is designed as a guide for directing the interview and organizing patient data.

Current health status

Chief complaint (CC). This usually is stated in the patient's own words and refers to the symptoms for which the patient is seeking treatment.

History of present illness (HPI). Signs and symptoms of the current problem should be described in this section, along with the location, onset, intensity, and duration of the problem. Additional probing questions may be in order to define and clarify the nature of the patient's needs, such as "When did this problem *first* occur?" "Describe the discomfort for me." "When does it bother you the most?"

Medications (Meds). It is important to note clearly the medications that the patient is currently taking. This includes over-the-counter remedies or preparations such as vitamins, aspirin, and weight control pills in addition to prescribed medications. State the reason for the medication and the dosage in which it is taken. The *Physicians' Desk Reference* (described later in the chapter) gives additional information. Note medication allergy or intolerance IN BOLD LETTERS. Inquiring into the patient's social habits, such as frequency of consumption of alcoholic beverages and coffee and tobacco use is appropriate at this time.

Review of systems (ROS). This allows information from the questionnaire and interview to be organized into physical systems. At this point, the professional is interested in the current (within 6 months) status of each system. The past medical/dental history will be summarized later.

Following are the signs and symptoms related to each system. The patient should be asked if he/she is bothered by any of these.

General constitution (Gen). Includes recent significant weight gain or loss, weakness, fatigue, fever, chills, insomnia, irritability, and change in general vigor.
If the patient has experienced any of these signs and symptoms, additional probing follow-up questions should be asked. The interviewer should summarize the patient's response. It is advisable to repeat the summary so that the patient can verify its content.

Otherwise, the interviewer may record "Patient denies" the specific symptoms.

Head, ears, eyes, nose, and throat (HEENT). Includes reports of headache, trauma, dizziness, disturbance of vision, loss of hearing acuity, ringing in ears, loss of balance, disturbances of smell, discharge, symptoms of obstruction, hoarseness, and difficulty in swallowing.

Respiratory (Resp). Includes difficulty in breathing, chest pain, coughing blood or sputum, wheezing, and effect of exercise.

Cardiovascular (CV). Includes chest pain, palpitation, difficulty in breathing when lying flat, murmurs, and blood pressure.

Gastrointestinal (GI). Includes abdominal pain, nausea, vomiting, indigestion, food intolerance, hernia, and change in bowel habits.

Genitourinary (GU). Includes painful urination, blood in urine, frequency of urination, flank pain, and change in menstrual cycle.

Muscles, bones, and joints (MBJ). Includes pain, stiffness, swelling, limitation of movement, arthritis, and back problem.

Central nervous system (CNS). Includes fainting, seizure, stroke, paralysis, spasm, tremor, and loss of feeling.

Endocrine (Endo). Includes change in growth or development, thyroid function, change in appetite or tolerance to temperature, diabetes, and excessive urination, thirst, or hunger.

Hemopoietic (Hemo). Includes tendency to bruise or bleed excessively after injury, recent blood transfusion, and exposure to radiation.

Medical/dental history

Past medical history (PMH). Summarize the medical status previous to current history. Include general health and vigor, childhood diseases, past infectious diseases, chronic diseases, injuries, accidents, hospitalizations (include name of hospital and dates), history of immunizations, allergies and type of allergic reactions, and service-related disability.

Family history (FH). Summarize data regarding the state of immediate family members, past hereditary diseases, and the presence of infectious or chronic disease in the family.

Past dental history (PDH). Summarize the nature of dental care the patient has had in the past. Include type of clinic, treatment by specialist, experience with local and general anesthetics, degree of preventive education, and satisfaction with past treatment.

MEDICALLY COMPROMISED PATIENTS

The following section provides the dental hygienist with information regarding common medical conditions that should be identified by the health history. A basic definition of the problem is presented, along with common signs or symptoms the patient may report. In some cases examples of medications the patient may be taking are given by generic name. The significance of the disease is presented followed by precautions recommended for dental treatment.

Heart disorders

Rheumatic heart disease. Rheumatic heart disease results from rheumatic fever and causes rigidity or deformity of the heart valves.

Patient reports: History of rheumatic fever or heart murmur. Patient may be taking antibiotics (e.g., penicillin) on a regular basis.
Significance: Patient is susceptible to subacute bacterial endocarditis.
Precautions:
1. Obtain consultation letter from physician concerning nature of heart involvement.
2. Antibiotic premedication necessary (Kaye, 1977; "Reports of Councils," 1977).
3. Be sure patient has taken antibiotic as prescribed before dental treatment.
4. Avoid unnecessary trauma to tissues during instrumentation.

Congenital heart defect. This term refers to structural defects of the heart (e.g., a hole in the common wall between heart chambers) that is present at birth.

Patient reports: History of heart murmur, "hole in heart," or other heart abnormality, corrective heart surgery, or valve replacement.
Significance: Patient is susceptible to subacute bacterial endocarditis.
Precautions:
1. Obtain letter from physician as to nature of defect and correction.
2. Antibiotic premedication may be necessary (Kaye, 1977; "Reports of Councils," 1977).

Surgical valve replacement. A diseased heart valve due to rheumatic heart disease or congenital heart defect is replaced with an artificial prosthesis.

Patient reports: History of heart surgery; may be taking anticoagulant.
Significance: Patient is susceptible to subacute bacterial endocarditis.
Precautions:
1. Obtain letter from physician as to heart status and surgical correction.
2. Antibiotic premedication necessary (Kaye, 1977; "Reports of Councils," 1977).
3. Patient may be taking anticoagulant (e.g., warfarin or coumarin). Consult physician. Test for bleeding time may be necessary before treatment, or patient may be advised to stop medication for a few days before appointment.

Coronary artery disease. Coronary circulation is inadequate for metabolic demands of the heart; this disease is secondary to hardening of arteries (arteriosclerosis) which causes blockage or narrowing of vessels.

Patient reports: Episodes of substernal pain (angina pectoris), typically radiating to left arm and jaw. Pain is precipitated by activity and anxiety and is relieved by rest and certain medications. Patient may be taking vasodilators, nitroglycerin, or propranolol.
Significance: Patient may have angina attack in dental office.
Precautions:
1. Obtain letter from physician to clarify medical status.
2. Have patient's vasodilator medication accessible.
3. Use local anesthetic without vasoconstrictor, or keep vasoconstrictor use to minimum (less than 0.04 mg vasoconstrictor (Bennett, 1984).
4. Keep appointments to reasonable length, avoiding unnecessary stress and anxiety.

Coronary thrombosis (myocardial infarction). The blood supply through the coronary arteries is insufficient to meet the metabolic demands of the heart; this differs from angina pectoris in that damage is irreversible (i.e., a portion of the heart muscle dies).

Patient reports: History of angina pectoris, previous heart attack, taking vasodilators.
Significance: Patient may have angina attack or myocardial infarction.
Precautions:
1. Obtain letter from physician as to severity of disease.
2. Do not treat patient if heart attack occurred within 6 months.
3. Have vasodilator medication ready.

4. Avoid vasoconstrictors in local anesthetic or keep to minimum.
5. Keep appointments short.
6. Be prepared to resuscitate patient; should cardiac arrest occur, call emergency rescue team.

Congestive heart failure. Blood backs up behind a failing chamber, causing congestion of circulation and pooling of blood in organs. For example, if the left ventricle fails, blood backs up in the pulmonary circulation and lungs. Forward flow from the failing chamber is also diminished.

Patient reports: Shortness of breath, swollen ankles, sleeping on two or more pillows; may be taking diuretics and/or digitalis.
Significance: Patient may have difficulty in breathing when supine in dental chair. If inhalation anesthetics are used, oxygenation of blood may be poor because of fluid in lungs.
Precautions:
1. Obtain letter from physician concerning severity of disease.
2. Keep patient in semiupright position.
3. Keep appointments short.
4. Possible need for supplemental oxygen.

Cardiac arrhythmias. This is a disturbance of the heart's electrical conduction system. The heart beats at too rapid or too slow a pace or at an irregular pace (either continuously or with occasional odd beats).

Patient reports: Fast or irregular heartbeat, palpitations (awareness of rapid heart beats), recurrent fainting, surgical implant of pacemaker; may be taking digitalis or other antiarrhythmic medication.
Significance: Patient may faint, a pacemaker device may be affected by electromagnetic interference (EMI). Dental office equipment such as ultrasonic scaling devices, pulp testers, electrodesensitizing equipment, electrosurgical instruments, and motorized dental chairs may adversely affect some devices.
Precautions:
1. Obtain letter from physician concerning severity of disease and/or surgical history. Inquire as to need for antibiotic premedication and type of pacemaker device implanted.
2. Avoid use of ultrasonic equipment or proximity to such equipment being used on other patients if pacemaker will be affected.

Hypertension

Hypertension is high arterial blood pressure (see Chapter 9).

Patient reports: History of elevated blood pressure, frequent dizziness, headaches, nosebleeds; may be taking antihypertensives or diuretics.
Significance: Patient may have a "stroke" (cerebrovascular accident). Disease can cause cardiac enlargement, impaired kidney function, and accelerate arteriosclerosis.
Precautions:
1. Take blood pressure at each appointment.
2. Obtain letter from physician if diastolic reading exceeds 95 mm Hg or systolic exceeds 160 mm Hg.
3. Do not provide dental treatment if diastolic blood pressure is greater than 115 mm Hg, or systolic blood pressure is greater than 160 mm Hg.
4. Determine if antihypertensive medication has been taken as prescribed.
5. Use local anesthetic without vasoconstrictor, or do not exceed 0.1 mg epinephrine (Bennett, 1984).
6. Avoid sitting patient up rapidly. This may cause fainting (orthostatic or postural hypotension), an effect of some antihypertensives.
7. Have patient remain sitting upright for several minutes before leaving the dental chair.

Diabetes mellitus (Zach, 1976)

Diabetes mellitus is a disorder of glucose intolerance manifested by hyperglycemia (increased blood glucose). In general, there are two types of diabetes mellitus. Insulin-dependent (type 1) diabetes has its onset in young people. Hyperglycemia is due to a lack of insulin normally produced by the pancreas. Adult-onset (type 2) diabetes occurs in older patients and is often associated with obesity. Although the amount of insulin produced by the pancreas is adequate, this type of diabetes is characterized by insulin insensitivity of the tissues.

Patient reports: Personal or family history of disease; excessive thirst, hunger, urination; high birth weight children; may be taking injectable insulin or oral hypoglycemics.
Significance: Patient has low resistance to infection; is prone to periodontal disease and poor healing; may have episode of insulin shock, especially if meal was missed prior to appointment.
Precautions:
1. Determine if disease is under control (frequency of urine testing, medication taken as prescribed, recent incidents of diabetic coma, insulin shock, or diabetes-related hospitalizations). Obtain letter

from physician to determine status of other diabetes-related conditions. Patient with severe diabetes may have compromised vascular system, renal impairment, or loss of vision.

2. Determine if patient has eaten. Schedule appointments around eating schedule.
3. Have sugar source available in case of impending shock, which patient can usually anticipate.

Epilepsy (Braham, 1977)

Epilepsy is a disorder characterized by convulsions (seizures) or disturbances of consciousness (e.g., momentary inattentive staring), usually associated with a disturbance of electrical activity of the brain.

Patient reports: History of seizures. Examples: petit mal (trancelike state, fixed posture, blinking); grand mal (twitching, seizing, loss of consciousness, incontinence). Patient may report a peculiar sensation, which heralds a seizure (aura), such as a specific odor or visual sensation; may be taking phenobarbital, phenytoin, or other anticonvulsant.
Significance: Patient may have a seizure. Phenytoin (Dilantin) may cause gingival hyperplasia or orofacial changes (Angelopoulous, 1975; Israel, 1974).
Precautions:
1. Determine if anticonvulsant medication has been taken.
2. Make appointments when patient is rested; keep them short.
3. If seizure occurs, do not try to restrict patient. Remove equipment from striking distance, and keep patient from injuring himself/herself. Keep airway open after the seizure when saliva, blood (from biting tongue), and/or dental materials may block airway, requiring suction or manual removal.

Allergies

Allergies are localized or systemic reactions caused by a variety of substances (allergens). The reaction may be mild, causing itching or a rash. A severe reaction may cause a rapid fall in blood pressure, airway obstruction from swelling of oral mucosa, and/or cardiac arrest (anaphylaxis).

Patient reports: Reaction to a known substance (e.g., penicillin).
Significance: Reaction may occur to substances used in dental treatment.
Precautions:
1. Determine exact cause and severity of previous reaction.
2. Avoid allergen or related substance.

3. Caution using anesthetics and antibiotics.
4. If patient is unsure of specific anesthetic agent that caused previous allergic reaction, request physician to perform skin patch test. (See Chapter 32 on local anesthesia.)
5. If anaphylaxis should occur, be prepared to support patient with cardiopulmonary resuscitation and to call emergency rescue team.

Kidney disease

In patients with kidney disease there is impairment of renal function with accumulation of waste products and fluid, resulting from congenital abnormalities, infection, diabetes, and other disease processes. The patient may be maintained on hemodialysis (an artificial kidney machine) or have a kidney transplant.

Patient reports: History of renal failure, hemodialysis, headache, swelling of extremities, fever, flank pain, nausea, mental dullness, excessive fatigue, easy bruising; or if kidney transplant, will be taking immunosuppressant medication.
Significance: Patient is prone to infection, poor healing, bleeds easily. Medications metabolized by kidney (e.g., local anesthetics of amide type) will remain in circulation longer.
Precautions:
1. Obtain letter from physician regarding extent of disease. If patient is immunosuppressed, obtain recommendations for precautions during dental treatment. These patients are susceptible to bacterial endocarditis at site of hemodialysis shunt or transplanted kidney graft, making prophylactic antibiotic coverage necessary.
2. If medication is to be administered, check with physician, *Physicians' Desk Reference*, or pharmacologist regarding renal metabolism.
3. Exercise care in instrumentation.

Infectious or contagious diseases

Hepatitis.* Hepatitis is an inflammation of the liver caused by several different viruses (see Chapter 3).

Patient reports: Past history of disease, fatigue, loss of appetite, nausea, fever, dark urine, tender liver, sore joints. Patient may appear jaundiced (yellow).
Significance: Patient may bleed excessively; may have impaired metabolism of drugs broken down in liver (e.g., local anesthetics of the ester type); excellent

---

*Hepatitis may be used as a model for other types of liver dysfunction (e.g., cirrhosis).

possibility for transfer of disease to dental professional or other patients.

Precautions:

1. Do not treat patient with active disease.
2. Wear gloves, face mask, and glasses; maintain strict sterilization and asepsis of all objects in contact with patient.
3. If medication is administered, consult physician, *Physicians' Desk Reference,* or pharmacologist regarding possible liver metabolism.
4. Determine status of office personnel for hepatitis B markers, (hepatitis B antibody or hepatitis B surface antigen).

Tuberculosis. Tuberculosis most commonly affects the lungs; it is caused by the organism *Mycobacterium tuberculosis.*

Patient reports: History of disease, positive TB test, fever, weight loss, night sweats, cough, blood in sputum, tender lymph nodes; may be taking streptomycin, ethambutol, isoniazid, or other antituberculosis medication.

Significance: Patient may transmit disease to others. Documented TB patients are generally followed yearly for a sputum culture and chest x-ray examination. If medical clearance is given for patient being noncontagious, no special precautions are required for treatment.

Precautions:

1. Obtain letter from physician determining if disease is active. Additional TB tests may be necessary.
2. Wear gloves, face mask, and glasses; maintain strict sterilization and asepsis of all objects in contact with patient.

Venereal disease. Venereal disease is an acute or chronic infectious disease such as syphilis or gonorrhea, typically acquired through sexual intercourse or other close physical contact.

Patient reports: Past history of disease, painful urination, urethral or vaginal discharge, sore throat, skin eruptions, painless ulcer with firm rolled edges involving oropharyngeal mucosa or genitalia (chancre), mucous patch in oral cavity (gumma).

Significance: Patient may transmit disease to others.

Precautions:

1. Wear gloves, face mask, and glasses; maintain strict sterilization and asepsis of all objects in contact with patient.

Blood diseases

Anemia. Anemia is a deficiency of red blood cells (erythrocytes) in the circulating blood. Anemia may result from a vitamin or iron deficiency, bone marrow problems, excessive loss of blood, or red cell destruction.

Patient reports: Fatigue, weakness; appears pale; may be taking iron and vitamin supplements.

Significance: Lowered resistance to infection; possibly delayed healing.

Precautions:

1. Exercise care in instrumentation.
2. Advise patient to consult physician for further investigation of problem.

Leukemia. In the patient with leukemia, there is an excessive number of white blood cells (leukocytes), which do not function normally; this disease is a type of blood cancer. Cells may overpopulate bone marrow and crowd out normal blood cells and other components such as red blood cells and platelets.

Patient reports: History of disease, fatigue and fever; bruises easily; may be taking medications directed at controlling proliferation of these abnormal leukocytes (chemotherapeutic agents).

Significance: Patient is extremely prone to infection; may have lesions of oral mucosa, xerostomia, more acidic saliva, and aggravated periodontal conditions as a result of chemotherapy. These conditions necessitate modifications in oral hygiene. Excessive bleeding due to bone marrow depression and decreased platelets may effect healing time. Consultation prior to periodontal treatment or extractions is indicated.

Precautions: Obtain letter from physician regarding disease status and recommended procedures for dental intervention.

Hemorrhagic disorders (hemophilia, other) (Grossman, 1975). Hemophilia is a hereditary disorder characterized by excessive bleeding due to lack or deficiency of a coagulation factor. Types include classical hemophilia, (factor VIII, hemophilia A), Christmas disease (factor IX, hemophilia B), and Von Willebrand's disease. Other hemorrhagic disorders include (1) clotting factor deficiency (vitamin K deficiency, for example, can cause depression in certain clotting factors, as do certain drugs such as warfarin and heparin) and (2) platelet dysfunction (platelets are crucial to clotting; aspirin and certain drugs, including dipyridamole, interfere with platelet aggregation).

Patient reports: Family history of hemophilia, spontaneous or excessive bleeding, tendency to bruise easily.

Significance: Failure of blood to clot, danger of patient aspirating blood or even bleeding to death if bleeding is not arrested; medical measures necessary when large quantity of blood is lost. Patient may have received blood plasma factor replacement therapy and may carry hepatitis B antigen or have history of hepatitis (Evans, 1977).

Precautions:
1. Obtain letter from physician concerning severity of disease, possible need for medication prior to treatment (e.g., transfusion of deficient factor).
2. Limit treatment to a specific area per appointment. If factor replacement therapy has been necessary prior to dental treatment, allow sufficient time for procedure to be completed in one visit/day to reduce risks and expense of multiple transfusions (Evans, 1977).
3. Do not prescribe aspirin or aspirin-related products for pain control. Substitute acetaminophen, codeine, propoxyphene hydrochloride, or other analgesic.
4. Wear gloves, face mask, and glasses; maintain strict sterilization because of hepatitis risk.

MEDICAL CLASSIFICATION

A medical classification system, as described in Table 8-1, is useful for identifying a patient's medical status. A standardized system of marking the medical classification in bold numbers on the chart provides a simple mechanism for conveying information quickly while preserving patient privacy.

UPDATING THE RECORD

A person's health is dynamic. Performing the comprehensive health history and classifying the medical status at the initial visit are only the first steps in providing safe treatment for the patient. Reviewing the chart at every visit is imperative. Should an emergency arise, precious time can be lost fumbling for information regarding medical problems or medications that would have been noted by a minute's review of the health history prior to beginning the day's treatment. Updating the chart at recall intervals is recommended. The dental professional should make a sincere inquiry about the patient's general health at every dental visit and note additional information.

Following are appropriate questions to ask the patient for updating the health history:
1. How has your health been lately?
2. What medications are you currently taking?
3. Have you been hospitalized for any reason since your last visit?

Table 8-1. Sample format for medical classification system

Classifi-cation	Description
1	*Minimal risk.* Patient in good health and all dental procedures may be carried out with no special precautions.
2	*Some precautions must be observed in treating this patient* (e.g., patients with drug allergies, rheumatic heart disease without decompensation, controlled diabetes, or controlled hypertension).
3	*Deferred classification.* Reserved for patients with questionable health status but who have given insufficient information regarding their ailment, abnormality, or treatment status. Consultation with local physician is usually required (e.g., patients taking unknown medications, patients with possible blood dyscrasias or with heart murmurs of unknown nature, and patients taking anticoagulants).
4	*Unable to withstand prolonged, difficult, or stressful dental procedures because of overall health status.* Ascertainment of degree of decompensation must be made on an individual basis.
5	*Should be hospitalized for treatment or referred for care by more qualified health care providers.* Experienced health care providers should exercise high-level precautions during treatment, preferably under hospital conditions (e.g., patients with uncontrolled hypertension, uncontrolled diabetes, severe congestive heart failure, or hemophilia).

4. How has your (name specific medical condition) been since the last appointment?
5. How did you get along with the dentistry we did last time?

These questions are direct, but open, to allow the patient to respond with as much information as possible.

The dental professional should take the blood pressure for the day and compare it to previous entries. The health history form should have a specific update summary area, since important information can be easily missed when one is looking through a long series of treatment notes.

THE MEDICAL RELEASE LETTER

A medical release form is used for the patient to give consent for health professionals to exchange otherwise confidential information. This is neces-

```
Dentist_____     Patient_____

Address_____     Address_____

Phone_____     Phone_____




REQUEST  Date_____

Dear Dr._____,


The patient named above was recently seen in our office as a new patient.
Before dental therapy is initiated, I would appreciate information
regarding the patient's health status in the following areas.  Thank you.




                                 _____

I,_____, hereby consent to the release of my medical/
dental records to the office of_____.

                                      (Patient signature)

REPLY  Date_____




                                      (Consultant signature)
```

Fig. 8-2. Sample medical release letter.

sary in acquiring pertinent medical details that the patient may be unable to provide regarding illness or medication. This is also useful in obtaining dental-related information when a patient transfers from one office or clinic to another.

A standard three–carbon copy format is practical (Fig. 8-2). A form such as this saves the staff from having to write individual letters. It allows the office to retain an original copy and the physician and/or dentist to mail back the reply copy and keep a copy for his/her own records.

PHYSICIANS' DESK REFERENCE

The *Physicians' Desk Reference (PDR)* is published annually and is used as a reference by health professionals when seeking information about medications. The *PDR* is used to check such information as drug dosage, composition, contraindications, and the interactions of one drug with another. Today, with the huge number of medications available, a drug dictionary of this nature is essential for providing information about current and newly released medicaments.

It is important for dental professionals to use the *PDR* to investigate medications being taken by their patients. In this way the dental professional will be familiar with the reason the patient is taking the medication and will be aware of possible contraindications or interactions between medication and dental treatment. For example, warfarin (Coumadin) is a blood anticoagulant, often prescribed for patients with phlebitis. Before a scaling procedure is performed, a consultation with the patient's physician may be necessary to change the patient's dosage to prevent prolonged bleeding during treatment.

Acetyl sulfisoxazole (Gantrisin) is an antibiotic used for the treatment of urinary tract infections. Procaine, once used as a primary dental local anesthetic, and sulfonamides (such as Gantrisin) are chemically related. Taken together, an antagonistic response occurs, rendering both medications ineffective.

Pharmacologic terms to be familiar with include *brand name*, *generic name*, and *drug classification*.

Brand name is the name given to a particular medication or product by its manufacturer. Many manufacturers make the same product but market it under their own brand name. *Generic name* is the chemical name of the product. The use of generic names is advised because these always remain the same, give more chemical information, and do not limit prescription to one commercial preparation.

Example: The product propoxyphene hydrochloride (generic name) is made by six manufacturers and marketed with these brand names: Darvon, Propoxyphene Compound 65 capsules, Propoxyphene Hydrochloride capsules, SK-65 capsules, Unigesic-A, Wygesic tablets.

Drug classification refers to the broad category to define drugs sharing similar actions.

Examples: Analgesics—products that alleviate pain
  Diuretics—products that promote urination
  Sedatives—products that induce a quiet, calm state

The *PDR* consists of cross-referenced indices of products arranged alphabetically by manufacturer, brand name, generic name, and drug classification. If a sample medication is available, a picture identification section is included. The largest portion of the book is the product information section. Each product is described as to its chemical composition, the form in which it is supplied, its action and suggested use, administration, recommended dosage, contraindications, precautions, and side effects. Other sections include information on diagnostic products and management of drug overdose. Between the yearly publication dates, quarterly supplements are issued to update product information or describe new products.

Procedure for using the *PDR*

Obtain as much information from the patient as possible. Perhaps the patient has brought the medication. Read the prescription; look at the product. Ask the following questions:

1. For what condition are you taking this medication?
2. How often do you take it?
3. How long ago was it prescribed for you?
4. Do you take the medication exactly as prescribed?
5. When did you last take the medication?
6. Besides the manner in which this medication helps you specifically, does it alter the way you feel in general?

Generally, patients are aware of the name and

nature of the medication and the prescribed regimen for administration. Knowing the dosage is not as common; follow-up by checking the prescription or the *PDR*.

Inquire whether the patient is taking the medication as directed by his/her physician. One may discover that the patient is altering the dosage in some way. This often happens when the patient "feels good" regardless of the state of his/her illness. Patient noncompliance in taking medications is a common problem. In a professional manner, reinforce the prescribed routine, and suggest that the patient check with his/her physician for approval of the alteration. Explain that not taking a medication as prescribed alters the control of the medical condition, which may create a risk to the individual and may affect reactions during dental treatment.

Often medications have minor effects that patients cope with readily. For example, antihistamines can make people sleepy; antibiotics can cause nausea; asthma medications can make people agitated or tremulous. The conditions may or may not affect dental therapy, but the clinician's understanding of these states may help put the patient at ease, making treatment more comfortable.

Following these questions, note the name of the medication, the reason for its prescription, and the patient's dosage in the appropriate history or update section. Check the *PDR* for drug action and any complication that might affect dental treatment.

SUMMARY

This chapter has discussed one part of the dental appointment: obtaining a comprehensive health history. It has been an introduction to some areas where medicine and dentistry are interrelated. Other courses such as anatomy/physiology and oral medicine/pathology will enrich the student's understanding of normal conditions and specific diseases in relation to dental care. In conclusion, the important points are recognizing the need for a thorough review of health conditions prior to dental treatment and detailing the contents of such a review to identify medical conditions that may necessitate changes in dental care. In addition, the history-taking experience provides an opportunity for the clinician and patient to interact in a way that can be the foundation of the professional relationship.

ACKNOWLEDGMENT

A special thanks to Donald C. Dafoe, M.D., for his critique and review of the information presented in this chapter.

ACTIVITIES

1. Provide sample health history information for small groups to discuss. Practice completing the patient write-up using this information.
2. Role play the medical interview. Discuss communication skills and hygienist/patient interactions observed.
3. Practice using the *Physicians' Desk Reference* by identifying medications, contraindications, side effects, and so on.
4. Observe and critique health histories (interviews or written documentation) completed by students during their final year of clinical education. Discuss the observations in small groups.
5. Complete a comprehensive health history for a student partner. Preserve the complete data for use in treatment planning (discussed in Chapter 18). Students should note that recording such data also ensures safe practice of intraoral procedures for a student partner.

REVIEW QUESTIONS

1. Respond to this situation: Mrs. Jones is a new patient. Partway through the health history interview she states, "This is just wasting time, I want my teeth checked."
2. Which of the following conditions should be followed up by a physician's consultation and why?
   a. Rheumatic heart disease
   b. History of myocardial infarction
   c. Blood pressure reading of 160/100
   d. Hemophilia
   e. All of the above
3. List the medical conditions that *require* antibiotic premedication prior to dental treatment to prevent bacterial endocarditis.
4. List several communication principles that help ensure a thorough medical history and a helping relationship with the patient.
5. How is the *Physicians' Desk Reference* useful to the dental hygienist?

REFERENCES

ADA Council on Dental Therapeutics. 1982. Accepted dental therapeutics, ed. 39. Chicago: American Dental Association.

Angelopoulous, A.P. 1975. Diphenylhydantoin gingival hyperplasia: a clinicopathological review. J. Can. Dent. Assoc. **41**:103.

Baltch, A.L., et al. 1982. Bacteremia following dental cleaning in patients with and without penicillin prophylaxis. Am. Heart J. **104**:1335.

Bennett, C.R. 1984. Monheim's local anesthesia and pain control in dental practice, ed. 7. St. Louis: The C.V. Mosby Co.

Bodak-Gyovai, L.Z. 1978. Diagnostic center manual. Philadelphia: Department of Oral Medicine, University of Pennsylvania School of Dental Medicine.

Braham, L., editor. 1977. The dental implications of epilepsy: report to the Commission for the Control and its Consequences, by the ad-hoc committee of the Academy of Dentistry for the Handicapped. DHEW Pub. No. (ASA) 78-5217. Washington, D.C.: Department of Health, Education, and Welfare.

Durack, D.T., Kaplan, E.L., and Bisno, A.L. 1983. Apparent failure of endocarditis prophylaxis: analysis of 52 cases submitted to a national registry. JAMA 250:2318.

Evans, B.E. 1977. Dental care in hemophilia. New York: Cutter Laboratories and The National Hemophilia Foundation.

Froelich, R.E., and Bishop, F.M. 1977. Clinical interviewing skills: a programmed manual for data gathering, evaluation, and patient management, ed. 3. St. Louis: The C.V. Mosby Co.

Grossman, R. 1975. Orthodontics and dentistry for the hemophilic patient. Am. J. Orthod. 68:391.

Israel, H. 1974. Abnormalities of bone and orofacial changes from anticonvulsant drugs. J. Public Health Dent. 34:104.

Kaye, D. Nov. 1977. New guidelines for preventing endocarditis. Drug Therapy (Hosp.); also Circulation 56:139A, 1977.

Kerr, D., and Ash, M., Jr. 1978. Oral pathology: an introduction to general and oral pathology for hygienists, ed. 4. Philadelphia: Lea & Febiger.

Physicians' desk reference, ed. 38. 1984. Onradell, N.J.: Medical Economics Co.

Reports of Councils and Bureaus, a committee report of the American Heart Association. 1977. Prevention of bacterial endocarditis. J. Am. Dent. Assoc. 95:600.

Small, I. 1971. Introduction to the clinical history, ed. 2. Flushing, N.Y.: Medical Examination Publishing Co., Inc.

Weinstein, L., and Schlesinger, J. 1974. Pathoanatomic, pathophysiologic, and clinical correlations in endocarditis, I and II. N. Engl. J. Med. 291:832; 1122.

Wintroke, M., et al. 1970. Harrison's principles of internal medicine, ed. 6. New York: McGraw-Hill Book Co.

Woodall, I.R., editor. 1975. Curriculum guidelines, ed. 3. Chicago: American Dental Hygienists' Association.

Zach, L. 1976. Diabetes and dentistry: a review of some correlates. N.Y. J. Dent. 46:229.

9

GENERAL PHYSICAL EVALUATION AND THE EXTRAORAL AND INTRAORAL EXAMINATION

OBJECTIVES: *The reader will be able to*

1. State the purposes and advantages of performing a complete general and oral examination for each patient.
2. Identify the characteristics to observe in assessing a patient's general appearance and state why they may be significant to treatment.
3. Identify the four vital signs.
4. Demonstrate the technique for obtaining a patient's vital signs.
5. Discuss the role dentistry plays in identifying and monitoring hypertension.
6. Describe the extraoral and intraoral examination, including:
   a. The names of all structures to be visually inspected and palpated
   b. Normal landmarks associated with these structures
   c. The prescribed method of palpation for each structure
   d. Common abnormalities that may be detected
7. Given an illustration of an abnormal lesion, describe its location in the mouth, size, and clinical characteristics using medical descriptions of the type of lesion represented.
8. Define the four different methods of examination: inspection, palpation, auscultation, and percussion and give an example of each method.

A complete head and neck examination is a vital component in the provision of comprehensive health services. The total procedure combines a subjective and an objective appraisal of the patient's health, an examination of extraoral structures of the head and neck, and a thorough clinical examination of all intraoral structures. In the appointment sequence, the clinical examination procedures described in this chapter should follow the gathering of all pertinent data in a comprehensive health history. Information recorded in the health history of the patient provides not only a summary of the patient's health background, but also valuable insight into potential health problems or clinical manifestations that might be detected during the head and neck examination.

The major objectives for performing a complete head and neck examination for each patient are as follows:

1. To thoroughly examine structures of the head and neck in an effort to gather accurate and comprehensive assessment data for diagnosis and treatment planning
   a. To determine the goals and priorities of treatment
   b. To determine the need for additional consultations and referrals
   c. To assist in planning preventive programs designed around patient needs
2. To provide early detection of oral diseases and thus improve the prognosis for recovery
3. To detect systemic disturbances that have oral manifestations
4. To detect contraindications for dental treatment
5. To provide baseline and continuing data of the patient's health status to aid in evaluating

the success of treatment and preventive education

6. To provide descriptions of the patient's health status in the charts for potential use as legal records

The treatment plan designed for the patient must be based on a thorough identification and description of all observed and suspected health problems. At this point in treatment, the health history has already provided information regarding past health experiences and insight into current problems of which the patient is aware. The clinical examination will *supplement and update this history* with identification and/or descriptions of the current health status of the patient. The clinical examination should assist in identifying the specific dental needs of the patient so that these needs can be discussed with the patient and an appropriate treatment plan can be designed. The information gathered in the examination will also help the clinician *assess* what *preventive methods* and *education* are most appropriate for each patient's needs.

The *need for further consultations* with dental or medical specialists is also identified through information gathered in the head and neck examination. Cooperative efforts among health professionals are necessary to provide comprehensive care for the patient. The clinical examination will provide clues as to whether the services of specialists such as pathologists, periodontists, endodontists, oral surgeons, or the patient's physician are needed.

Total patient care involves a responsibility for more than just the patient's teeth and gums. It includes an awareness of other health problems that may be manifested during the head and neck examination. Often, systemic disorders can be identified through signs and symptoms that occur extraorally or intraorally. The complete examination may reveal signs of nutritional deficiencies or imbalances that may have dental implications.

Early detection of diseases that are progressive and irreversibly destructive in nature is a critical factor in determining the extent of the destruction that they might cause. This is especially true of oral cancer. A thorough head and neck examination performed at regular intervals could greatly reduce the incidence of deaths from oral cancer. It is estimated that in 1983 there were 27,100 new cases of oral cancer, 11,000 cases of cancer of the larynx, and 17,400 cases of skin cancer (some of which may have been manifested on the head and neck area) (American Cancer Society, 1983). Early detection and diagnosis of these malignancies are critical to reduce deaths caused by oral and other cancers.

It is the responsibility of every practitioner to apply the necessary skills and knowledge to ensure that all patients are not only examined thoroughly, but also educated to perform frequent and effective self-examination to increase the chances of early detection of cancer. This self-examination procedure is discussed in greater detail later in this text. Since each patient will be seen at regular recall intervals, it is likely that the clinician will be able to detect health or tissue changes from one appointment to another and thus identify the need for prompt and early treatment of disease or malignancies. The clinician can also use this opportunity to revise or reinforce patient education and self-care methods based on new information gathered from each updated clinical examination. Frequent examinations enable the clinician to become more familiar with a patient's normal oral manifestations. This will make it easier for deviations to be identified.

Throughout the clinical examination, the clinician should *identify contraindications* to dental treatment that would affect the health of the patient, the clinician, or both. Clinical signs of contagious diseases such as syphilis, hepatitis, or severe sore throat may be apparent at the time of the examination, even though they were not discussed in the health history. By referring these patients back to their physicians for care, both the patient's health and that of the dental team are protected.

The information gathered from the initial head and neck examination serves as valuable *baseline data* describing the patient's health status at the time of the initial appointment. These data form a standard by which the patient's progress through treatment and preventive procedures can be measured. It is the primary starting point from which the dental professional can measure effectiveness in treatment. If those problems identified in the clinical examination are not resolved through treatment and home care, the professional must reevaluate the current treatment plan to determine what factors may be causing the lack of success and whether or not those factors can be alleviated. Clinical examinations at recall appointments will provide additional data to be added to the patient's overall health profile and will ensure a constant reevaluation of present oral conditions.

It is important that the description of the patient's general health and oral conditions be noted as completely as possible in the patient's chart to facilitate the chart's use as a *legal record* if it should become necessary. Evaluation of information recorded in patient records is also becoming more and more prevalent in situations in which *third-party insurance carriers* are involved or in situations in which *peer review* is used to evaluate treatment.

In summary, the clinical head and neck examination is a necessary component of the total assessment of patient health care needs. It provides detailed information of disease, malignancy, or dysfunction that will help determine treatment planning and priorities. It identifies problems that necessitate further laboratory tests or consultation with other health practitioners. It provides data that will assist in patient education and self-care. When the clinical examination occurs frequently and regularly at recall appointments, continual monitoring of the patient's oral health care status and early detection of new disease processes are possible.

A thorough knowledge of head and neck anatomy and physiology, coupled with the mastery of comprehensive examination techniques as described in this chapter, will enable the clinician to identify deviations from normal and accurately report them for diagnosis. Since the health history data has already been gathered and recorded, that information can be correlated with clinical findings to provide a comprehensive review of all pertinent findings.

CLINICAL HEAD AND NECK EXAMINATION

The clinical head and neck examination is divided into four basic components: (1) general appraisal, (2) vital signs, (3) extraoral examination, and (4) intraoral examination.

In the following descriptions of each component, the tissues, structures, or functions to be examined are given, along with the suggested examination technique and sequence and possible significant findings that might be encountered during the examination. In most cases one of the following four methods of examination will be used to gather clinical information:

inspection A systematic visual assessment of body tissues, structures, or systems to identify normal and abnormal appearances and/or functioning.
palpation The use of the fingers or hands to examine the texture, form, and function of soft and hard tissue structures.
auscultation Listening for sounds produced within the body (e.g., clicking of the temporomandibular joint [TMJ], abnormal breathing sounds, vocal fremitus).
percussion Striking tissues with the fingers or an instrument to hear the resulting sounds and patient response.

Information from one or more of these methods and the patient's subjective responses provide a complete description of clinical findings.

General appraisal

There are many aspects of the patient's health and general disposition that may be detected from simple observation of overall appearance, movements, and responses. The examination methods used are inspection and auscultation. As the patient enters the office or operatory, *observe the general body weight, height, posture, and gait* for abnormal signs. Obesity, for example, or excessive height deviations not only may provide clues to possible nutritional or endocrine disorders, but also may indicate necessary alterations in patient positioning. The posture and gait may signal back problems or other handicaps that would also affect patient positioning in the chair. Does the patient limp or seem uncoordinated? Deficiencies of motor or sensory functions that include hand or arm movements would affect the type of home care the patient is capable of performing. Are there additional signs of paralysis, tremors, or other dysfunctions that will affect the patient's needs or treatment? What do the rate and character of the gait or gestures indicate about the patient's level of anxiety? While looking at the extremities, glance at the patient's legs and ankles for signs of swelling or other indications of poor circulation.

Observe the patient's face. Is the skin color normal, pale, or flushed? Does it appear dry or sweaty? What might the patient's facial expression indicate about his/her general attitude? Are there any signs of facial paralysis, tremors, asymmetry, or other abnormalities?

Monitor the patient's respiration rate. Is it shallow or deep? Is it fast or slow? Is it regular or punctuated with gasps, puffs, or wheezes? Are there signs that the patient experiences difficulty in breathing through either the nose or mouth? Does the chest cavity appear particularly shallow (caved in), or is the patient barrel chested? Any deviation from normal breathing may be an indication of respiratory or cardiac problems, or of an anxiety response to the dental appointment.

Once the patient is seated and engaged in a conversation, the clinician can take a closer look at the appearance of the skin, hair, eyes, and nose for signs of abnormalities. The clinician should also *evaluate the speech* for hoarseness, rate, pitch, and general quality. This may assist in the recognition of problems of the larynx (voice box), and, again, the patient's anxiety level. A nervous patient may speak at a pitch and rate higher than normal.

Observe the patient's hands to acquire valuable information about general health and attitude. Does the patient bite or chew the nails? Are the palms dry or sweaty? Are the hands fidgeting and gesturing nervously? Look between the first and second fingers for signs of tobacco stain from cigarettes. A constant tremor or paralysis of the hands or fingers may indicate nerve damage. The hands may also manifest signs of systemic or local diseases. For instance, a patient with anemia may exhibit spoon-shaped nails. Clubbing of the fingers may be associated with cardiac or pulmonary disorders. Swollen, painful finger joints are observed in the arthritic patient. Any of these specific conditions of the hands would likely have an effect on the overall treatment plan and should be noted.

Since this general appraisal is the first clinical introduction to the patient, it is important to retain the impressions and information that are accumulated and use them to guide later discussion with the patient concerning the health history and reactions to dental treatment. As subjective observations become confirmed through the health questionnaire or discussion with the patient, the final objective findings should be recorded in the patient's chart.

After reviewing the health history with the patient and not finding any obvious contraindication to proceeding (e.g., current contagious disease), the hygienist should explain the content and purpose of the clinical examination. Hopefully, the patient-hygienist rapport will have developed into a feeling of mutual trust and confidence such that patients will feel free to ask questions they have about the procedures and will share responsibility for the information gathering by reporting any symptoms that occur as the examination progresses. When all examination procedures have been explained and agreed to by the patient and assuming there are no contraindications to treating the patient at this point, the hygienist is ready to proceed with the next portion of the examination—taking the vital signs.

Vital signs

Pulse rate, respiration rate, temperature, and arterial blood pressure constitute the patient's vital signs. Usually this part of the physical examination is performed as one of the initial procedures in the appointment. For some patients, however, apprehension about the dental appointment or rushing to be on time may increase the vital signs. An attempt should be made to relax the patient through conversation or a calm atmosphere to ensure accuracy of the findings. Repeating the pulse and blood pressure measurements near the end of the appointment may be helpful to ensure accuracy.

Pulse rate. An arterial pulse that reflects the count of heartbeats may be palpated at several locations. Of practical use to the clinician is the location of the pulses in the following arteries:

radial Located on the thumb side of the patient's wrist over the radial bone.
brachial Located in the antecubital fossa before the brachial artery branches into the radial and ulnar arteries in the lower arm.
carotid Located on the lateral aspect of the neck on either side of the trachea.
temporal Located slightly above and in front of the ear.
facial Located at the border of the mandible in the mandibular notch.

Because of its accessibility, the radial pulse in the wrist area is most commonly used for determining the pulse rate during the physical examination. The pulse rate may be affected by age, exercise, and emotional status. Generally, a rate of 60 to 80 beats per minute is considered normal for the adult. Patients accustomed to regular exercise may exhibit lower pulse rates because of the strength and efficiency of the heart muscle's pumping ability. The normal pulse rate for children is 90 to 120 beats per minute.

Technique (Castano and Alden, 1973; Miller, Grainger, and Gagliardi, 1973). Seat the patient

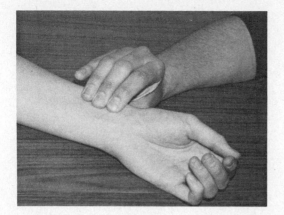

Fig. 9-1. Technique for pulse determination. Place fingers on radial artery. Gently compress artery against bone. Count pulse for 1 minute.

with the arm supported comfortably at the patient's side. Place the first three fingers on the patient's radial artery. The clincian's thumb is not used to determine the pulse, since it contains a pulse and may create confusion when determining the patient's pulse rate. Gently compress the artery against the underlying bone. Count the pulse for 1 minute while noting the rate, rhythm, and character of the beats (Fig. 9-1). If a pulse rate is abnormally fast, slow, irregular, or inconsistent in character, note this in the chart. Repeat the procedure a few minutes later to confirm the previous measurement. Alert the dentist to unusual findings, and discuss the situation with the patient. A physician's consultation may be suggested.

Respiration rate. The hygienist notes the quality and rate of respirations. This may be particularly important for patients reporting a health history of respiratory symptoms such as asthma, congestive heart failure, or allergic reactions, or for apprehensive patients prone to hyperventilation.

Technique. With the patient relaxed and sitting, observe the rate of respirations per minute. The normal respiration rate for the adult is 14 to 20 breaths per minute. The respiration rate usually increases with fever, pain, and excitement. Since the breathing rate may be altered by the patient's awareness of the procedure, counting respirations immediately after taking the pulse is suggested. Keeping the fingers on the wrist is a distraction.

Count the inspiration and expiration of air as one breath. Note the rate, rhythm (regular, irregular), type (strong, labored, weak), and depth (shallow, deep) of the patient's quiet breathing. Listen for wheezing sounds, and observe whether breathing occurs primarily through the nose or the mouth.

Record the findings on the chart. Notify the dentist of unusual or abnormal recordings.

Temperature. The average temperature of the body is 98.6° F or 37° C. Although slightly influenced by the time of day or imposed conditions such as exercise, the temperature is quite stable. When the temperature rises a full degree or more to 99.6° F or greater, the patient is said to have a fever. This usually is an indication of infection or tissue injury. Temperatures below 98.6° F may occur with shock or when the patient has been overly exposed to cold. The accepted normal temperature has been established by the oral method, but body temperature can be taken rectally or externally in the axillary or groin areas if the oral method is contraindicated (Kerr, Ash, and Millard, 1983). Standard normal temperature by the rectal method is 99.6° F and by the external methods is 97.6° F. The oral temperature method is contraindicated for infants, unconscious patients, those unable to breathe through the nose, or patients unable to hold the thermometer or understand the procedure.

Technique. Using an oral thermometer, shake the mercury indicator to below 96° F. Insert the thermometer under the patient's tongue. Ask the patient to hold the thermometer with the lips. Avoid taking the temperature immediately after the mouth has been rinsed with hot or cold liquids. Do not engage the patient in conversation when determining the temperature. Remove the thermometer after 3 minutes. Read the thermometer, and repeat the procedure if the accuracy of the reading is in doubt. Record the temperature in the chart. Unless the thermometer is disposable, wash it with detergent and water and disinfect it properly.

As an efficiency measure, the pulse and respiration rate may be recorded while the thermometer is in the patient's mouth.

Arterial blood pressure. Blood pressure is the measurement of the force of the blood pushing against the walls of the blood vessels. The pressure is influenced by the physical condition of the heart, the volume of blood being pumped, and the nature of the peripheral vessels. The blood vessel used

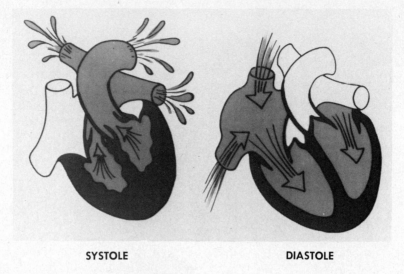

SYSTOLE   DIASTOLE

Fig. 9-2. Heart chamber during ventricular contraction (systole) and during ventricular relaxation (diastole). (From Anderson, J., and Geistfeld, N.C. Hypertension . . . the silent killer, slide No. 14, self-instructional package. Minneapolis: University of Minnesota.)

most commonly for blood pressure determination is the brachial artery in the arm. The normal adult blood pressure is 120/80 mm Hg. The top number refers to *systolic pressure,* the pressure in the blood vessel at the point of ventricular contraction of the heart. The bottom number refers to *diastolic pressure,* the pressure in the blood vessel during ventricular relaxation (Fig. 9-2). Generally, when the systolic blood pressure is greater than 160 mm or the diastolic pressure is greater than 95 mm Hg, the patient is considered to have hypertension (excessive pressure in the blood vessels) (Silverberg, 1976). The diagnosis of this condition is made when the patient sustains high blood pressure readings taken several times over a period of days. Because an increase in diastolic pressure generally results from a narrowing of the arterioles throughout the body, this figure is considered more significant. A diastolic blood pressure of 90 to 104 mm Hg is considered mild hypertension, a diastolic pressure of 104 to 114 mm Hg is considered moderate hypertension, and a diastolic pressure greater than 114 mm Hg is considered severe hypertension (Joint National Committee, 1980). External factors that influence blood pressure include exercise, emotional status, ingestion of stimulants (e.g., coffee) and depressants (e.g., alcohol). Systolic pressure tends to be more influenced by external factors. Because of the significance of screening for hypertension in the dental office and the need for modifications in dental treatment for these patients, following is a discussion of hypertension.

Hypertension. Hypertension is a common disorder affecting between 10% to 20% of the population (Gaynor, 1983). Half this number are experiencing hypertensive heart disease. Although not often stated as the cause of death, chronic hypertension is the principal risk factor in congestive heart failure, stroke, and kidney failure and is related to coronary heart disease as a predisposing factor in the acceleration of arteriosclerosis (Laragh, 1974). Undiagnosed or untreated hypertension can shorten a person's life by 10 to 30 years (Silverberg, 1976).

Since hypertension is prevalant among the population of the United States, screening patients for high blood pressure is important. Many patients visit the dentist more frequently than they do the physician, making the dental office a prime location for detecting patients who may require medical consultation and treatment (Abbey, 1976; Silwitz, 1977). In 1976 the American Dental Association adopted guidelines stating that blood pressure measurement for screening purposes would be appropriate for all new patients, including children, and for recall patients once a year. The procedure could be included in the office routine as part of taking or updating a health history (Joint National Committee, 1980).

Singer et al. (1983) report that during dental hygiene treatment diastolic pressure demonstrate average fluctuations of 2.1 mm Hg for normotensive patients, fluctuations of 1.0 mm Hg for nonmedicated hypertensive patients, and fluctuations of 0.1 mm Hg for medicated hypertensive patients. These findings indicate that anticipated stress over dental treatment does not significantly increase blood pressure and that blood pressure readings taken in the dental office are quite reliable.

REFERRAL. (Longenecker and Beck, 1983). If the patient's diastolic blood pressure is between 90 and 94 mm Hg, the patient should be informed that this reading is above normal. Although the day's dental treatment need not be affected, the patient should be referred to have this reading confirmed medically within 3 month's time. When the diastolic blood pressure is between 95 and 114 mm Hg, the patient should be referred for a medical confirmation within 1 month's time. A telephone consultation with the patient's family physician would be appropriate to determine whether dental treatment should be continued for the day and to establish communication for following the patient's medical status. If a diastolic blood pressure greater then 115 mm Hg is recorded, the patient should be allowed to remain quiet for at least 5 minutes and the reading should be confirmed by the dentist. If the diastolic blood pressure is still in this range, dental treatment should be delayed, with immediate medical referral and confirmation obtained.

When a medical referral is made, the patient should understand that (1) his/her blood pressure exceeds normal limits, (2) hypertension is often asymptomatic, (3) uncontrolled high blood pressure has serious consequences, (4) long-term follow-up and therapy are necessary, and (5) therapy will control but not cure high blood pressure (Joint National Committee, 1980).

When screening of dental patients is performed routinely, between 5% and 6% of the patients can be expected to be referred to a physician. Of the patients referred, five of every six patients will actually be positively diagnosed as having hypertension. Four of these will be previously undi-

agnosed, and one will be delinquent or not following prescribed treatment (Abbey, 1976).

In addition to the role of screening patients for untreated hypertension, the dental professional must consider the implications of this disease for dental treatment (Argentieri, 1978). Often the diagnosed hypertensive patient may not be adhering to the prescribed treatment regimen. Taking the blood pressure at each visit is critical. Although it is not the dentist's role to diagnose or treat hypertension, referral may be necessary to ensure that dental treatment can be provided safely.

In a case tried by the New Jersey Supreme Court, a dentist administered a local anesthetic with epinephrine vasoconstrictor to a patient for a routine filling. The patient collapsed with a stroke and died a few days later. Negligence was alleged in this case on the dentist's failure to make a physical evaluation or complete a medical history prior to administering anesthesia. Therefore the clinician was unaware of the patient's cardiovascular status. The court upheld the case of negligence. This is probably the most specific case on a dentist's failure to conduct a physical exam (Conway, 1980).

TREATMENT. In mild cases of hypertension, weight reduction and control of sodium intake may bring the blood pressure into normal range. When drug therapy is necessary, a stepped-care program is advisable. This entails initiating therapy with a small dose of antihypertensive medication, increasing the dosage of that drug, and adding sequentially one medication after another gradually as needed until the goal blood pressure is achieved, side effects become intolerable, or the maximum dose is reached (Joint National Committee, 1980). Depending on the patient, several medications may be necessary, making medical follow-up an important part of ongoing care. Generally, the need for treatment continues for life (Silverberg, 1976).

Diuretics are the first drug of choice for treating mild hypertension. These medications promote the renal excretion of water and sodium ions. Positive results occur in about 50% of mild hypertensive patients (Gaynor, 1983). Common diuretics include hydrochlorothiazide, furosemide, and spironolactone. The second step after diuretics is to prescribe adrenergic inhibiting agents, such as reserpine, methyldopa, clonidine, and propranolol hydrochloride. These agents deplete or inhibit norepinephrine. A vasodilator such as hydralazine may be added as the third step in medical therapy. For severe hypertension, the fourth step would include an additional adrenergic inhibiting agent such as guanethidine sulfate.

IMPLICATIONS FOR DENTAL TREATMENT. Antihypertensive medications often cause postural hypotension (positional low blood pressure), necessitating raising the patient slowly from the supine position to prevent dizziness or syncope. Antihypertensive medications may affect the fluid balance in the oral cavity, causing a dry mouth with resultant dental complications. Analgesic agents (cyclopropane, halothane) may produce a decrease in oxygen in the blood and cause a rapid increase in blood pressure for these patients (Chue, 1975). Local and general anesthetics and vasopressor substances may potentiate the hypotensive effects of the antihypertensive medication, possibly causing cardiovascular collapse and shock. Epinephrine in the form of a gingival retraction cord or in a local anesthetic is contraindicated in patients taking guanethidine, reserpine, or methyldopa. It may potentiate the pressor effects of catecholamine, possibly causing a rapid increase in blood pressure. In a well-controlled hypertensive patient, 0.1 mg of epinephrine is allowed if necessary.

The dental team and physician need to work cooperatively in detecting, treating, and following the hypertensive patient. Noting the blood pressure at each dental visit is a preventive health service that cannot be overlooked. For the patient with a history of hypertension, the medical history should be updated at recall intervals by inquiring about the patient's current medications and recent visits to the physician in addition to recording the blood pressure for the day.

Technique. Obtain a stethoscope and a sphygmomanometer (blood pressure apparatus). This usually includes an inflatable bladder enclosed in an unyielding cuff, which will be wrapped around the patient's arm. The cuff must be the correct width for the diameter of the patient's arm. If the cuff is too narrow, the blood pressure reading will be erroneously high; if it is too wide, the reading may be too low. For the average adult arm, a cuff 12 to 14 cm wide has been found to be satisfactory (Kirkendall et al., 1980). Several sizes of cuffs are available to fit small to obese patients. The circumference of the arm, not the age of the patient, is the determining factor in selecting the proper

sphygmomanometer. Attached to the cuff is a rubber bulb to pump air into the bladder and a gauge (aneroid dial or mercury column) that reflects the pressure in the blood vessel as the air in the bladder is deflated by regulation of the air-release clamp. Equipment is also available that inflates and deflates the cuff automatically and displays a computerized digital readout of the blood pressure.

1. Seat the patient in a comfortable position in which the arm can be easily supported. Ask the patient to roll up a sleeve or to slip the arm out of the clothing to permit access to the brachial artery. Rest the arm in a slightly flexed position with the hand open and relaxed.
2. Wrap the sphygmomanometer cuff around the patient's arm. The lower border of the cuff should be ¾ to 1 inch above the bend in the arm. Place the gauge in a position to be easily viewed (Fig. 9-3).
3. Find the radial pulse in the wrist. Lock the air-release clamp, and inflate the cuff until the pulse is no longer felt. Note the pressure registering on the gauge. Open the air-release clamp until the cuff is completely deflated. Allow the patient a few moments to rest the arm and exercise the hand.
4. Place the stethoscope comfortably in the ears, with the earpieces directed forward. Place the diaphragm of the stethoscope over the branch of the brachial artery (Blozis, 1979) (approximately 1 inch from the bend in the arm, toward the hand, and close to the inner aspect of the forearm) (Fig. 9-4).
5. Inflate the cuff 20 to 30 mm Hg higher than the pressure at which the radial pulse disappeared, as noted in step 3.
6. Using the air-release clamp, slowly deflate the cuff. Note the pressure at which the first pulse beat is heard. This is the systolic pressure. Continue to release the air in the cuff. The pulse sound will increase in intensity, then become muffled and disappear. Note the pressure at which the last sound occurred. This is the diastolic pressure. Release the remaining air in the cuff.
7. Record the blood pressure as a fraction:

Systolic pressure
―――――――――――
Diastolic pressure

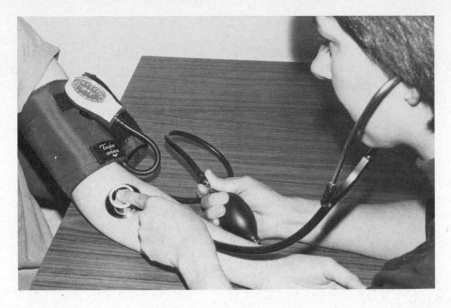

Fig. 9-3. Place cuff 1 inch above bend in arm with gauge in position for easy viewing.

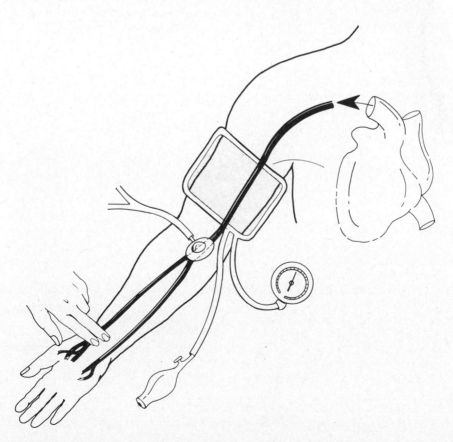

Fig. 9-4. Place diaphragm of stethoscope over branch of brachial artery. This is approximately 1 inch from bend in arm toward hand and close to inner aspect of forearm. (From Boundy, S.S., and Reynolds, N.J. 1979. Current concepts in dental hygiene, vol. 2. St. Louis: The C.V. Mosby Co.)

Note the arm position of the patient (i.e., 120/80 RAS—(right arm, sitting).

8. Let the patient relax the arm once again before repeating the procedure for confirmation of the reading. Avoid repeating the procedure several times in a row without allowing the patient's circulation to return to normal. This may arouse anxiety in the patient and affect the reading, and the arm may become quite uncomfortable.

9. Compare the current reading with past blood pressure readings (if available). Consult the dentist and physician when the systolic pressure is greater than 160 mm Hg or the diastolic pressure is greater than 95 mm Hg. Note any unusual findings or changes in the pattern of blood pressure recordings as compared with past visits.

• • •

Once vital signs are recorded, the hygienist begins the extraoral examination.

Extraoral examination

For this part of the head and neck examination, the patient should be seated in an upright or semi-supine position. It is difficult to examine the deeper structures of the neck and submandibular area when the patient is in a full supine position because many of the soft tissue structures tend to fall back into the deeper structures of the head and neck and are less accessible for examination and palpation. The clinician will be working either in front of or behind the patient, depending on which structures are being examined. At all times, the patient should be positioned for maximum visibility. All necessary supplies that are needed for the examination procedure should be assembled and accessible to the clinician. Fig. 9-5 shows a suggested tray setup for the extraoral and intraoral examination procedures.

The following guidelines should be considered while the examination is being performed:

1. The clinician should be able to locate each structure in the head and neck region that will be examined.

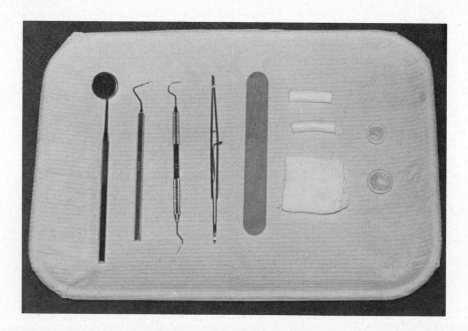

Fig. 9-5. Suggested tray setup for performing oral examination. *From left to right:* Mouth mirror, probe, explorer, college pliers, tongue blade, cotton rolls for isolation of teeth, gauze, and finger cots.

2. All structures being examined should be accessible for observation or palpation.
3. The clinician should use a thorough technique to examine each structure.
4. The clinician should use a sequence of examination that is systematic and time/motion efficient.

Patient considerations. The clinician should give careful consideration to each patient's need for privacy and comfort. This need exists in all patients regardless of the type of procedure that is being performed. During the head and neck examination, the clinician should carefully explain the purpose of the examination and its value as an assessment tool that will be used to help the patient and the dental professional create a treatment plan that will be comprehensive and acceptable to the patient. Patients appreciate a clinical attitude that demonstrates professional interest in their feelings and concerns. The clinician should speak in a quiet and friendly voice so that the conversation will not be overheard by other patients or personnel outside the operatory. Patients deserve to have all procedures explained to them and to be considered as a partner in care rather than an object of care. During the head and neck examination, the clinician should display a confident attitude and approach to the examination that demonstrates competence. Patients may not be used to being touched and examined in so close a manner and may feel some shyness or embarrassment until the clinician can put them at ease. Many patients may avoid any type of physical examination because they fear the results of the procedure. The clinician can ease this apprehension by explaining the importance of regular professional examinations and self-examinations and by reinforcing this behavior in the patient. These same patient fears can be heightened if the clinician verbalizes clinical findings using technical jargon that the patient cannot understand. The clinician can accomplish a great deal of patient education on self-assessment of oral conditions if language is used that is easily understood and if the significance of diagnoses are carefully and thoroughly discussed with the patient in lay terms. For instance, while examining the extraoral and intraoral structures, the clinician can describe what is being examined and why. This eliminates any guesswork and potential misunderstanding by the patient. An excerpt from such a conversation might sound like this:

Mrs. Willis, the next thing I will be examining is your tongue. Have you ever looked closely at your tongue? If you will watch me in the mirror you're holding, I'll show you how it can be examined and what to look for. First, I'd like you to place the tip of your tongue on this gauze square so that I can move it easily. Good! Now, as I look at the top of the tongue, I can see that it has a slight coating. This can be easily removed by brushing the tongue with a toothbrush. Otherwise, your tongue looks very pink and healthy. These bumps back here are normal papillae. Now I'm going to check the sides of the tongue for any areas that look or feel like sores or for any white or red patchy areas. The sides of the tongue and the floor of the mouth are two areas where oral cancer may sometimes occur, so you will want to take the opportunity to inspect these surfaces yourself at home. After seeing them here and at home, you'll have a good idea of what they normally look like and it will be easier for you to recognize any changes that might occur. These structures in the back of your tongue are also normal. They are the lingual tonsils. Now I'm going to feel your tongue for lumps or hard areas. Everything looks and feels fine, Mrs. Willis. Do you have any questions about what I've shown you?

In this way the patient will gain an understanding of the normal structures of the mouth while observing the clinician's examination and listening to the clinician's explanations. In addition, patients should be given the following instructions regarding their own oral self-assessments: (1) they should be looking for unusual lumps or bumps in the mouth; (2) they should check for unusual color changes that may appear as white, red, or bluish patches, or areas that appear to be speckled with both white and red areas; (3) they should establish a sequence for examining all parts of the mouth; (4) they should perform their own oral examination on a monthly basis; and (5) they should observe any unusual lesion for 2 weeks to see if it heals; if not, then it should be reported to a dentist or physician promptly (Glass et al., 1975).

Patients will not only benefit from the health information you have provided them about their own mouths, but they will also appreciate your interest in taking the time to answer their questions and discuss their concerns. This process will help make each patient a more educated and prevention-oriented health consumer. A more detailed explanation of self-assessment techniques for dental patients is contained in Chapter 19.

Visual inspection. The extraoral examination

includes two components. The first is a visual inspection of each structure. It is followed by palpation and auscultation.

For the visual inspection the patient should be seated in an upright or semisupine position with the clinician seated facing the patient. Glasses should be removed if worn, and clothing that restricts access to the neck (e.g., tight-fitting collars and ties) should be loosened. Starting from the top of the head and neck area and moving downward, *examine the hair* for texture, amount, and distribution. Note any apparent *scalp lesion,* such as scars, sores, or growths. Examine for the presence of lice or other transmittable conditions within the hair.

Next *examine the face* for symmetry, form, and profile. Observe the skin of the face for abnormal pigmentation, hair, texture, scars, or lesions. Facial asymmetry may be indicative of inflammatory conditions such as dental abscesses or mumps. Stroke victims or others who suffer from unilateral paralysis of facial muscles demonstrate an inability to produce normal facial expressions on the affected side. The muscles and soft tissues of the affected side may have a drooping or flaccid appearance.

Note the general color of the skin. An abnormal redness may indicate the presence of inflammation, fever, sunburn, or increased vascularity due to excitement or exertion. Abnormal paleness could indicate anemia, systemic illness, or shock. Patients with a history of heart or pulmonary disorders may exhibit a slightly bluish cast to their skin. Jaundice or yellow skin may be indicative of liver disease (hepatitis), red blood cell disorders, or drug toxicity (Kutcher et al., 1981).

Question the patient about the presence of any raised lesions, such as moles, to determine how long they have been present and whether they have undergone any changes in size, texture, color, or tendency to bleed. Scars are indications of past trauma to the head or face. Discuss the cause of the trauma to determine its relevance to the patient's medical and dental history.

While examining the *eyes,* observe the following structures:

Scleras. Note color and signs of irritation.
Pupils. Note size and reactivity to stimuli such as light.
Eyelids. Note texture, form, color, and habits (blinking).
Conjunctiva. Note color, degree of moisture, and presence of foreign bodies; examine by retracting the lower lid in a downward direction with the tip of the index finger

Examine the *nose* for form, symmetry, and obstructions. The airflow can be examined by placing the dental mirror underneath the patient's nostrils during normal respiration.

Examine the *lips* for symmetry, form, texture, color, and habits. Note signs of irritation, chapping, or breaks in the skin, especially at the corners of the mouth. Chapped lips should be protected with a coating of petroleum jelly or other lubricant to prevent the dried tissues from breaking open during the examination. Mouth ulcers or intact and healing vesicles on the lips should never be touched with unprotected hands. Herpes simplex virus can be transmitted from infected lesions to small breaks in the skin of the clinician, such as hangnails or torn cuticles. A recurrent viral infection, herpetic whitlow, can be established in the fingers of the clinician in this manner. Examine the function of the lips by asking the patient to open and close the mouth. Note lack of closure or mouth-breathing tendencies.

Examine the *ears* for form, texture, hair, symmetry, and color. Be sure to look behind the ears for possible lesions that would normally be shielded from view.

Check the *neck* area for symmetry of the structures in the neck. Examine the skin of the neck for pigmentation, texture, scars, obvious swellings, or lesions.

All findings from the visual inspection, either normal or abnormal, should be noted in the patient's chart. Any suspicious lesions should be recorded with complete descriptions of their appearance, size, location, duration, and any other symptoms related to their presence. The following terms may aid in describing the appearance of tissues or lesions:

discrete Separate, not blending or occurring together.
confluent Blending or occurring together; originally separate, but subsequently combined.
verrucose Covered with wartlike lesions.
erythema Red area of variable size or shape.
petechia(e) Minute round red spot(s).
induration Hardened area of tissue.
pedunculated Elevated papillary type lesion attached to underlying tissue by a stem or narrow connector.
sessile Attachment of a lesion by a broad base.

Lesions that are detected during the examination should be described using the following descriptive categories:

macules Flat areas that are differentiated from surrounding tissues by color; they may vary in size, shape, and color. Examples are petechiae, ecchymosis, freckles, and melanosis.

papules Small (pinhead to 5 mm) superficial elevated areas of tissue, which may appear flattened, rounded, or pointed; color may vary. Examples are found in lichen planus and traumatic hyperplasia.

nodules Enlarged papules that are deep seated into submucosa or lower dermis of the skin. Examples are traumatic fibromas, gumboils, and lesions associated with rheumatoid arthritis, leprosy, and syphilis.

vesicles Small elevations containing fluid with a thin surface covering of epithelium or mucosa (e.g., blisters); they may occur singly or in clusters. Examples are herpes simplex, primary herpes, and herpes zoster.

pustules Vesicles that contain pus.

bullae Large (5 mm to several centimeters) vesicles that are relatively deep seated and less prone to rupture. Examples occur in pemphigus and as the result of traumatic injuries.

erosion Shallow surface defect that does not extend through the epithelium into underlying tissues.

ulcer Defect in the skin or mucosa that extends beyond the surface epithelium and into the underlying tissues. Reddened border may be ragged or punched out; depressed bases may appear soft or indurated with a floor that is smooth, granular, glazed, pus covered, or hemorrhagic; may be painless or extremely sensitive. Examples are found in acute necrotizing ulcerative gingivitis and herpes simplex (beneath ruptured vesicle) and also result from trauma to the tissues.

tumor Solid growth of hard or soft tissue; swelling or overgrowth of cells independent of normal tissue; may be reactive or neoplastic; can be identified clinically in terms of size, shape, type of base (sessile or pedunculated), surface texture, and form. Examples are papillomas, polyps, and tori.

keratosis Abnormal thickening of the outer layers of skin or mucosa that may appear as white, greyish white, or brown lesions; may occur as localized or diffuse areas. Examples are linea alba, cheek biting, nicotine stomatitis, certain lesions of lichen planus, and leukoplakia.

Extraoral palpation. The clinician is now ready to continue the extraoral examination by palpating all extraoral structures. One of the following methods of palpation will be indicated for each structure, or several techniques may be combined:

digital palpation Use of a finger to examine tissues.

bidigital palpation Use of one or more fingers and the thumb to examine tissues by grasping the tissue between thumb and fingers.

manual palpation Use of all the fingers of one hand to examine tissues.

bimanual palpation Use of both hands by grasping tissues between them for examination.

bilateral palpation Examination of structures on both sides of the face or neck simultaneously to detect differences between the two sides.

circular compression Moving the fingertips in a circular pattern over a structure while simultaneously applying pressure to the tissue.

It is important for the clinician to palpate soft tissue structures against a harder structure such as underlying bone, other fingers, or hands. If the soft tissues are not supported by some means, there is greater possibility that abnormal masses might be displaced away from the examining fingers and not detected.

Sequencing the palpation. The following sequence of the palpation procedure is designed so that all structures are examined in a logical and systematic order that avoids ''hopping'' from one area of the head to another. By following a set pattern of examination such as the one recommended, the clinician always knows which structures have or have not been examined in case the procedure is interrupted and at the same time has assured efficient time and motion management. Although the following sequence meets these criteria, other patterns of examination might be equally as effective and efficient as long as the aforementioned criteria are applied.

The first structure to be palpated is the *mentalis muscle*. This muscle attaches to the lower lip and inserts into the symphysis of the mandible. Palpate it with digital compression, rolling the tissue over the mandible. Have the patient swallow and observe the function of this muscle in swallowing. Patients with abnormal swallowing habits often will grimace and use this muscle to assist in swallowing by wrinkling the chin. (A glass of water may be useful to assist the patient in swallowing at various points during the examination.)

Examine the *anterior border of the mandible* next. From a position behind the patient, use bidigital and circular compression on the soft tissues, starting at the symphysis of the mandible and moving posteriorly along the borders of the mandible

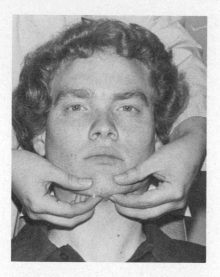

Fig. 9-6. Anterior border of mandible as it is palpated using bidigital compression and circular motion of soft tissues against bone.

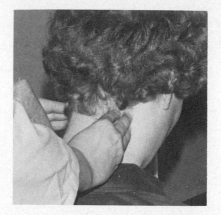

Fig. 9-7. Occipital nodes are being examined. Circular compression is applied at base of skull.

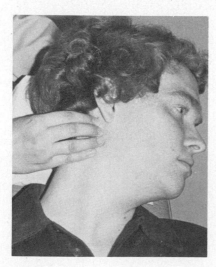

Fig. 9-8. Inferior auricular nodes are being examined by circular compression against tissues. Both anterior and posterior auricular nodes are examined in same manner.

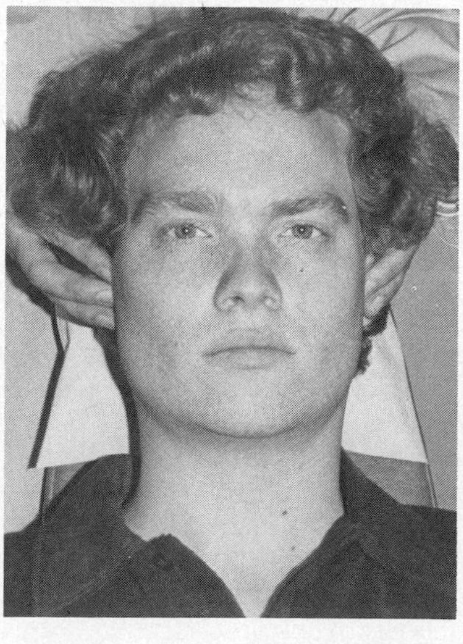

Fig. 9-9. Palpation of temporomandibular joint occurs when fingertips are placed bilaterally just anterior to outer opening of ear.

(Fig. 9-6). Through palpation, examine the soft tissues and underlying bone to locate normal bony landmarks, deviations in symmetry, tenderness, and crepitus (cracking sounds). Continue this method of palpation bilaterally until the angle of the mandible is reached.

The *occipital lymph nodes* are located at the base of the skull at the back of the head. Ask the patient to lean his/her head forward, and apply digital circular compression bilaterally with the fingertips. The palpation should begin at the back of the neck and extend horizontally to the sternocleidomastoid muscle (Fig. 9-7).

The *auricular lymph nodes* are located behind (posterior auricular), beneath (inferior auricular), and in front (anterior auricular) of the ears. Begin by applying the fingertips in digital compression and circular movement to the area of the posterior auricular nodes. The palpation should be done bilaterally to identify deviations from one side to another. Continue this palpation to the *inferior auricular nodes* and the *anterior auricular nodes,* located anterior to the tragus of the ear. Note enlargements, tenderness, degree of mobility, and firmness of nodes (Fig. 9-8).

Palpate the *temporomandibular joint* bilaterally by placing the index fingers of each hand just anterior to the outer meatus of the ear and asking the patient to open and close the mouth slowly several times. Also ask the patient to do the following: perform right and left lateral movements with the teeth apart, and make protrusive movements with the teeth together and then apart. Feel for abnormal function of the joints and differences in function between the right and left sides. Question the patient about any painful symptoms associated with these jaw movements. Auscultation of the joint during movement is used to detect the presence of clicking, popping, or grating sounds (Figs. 9-9 and 9-10).

Palpate the *parotid gland* (including the parotid nodes) bilaterally using digital compression and circular movement. Begin anterior to the tragus of the ear, and extend the palpation inferiorly to the angle of the mandible. Note any deviations in form, density, or size, or any complaints by the patient of tenderness in the area (Fig. 9-11).

Palpate the *masseter muscle* by placing the fingers of each hand over the angle of the mandible and extending the hand up onto the cheek. Then

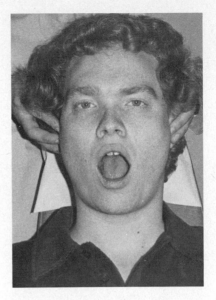

Fig. 9-10. Patient is asked to perform a variety of jaw movements as temporomandibular joint is palpated. Here patient is slowly opening his mouth as far as is comfortable while clinician feels for abnormal movement or clicking in joint.

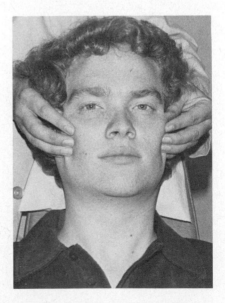

Fig. 9-11. Area of parotid gland is palpated with circular compression over entire area of gland. This is a large gland and extends from in front of ear to cheek area and down to angle of mandible.

ask the patient to clench the teeth together several times, and examine the muscle bilaterally for size, function, and deviations between the two sides.

Examine the *temporalis muscle* in much the same way as the masseter muscle; place the hands bilaterally across the muscle on the patient's temples, and ask the patient to clench the teeth together several times. Check for muscle function and tenderness.

Examine the *submental region* (including lymph nodes) using digital compression and circular motion behind and beneath the symphysis of the mandible. Examine for swelling, enlargements, tenderness, firmness, and mobility of lymph nodes (Fig. 9-12).

Palpate the *submandibular region* (including glands and nodes) using bidigital compression and circular movements. Ask the patient to lower the head so that the skin and muscles beneath the chin are not taut. This adjustment will make it easier to gain access to the deeper soft tissues of the submandibular area. Starting at the anterior border of the mandible, push the tissue from the left submandibular area over to the right and grasp it with the fingertips of the right hand. The examining fingers should be cupped slightly to effectively grasp the tissues. Then use the fingertips to roll the soft tissue over the right border of the mandible, feeling for swelling or enlargements, tenderness,

mobility, and firmness of lymph nodes. Reverse this procedure for the left submandibular area. Finally, use the fingertips to compress bilaterally the soft tissues of the submandibular region. Start this palpation at the midline of the submandibular area, and proceed outward to the borders of the mandible and posteriorly to the angle (Fig. 9-13).

To examine the structures of the neck, start with the *sternocleidomastoid muscle*. Ask the patient to turn the head to the left and lower the chin. This will cause the muscle on the right side of the neck to be more prominent and increase its accessibility for the examination. The left hand of the clinician should support the patient's head at the chin, and the right hand should grasp the muscle between the thumb and fingers.

Begin bidigital palpation, starting from behind the ear and continuing all the way down the muscle until you reach the clavicle. Remember that for thorough examination of the structures of the neck, the patient should have loosened tight collars or ties so that the neck area is exposed. Repeat the examination on the left side of the neck. Examine the muscle for rigidity, tenderness, induration, presence of masses, and difference in function from one side to the other (Fig. 9-14).

The *superficial cervical lymph nodes* are located anterior and posterior to the sternocleidomastoid muscle. Apply digital compression and circular

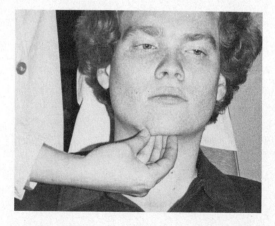

Fig. 9-12. Palpation of submental region using circular compression and digital compression against anterior portion of mandible. This area will also be examined along with the floor of the mouth.

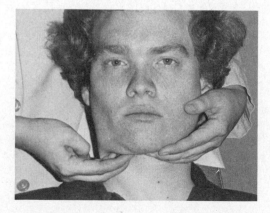

Fig. 9-13. Palpation of submandibular area. Note that clinician has pushed tissue from patient's left side over to opposite side, where it is being grasped and rolled over angle of mandible. Opposite side will be examined in same way.

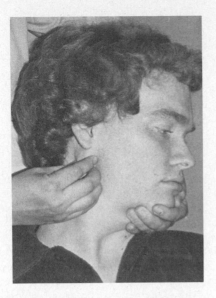

Fig. 9-14. Note patient positioning for palpation of sternocleidomastoid muscle. His head is turned to side and slightly down while chin rests in clinician's free hand. This causes muscle to protrude so that it is easily seen. Palpation is bidigital compression starting from below ear and continuing whole length of muscle to clavicle.

movement to this area, extending from the angle of the mandible in a downward direction along the anterior and posterior aspects of this muscle (Fig. 9-15). The patient's head should be in an upright and forward position. Palpate the area bilaterally to examine for deviations from normal. Look for enlarged lymph nodes, and note their tenderness, degree of mobility, and firmness.

The *deep cervical lymph nodes* are located along and behind the sternocleidomastoid muscle. The technique of palpation is the same as for the anterior cervical lymph nodes, with an increased effort being made to locate the thumb and fingers behind the muscle to locate nodes in the deeper, less accessible tissues.

The *thyroid gland* is normally not visible. It is located vertically between the cricothyroid ligament and the fourth tracheal ring and horizontally between the sternocleidomastoid muscle and the trachea. It can be palpated from behind or in front of the patient. With one hand place the fingers on one side of the trachea and gently displace the thyroid tissue over to the other side of the neck. With the opposite hand apply gentle circular digital compression to the tissues. Palpate the thyroid gland for enlargements, tenderness, and mobility. Ask the patient to swallow, and examine the gland for signs of masses or lack of movement during swallowing (Fig. 9-16).

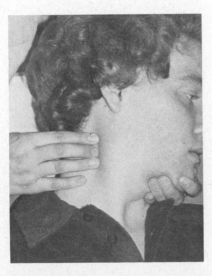

Fig. 9-15. Circular, digital compression is used to examine cervical chain of lymph nodes anteriorly and posteriorly to sternocleidomastoid muscle.

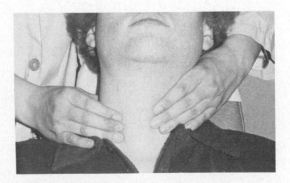

Fig. 9-16. Thyroid is being palpated from rear of patient. One hand gently displaces tissue to one side while fingers of other hand carefully feel for enlargements or abnormal masses.

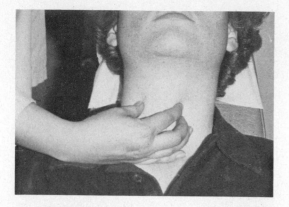

Fig. 9-17. Gentle medial pressure is used in area of larynx to check for mobility of larynx and trachea. Inability to move this structure slightly might indicate problems.

Examine the *larynx* by placing the fingertips of one hand bilaterally over the larynx and applying alternate pressure in a medial direction against the structure. A normal larynx should be freely movable and should ascend and descend during the process of swallowing. A slight fremitus (palpable vibration or movement) may be noted when the normal larynx is displaced during palpation (Fig. 9-17).

This completes the description of the extraoral examination. All significant findings should be described and recorded in the patient's chart to aid in diagnosis and treatment planning. Significant inclusions in the chart may be summarized from the palpation as follows:

Boney structures. Record abnormal anatomy, growths, fractures, crepitus, and pain.
Muscles. Record hyperfunction or hypofunction, deviations between the two sides, swellings, masses, indurations, and tenderness.
Glands. Record abnormal swellings, tenderness, and hard masses.
Lymph nodes. Record palpable nodes and describe their size (estimate diameter), firmness (hard or soft), mobility (fixed or freely movable), tenderness (sensitive or painless), and how long they have been present. Determine if presence of lymph nodes can be traced to current manifestations of disease or recent history of disease.
Skin. Describe all lesions using the terminology discussed earlier.

Significance of lymph node examination

Normal lymph nodes are not visible or palpable during the head and neck examination. When the presence of swollen lymph nodes can be detected by either of these methods, the clinician should continue the evaluation of the patient to determine what the cause of the abnormality might be. Lymph nodes of the head and neck area can become swollen and tender from infections that originate in the areas that they are draining. The clinician must have a clear understanding of human anatomy and the lymph node system in order to trace a detectable lymph node back to its associated cause. Enlargement of lymph nodes as a result of acute or chronic infections is known as *lymphadenitis*. Lymph nodes may become temporarily enlarged because of localized infections such as a dental abscess, regional infections such as tonsillitis, or systemic infections such as tuberculosis or syphilis. In most cases of acute inflammation, resolution of the infection allows the lymph nodes to return to their normal state. In some cases chronic infections will cause enlargement of affected lymph nodes because of the presence of scar tissue, so that they remain palpable as nontender firm or fibrotic single masses even after the source of the infection has been removed. Since many of these same characteristics might be found in nodes associated with malignant or metastatic diseases (cancer), the patient's medical history should be explored and the patient should be interviewed to determine possible explanations for the presence of these nodes. In general, nodes that arise from acute inflammatory conditions are tender, soft, enlarged, and freely movable.

Lymph node involvement due to malignant diseases may display different characteristics. Detection and examination of these nodes reveals that they are often very hard, nontender, and fixed to underlying tissues, and they may involve multiple nodes that are matted together. The patient may indicate no recent history of local or systemic infection in these cases to explain the presence of the detectable nodes. Bilaterally enlarged nodes may indicate the presence of systemic infection or an advanced malignancy. The presence of unilateral node enlargement may indicate either localized infection or possibly early metastatic disease. The alert clinician will combine information from the patient's medical and dental history, the oral examination, the lymph node examination, and an up-to-date knowledge of the demographics of patients who are at high risk for malignant diseases in order to evaluate the potential significance of detectable lymph nodes. When lymph node involvement suggests malignant changes, the clinician should examine the areas served by those nodes for signs of abnormal tissues. Although many detectable nodes may be easily explained by the presence of local, regional, or systemic infections, the dental professional should refer all questionable findings to the patient's physician or a specialist for a definitive diagnosis (Kerr, Ash, and Millard, 1983; Kutcher et al., 1981).

Intraoral examination

The supplies and instruments that are needed for the intraoral examination include a mirror, explorer, probe, gauze squares, and a tongue depressor. For this treatment procedure and all other intraoral procedures, the clinician should wear disposable gloves, a face mask, and safety glasses to prevent disease transmission.

The following factors will help ensure optimal examination technique: (1) lighting, (2) positioning, (3) tissue retraction, and (4) sequence. A complete and thorough examination cannot be performed without optimal consideration of all of these factors.

Direct lighting is provided by directing the central beam of the overhead light onto the area being examined. Care should be taken not to direct the light into the patient's eyes. Readjustment of the light beam is necessary as different areas of the mouth are examined. This responsibility should be assumed by the chairside assistant if one is present. Supplementary *indirect lighting* is also provided by the mouth mirror. This is especially useful for the posterior parts of the mouth, where it is difficult to use the direct beam of the overhead light.

Patient and clinician positioning should be such that both parties are comfortable and all areas are accessible to the clinician for complete examination. When necessary, the patient must be given instructions as to where to turn the head or place the tongue so that all areas are visible. The clinician should follow the principles of good positioning, discussed in previous chapters, and make sure that there is a direct view of the structure to be examined. If a direct view cannot be obtained without

violating the principles of effective positioning, such as in the maxillary tuberosity area, the dental mirror should be used to examine that area thoroughly.

The third factor for good examination technique is thorough, but gentle, *retraction* of soft tissues so that their entire area can be observed. There is no guarantee that lesions will not occur behind folds of tissue or at the hidden corners of the mouth. Failure to examine completely all tissues regardless of their accessibility can only be considered negligent.

The establishment of an efficient *sequence* is also an important factor. Optimal time and motion management, use of a logical order, and asepsis should all be considered in determining the sequence of examination. Since the examination of some intraoral structures such as the labial and buccal mucosa and the floor of the mouth requires external retraction or palpation technique, these structures should be done consecutively as a group. In this way the need for repeated handwashing can be minimized. Thus the sequence presented in this chapter will be as logical and efficient as possible while still preserving maximal asepsis.

The clinician must be fully acquainted with the hard and soft tissue anatomy of the head and neck and especially of the oral cavity. To perform an examination that is comprehensive, it is necessary to be able to discriminate normal appearances from abnormal ones. For records to be universally understandable, the clinician must be well acquainted with the specific names and terminology associated with the structures to be examined and record all findings accurately.

To begin the intraoral examination procedure, the back of the dental chair should be lowered to a semisupine position. The clinician should be seated at the 9 o'clock (3 o'clock for left-handed clinician) position, where a direct view of the oral cavity and structures can be obtained. The patient should be asked to *remove all dental appliances* that are not permanent, and they are placed in appropriate containers until they can be examined. Radiographs should have been reviewed prior to the appointment, if they were available. Information from the radiographs will be correlated with the head and neck examination to aid in the detection of clinical findings. All necessary forms and supplies should be assembled and placed within easy reach of the clinician and assistant. Since this is the first intraoral procedure that the clinician is likely to perform, the hands should have been thoroughly scrubbed and gloved prior to the examination.

Before beginning a detailed examination of each structure, it is wise to *perform a cursory screening* of the intraoral tissues with the mouth mirror or a tongue blade. This screening is to determine whether or not there are contagious lesions present that should not be contacted because of the risk of disease transmission (e.g., herpes simplex, syphilis) or patient discomfort (e.g., mouth ulcers, other traumatic lesions). The clinician should briefly inspect the following structures: lips, labial mucosa, buccal mucosa, hard palate, soft palate, tongue, floor of mouth, and alveolar ridges (Figs. 9-18 and 9-19). The clinician should also check the throat for signs of severe sore throat or other manifestations that would suggest that the patient should be seen or treated by a physician before any intraoral procedures are performed. A serious sequela of performing an examination of oral tissues in the presence of a severe sore throat could be the introduction of multitudes of streptococci into the bloodstream. If the patient has a history of heart disease, a subacute bacterial endocarditis could result. The dental professional should postpone additional treatment until any acute infections have subsided or until infective leasions have healed. This will provide protection not only for the patient, but also for the dental personnel and other patients who could encounter the disease pathogens indirectly from contaminated surfaces or supplies.

Once the initial screening is complete and no contraindications to continuing treatment have been detected, the clinician should start the inspection and palpation of all intraoral structures using the following sequence:

1. *Lips.* Inspect the clinical appearance of the lips before retracting them. The skin should be intact and have a semimoist, firm texture. They should be free of all lesions, discolorations, growths, or swellings. Common abnormalities that might be detected include chapped lips, cracks at the corners of the mouth, traumatic lesions such as from lip biting and blisters, ulcers, and cold sores. Protect dry and cracked areas from further trauma by applying petroleum jelly to lubricate the area during retraction. Avoid touching ulcers or blisters. The wearing of gloves is advised.

2. *Labial mucosa.* Retract the mandibular labial mucosa down and away from the teeth. Grasp the tissues so that the thumb is placed intraorally and the fingers are kept extraorally. Always try to use

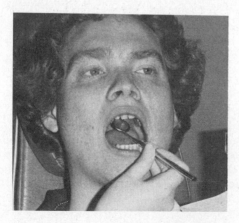

Fig. 9-18. A quick but thorough initial inspection of all areas of the mouth should be made before clinician begins more comprehensive examination of intraoral structures. In this view, a mirror is being used to examine palate and back of mouth.

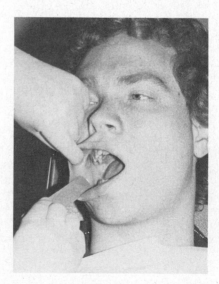

Fig. 9-19. A tongue blade may also be used to assist in tissue retraction during intraoral inspection.

this same arrangement so that the fingers used extraorally do not go back inside the mouth at any time unless the hands have been washed again. This will help reduce contamination during the examination. On the labial mucosa check for a moist red surface that does not demonstrate any abnormal lesions, masses, or color deviation. You might notice small white or yellowish bumps located just below the mucosal lining. These are probably the labial sebaceous glands and are normal for this tissue. Examine the labial frenum for any tissue

tags or lesions. Check also to make sure that this muscle attachment is not pulling on the gingival tissues and causing recession. Continue this inspection and retraction around the corners of the mouth and up onto the maxillary labial mucosa. Palpate this tissue using bilateral, bidigital compression, feeling the tissues between the thumb and fingers. Note any swelling, hard masses, or tenderness (Figs. 9-20 to 9-22).

3. *Buccal mucosa.* Retract the buccal mucosa out and slightly away from the teeth so that its surface can be inspected from the labial mucosa back to the retromolar area. Alternately extend and examine the vestibular areas. As with the labial mucosa, the tissue should be moist and red. The soft tissue structure visible opposite the maxillary molar area is the parotid papilla. It houses the opening of Stensen's duct of the parotid salivary gland. Check the salivary flow by drying the duct opening with a gauze square and applying light, intermittent external pressure to the parotid gland. Watch for evidence of salivary flow from the duct opening. Examine the tissues for swelling, lesions, breaks in the mucosa, or abnormal color changes, including white or red patches. There will be variable amounts of brown melanin pigmentation in this tissue, depending on the race of the patient. Increased pigmentation is prevalent in members of the black race. Palpate this area bimanually by placing the fingers of one hand intraorally against

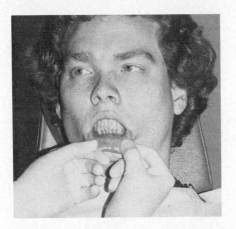

Fig. 9-20. Mandibular labial mucosa is retracted and examined. General appearance of gingiva and frenum attachments are also assessed.

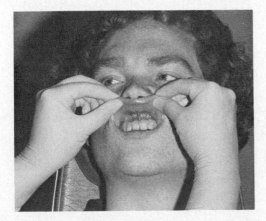

Fig. 9-21. Maxillary labial mucosa is retracted; clinician should try to use same fingers intraorally at all times if possible, or wash hands before proceeding.

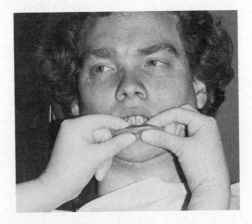

Fig. 9-22. Labial mucosa is palpated with bilateral bidigital compression, moving from midline to corners of mouth.

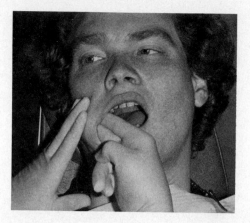

Fig. 9-23. Buccal mucosa is palpated bimanually with fingers of one hand inside mouth and fingers of other hand supporting tissues extraorally.

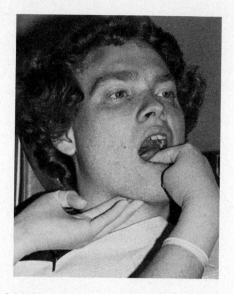

Fig. 9-24. Floor of mouth is palpated bimanually by placing one hand intraorally and supporting tissues against extraoral hand. Entire floor of mouth should be examined in this way.

the tissues while the other hand supports the tissues extraorally. Palpate the tissue between the two hands from the front of the mouth all the way back to the retromolar area. Note all abnormal swellings, masses, or tenderness (Fig. 9-23). Common findings may include Fordyce's granules, xerostomia, scarring, cheek biting, and linea alba.

4. *Floor of the mouth.* Before washing hands and proceeding with the rest of the intraoral examination, examine the floor of the mouth. Ask the patient to lift the tongue to the roof of the mouth. This area should appear moist and extremely vascular. Examine the following structures of the floor of the mouth:

Lingual vein. This vein courses up either side of the ventral surface of the tongue. Varicosities may be seen in the older patient.

Plica fimbriata. These are small hairlike projections of tissue that lie along the lingual vein.

Lingual frenum. This is the muscle attachment between the tongue and the floor of the mouth. An extremely short lingual frenum will restrict the movement of the tongue (ankyloglossia or "tongue-tied"). This is often detected when the tongue cannot touch the palate. It may also be manifested in abnormal speech patterns.

Sublingual caruncle. This is located at the base of the frenum and appears as a small rounded projection. It houses the opening of Wharton's duct for the submandibular salivary gland. Test the action of this duct by drying the floor of the mouth with a gauze square and then applying intermittent compression to the sub-

mandibular tissue between the ducts. Observe the floor of the mouth for the rate and amount of saliva flow entering the area.

Sublingual folds. These appear as two elevations or ridges that run along the floor of the mouth on either side of the tongue. These tissues house the ducts of Rivinus that service the minor sublingual salivary gland in the floor of the mouth.

Plica lingualis. These are small hairlike projections of tissue that lie along the crest of the sublingual folds.

While inspecting these structures, inspect the floor of the mouth for lesions or abnormal color changes. Palpate the area by placing the right hand intraorally and the left hand extraorally and feeling the tissues between the two hands (bimanual palpation) (Fig. 9-24). Note any swellings, masses, white or red patches, the comparative size of glands, and any tenderness described by the patient.

Since the remainder of the examination will involve only intraoral structures, the clinician should now stop and wash both hands before proceeding.

The next area to be examined is the *hard palate.* With the light source directed up onto the palate, inspect the surface for lesions, swellings, and color deviations. A normal palatal surface will appear light pink and will have the following anatomic structures:

incisive papilla A protuberance of soft, firm tissue located between the two central incisors. It covers the incisive foramen, which is the opening for the blood and nerve supply to this area of the palate. This papilla is normally slightly redder than the surrounding palatal tissue because of increased blood supply.

medial palatal raphe A white line extending from the incisive papilla to the soft palate.

palatal rugae Irregular ridges of tissue irradiating from either side of the raphe.

palatine foveae Two small depressions, one on either side of the midline, at the junction of the hard and soft palate.

Inspection of these structures may reveal abnormalities such as nicotine stomatitis, inflamed incisive papilla, ulcerations, palatal tori, or redness and irritation due to dentures.

Palpate the palate using digital compression of one or two fingers against the palatal surface (Fig. 9-25). Take care not to extend this technique onto the soft palate, since this could initiate gagging in some patients. It should also be noted that firm on and off pressure against the tissue is more comfortable than light circular pressure, which tends to "tickle" the palate. Palpate for swellings or hard masses (e.g., palatal tori), tenderness, and continuity of the underlying bone.

Next inspect the back of the mouth and examine the *soft* palate for color and lesions (Fig. 9-26). Observe the *palatine uvula* for deviations in form or color. To examine the oral pharynx, place a tongue depressor on the middle third of the dorsum of the tongue and ask the patient to say "ah." As the patient does this, the posterior third of the tongue should lower, providing a full view of the entire area. Observe also the movement of the uvula as the patient is saying "ah." Note any deviation of movement to either the right or the left. With the pharynx clearly visible, locate the following structures and examine them for color and signs of abnormal lesions or form: posterior wall of the pharynx, posterior pillars, palatine tonsils, and anterior pillars. Note any redness, signs of exudation, lesions, or tenderness.

The examination of the tongue is specific for each of four surfaces: the dorsal (top), ventral (bottom), and the two lateral borders. Examine the

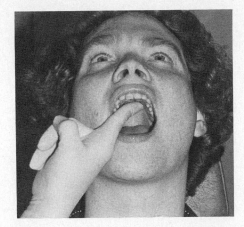

Fig. 9-25. Hard palate is palpated using firm digital pressure against hard tissues.

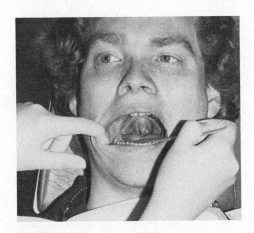

Fig. 9-26. Since the tongue normally shields the oral pharynx from view, this area is examined by placing a mirror or tongue blade on anterior third of tongue and asking patient to say "ah."

dorsal surface first for color, lesions, symmetry, and form. The normal structures of this surface of the tongue include:

filiform papillae Plentiful hairlike papillae covering the dorsal surface of the tongue. These generally have a whitish color, although they often are stained extrinsically from food, tobacco, or medication.

fungiform papillae Flat, broad papillae that appear as red, mushroom-shaped elevations and are scattered among the filiform papillae. They house taste buds for sweet, sour, or salty stimuli.

circumvallate papillae A series of large papillae located in a V-formation on the posterior dorsal surface. They contain taste buds that respond to bitter stimuli only.

Retract the tongue by wrapping a gauze square around the anterior third to obtain a firm grasp and pulling it anteriorly as far as it will extend comfortably. Palpate the dorsal surface using digital compression over the entire surface (Figs. 9-27 and 9-28). Feel for abnormal masses, indurations, or swellings. Common abnormalities that may be detected on the dorsal surface of the tongue include a coated tongue, black hairy tongue, geographic tongue, and fissured tongue.

While still retracting the tongue out from the mouth, inspect the lateral borders by turning the tongue slightly over on its side so that a full view of the border can be seen (Fig. 9-29). Examine this area carefully for abnormal redness, red or white patches, swellings, ulcerations, or masses, since it is a common site for oral cancer. The normal structures found on the lateral borders of the tongue are the foliate papillae, which appear as a series of vertical ridges on the posterior borders. These papillae house taste buds for sour and acidic stimuli. Inspect the other side of the tongue in the same way. Palpate the lateral borders using bidigital compression of the tissue between the thumb and fingers, beginning at the posterior borders and moving to the anterior borders after removing the gauze (Fig. 9-30). Inspect and palpate the entire ventral surface of the tongue using digital compression (Fig. 9-31).

Use the mirror to aid in the inspection of the maxillary tuberosity and retromolar area. Note any deviations in form, color, or size; presence of abnormal growths of tissue; or lesions. Palpate the retromolar areas and maxillary tuberosities using digital compression. Common findings may include scarring from third molar extractions, overgrowth of tissue, inflammation, and tenderness due to erupting third molars.

Thoroughly examine the *alveolar ridges* for signs of redness, color deviations, swellings, or lesions. Retraction of the buccal mucosa and tongue is necessary for good visibility of these structures. Palpate the ridges using bidigital compression with thumb and index finger opposing each other. Examine the ridges for hard masses (tori), swellings, or crepitus, and note any tenderness experienced by the patient (Fig. 9-32).

• • •

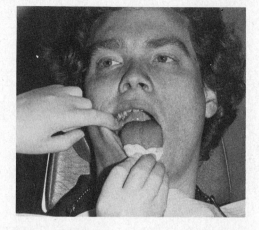

Fig. 9-27. Tongue is grasped by holding it with a folded gauze square and retracted so that entire dorsal surface can be examined.

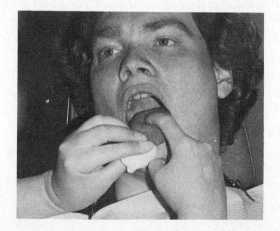

Fig. 9-28. Palpation of dorsal surface of tongue is done with digital compression over entire surface.

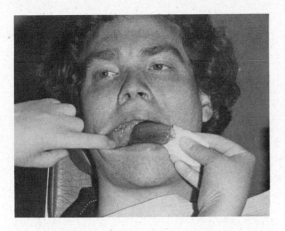

Fig. 9-29. Inspection of lateral borders of tongue involves retracting tongue out using a gauze square and turning it slightly over on its side so that entire lateral border can be closely examined. This is a common site for oral cancer.

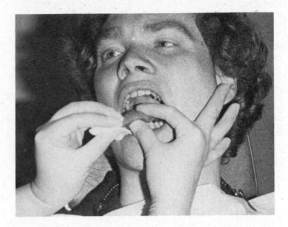

Fig. 9-30. Lateral borders of tongue are palpated with bidigital compression. While one hand stabilizes tongue, the other palpates. This procedure is repeated for other side.

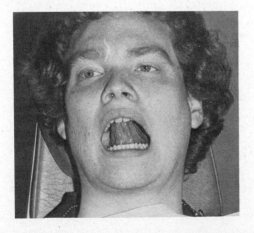

Fig. 9-31. Ventral surface is inspected by asking patient to lift tip of tongue to roof of mouth. With use of a mirror or tongue blade, the floor of the mouth can be examined simultaneously.

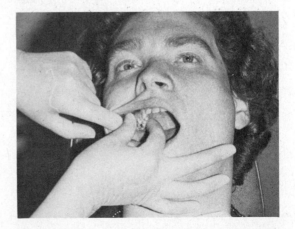

Fig. 9-32. Alveolar ridges are shown being palpated with bidigital compression. Any signs of abnormal masses or lack of continuity in the bone should be noted. Patient should also be requested to report any symptoms experienced during palpation.

This completes the description of the general and oral examination of the patient. After all significant findings are recognized and recorded, the clinician can continue the examination and assessment of the patient with more specific assessments of the dental and periodontal structures in the mouth. These are explained in later chapters, and, together with the information obtained from this portion of the examination, will be used to construct a total picture of the patient's needs so that treatment planning and implementation can be accomplished.

IDENTIFICATION OF PATIENTS WITH SPECIAL NEEDS

During the course of the examination of patients for dental treatment planning, the dental professional may encounter signs and symptoms of conditions that demand the attention of medical and other professionals. As health professionals, the dentist, hygienist, and dental assistant should be alert to the presence of conditions that require referrals. Specific situations discussed in this chapter include nutritional disorders, anorexia nervosa, and child neglect or abuse.

Nutritional disorders

A number of conditions that may be observed during the physical evaluation of the patient may be indicative of nutritional disorders. For example, the hair may lack luster and be thin and sparse; the fingernails may appear spoon shaped, dry, and brittle; the skin may lack color and appear dry and flakey; bruised areas may be visible under the skin because of subdermal bleeding; in general, there is an abnormal lack of body fat; the face may appear red and swollen; areas under the eyes may appear dark and shadowed; the eyes may appear dull or bloodshot; and the corners of the eyes and lips may be dry, red, and fissured.

Intraoral signs that may indicate nutritional deficiencies include gums that bleed easily and a tongue that appears deep red and raw, abnormally smooth and glossy. The tongue may also exhibit sores or hypertrophy of papillae on the dorsal surface. The teeth may show evidence of decay or abnormal eruption patterns.

Other signs that the nutritionally deficient patient may exhibit include an increased heart rate, hypertension, enlargement of the abdominal cavity due to liver or spleen enlargement, mental irritability, loss of normal reflexes in the knees and ankles, and muscle weakness. This list of signs and symptoms is by no means specific only to nutritional disorders, since other medical conditions could produce similar effects. The clinician should combine these findings with information gathered during the patient interview, however, to assess the need for including a nutritional survey in the preventive treatment plan. Additional data from that survey may provide sufficient information that will allow the dental professional to ascertain the role of nutrition in contributing to these conditions (Christokis, 1973).

Anorexia nervosa/bulimia

Patients suffering from anorexia nervosa may be encountered in the dental office for treatment. In general, these patients do not recognize their condition as a health hazard and need the support and understanding of those around them to encourage them to seek professional help. The high-risk group for this condition generally includes adolescents or young women who have a poor self-image and respond by depriving themselves nutritionally in an effort to improve their body image. The results are that these patients show a significant loss of body weight in the absence of any apparent medical problem. Patients with bulimia often go on eating binges and then "purge" themselves by vomiting.

The frequent vomiting has a number of medical and dental implications. Medically, it can lead to cardiac abnormalities, endocrine imbalances, and electrolytic disturbances. Dentally, the patient may exhibit signs of chemical erosion of the teeth and dentinal hypersensitivity, and amalgams may have a "raised" appearance because of the loss of surrounding tooth structure. Patients suffering from this problem will deny its existence and deny vomiting. They do not respond positively to criticism, so an empathetic, yet direct approach to the problem is needed. The treatment of this condition is not within the dental professional's purview; referral for treatment is necessary. The dental professional, however, must consider the oral manifestations of the condition and incorporate effective preventive measures to prevent further loss of tooth structure. Daily fluoride rinses or tray applications of gel can help treat the hypersensitivity and prevent future erosion. In addition, patients should be instructed not to brush immediately after vomiting, since this might increase the eroding effect. Instead, the patient should be instructed to rinse with an alkaline or 0.05% fluoride rinse after vomiting to counteract the acidic effect. Patients who are undergoing treatment for the condition are likely to be on a highly caloric diet, so plaque control measures must be stressed to prevent an increased decay rate (Barkmeier et al., 1982).

Child neglect or abuse

The performance of the general appraisal and head and neck examination of children may lead to suspicions regarding the presence of child neglect or abuse. Dental professionals are obliged legally and ethically to report all cases of suspected abuse or neglect to the appropriate state agency for investigation. In most states failure to report such cases is a punishable offense. Dental professionals are likely to detect the signs and symptoms of an abused child during their examinations, since it is estimated that 50% of the injuries occur to the head, face, and intraoral areas (Becker et al., 1978; Kittle et al., 1981).

There is a difference in the meaning of the terms *child neglect* and *child abuse*. *Child neglect* refers to physical or emotional negligence relative to a child. These are usually cases of omission (failure to provide shelter, food, and medical and dental care). Child neglect in terms of dental care might include such findings as untreated rampant caries, untreated dental pain or infection, or a lack of continuity of dental care in the presence of known pathology (Davis et al., 1979).

Child abuse includes any physical, sexual, or emotional act that is directed against a child. During the general appraisal of the patient, the dental professional might notice that the child appears fearful, withdrawn, watchful, and provides no eye contact or spontaneous smiles. There may be signs of malnutrition, uncleanliness, limping, or a slumped or withdrawn posture. During the extraoral examination signs of bruises, slap marks, bite marks, black eyes, cigarette burns, or abrasions and lacerations in unusual places should be noted. The ears should be examined for signs of trauma that might have been caused by twisting, pulling, or pinching. Marks on the neck that might have been caused by strangling may be detected (Davis et al., 1979).

Intraorally, signs of child abuse may include

teeth that have been fractured or displaced; scars on the lips, mucosa, or tongue; binding marks at the corners or the mouth where the child had been gagged; darkened or nonvital teeth; or laceration to the maxillary frenum. Jaw fractures might also result from abuse.

Surveys of abused children have shown that there are no reliable predictors for its occurrence. The age distribution varies from birth to 17 years. Children from all socioeconomic groups are affected (Davis et al., 1979; Kittle et al., 1981). Swartz et al. (1977) have noted little difference in the incidence of the problem based on racial, religious, economic, or educational grounds. In the United States over 1 million cases are reported each year (Kittle et al., 1981), and it is difficult to estimate how many cases escape detection. This is a serious problem that deserves the attention and action of the dental community to assist in its detection and solution.

The responsibility of the dental professional is to diagnose the problem through a number of steps. The professional must first recognize the presence of traumatic injuries and then attempt to relate them to the explanations that are supplied by both the child and the parents. If the explanations seem unsatisfactory in explaining the nature of the injuries, the dental professional may seek assistance through consultation with the family's physician or with special agencies set up to deal with these problems. As stated previously, if child abuse or neglect is suspected, the dental professional has both a legal and an ethical responsibility to report the case to the appropriate state agency for investigation (Swartz et al., 1977).

ACTIVITIES

1. Obtain a presentation designed to teach the concepts of blood pressure screening and hypertension such as *Hypertension . . . The Silent Killer:* "Screening" (14:41) B-1460 and "Practice in Blood Pressure Reading" (13:40) B-1315.*
2. Practice the procedures for determining each of the four vital signs on a lab partner or clinic patient.
3. Practice the procedures for intraoral and extraoral examination on a lab partner or clinic patient. To

*Written by Jane Anderson, G.D.H., B.S., and Nancy Champlin Geistfeld, G.D.H., B.S. Produced by Health Sciences Learning Resources, Dental Audio-Visual, Biomedical Graphic Communications, University of Minnesota, Minneapolis.

sharpen tactile perceptions during the palpation of hard and soft tissues, work in pairs and practice palpating individual structures on a lab partner with your eyes closed. Concentrate on the different anatomic structures and textures that you feel and describe these to your partner.

4. Arrange for a guest speaker from the oncologic department of a nearby hospital to speak on the incidence of oral cancer in your area; check with the local American Cancer Society to get the latest pamphlets, statistics, and public information on oral cancer.

5. Have a group discussion about students' feelings regarding touching another person's body as in the head and neck examination. Some students react at first with embarrassment at having to perform this procedure on strangers. Discuss ways in which these feelings might be dealt with. Role play explaining the purpose and use of the oral examination to a patient. Include in the role play a situation in which a suspicious lesion that might be cancerous is detected. What would be said to the patient in that situation? When discussing the role play, ask the "patient" what feelings or reactions he/she had to a thorough examination.

6. Contact the state or local child welfare department to find out the exact procedures required for reporting child neglect or abuse in your state.

7. Show slides of a variety of intraoral and extraoral lesions and have students write a clinical description of each lesion.

REVIEW QUESTIONS

1. State five reasons for performing a complete general and oral examination.
2. List the four vital signs.
3. State the normal range for each of the following:
   a. Adult pulse
   b. Adult respiration rate
   c. Adult temperature
   d. Adult blood pressure
   e. Borderline temperature for fever
   f. Borderline blood pressure for hypertension
4. Describe the procedure for obtaining a patient's:
   a. Pulse rate
   b. Blood pressure
5. State the four methods of examination described in the text and give an example of how each method is used.
6. Describe the palpation technique recommended for the following structures:
   a. Submandibular lymph nodes
   b. Floor of the mouth
   c. Buccal mucosa

7. Why is the initial inspection of the mouth necessary before the clinician's hands enter the mouth?
8. What chain of lymph nodes is located near each of the following structures?
   a. Ear
   b. Sternocleidomastoid muscle
   c. Base of the skull
   d. Floor of the mouth

REFERENCES

Abbey, L.M., et al. 1976. A resurvey of hypertensive patients detected in a dental office screening program. J. Public Health Dent. **36**:244. (a)

Abbey, L.M., et al. 1976. Hypertension screening among dental patients. J. Am. Dent. Assoc. **93**:996. (b)

American Cancer Society. 1983. Cancer statistics 1983. CA **33**:9.

Argentieri, R. 1978. Dental care for the hypertensive patient. N.Y. State Dent. J. **44**:55.

Barkmeier, W.W., et al. 1982. Anorexia nervosa: recognition and management. J. Oral Med. **37**:33.

Bates, B. 1982. A guide to physical examination, ed. 3. Philadelphia: J.B. Lippincott Co.

Becker, D.B., et al. 1978. Child abuse and dentistry: orofacial trauma and its recognition by dentists. J. Am. Dent. Assoc. **97**:24.

Bennett, C.R. 1984. Monheim's local anesthesia and pain control in dental practice, ed. 7. St. Louis: The C.V. Mosby Co.

Blozis, G.G. 1979. Blood pressure. In Boundy, S.S., and Reynolds, N.J., editors. Current concepts in dental hygiene, vol. 2. St. Louis: The C.V. Mosby Co.

Bodak-Gyovai, L., and Manzione, G.V. 1980. Oral medicine: patient evaluation and management. Baltimore: Williams & Wilkins.

Bowen, P.L. Feb. 1980. Child neglect identification: the hygienist and child advocacy. Dent. Hyg. **54**:71.

1979 Cancer facts and figures. 1978. New York: American Cancer Society, Inc.

Castano, F.A., and Alden, B.A. 1973. Handbook of expanded dental auxiliary practice. Philadelphia: J.B. Lippincott Co.

Christokis, G., editor. Nov. 1973. Clinical assessment of nutritional status, Am. J. Publ. Health (Suppl.) **63**:18.

Chue, P.N.Y. 1975. Hypertension: implications for dentistry. Dent. Surv. **51**:25.

Conway, B.J. Dec. 1980. High blood pressure screening and referral by dentists: legal implications of blood pressure measurement in the dental practice. R. I. Dent. J. **13**:16.

Cooley, R.L., and Lubow, R.M. 1983. AIDS: an occupational hazard, J. Am. Dent. Assoc. **107**:28.

Davis, G.R., et al. 1979. The dentist's role in child abuse and neglect. J. Dent. Child. **46**:185.

Engelman, M.A., and Schackner, S.J. 1966. Oral cancer examination procedure. Poughkeepsie, N.Y.: Oral Diagnostic Center, St. Francis Hospital.

Freis, E.D. 1973. Age, race, sex and other indices of risk in hypertension. Am. J. Med. **55**:275.

Gaynor, A.M. Jan. 1983. Commonly used drugs in dentistry and the hypertensive patient. W. Va. Dent. J. **57**:18.

Glass, R.T., et al. 1975. Teaching self-examination of the head and neck: another aspect of preventive dentistry. J. Am. Dent. Assoc. **90:**1265.

Halstead, C.L., et al. 1982. Physical evaluation of the dental patient. St. Louis: The C.V. Mosby Co.

Joint National Committee on Detection, Evaluation, and Treatment of High Blood Pressure. 1980 Report. Dec. 1980. U.S. Department of Health and Human Services, Public Health Service–National Institutes of Health, NIH Pub. No. 81-1088. (Also published in Arch. Intern. Med. **140:**1280, Oct. 1980.)

Kerr, D.A., Ash, M.M, and Millard, H.D. 1983. Oral diagnosis, ed. 6. St. Louis: The C.V. Mosby Co.

Kirkendall, W.M., et al. 1980. Recommendations for human blood pressure determination by sphygmomonometers. Circulation **62:**1146A.

Kittle, P.E., et al. 1981. Two child abuse/child neglect examinations for the dentist. J. Dent. Child. **48:**175.

Kutcher, M.J., et al. 1981. Oral medicine in general dental practice. I. Physical evaluation of the dental patient. Compend. Contin. Educ. Dent. **2:**79.

Laragh, J.H. 1974. An approach to the classification of hypertensive state. Hosp. Pract. **9:**61.

Longenecker, S., and Beck, F. Aug. 1983. Blood pressure measurement—referral of suspected hypertensive dental patients. Dent. Hyg. **57:**18.

Mashberg, A. 1978. Erythroplasia: the earliest sign of asymptomatic oral cancer. J. Am. Dent. Assoc. **96:**615.

Miller, D., Grainger, D., and Gagliardi, H. 1973. Expanded functions manual for on the job training. Florida Department of Education and Florida Dental Journal.

Newkirk, C. 1977. The hypertensive dental patient: detection and treatment. Dent. Hyg. **51:**205.

Silverberg, D.S. 1976. The dentist's role in hypertension detection. J. Can. Dent. Assoc. **42:**549.

Silwitz, R.H. 1977. The dental professional's role in programs for detection of high blood pressure. J. Public Health Dent. **37:**253.

Singer, J., et al. Aug. 1983. Blood pressure fluctuations during dental hygiene treatment. Dent. Hyg. **57:**24.

Swartz, S, et al. 1977. Oral manifestations and legal aspects of child abuse. J. Am. Dent. Assoc. **95:**586.

Weedman, B., and Warman, E. 1980. Lymph nodes of the head and neck, J. Oral Med. **35:**39.

10 BASIC EMERGENCY PROCEDURES

OBJECTIVES: *The reader will be able to*

1. Explain briefly why a dental hygienist should:
   a. Be able to identify basic emergency signs and symptoms
   b. Follow a predetermined pattern of procedures in response to any emergency situation
   c. Successfully complete a comprehensive course of study in first aid and basic life support
2. Identify the location and contents of the medical emergency kit in a given clinical setting.
3. Locate and operate the oxygen supply and equipment in a given clinical setting.
4. Maintain a complete, current medical emergency armamentarium for use in a dental clinical setting.
5. Describe the basic signs of medical emergencies likely to occur in a dental office.
6. Given signs and symptoms of medical emergencies, specify the proper responses to each situation.
7. Identify how a complete, reviewed medical history and preoperative vital signs can function in preventing and identifying medical emergencies.
8. Develop and rehearse a plan of action among clinical team members for each medical emergency sign.
9. Identify basic fire, accident, and personal injury prevention guidelines for a clinical setting.

Prior to beginning clinical practice, it is essential that a dental hygiene student be able to identify and respond to basic emergency signs, which may occur while providing care for patients. It is also important for the student to recall significant assessment data that may indicate the likelihood and nature of an emergency situation for the patient. This chapter serves to alert the student to the rudiments of responsible attention to safety in practice. *A complete course in first aid and in basic life support, including cardiopulmonary resuscitation (CPR) and techniques for clearing the airway, is essential.*

THE HYGIENIST'S ROLE

A dental hygienist often works in situations in which he/she is the first to recognize the potential for a medical emergency, since the dental hygienist may be the one to perform the medical history and record vital signs. Likewise, working with a patient in a private or semiprivate operatory frequently makes the hygienist the sole observer of the patient's condition and responses to various phases of care. It is the competent hygienist's responsibility to *monitor the patient's responses* throughout care, being constantly aware of changes in expression, skin tone, muscle tonus, respirations, and verbal expression. As intraoral procedures are performed, the clinician's peripheral vision should watch for signs of distress, relaxation, puzzlement, and other indications of the patient's state.

An additional responsibility is to be able to *classify the kinds of responses* and identify when an emergecy situation seems imminent. Prompt, appropriate reaction to a patient showing signs of distress may avert an emergeny and even save a life. Being able to provide complete descriptions of signs of distress to the dentist or attending medical team can hasten the provision of appropriate care.

A further responsibility that may be assumed following a comprehensive first aid and life-support course is that of *administering care to reverse an emergency or to sustain life* until help can be secured. This role is essential for hygienists who function under general supervision when a dentist or physician may or may not be present and for hygienists who work as part of a team on which only one person, such as the dentist, has training in managing emergencies. The one person who is trained to manage such a situation may be the one in distress, or that person may "freeze" under the pressure of the emergency and be unable to respond quickly and appropriately. Ideally, all members of the dental team should be qualified to administer oxygen, record vital signs, perform basic procedures to open an airway, and perform CPR. As a primary provider of care, the dental hygienist certainly has this responsibility.

Once the signs of distress are noted, the clinician should be able to *follow a logical, rehearsed pattern of behavior* in response to the signs. The response may be simply to move instruments and other pieces of potentially harmful equipment away from the patient, to raise the back of the chair, to lower the back for a full supine position, to calmly go for help or push the emergency signal button, or to let the patient rest quietly for a moment. It may also include preparing a syringe for an intramuscular (IM), intravenous (IV), or subcutaneous injection; performing CPR; or directing an emergency squad to the right location. For each possible situation, the clinician should be prepared to respond in a predetermined fashion, since there may be little time for contemplation or turning to references for suggested behavior.

BEING PREPARED TO ACT

Responding to a medical emergency involves many steps that can and should be divided among dental team members according to their skill levels and ability to react quickly and appropriately under stress. All team members should be aware of the possible problems and the proper responses to ensure that everyone participates knowledgeably and according to a well-rehearsed plan. While procedures should be divided and delegated to individual team members, the division should be flexible enough to ensure that all steps are taken even when a team member is missing, or worse yet, is the subject of the emergency care.

A rehearsal of who performs what functions for one of the variety of anticipated emergencies should be held monthly, according to a carefully delineated script. For instance, in the event of aspiration of a foreign object into the lung, the cli-

nician would follow predetermined steps to assist the patient and alert another team member to notify the dentist and the emergency squad.

Examples of more specific common emergency procedures performed by team members and the speed and competence at which they must be performed are (Kinne, 1982):

1. Remove the oxygen mask from storage, attach to the oxygen unit, obtain a tight fit to the patient's face, and start the oxygen flow within 30 seconds.
2. Remove the stethoscope from storage, and obtain breath sounds at four locations and heart sounds at one location within 45 seconds. (NOTE: Use the stethoscope on the larynx first.)
3. Expose the neck, locate and palpate the carotid pulse for a period of 15 seconds, and calculate the pulse rate within 20 seconds.
4. Select and remove from storage the correct blood pressure cuff, place it correctly on the patient's arm, palpate the brachial artery, raise the pressure until the pulse is no longer palpable, and call out the level within 20 seconds.
5. With the appropriate-size blood pressure cuff in place in the correct position on the patient's arm, palpate the brachial artery, position the diaphragm of the stethoscope, inflate the cuff, and call out the systolic and diastolic levels within 60 seconds.
6. Move the patient to the floor for CPR, without harming the patient, within 10 seconds.
7. Locate lidocaine in the emergency drug kit and the appropriate syringe, determine the patient's weight, calculate and call out the correct dosage, and load the syringe and remove air bubbles within 35 seconds.

Emergency phone numbers must be readily accessible and ideally are attached to the phone itself. Procedures for alerting other team members of the occurrence of an emergency should be unmistakable, but, as much as possible, a calm atmosphere should be preserved.

There are many tasks to be performed that must be assigned and rehearsed. Eleven generic functions described by Kinne (1982) that are a part of any emergency are:

1. Evaluate the vital signs.
2. Diagnose the nature of the emergency.

3. Decide on the appropriate treatment.
4. Instruct others on what to do.
5. Phone for help.
6. Prepare for treatment administration.
7. Administer treatment.
8. Monitor vital signs.
9. Reassure the patient.
10. Record events that occur.
11. Ensure privacy and/or manage other patients.

EMERGENCY SUPPLIES AND EQUIPMENT

The dental clinical setting must include standard supplies if the clinician is to be adequately prepared to respond to emergency situations. The contents of an emergency "kit" should include injectable drugs such as epinephrine, diazepam, and others; and noninjectable drugs such as aromatic ammonia, oxygen, and others (Table 10-1).

Additional emergency supplies include an oxygen delivery system, suction and suction tips, syringes, tourniquets, an airway, a blood pressure cuff, and a stethoscope. Materials for an eyewash, such as boric acid crystals and an eye cup should be available for rinsing a foreign object or chemical from the eye. Orange juice should be available for ready administration to a patient suffering from hypoglycemia (low blood sugar). A blanket should be available to cover a patient who is in shock or who is having chills or to smother flames. Bandages and an antiseptic are useful for minor cuts and scrapes.

A portable or wall-connected oxygen supply is also an indispensable item. Many emergency situations require support or assistance for the respiratory function of the patient. Syncope (simple fainting), cardiac problems, vasodepression, and many other maladies require the use of pulmonary support, ideally with a higher concentration of oxygen than regular air. Even if fixed wall units are used, one portable unit should be available for use in a remote site such as the reception area (Malamed, 1982).

The oxygen can be delivered to the patient through a positive pressure oxygen mask that forces 100% oxygen into the patient's lungs (Malamed, 1982). The ability to force oxygen into the patient's lungs is important for unconscious patients who cannot breathe on their own. A clear face mask is best because the clinician can observe the patient's mouth for vomitus, blood, or other secretions through the mask. The mask should fit over the patient's nose and mouth. An expiration valve allows expired air to be released.

Oxygen can also be delivered through a portable self-inflating resuscitation bag (i.e., an Ambu bag that is attached to a face mask). The mask is placed over the patient's nose and mouth, and the bag is squeezed to force room air (about 20% oxygen) into the patient's lungs. This bag and mask system is a wise addition to emergency equipment, since a patient may require resuscitation in a waiting room, hallway, or rest room. This bag system may be attached to a portable oxygen tank system to force 100% oxygen into the patient's lungs if necessary.

Oxygen can be delivered to patients from equipment such as a nitrous oxide and oxygen sedation system. This system does not force the oxygen into the patient's lungs unless it has a special positive pressure attachment. This oxygen delivery system

Table 10-1. Emergency drugs

Category	Examples
Injectable	
For acute allergic reactions	Epinephrine (Adrenalin)
Anticonvulsant	Diazepam (Valium)
Antihistaminic	Chlorpheniramine (Chlor-Trimeton) maleate
Analgesic	Morphine sulfate
Vasopressor	Methoxamine (Vasoxyl) hydrochloride
Corticosteroids	Hydrocortisone succinate (Solu-Cortef)
Antihypoglycemic	50% dextrose, glucagon
Narcotic antagonist	Naloxone (Narcan)
Noninjectable	
Oxygen	—
Respiratory stimulant	Aromatic ammonia
Antihypoglygemic	Carbohydrate (i.e., sugar packets or orange juice)
Bronchodilator	Epinephrine (i.e., an inhalant)
Vasodilator	Nitroglycerin

Data from Malamed, S.F. 1982. Handbook of medical emergencies in the dental office, ed. 2. St. Louis: The C.V. Mosby Co.

is appropriate for a patient in distress who is able to breathe on his/her own, such as a patient suffering from syncope.

Practice in using the available oxygen supply and mask is an important exercise in achieving baseline competence in providing emergency care.

Since recording vital signs at frequent intervals is the recommended procedure for most emergencies requiring the administration of oxygen, a clipboard with a form for entering readings at 5-minute intervals can be attached directly to the oxygen apparatus (Blitz, 1979; Malamed, 1982). This record can then accompany the patient to the hospital.

The tanks that store the oxygen should be maintained so that at least a 1-hour supply is available for an emergency situation; 1 hour should allow time for the arrival of emergency assistance and transport to the hospital, if necessary. Malamed (1982) recommends that portable tanks with at least a 30-minute supply (size E) be used in dental offices. At least one extra full tank should be available to provide a 1-hour supply of oxygen. A clear and precise record should be kept on the tanks in use, which indicates the date of each use and the amount of time the tank was used. When less than 10 minutes remain on an oxygen tank that is to be used in emergency situations, the clinician should consider changing the tank. Full backup tanks should *always* be available.

All emergency equipment should be readily accessible to staff and centrally located. As with any program designed for an emergency, all supplies and equipment should be regularly inspected. Out-of-date (expired) drugs must be replaced; malfunctioning equipment must be repaired or replaced.

MEDICAL EMERGENCIES IN THE DENTAL ENVIRONMENT

Any medical emergency can occur in the dental office. Patients with a predisposition to a medical emergency (such as patients with high blood pressure, cardiac insufficiency, asthma, or angina) may be more likely to experience such an occurrence in a dental office, since anxiety levels may be high for a patient anticipating or experiencing dental care. The combination of a medical problem and the anxiety may trigger a physical response that can be classified as an emergency (Trieger, 1982).

Table 10-2 summarizes the signs, symptoms, and treatments for the medical emergencies presented in this section. The emergency situations presented here are by disease or emergency (e.g., syncope, cardiac arrest, angina pectoris). But when a medical emergency occurs, the clinician will be faced with the signs and symptoms of a patient experiencing a medical emergency, such as an unconscious or convulsing patient. It is strongly suggested that the reader complete activities 8 and 9 on p. 175 to prepare for responding to a medical emergency.

Syncope, or simple fainting, can occur if the patient's brain fails to receive adequate oxygen and glucose as the result of vasodilation or loss of vasomotor tone. The signs of simple syncope are loss of color from the skin (pallor), perspiration, slight confusion, complaints of nausea or dizziness, and sometimes loss of consciousness from which the patient can be roused; in coma, the patient cannot be roused (Miller, 1982). Since most dental procedures are performed with the patient in the supine position, which facilitates adequate blood flow to the brain, syncope is probably a less likely occurrence now than in the era of the upright position (Miller, 1982).

Sitting up rapidly after being in a supine or recumbent position can, however, bring on syncope.

If a patient does exhibit signs of syncope and complains of discomfort, instruments should be moved away, the chair should be adjusted to the full supine position and another team member should be alerted. Oxygen should be readied for administration, a cool cloth may be applied to the patient's forehead, and an ammonia ampule should be ready for wafting under the patient's nose.

Many times, prompt action such as described can avert loss of consciousness. If the patient does retain consciousness, he/she should be allowed to rest comfortably, essential procedures such as suturing an area should be completed, and the patient should be allowed to leave when fully recovered.

If the patient does lose consciousness, an ammonia ampule can be broken and placed momentarily under the patient's nose (Dunn and Booth, 1975; Malamed, 1982; Miller, 1982). A quick whiff will usually restore consciousness. Oxygen can then be administered along with comforting words. When fully recovered, the patient should be allowed to leave. It may be necessary to escort the patient home.

Table 10-2. Emergencies: signs, symptoms, and treatments

Emergency	Signs and symptoms	Treatment
Syncope (vasopressor syncope; faint)	Pallor Perspiration Slight confusion Nausea Dizziness Sometimes loss of consciousness	Stop treatment; alert team members Place patient in supine position; elevate patient's legs Ensure an open airway; tilt patient's head back Check breathing Monitor vital signs Waft ammonia ample under patient's nose Administer oxygen if needed Place cool towel on patient's forehead Reassure patient

Acute adrenal insufficiency (adrenal crisis)	Confusion
	Weakness
	Extreme fatigue
	Nausea, vomiting
	Decreased blood pressure; pulse may be elevated
	High fever
	Severe pain in abdomen, lower back, legs
	Syncope
	Loss of consciousness
	Coma
		Stop treatment; alert team members
		If conscious:
		   Monitor vital signs
		   Place patient in supine position
		   Administer oxygen
		If unconscious:
		   Place patient in supine position
		   Ensure an open airway
		   Begin CPR
		   Summon emergency medical assistance

Insulin shock (insulin reaction; hypoglycemia)	Loss of consciousness (sometimes)
	Sudden onset of confusion
	Nervousness, agitation
	Cool moist skin
	Hunger
	No alcohol on breath
		Stop treatment; alert team members
		If conscious:
		   Give sugar or orange juice
		If unconscious:
		   Administer glucose by IV or IM

Diabetic coma (hyperglycemia)	Loss of consciousness (sometimes) Gradual onset of confusion Dry skin, flushed Rapid breathing Very thirsty Acetone breath Nausea, vomiting	Stop treatment: alert team members Patient needs insulin; summon medical assistance Transport to hospital Maintain patient

Respiratory problems
  Choking (aspiration)
	Choking
	Coughing
	Panic
	Inability to breathe
	Loss of consciousness
		Stop treatment; alert team members
		If able to cough:
		   Place patient in upright position
		   Allow patient to cough, clearing own airway
		If unable to cough:
		   Place patient in upright position
		   Administer several blows between shoulder blades
		   Administer Heimlich maneuver
		   May need further emergency medical assistance

Data from Howell (1979); Malamed (1982); McCarthy (1982); Woodworth and Woodworth (1978).

Table 10-2. Emergencies: signs, symptoms, and treatments—cont'd

Emergency	Signs and symptoms	Treatment
Hyperventilation	Tingling fingers, toes, perioral area Light-headedness Acute anxiety Rapid breathing Shortness of breath Palpitations Increased pulse rate	Stop treatment; alert team members Assist patient into comfortable position Have patient breathe in and out of a paper bag or headrest cover to increase CO_2 supply Reassure, calm patient
Acute asthmatic attack	Feeling of thickness in chest Coughing Wheezing Increased efforts to breathe Increased anxiety	Stop treatment; alert team members Place patient in comfortable position, usually standing or sitting Administer aerosol spray of epinephrine or similar agent; usually patient has own Administer oxygen Administer IM epinephrine Summon further medical assistance if needed
Chest pain Heart failure	Chest pain Palpitation Feeling of suffocation Coughing, perhaps bloody sputum Possible cyanosis	Stop treatment; alert team members Place patient in upright position Administer oxygen Monitor vital signs Summon emergency medical assistance

Angina pectoris	Mild to severe pain, often radiates to left shoulder and arm
	Patient will remain still to lessen pain
		Stop treatment; alert team members
		Place nitroglycerin tablet under patient's tongue
		Observe patient for pain relief
		If no pain relief:
		  Summon emergency medical assistance
		  Administer oxygen
		  Monitor vital signs

Myocardial infarction	Severe crushing pain
	Pain unrelieved by nitroglycerin
	Cold sweat
	Weakness
	Light-headness
	Restlessness
	Nausea
	Coughing, wheezing
	Abdominal bloating
		Stop treatment; alert team members
		Place nitroglycerin tablet under patient's tongue
		Observe patient for pain relief
		If myocardial infarction, pain continues or increases:
		  Summon emergency medical assistance
		  Administer oxygen
		  Monitor vital signs
		  An analgesic may be given to relieve pain
		  Cardiac arrest is possible; be prepared to begin CPR

Cardiac arrest	May occur as a complication to another emergency (e.g., airway obstruction, drug overdose, anaphylaxis, seizure disorder, acute adrenal insufficiency, myocardial infarction) Cessation of pulse Cessation of respiration	Stop treatment; alert team members Begin CPR Summon emergency medical assistance Monitor vital signs if possible

Continued.

Table 10-2. Emergencies: signs, symptoms, and treatments—cont'd

Emergency	Signs and symptoms	Treatment
Altered consciousness		
Intoxication	Alcohol breath	Stop treatment; alert team members
	Confused, "drunk" appearance	Arrange for patient to be taken home
Hypoglycemia	See insulin shock	
Hyperglycemia	See diabetic coma	
Hypothyroidism	Confused, altered behavior	Stop treatment; alert team members
	Slow speech	Monitor patient
	Lethargy	Summon assistance; consult physician
	Dry skin	
	Puffy face, eyelids	
	Decreased heart rate	
Hyperthyroidism	Unusual, confused behavior	Stop treatment; alert team members
	Anxiousness	Monitor patient
	Slight tremor	Summon assistance; consult physician
	Sweating	
	Rapid speech	
	Increased blood pressure	
	Increased heart rate	
	Flushed skin	
Convulsive state (seizure, epilepsy)	Aura	Stop treatment; alert team members
	May lose consciousness	Place patient in supine position
	May fall	Protect patient from being hurt
	Seizure activity	Establish an airway if necessary
	May lose bowel, urinary control	Prevent aspiration of foreign objects or tongue
	Brief cessation of respiration	Summon assistance
Cerebral vascular accident	Confused, unusual behavior	Stop treatment; alert team members
	Intense headache	Place patient in semierect position
	Weakness or paralysis of speech, extremities	Manage symptoms
		Monitor vital signs
	Dizziness	Summon emergency medical assistance
	Nausea, vomiting	
Allergic reaction		
Mild, transient reaction	Itching	Stop treatment; alert team members
	Urticaria	Place patient in supine position
	Wheezing	Administer antihistimine
		Consult/refer to physician
Severe, immediate reaction (anaphylaxis)	Itching	Stop treatment; alert team members
	Urticaria	Place patient in supine position
	Muscle spasms	Check vital signs
	Fluid accumulation	Summon emergency medical assistance
	Swelling in throat	Give epinephrine IM, IV
	Inability to breathe	Give antihistimine
	May lose consciousness	Begin CPR if needed
Toxic reaction to local anesthesia or vasoconstrictor		
Mild reaction	Restlessness	Stop treatment; alert team members
	Talkativeness	Allow patient's system to remove agent
	Agitation	Treat symptoms
		Observe patient
		Reassure patient
Severe reaction	Agitation	Stop treatment; alert team members
	Excitation, perhaps convulsions followed by:	Check vital signs
		Begin CPR if needed
	Depression of CNS	Summon emergency medical assistance
	May lose consciousness	

Data from Howell (1979); Malamed (1982); McCarthy (1982); Woodworth and Woodworth (1978).

If a woman in the late stages of pregnancy loses consciousness, the back of the chair should be lowered and the patient should be turned onto her side (Malamed, 1982). Placing a woman in the third trimester of pregnancy on her back, especially on a hard surface, can cut off circulation in the venous system; the weight of the uterus impinging on the vena cava can encourage loss of consciousness.

A patient recovering from syncope (or another emergency) may be frightened or even embarrassed. Caring and comforting without being overly solicitous may be appreciated by the patient during the recovery stages.

Syncope is only one of the possible reasons for a patient lapsing into unconsciousness. In the beginning stages of syncope, the patient has a lowered blood pressure and increased pulse. Recovery is usually rapid if the previously mentioned actions are taken. If the recovery is not immediate, the clinician should check for respirations. The mouth mirror can be placed close to the mouth or nose to check for fogging, or the clinician can listen for sounds of respiration by placing his/her ear close to the patient's mouth. The pulse can be checked by placing the fingers in the area of the carotid artery between the larynx and the anterior border of the sternocleidomastoid muscle. If either sign is absent, help should be summoned immediately. Someone should be directed to call a rescue team. Then the procedures of basic life support are begun by the clinician clearing and maintaining an airway, forcing oxygen into the lungs, and performing external cardiac massage if there is no pulse. (Dunn and Booth 1975; Malamed, 1982; McCarthy, 1982).

Acute adrenal insufficiency, wherein the adrenal gland does not produce sufficient amounts of cortisol, rendering the body incapable of coping with stress, is another possible cause of loss of consciousness. Patients likely to experience acute adrenal insufficiency fall into three groups: persons in the late stages of Addison's disease (adrenocortical insufficiency) who have not yet been diagnosed and are not yet taking medication, persons who are suddenly withdrawn from steroid hormones, and persons experiencing stress, particularly those with compromised functioning of the adrenal or pituitary glands (patients receiving corticosteroids) (Malamed, 1982). Many diseases (e.g., Addison's disease, asthma, herpes zoster,

ulcerative colitis, rheumatoid arthritis, lichen planus, to name only a few) are treated with steroid hormones. A thorough review of the patient's medical history, including medications being taken or recently stopped, is imperative so that the clinician can be aware of factors that may predispose a patient to acute adrenal insufficiency. A patient experiencing acute adrenal insufficiency is in danger of death from shock and cardiac arrest. The hygienist should summon assistance, initiate CPR, and relate the symptoms to the dentist or physician, who may administer cortisone to counteract the crisis.

A person with *diabetes mellitus* may lose consciousness as a result of low blood sugar levels (*hypoglycemia*) secondary to a relative excess of insulin. This can happen if a meal is omitted, if the patient exercises heavily and uses available blood glucose, or if there is an overdose of insulin (insulin shock). For the conscious patient, orange juice can reverse the condition. For the unconscious patient, IV or IM glucose is indicated.

Hypoglycemia can occur in patients who do not have diabetes. Patients who skip meals prior to dental treatment and who are anxious about the dental visit may experience a drop in the blood glucose level. Alcoholics suffer from hypoglycemia because of a lack of stored glycogen in the liver and poor nutrition.

Hyperglycemia is a possible cause of loss of consciousness for the diabetic. In this case insulin levels are insufficient; the blood sugar rises above safe levels. Insulin is necessary to reverse this situation. If the patient has a history of insulin shock, this information should be available in the medical history. The patient may carry a supply of insulin for injection, of which the clinician should be aware. Coma associated with hyperglycemia occurs most frequently in juvenile diabetics, usually when the case is first diagnosed. In most cases a comatose patient is hypoglycemic and needs glucose. The response to glucose should be immediate. The hyperglycemic patient will not improve with glucose.

Patients may experience respiratory difficulty in a number of ways. A patient may be *choking* on excess saliva, water, or a foreign object or need to cough for some other reason. If the patient is able to cough, little assistance is necessary other than to position the patient upright so that the foreign material can be cleared from the throat. If the patient cannot cough and begins to express panic, assistance may be necessary to free the air passage, such as with several blows between the shoulder blades or the Heimlich maneuver, in which the air in the lungs is forced out by upward compression on the diaphragm. This technique should be learned under supervision as part of a life-support course.

A second form of respiratory difficulty is *hyperventilation* (Dunn and Booth, 1975; Malamed, 1982), usually due to anxiety, in which insufficient carbon dioxide is present in the bloodstream because of prolonged rapid breathing. It is characterized by tingling fingers and toes, light-headedness, acute anxiety, and rapid breathing. Perioral tingling or numbness is characteristic also of hyperventilation. Usually, having the patient breathe in and out of a bag (a headrest cover, perhaps) will permit the patient to inhale sufficient amounts of carbon dioxide to reverse the problem. The patient should be calmed. A tranquilizer may be necessary in severe cases.

There are two kinds of *asthmatic attacks*. The mild form is more typical and is characterized by a feeling of thickness in the chest, coughing, wheezing, slow and labored breathing, heightened anxiety, a slightly elevated blood pressure, and an elevated heart rate. Treatment for a mild attack includes steps 1 to 3 (see below), which will usually be effective; steps 4 and onward can be taken in the case of a severe attack or if relief is incomplete (Malamed, 1982).

1. Terminate dental therapy.
2. Position the patient comfortably (usually either sitting up or standing.
3. Administer an aerosol spray of epinephrine or similar drug. (Most patients who suffer from these attacks carry a bronchodilator for such emergencies.)
4. Administer oxygen.
5. Give IM or subcutaneous injection of aqueous epinephrine if necessary.
6. Give IV medication if necessary.
7. Summon medical assistance if steps 1 to 6 are ineffective.
8. After recuperation, reevaluate for continued therapy, recovery, and eventual dismissal.

Chest pain associated with cardiovascular problems can be caused by heart failure, angina pectoris, or myocardial infarction. Further discussion of these diseases is found in Chapter 8.

Heart failure will cause respiratory difficulty (Malamed, 1982). The signs of onset include chest pain and palpitation, a feeling of suffocation, coughing including bloody sputum, and possible cyanosis. The difficulty in breathing is due to the filling of the interstitial tissues of the lungs with serous fluid. The patient should be positioned in an upright position as long as the patient is conscious, which allows the excess lung fluid to settle in the lower lung areas so that there can be some exchange of air in the tissues. Oxygen should be administered, avoiding a mask if possible to minimize the patient's sensation of suffocation. Emergency assistance and hospital transport must be summoned. Diuretics to reduce the fluid and digitalis to improve heart contractility may be administered as a part of medical treatment.

Angina pectoris is a temporary lack of oxygen in the heart muscle due to narrowed coronary arteries; exertion, excitement, or eating a heavy meal; or an increased work load. The pain ranges from mild to severe and often radiates to the left shoulder or arm. It usually is not as intense as the pain caused by an infarction, wherein blood supply is cut off to a portion of muscle, causing tissue death. The patient with angina should place a nitroglycerin tablet under the tongue. The nitroglycerin allows the circulatory capacity of the heart muscle to dilate, improving flow and reducing the work load and, thus, pain. Aid should be summoned if the pain persists (McCarthy, 1982).

Myocardial infarction results when the coronary artery flow to some portion of the heart muscle is stopped. It is also called coronary occlusion. The affected muscle dies from lack of oxygen. About 75% of cases are caused by a thrombosis (blood clot). Symptoms are similar to those of angina pectoris, but the pain is more crushing and is not relieved by nitroglycerin. The patient is often in a cold sweat, weak, and restless. In contrast, the patient with angina stays still, knowing movement heightens the pain. An infarction often is accompanied by nausea, light-headedness, coughing, wheezing, and abdominal bloating (which may cause the patient to erroneously infer that the problem is indigestion) (McCarthy, 1982).

A first step is to administer nitroglycerin and

watch for pain relief. If the pain continues or increases, summon emergency assistance, administer oxygen, and monitor vital signs. Drugs for relief of pain can be administered. The emergency medical team should manage complications such as arrhythmia. In the event of cardiac arrest, CPR must be begun to prevent death (Blair, 1982; Malamed, 1982; McCarthy, 1982).

Cardiac arrest occurs when the heart has stopped beating or "circulation of blood is absent or inadequate to maintain life" (Malamed, 1982). Myocardial infarction is only one cause. Others are airway obstruction, drug overdose, anaphylaxis, seizure disorders, and acute adrenal insufficiency. The treatment is to restore circulation. In a dental office CPR, where a heartbeat and respiration are created for the patient through external cardiac compression and compression of oxygen into the lungs, is the method of choice.

All dental health care providers must complete a course in CPR and participate in regular refresher courses.

Altered consciousness can be observed in patients who are intoxicated, patients in early stages of hypoglycemia or hyperglycemia, patients with hypothyroidism or hyperthyroidism, or patients entering a convulsive state, such as epilepsy. The patients should be protected from injuring themselves, should be monitored to ensure they do not lose vital signs, and should be escorted home (in the case of excess alcohol) or taken for physical evaluation by a physician. In severe cases hospitalization may be indicated. In the case of epilepsy, it is important to ensure that the airway is not obstructed by the person biting the tongue (bleeding) or the presence of removable dental appliances.

An additional cause of altered consciousness is a *cerebral vascular accident* in which a blood vessel in the brain breaks or is occluded, preventing adequate blood supply to the brain. Accompanying signs are intense headache, weakness or paralysis of speech and extremities, dizziness, and nausea. The patient should be positioned in a semierect position. The symptoms should be managed until assistance can be summoned.

Reactions to a local anesthetic

Patients can have a reaction to a local anesthetic ranging from syncope to a toxic reaction to an allergic reaction (Malamed, 1982). It is extremely important that a member of the dental team capable of recognizing an emergency situation remain with a patient after he/she has received an injection, since a minor or severe immediate reaction can occur. Most patients are anxious before and during an injection. Syncope is the most common reaction to a local anesthetic injection; its signs and symptoms and the methods for treating it have been described. Another stress-related reaction that can occur is hyperventilation, which has also been described previously.

A *toxic reaction* is due to an overdose of a local anesthetic agent or a vasoconstrictor. It is caused by the clinician injecting more solution that the patient's body can metabolize and excrete. This reaction can be prevented by injecting the solution slowly, injecting only the recommended amount according to body weight, and checking the patient's history for liver or plasma complications. During a mild toxic reaction the patient will appear restless, talkative, and agitated. The clinician should stop administering the agent and allow the patient's system to remove some of the anesthetic; a mild toxic reaction will reverse itself. A severe toxic reaction is characterized by an excitatory stage (agitation or possibly convulsions), followed by a corresponding depression. A patient suffering from such an attack needs immediate medical attention. The clinician should begin life-support measures, alert the supervising dentist immediately, and have someone notify a rescue squad.

Another possible reaction is an *allergic reaction*, which can be a delayed mild reaction or an immediate severe reaction.

The immediate and severe reaction, called *anaphylaxis*, begins with itching and urticaria but rapidly progresses to a life-threatening stage including muscle spasms, fluid accumulation, swelling in the throat causing inability to breathe, and cardiovascular collapse and death (Stroh and Johnson, 1982). Anaphylaxis requires immediate attention, including epinephrine IM or IV, an antihistaminic IM or IV, and a corticosteroid IM or IV. Further assistance from a medical team should be sought.

At the first signs of itching or urticaria, the clinician should stop dental treatment and prepare epinephrine (0.3 ml. of 1:1000 aqueous) for subcutaneous injection. If the reaction progresses, this agent should be administered immediately. If the patient is already in shock, the quickest route for distribution of the drug is IV. Since peripheral veins may be collapsed at this stage, injection is best accomplished by injecting into the highly vascular underside of the tongue. Such injections have been shown to assist resuscitation (Stroh and Johnson, 1982; Shaber and Smith, 1982).

Following injection, the clinician should ensure that the airway is maintained, which may require an emergency tracheostomy. Since the throat is occluded, and no air can circulate, an alternative airway can be created by penetrating the neck with a large-bore needle into the trachea through the cricothyroid cartilage. As soon as the opening is created, the tubeway should be firmly stabilized and oxygen administered via that route.

A mild allergic reaction is characterized by a skin rash and itching; usually this will be a delayed reaction. The patient may call the office several hours after the injection, complaining of a rash and itching. A mild allergic reaction is treated by administering an antihistaminic; the patient should be referred for further medical care.

It is extremely important to accurately record any untoward reaction of a patient during treatment. Many of the medical emergencies described could recur or may indicate a severe physical condition that needs prompt medical attention. The supervising dentist should refer a patient for a medical evaluation if a previously indicated medical condition seems apparent.

In addition to the patient's safety, accurate records are necessary in the case of ensuing legal proceedings. Thorough, objective, accurate progress notes about a medical emergency are part of the dental personnel's best defense.

Accident, personal injury, and fire prevention

Although many emergencies in the dental office relate to the disposition of patient medical emergencies, other kinds of emergencies can be precipitated by negligence, carelessness, or unforeseeable circumstances.

To prevent accidents, it is important to ensure that all equipment is safe and functioning properly. A loose hinge, a missing bolt, or a short circuit can lead to unfortunate accidents that can harm the patient and the dental professional. It is the dental professional's responsibility to protect the patient from harm due to faulty equipment and to eliminate hazards that could cause harm, such as a tangle of cords in the patient's pathway or a wet, slippery floor.

Personal injury can result from criminal acts of intruders as well as from physical hazards in the office. It is always wise to have a co-worker available to summon assistance in the case of a medical emergency and to dissuade persons (including, perhaps, a patient) from assaulting the dental professional. Working alone in a quiet office in close proximity with a patient may stimulate a normal patient and may provoke erratic behavior in an emotionally disturbed patient.

Drugs and cash or checks should be locked away in an unnoticeable place to reduce the likelihood of robbery during or after office hours.

Fire prevention is an additional factor in preventing emergencies. Flammable substances should be kept clear from the flame of a Bunsen burner and from the heat of a radiator. The laboratory, in particular, is a hazardous area, since the open flame of a Bunsen burner may ignite hair, electrical wiring, papers, or other materials. A fire extinguisher should be kept in the laboratory for prompt response to such occurrences. The natural gas supplied to operatories and the laboratory is a potential hazard if there is a leak or if a gas jet is left open. Simply turning on a light switch and producing a spark or static electricity can cause a sudden explosion if such a leak goes undetected and fills the room.

Preparing for emergencies

Once the entire dental team has completed life-support and first aid courses, the team should write out specific protocols for action in the event of medical emergencies. Specific assignments should be made to individuals to ensure that all designated procedures are completed. The protocols should be posted, reviewed monthly, and rehearsed.

Routes for fire escape, procedures for extinguishing fires that are contained, and procedures for summoning assistance should be drafted by the team, reviewed, and rehearsed. Smoke detectors should be installed. A main valve for natural gas should be installed and should be closed at the end of each working day. Again, procedures in the event of a police or fire emergency should be rehearsed. This preparation could save a person's life.

ACTIVITIES

1. Identify the location of the emergency kit in the clinic. Note the contents and purposes of each item included. Also note the expiration date of each drug. Discuss the security system for guarding against theft of drugs while ensuring ready access to drugs during an emergency.
2. Locate and operate the oxygen mask and supply for the conscious and the unconscious patient.
3. Role play various emergency situations, including:
   a. Cardiac arrest
   b. Syncope
   c. Hypoglycemia
   d. Respiratory difficulty
4. Discuss procedures for epileptic seizure and cerebral hemorrhage emergencies.
5. Review a variety of medical histories of medically compromised patients. In groups of three or four, plan for potential medical emergencies and simulate the proper emergency responses for the entire class.
6. Discuss procedures to follow if the dentist or physician in charge is suddenly unable to cope with the emergency situation (i.e., "freezes" in the face of the emergency, faints, or suffers some other unexpected reaction).
7. Simulate a fire emergency evacuation from the clinical setting.
8. Refer to Malamed (1982): "Appendix/Quick-reference Section to Life-threatening Situations," pp. 377-382. Discuss each of the emergency situations contained in this appendix among your emergency team.
9. Refer to Blair (1982), and discuss each of the errors shown and described, among your emergency team.
10. Locate your own carotid pulse by palpating with your fingers between your larynx and the anterior border of the sternocleidomastoid muscle. Check for respirations by using a stethoscope on a partner's larynx and by placing a dental mirror under the nose.

REVIEW QUESTIONS

1. Why is it essential for a dental hygienist to have completed a comprehensive course in first aid and in basic life support?
2. List at least seven important drugs to maintain in a medical emergency kit.
3. How can the dental team prepare for an emergency?

4. What do you do if:
   a. Your patient becomes ashen and agitated and complains of nausea and dizziness?
   b. Your patient complains of severe chest pain?
   c. Your patient suddenly loses consciousness?

REFERENCES

ADA Council on Dental Therapeutics. 1982. Accepted dental therapeutics, ed. 39. Chicago: American Dental Association.

ADA Council on Dental Materials, Instruments, and Equipment. 1981. Dentist's Desk Reference: materials, instruments and equipment. Chicago: American Dental Association.

Blair, D.M. 1982. Cardiac emergencies. Dent. Clin. North Am. **26:**49.

Blair, D.M. 1982. Common errors in handling medical emergencies. Dent. Clin. North Am. **26:**163.

Blitz, P. 1979. Personal communication.

Bodak-Gyovai, L.Z. 1980. Oral medicine: patient evaluation and management. Baltimore: Williams & Wilkins.

Capello, J., et al. Aug. 1977. Medical emergencies: the dental team approach. Dent. Surv. **53:**24.

Dunn, M.J., and Booth, D.F. 1975. Dental auxiliary practice: internal medicine and systemic emergencies. Baltimore: Williams & Wilkins.

Freeman, N.S., et al. Oct. 1977. Office emergencies: causes, symptoms, treatment. Oral Health **67:**60.

Howell, R.B. 1979. Office emergency procedures: a self-study course. Chicago: American Dental Hygienists' Association.

Jaffe, M. 1982. Teaching medical emergencies in a dental hygiene program. N.Y. State Dent. J. **48:**456.

Kinne, R.D. 1982. Training for the effective management of medical emergencies. Dent. Clin. North Am. **26:**147.

Maitland, R.I. 1978. Patient assessment in the dental office emergency. N.Y. State Dent. J. **48:**442.

Malamed, S.F. 1982. Handbook of medical emergencies in the dental office, ed. 2. St. Louis: The C.V. Mosby Co.

McCarthy, F.M. 1982. Medical emergencies in dentistry, ed. 8. Philadelphia: The W.B. Saunders Co.

Miller, A.G., Jr. 1982. Syncope. Dent. Clin. North Am. **26:**119.

Morrow, G.T. 1982. Designing a drug kit. Dent. Clin. North Am. **26:**21.

Perks, E.R. Sept. 1977. The diagnosis and management of sudden collapse in dental practice. I. Br. Dent. J. **143:**196.

Proy, H.G., et al. 1982. Minicomputer simulation of medical emergencies and advanced life support. J. Dent. Educ. **46:**657.

Rose, L. 1977. Diagnosis and management of medical emergencies in the dental office. Contin. Dent. Educ. (Self-instruction Series) **1:**3.

Rose, L.M., and Hendler, B.H. 1981. Medical emergencies in dental practice, Chicago: Quintessence Publishing Co., Inc.

Ryan, D.E., and Bronstein, S.L. 1982. Dentistry and the diabetic patient. Dent. Clin. North Am. **26:**105.

Safar, P. 1981. Cardiopulmonary cerebral resuscitation. Stavanger, Norway: Asmund S. Laerdal.

Sanger, R.G., et al. 1979. Training program in emergency medical service for the dental profession. J. Am. Dent. Assoc. **98:**695.

Shaber, E.P., and Smith, R.A. 1982. Techniques of drug administration. Dent. Clin. North Am. **26**:35.

Shannon, M.E. 1982. Strokes. Dent. Clin. North Am. **26**:99.

Shijatshky, M. 1975. Life threatening emergencies in the dental practice. Translated by Koehler, H.M. Chicago: Quintessence Publishing Co., Inc.

Solomon, A.L. 1982. Emergency treatment: local and general anesthesia. N.Y. State Dent. J. **48**:447.

Standards and guidelines for cardiopulmonary resuscitation and emergency cardiac care. 1980. JAMA **244**:453.

Stroh, J.E., Jr., and Johnson, R.L. 1982. Allergy-related emergencies in dental practice. Dent. Clin. North. Am. **26**:87.

Trieger, N. 1982. Special care of the medically compromised patient. N.Y. State Dent. J. **48**:451.

Woodworth, J.V., and Woodworth, C.E. May-June 1978. Emergency! The dentist's role in prevention and treatment, I. Gen. Dent. **26**:35.

Woodworth, J.V., and Woodworth, C.E. July-Aug. 1978. Emergency! The dentist's role in prevention and treatment, II. Gen. Dent. **26**:46.

Woodworth, J.V., and Woodworth, C.E. Sept.-Oct. 1978. Emergency! The dentist's role in prevention and treatment, III. Gen. Dent. **26**:56.

Zinman, E.J. Aug. 1979. Emergency care: some legal implications, Dent. Sur. **55**:46.

11 COMPREHENSIVE CARIES, RESTORATIVE, TOOTH CHARACTERISTIC, AND RADIOGRAPHIC CHARTING

OBJECTIVES: *The reader will be able to*

1. Identify the basic purposes of preparing dental chartings.
2. Describe the advantages and disadvantages of anatomic, geometric, and numerically coded charting forms.
3. Given examples of tooth numbering systems, including universal, international, and Palmer's notation, identify which tooth is being referred to and specify from which system the notation is derived.
4. Complete comprehensive chartings for a variety of patients, including identifying and recording the following from clinical and radiographic findings:
   a. Sound teeth
   b. Missing or unerupted teeth
   c. Removable prostheses
   d. Restorations (including all classifications of single-tooth restorations, crowns, bridgework, sealants, and endodontic treatment
   e. Caries
   f. Decalcification and hypocalcification
   g. Developmental anomalies
   h. Attrition, abrasion, erosion
   i. Malposed teeth
   j. Periapical pathology
   k. Calculus
   l. Changes in supporting bone
5. Read aloud recorded notations concisely, accurately, and using proper dental terminology for verification by a second clinician.

A comprehensive dental charting provides an accurate description of the patient's dental status. It is a valuable tool in the assessment phase of care, since it provides, in most instances, a graphic representation of the active or repaired disease process and the unique clinical problems related to the patient's teeth. As a combined record of clinical and radiographic findings, it is a comprehensive diagnostic tool. Dental chartings are valuable legal records, since they show the dental conditions of the patient at the beginning of care and a pictorial review of how those conditions changed over a period of months and years.

Depending on the format and manner in which a patient's treatment is documented, the dental charting can depict the maintenance of health in some instances or the progression of disease.

It also provides a useful check against financial records. Entries in financial records indicating the placement of specific restorations should be reflected in the updated charting of the patient's teeth.

Since the comprehensive charting is most often used in establishing a basis of entering needs for purposes of treatment planning, the most comprehensive charting procedures occur at the initial pa-

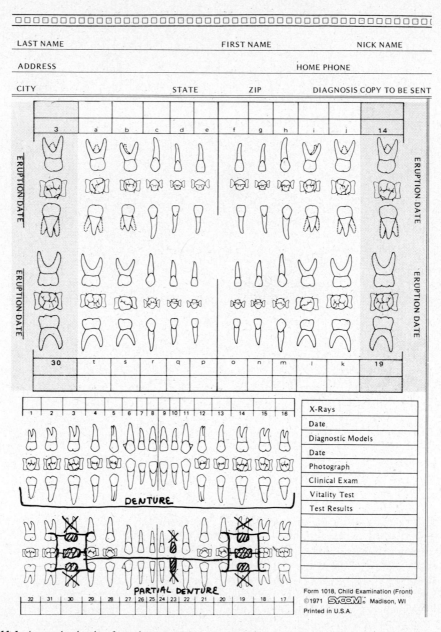

Fig. 11-1. Anatomic charting form that accommodates chartings of adult, primary, and mixed dentitions. A complete maxillary denture and mandibular partial denture are charted to illustrate one method of symbol use. (Courtesy Sycom, Madison, Wis.)

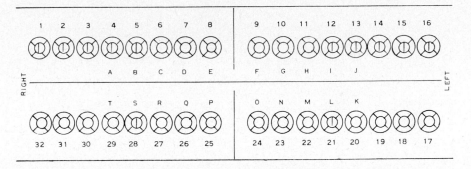

Fig. 11-2. Geometric charting form with stylized teeth. This form accommodates charting adult, primary, and mixed dentition.

tient visit. The initial data should be updated as treatment progresses and at subsequent recall visits when the patient returns for periodic diagnosis of new needs.

CHARTING FORMS

Fig. 11-1 is an example of an anatomic charting form. The anatomy of the crown and root(s) of each tooth is shown with facial, occlusal, and lingual views. Anatomic charting provides the most realistic graphic description, since the anatomic features of each tooth can be used to more specifically denote the presence of lesions and restorations. This particular form allows for charting both permanent and primary teeth.

Fig. 11-2 provides an example of a geometric charting, with stylized "anatomy." The tooth surfaces are divided by lines to indicate marginal ridges and line angles so that the extent of disease or a restoration can be shown without attempting to replicate the exact design. Since precise anatomy is not required, it is usually a neater, more easily read charting.

To follow the patient's progress, a comprehensive charting must be completely redone at each visit, or changes at each 6-month visit will become lost in the original charting. The original generally becomes increasingly cluttered and unreadable if there are many clinical changes. One way to preserve the original charting, to show progress at each assessment visit, and to avoid the time-consuming and tedious process of recharting the entire dentition is to photocopy the original charting. Findings at the second visit can be marked in colored pencil or pen on the photocopy to highlight recent changes. At the beginning of a third course of treatment in which a charting is indicated, the charting from the second course is photocopied with the new photocopy updated in color. This procedure results in a highly specific time line of conditions and care. It also results in many additional pages in the patient record. Eventually, microfilm or microfiche will be necessary to permit long-term storage.

The numeric coding system requires less paper for showing progress through time. Since number codes rather than drawings are used to indicate conditions of the teeth, the pictorial quality of anatomic/geometric chartings is lost. Fig. 11-3 shows a numeric code charting. As conditions change, markings are made in the next line above (for the maxillary teeth) or below (for the mandibular teeth). The lines are dated so that changes are identified along a time line.

TYPES OF CHARTINGS

The vast majority of chartings focus on the presence of caries, restorations, and missing teeth. Depending on treatment protocols in a given practice setting, the routine charting may be limited to these three conditions or may be expanded to include malposed teeth, attrition, erosion, abrasion, developmental anomalies, and other findings.

In addition to chartings of the clinical and radiographic conditions of the teeth, protocols may call for charting calculus deposits, periodontal conditions, plaque and hemorrhage points, and occlusal assessment. This section focuses on charting clinical and radiographic findings of the teeth. Charting the other conditions is explained in subsequent chapters.

Date	1	2	3	4	5	6	7	8	9	10	11	12	13	14	15	16
1-29-85							M TC	M TC		D TC						
7-16-84	M						M- C	M- C	D TC	D-C		DO A				M
Maxilla	1	2	3	4 a	5 b	6 c	7 d	8 e	9 f	10 g	11 h	12 i	13 j	14	15	16
Mandible	32	31	30	29 t	28 s	27 r	26 q	25 p	24 o	23 n	22 m	21 l	20 k	19	18	17
7-16-84		DO C	MO A	OC	M									M,D C	M	M
1-29-85		DO A		Occ A										MOD A		

Fig. 11-3. As each examination is performed, entries of charting symbols are made in the boxes above the maxilla entry and below the mandible entry. As defects are treated, corrections are entered in the next row of boxes above or below the corresponding teeth needing treatment. Since no anatomic drawings of caries and restorations are used, charting symbols need to be explicit regarding location of specific condition.

TOOTH NUMBERING SYSTEMS

Regardless of the selection of anatomic, geometric, or numerically coded chartings, it is essential that a consistent method of denoting each of the teeth be adopted. The *universal* system numbers each of the permanent teeth from *1* to *32* and the primary teeth from *a* to *t,* beginning with the last molar on the maxillary right quadrant and progressing sequentially around the arch to the last molar (Project ACORDE, 1974). The next tooth counted (or lettered) is the last molar on the mandibular left quadrant, progressing sequentially around the mandible to the last molar on the mandibular right. The "last molar" for permanent dentition (1 to 32) is the third molar; for children (a to t) it is the second primary molar. This system is widely accepted in the United States and is frequently used in denoting teeth. (See Figs. 11-1 and 11-2 for the numbering of each tooth.)

An older system, *Palmer's notation,* numbers or letters each of the teeth in the quadrant from *1* to *8* for permanent dentition and from *a* to *e* for primary teeth. Therefore a permanent central is always No. 1. A permanent cuspid in any quadrant is labeled No. 3. The quadrant position of the tooth under consideration is identified by using the appropriate quadrant of a graph created by two intersecting perpendicular axes. Using the quadrant denotation, the second permanent premolar in the maxillary left quadrant would be written |5. The second primary molar on the mandibular right would be written e̅| (Kraus, 1969).

The *international system* is similar to Palmer's notation, since each tooth in the quadrant is numbered *1* to *8* from central to third molar. However, the quadrant location is designated by a prefix number *1, 2, 3,* or *4* for the maxillary right, maxillary left, mandibular left, and mandibular right, respectively. The quadrant prefix is followed by the tooth number (Project ACORDE, 1974). Thus the second permanent premolar in the maxillary left quadrant shown as an example in the previous paragraph would be written 25. For distinguishing primary and permanent teeth, primary quadrants are numbered *5, 6, 7,* or *8,* respectively, with numbers (not letters) used for primary teeth. Therefore the second primary molar on the mandibular right, shown as an example in the previous paragraph, would be written 85.

Table 11-1 summarizes the differences among

Table 11-1. Summary of tooth numbering systems

System	Permanent dentition	Primary dentition
Universal	Each tooth is designated by a number (*1* to *32*)	Each tooth is designated by a letter (*a* to *t*)
International	Each tooth is designated by a quadrant number prefix (*1* to *4*) and a tooth number suffix (*1* to *8*) $$\frac{1\ \vert\ 2}{3\ \vert\ 4}$$	Each tooth is designated by a quadrant number (*5* to *8*) and a tooth number (*1* to *5*) $$\frac{5\ \vert\ 6}{8\ \vert\ 7}$$
Palmer's notation	Each tooth is numbered (*1* to *8*) and positioned within intersecting axes to designate the quadrant	Each tooth is lettered (*a* to *e*) and positioned within intersecting axes to designate the quadrant

the three numbering systems. In practice it is important to determine what system has been adopted to enable all co-workers to accurately communicate the tooth under discussion. Since the universal system is still the most widely understood and used, the detailed procedures for preparing a charting are described with *1* to *32* and *a* to *t* tooth designations. To ensure an accurate, complete charting, a sequence moving from the maxillary right third molar to the mandibular right molar (1 to 32) will be adhered to.

PROCEDURE FOR CHARTING

To prevent confusion and error, the first condition that should be charted is *missing teeth*. The teeth may have been extracted, or they may not have erupted yet. It is also possible that the tooth buds for the teeth were missing congenitally. In most instances it is not possible, with clinical data alone, to determine why the tooth is not present. A radiographic series can add data; a patient's dental history also provides information to help determine the cause of missing teeth.

Missing teeth should be crossed out with a single vertical line or an *X*. Some practitioners prefer to box or color in missing teeth.

Fig. 11-4 shows three ways in which No. 32 can be marked as missing. A partially erupted tooth

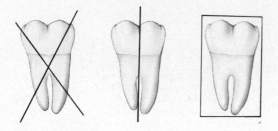

Fig. 11-4. Three symbols to indicate a missing tooth.

can be marked so that it is obvious which portion of the tooth is exposed clinically. (See tooth No. 16 in Fig. 11-5.) Marking *all missing teeth first* is especially important when charting mixed dentition.

Once all missing teeth are marked, removable prostheses, such as partial dentures, complete dentures, and removable bridges should be marked with brackets. Fig. 11-1 (on the adult dentition) shows a maxillary denture and a mandibular partial denture replacing Nos. 23, 30, and 19. The clasps are shown on Nos. 31, 29, 18, and 20.

After marking all missing teeth and removable prostheses, the clinician should return to the first chartable tooth in the maxillary right quadrant. The tooth number should be identified, and the tooth should be examined for existing restorations.

Marking restorations

The basic shape of the restoration should be drawn on the appropriate tooth on the charting form. There are a number of ways to further designate that the area defined is an existing restoration—including filling in the area with a designated color or simply leaving the restoration outlined with a letter code for labeling the area according to the material used in the restoration, such as amalgam, resin, gold foil, cast gold, or silicate.

For a precise charting, these letter designations for the type of restorative material may be used even if shading or otherwise filling in the outline is the preferred method. Thus an amalgam restoration may be designated by an anatomic outline of its shape, which is shaded in a color and marked *A* for amalgam. (See tooth No. 2 in Fig. 11-5 for an example.)

To draw and identify single-tooth restorations, a knowledge of G.V. Black's classification system is helpful. Fig. 11-6 provides a summary of the system. In identifying restorations for chartings, the classification of restoration (I, II, III, IV, V, VI) may also be noted, especially where idealized drawings are used. When orally describing the restorations to an assistant who is recording the data on the charting, describing the classification of restorations helps the recorder picture the likely shape.

Fig. 11-5. Composite charting of most commonly used charting symbols with provisions for clinical and radiographic findings. (Courtesy Sycom, Madison, Wis.)

Key to symbols (numbers refer to teeth):
1—Facially inclined; drifted mesially
2—Occlusal amalgam; drifted mesially
3—Mesioocclusal gold inlay; caries on distobuccal margin; mesially inclined and drifted mesially
4—Missing
5—Three-quarter gold crown; distally inclined
6—Class III, mesial gold foil
7—Class III, distal tooth-colored restoration
8—Porcelain jacket crown; periapical disease
9—Temporary crown; root canal
10—Peg lateral
11—Lingually inclined; watch for distal caries
12—Distal pit caries
13—Decalcification in gingival third on facial aspect; supernumerary tooth between 13 and 14
14—Decalcification in gingival third on facial aspect
15—Full gold crown
16—Partially erupted
17—Abutment tooth for fixed bridge; full gold crown
18—Pontic
19—Pontic with porcelain facing
20—Full gold crown with porcelain facing
21—Full gold crown with porcelain facing
22—Attrition; loss of continuity of lamina dura
23—Attrition; erosion
24—Attrition; erosion
25—Attrition; erosion
26—Attrition; erosion
27—Facet on distal third of facial surface; distal surface rotated toward facial; widened periodontal ligament (PDL)
28—Abrasion
29—Abrasion; mesioocclusal amalgam; overhang on mesial surface
30—Mesioocclusodistal gold onlay
31—Sealant
32—Unerupted

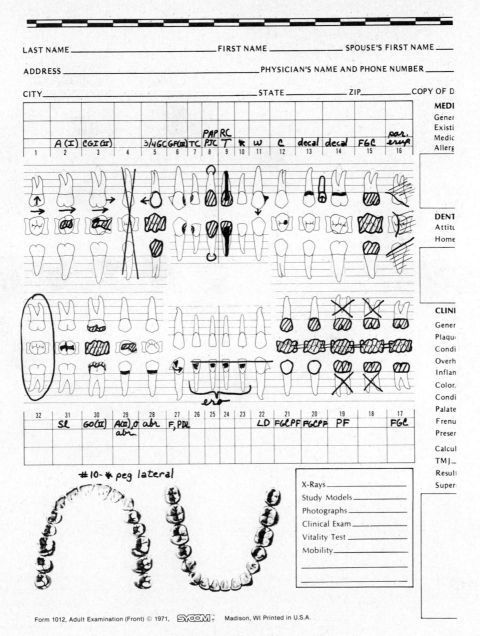

LAST NAME_____ FIRST NAME _____ SPOUSE'S FIRST NAME_____

ADDRESS_____ PHYSICIAN'S NAME AND PHONE NUMBER_____

CITY_____ STATE_____ ZIP_____ COPY OF D

Fig. 11-5. For legend see opposite page.

Form 1012, Adult Examination (Front) © 1971, **SYCOM** · Madison, WI Printed in U.S.A.

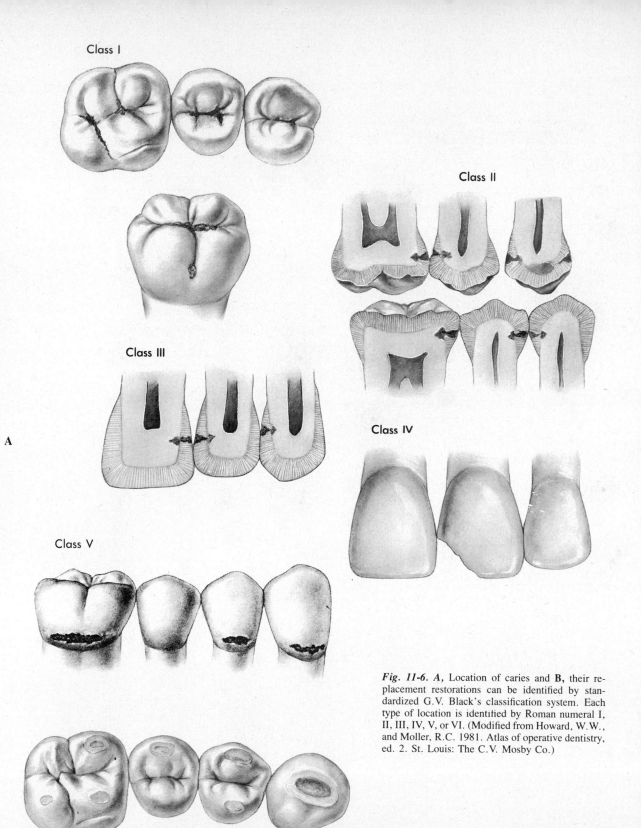

Class I

Class II

Class III

Class IV

Class V

A

Fig. 11-6. A, Location of caries and **B,** their replacement restorations can be identified by standardized G.V. Black's classification system. Each type of location is identified by Roman numeral I, II, III, IV, V, or VI. (Modified from Howard, W.W., and Moller, R.C. 1981. Atlas of operative dentistry, ed. 2. St. Louis: The C.V. Mosby Co.)

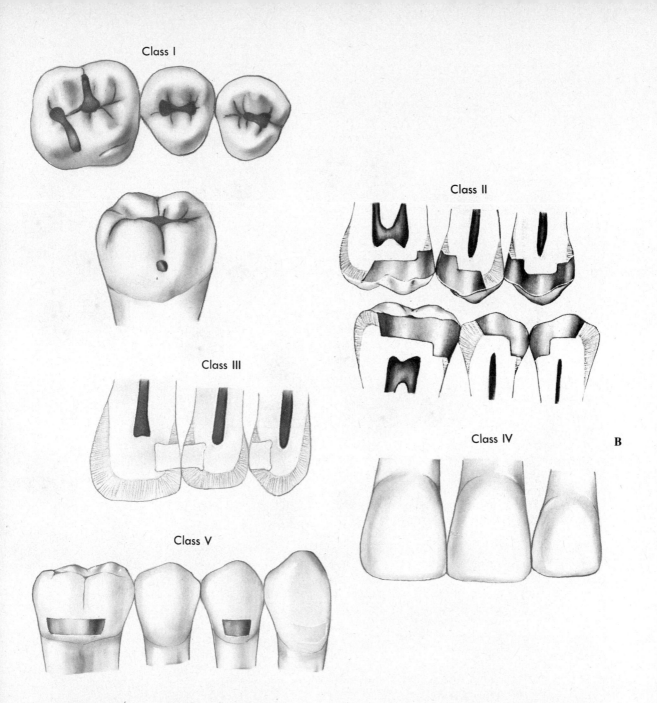

Class I

Class II

Class III

Class IV

B

Class V

Class VI

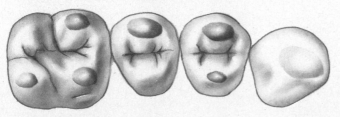

Fig. 11-6, cont'd. For legend see opposite page.

Since restoration shape and size is dependent largely on the physics of retention and resistance to masticatory stress and strain as well as maintenance of esthetics, restorations follow predictable patterns, most of which are shown in the comprehensive charting (Fig. 11-5) and in Fig. 11-6.

Therefore the procedure for marking a restoration is to outline its shape according to G.V. Black's classification system, to shade in the outline carefully, and to label it according to the type of restorative material.

Amalgam restorations. See Plate 3, *F* through *G*, for a variety of amalgam restorations. They are identifiable by their dark grey (unpolished) or bright silver (polished) appearance. Amalgam is commonly used for Class I, II, and V restorations. There may be times when a restoration with most of the characteristics of silver amalgam has a gold or orange cast to it. This restoration may be an example of a copper amalgam alloy. The proper designation for this type is *CuA*.

Gold restorations. Gold is easily distinguished from amalgam and copper amalgam by the obvious color difference. Gold has no grey cast to it; it resembles gold jewelry in color and shine. It is designated with a *G*. (Compare the restorations in Plate 3, *E* and *F*.

The most frequently seen gold restoration is cast gold. A wax pattern of the exact shape and size of the needed restoration is prepared and then replaced by molten gold alloy in a laboratory process of casting similar to the manner in which jewelry is made. The result is a solid piece of gold that fits exactly into the prepared tooth. It is polished in the laboratory and cemented into the tooth as a permanent restoration when the fit is exact.

Such a cast gold restoration feels hard to the touch of the explorer. As with the amalgam restoration, the outline is drawn to match the shape and size of the restoration, and it is shaded and labeled, in this case with a *G*.

Since a single-tooth cast gold restoration can be either an *inlay (GI)* or an *onlay (GO)*, more detail is necessary to differentiate gold restorations. Tooth No. 3 in Fig. 11-5 has a gold inlay. It lies within the marginal ridges of the occlusal table, except where it crosses the mesial marginal ridge to include the mesial surface. It is a Class II gold inlay. Tooth No. 30 shows a Class II *mesioocclusodistal (MOD)* gold onlay, which includes all cusp tips and thus covers all the marginal ridges of the tooth. However, the onlay rarely extends below the occlusal third of the facial or lingual surfaces of the tooth. (See Plate 3, *J*, for two gold onlays, a DO inlay, and an MO amalgam.)

The three-quarter crown, in contrast, includes the full occlusal table and extends to the gingiva on the mesial, distal, and lingual aspects of the tooth. The facial marginal ridge is included, along with a small portion of the facial surface, to ensure strength and retention while allowing the natural tooth structure on the facial aspect to preserve esthetics.

The three-quarter gold crown is designated with an outline, shading, and the label *3/4 GC,* as is shown for tooth No. 5 in Fig. 11-5.

The three-quarter gold crown should be differentiated from the full gold crown with a porcelain or acrylic facing. The full gold crown covers and replaces all visible enamel tooth structure and considerable underlying dentin. It is used to restore badly broken-down teeth. Although it is stronger than the three-quarter gold crown, it may result in less than desirable esthetics if the facial aspect is visible when the patient speaks or smiles. Thus when the crown is cast, an area is created on the facial aspect where white porcelain or acrylic may be added to simulate white tooth structure. A full gold crown is outlined, shaded, and labeled *FGC*. (See tooth No. 15 in Fig. 11-5.) A gold crown with a facing is labeled *GCPF* for porcelain and *GCAF* for acrylic.

Another type of single-tooth gold restoration is *gold foil*. This restoration material is quite different from cast gold. It lacks the strengthening alloys that make cast gold hard and able to endure stress and strain. Gold foil is soft and is condensed or packed into the tooth preparation until the void area is completely filled and the anatomy can be carved. The material (1) feels softer to the touch of an explorer than does cast gold, (2) is a lighter or more yellow gold color because of the purity of the material, and (3) is used in Class I, III, IV, V, or VI restorations where occlusal forces would be unlikely to shear away or fracture the restoration. When identified on a tooth, the outline should be drawn, shaded, and labeled *GF*. (See tooth No. 6 in Fig. 11-5.)

Gold is also used for multiple-tooth restorations such as *fixed bridges* (fixed partial dentures) that replace one or more missing teeth or *splints* that join several teeth together with a series of soldered or cast-together gold crowns intended to strengthen the ability of individual teeth to absorb occlusal forces. The teeth absorb the forces collectively by virtue of their joined crowns.

A bridge enables two or more healthy adjacent teeth to support a *pontic* (dummy tooth) so that an open space in the arch can be preserved with a functional tooth replacement. Usually the supporting teeth have full crowns or three-quarter crowns. They are called *abutment* teeth. The pontics are made of cast gold also; they can be distinguished from the abutment teeth because they have no roots. They are either cast in one piece with the abutments or soldered to the abutment teeth. In either case, the contacts are sealed together.

The easiest way to locate and chart a bridge is to first identify the location of the missing teeth. The roots of the missing teeth should be charted as absent (by a vertical line, an *x,* or boxing the roots). The crowns replaced by pontics can be outlined and shaded. The abutment teeth are then identified by examining the location of permanently joined contacts. The crown restorations on the abutment teeth are outlined, shaded, and labeled (3/4 GC, FGC, GCPF, etc.). Then horizontal lines should be drawn between the attached abutments and pontics to show the size and location of the entire bridge. Fig. 11-5 shows a five-unit bridge (three abutments and two pontics) extending from Nos. 17 to 21. No. 17 has a full gold crown; Nos. 18 and 19 are pontics, with No. 19 having a porcelain facing; and Nos. 20 and 21 are full gold crowns with porcelain facings.

If the pontics are in close contact with the gingiva and cannot easily be differentiated clinically from rooted teeth, reference to a radiographic survey will quickly identify pontics and abutments. Also, threading dental floss underneath one of the closed contacts should enable the clinician to pass the floss under the pontics and to identify the presence or absence of the root structure. Palpating the alveolar process should also help distinguish between edentulous areas where pontics replace the teeth and areas where abutments are present. The shape of the roots of the natural teeth can be felt in the alveolar bone.

Tooth colored restorations. Tooth-colored restoration (designated *TC*) is the generic term for silicate, composite, and resin single-tooth restorations that restore the tooth functionally and esthetically. They are used primarily in anterior teeth but are also found in Class I or V restorations, depending on the location and size of the area to be restored. If it is possible and desirable to distinguish the material used, the labels *S* for silicate, *R* for resin, and *CR* for composite resin can be used in conjunction with the shaded-in outline of the restoration. Otherwise, the label *TC* is sufficient. (See tooth No. 7 in Fig. 11-5.)

In addition to tooth-colored restorations that restore a portion of a tooth, there are porcelain and acrylic jacket crowns (designated *PJC* and *AJC*) that provide full coverage of teeth, usually where maintenance of esthetics is critical. (See tooth No. 8 in Fig. 11-5; for a radiographic example, see tooth No. 9 in Fig. 11-7; and for a clinical example, see tooth No. 9 in Plate 3, *A, B,* and *D.*)

Temporary restorations. Temporary restorations are usually easily identified as a chalky yellow, white-tone, or pink substance placed in a prepared tooth or by an aluminum preformed or nonanatomic "can" fitted over a posterior tooth prepared for a full crown. Sometimes relatively crude-looking acrylic crowns are used as temporary restorations also, particularly for anterior teeth undergoing crown preparation. The label *T* is used to designate a temporary restoration. It is usually outlined and shaded as a permanent restoration would be. (See tooth No. 9 in Fig. 11-5.)

Sealants. Sealants are thin, transparent plastic coatings that are chemically and physically bonded to posterior teeth that have pits and fissures that would be highly susceptible to decay (caries). Therefore they are usually found on occlusal surfaces of posterior teeth. They are detected as a shiny narrow clear filling when felt with the tip of an explorer. When detected, they should be outlined, shaded, and labeled *Sl.*

Sealants are being used more frequently, both for purposes of preventing caries and for restoration of areas that have beginning caries. The clinician can simply remove the carious portion of the tooth, without having to remove any additional tooth structure, to make a boxlike preparation as is commonly done for the previously introduced restorations. Research has shown that these restorations, if the teeth and type of sealant are carefully selected, give excellent results. Small restorations where little wear is expected are usually pit and fissure sealants, as discussed in Chapter 30. These are termed Group A preventive resin restorations (PRR). Filler is added to the unfilled resin when

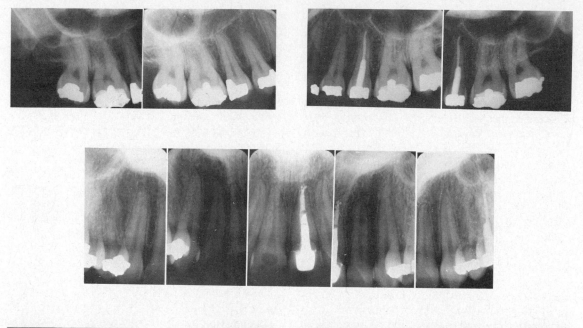

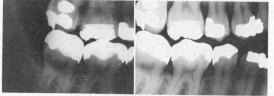

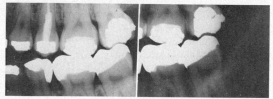

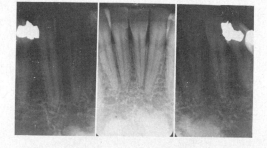

Fig. 11-7. Complete set of radiographs, including 4 bitewing films (teeth occluded, apices not visible) and 16 periapical views.

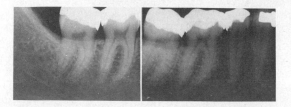

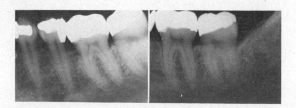

preparation size, location, or number predicts greater wear of the resin. These are termed Group B PRRs. Group C PRRs use undiluted filled resin on top of a thin intermediate layer of unfilled resin and are found where the factors of size and location indicate substantial occlusal wear (Simonson, 1980, 1982). Such restorations should be carefully recorded so that the clinician can follow the success of the sealant over many years' time.

• • •

Using the abbreviations described and being anatomically specific about the size and location of restorations and sealants create an accurate, detailed charting of the clinical conditions of the teeth.

Charting for other conditions

As each tooth is charted for the presence of restorations, the margins of each restoration should be explored to evaluate for the presence of *recurrent caries* or an open area that may eventually become carious. *Overhanging margins* should be identified (with an *O*), since the overhangs should be removed or the restoration replaced. The prefix of *C* for caries and *D* for defective should be added to the letter label for the restoration. Therefore a carious amalgam would be labeled *C-A*. (See tooth No. 3 in Fig. 11-5 for a carious gold inlay.) A defective composite resin would be labeled *DCR*. When colored pencils are used to differentiate carious areas from existing restorations, the carious margin can be marked simply with the color designated for caries, and the prefix letter is then unnecessary.

Likewise, all the exposed surfaces of the teeth should be felt for soft, *carious areas,* particularly in pits and grooves, at contact points, and on exposed root surfaces. If the sharp explorer tip sticks in a pit (i.e., it seems to be retained by the pit or groove) and the area feels soft, then it should be marked for caries with either the designated color or by outlining the area of caries, shading it in, and marking it *C.* Incipient or beginning caries or suspicious pits and grooves can be marked "watch," *W.* (See Nos. 11 and 12 in Fig. 11-5.)

Obvious areas of tooth breakdown, such as large craters, do not require exploration, and exploring them may cause the patient considerable pain.

Closely related to caries are areas of *decalcification.* In these areas there is evidence of demineralization of the tooth structure with an enamel surface that is whiter than the surrounding tooth and that may be chalky and soft. If such an area is likely to become carious or needs to be noted for some other reason, such as esthetics, it can be noted on the chart by shading in the area and labeling it *decal. Hypocalcification,* which rarely is clinically significant and thus is rarely charted, can be labeled *hycal.* (See Plate 1, *D,* for a clinical example.)

A *supernumerary tooth* can be drawn in its general location. (See Fig. 11-5 in the maxillary left quadrant.) Other developmental *anomalies* are usually marked with an asterisk near the tooth involved, with a full notation included on the charting page to explain the observed characteristics. (See tooth No. 10 in Fig. 11-5.)

Attrition, the loss of tooth structure due to normal mastication, is often seen on the incisal edges of anterior teeth (Fig. 11-5). This can be noted with a horizontal line drawn across the facial aspect of the drawings of the teeth to illustrate the amount of lost tooth structure. (See the mandibular anterior teeth in Plate 4 for a clinical example.) Closely related to attrition, but far more clinically significant, is the presence of *wear facets.* These highly polished wear areas often show the pattern of wear associated with malocclusion. Wear facets are boxed in to show the plane of wear on each tooth. They are marked with an *F.*

Abrasion is caused by mechanical wear other than that associated with mastication. Vigorous horizontal strokes with a toothbrush cause abrasion, as does improper flossing, opening hairpins with the teeth, and other habits that wear the tooth structure. The area is outlined and shaded and marked *abr.* Colored pencils are useful to distinguish this characteristic from a Class V restoration or other defect. (See Plate 2, *H,* especially the maxillary right quadrant, for a clinical example.)

Erosion, in contrast to attrition and abrasion, is caused by chemical wear of the teeth. Sucking lemons, for instance, can cause generalized erosion of the anterior facial surfaces. Since this feature is more generalized over a broad surface and involves several teeth, the teeth involved can be bracketed and marked *ero.* (See Fig. 11-5 for a graphic description of these characteristics on Nos. 22 to 29.)

Malposed teeth should be charted on a comprehensive dental charting including rotated, extruded, and inclined teeth. Rotated teeth are marked by drawing an arrow on the proximal surface that is rotated toward the facial. The arrow is then arced across the facial view of the tooth to suggest the direction of rotation of the tooth. Fig. 11-5 shows No. 27 as having the distal surface rotated toward the facial. The arrow starts on the distal and arcs across the facial surface. It would be just as valid to show an arrow starting on the mesial surface and arcing across the lingual view. For purposes of consistency, facial views are used for rotations. Because of the different perceptions persons have when viewing a two-dimensional drawing and attempting to visualize a three-dimensional characteristic, it is best for all persons who may record or interpret a dental charting to agree on one way to chart malpositions.

This is true not only for axial rotations, but also for lingual and labial versions (inclinations), which may cause equal confusion if a variety of methods are used to chart the condition. One easily understood rule is to mark a vertical arrow pointed from the incisal edge away from the facial aspect of the tooth to show *lingual version* (see tooth No. 11 in Fig. 11-5) and to show the vertical arrow starting at the incisal edge and traveling vertically up or down the facial aspect of the drawing of the tooth to depict *labial version*. Mesial or distal inclination is shown with a straight, horizontal arrow pointing toward the midline of the arch from the mesial surface to show mesial inclination and pointing posteriorly from the distal surface to show distal inclination.

Drifting of the teeth either mesially or distally with or without rotation or inclination is shown with a horizontal arrow pointed in the direction of the drift, above the occlusal table or incisal edge. Fig. 11-5 shows the distinction in recording version and drifting. Tooth No. 5 is distally inclined; tooth No. 3 is mesially inclined and drifted; and Nos. 1 and 2 are positioned mesial to their usual locations but are not inclined. This is probably due to the loss of tooth No. 4.

Locating all these malpositions is accomplished best by sitting in a rear position (11 o'clock, for instance) and observing the curve of the maxillary arch in the dental mirror. Careful observation should help contrast rotations and versions from the natural curvature of the maxillary arch. Likewise the curve of the arch on the mandible should reveal deviations from normal arch curve. (See the anterior rotations evident in Plate 3, *C,* and the more obvious malpositions in Plate 2, *G.*) Having the patient close his/her teeth and retracting the cheeks should reveal patterns of drift and version.

Radiographic chartings

Radiographs are a necessary and helpful adjunct to the clinical examination. The radiographs provide information about the teeth and supporting structures that cannot be collected during a clinical examination. Most practitioners require a complete series of radiographs consisting of 16 to 18 periapical views or a panoramic radiograph and bitewing radiographs at the beginning of treatment (Wuehrmann and Manson-Hing, 1981). (See Fig. 11-7 for a complete set of radiographs.) The radiographs are updated according to the dental care practice's policies, individual patients needs, and the legal constraints of the state.

Ideally, the radiographs should be reviewed prior to the clinical examination to reduce the chance of reading into the radiographs findings suspected by the clinical examination (Wuehrmann and Manson-Hing, 1981) (Fig. 11-8). If the radiographs are viewed chairside, the clinician's eye movements between the radiographs and the patient should be minimized, since the change in lighting can be a physical strain on the clinician's eye and reduce the ability to detect subtle contrast differences in the radiographs (Wuehrmann and Manson-Hing, 1981).

The *radiographic findings* are charted on the comprehensive charting form using the same symbols and codes explained earlier in this section. Several additional symbols and codes, which are unique to a radiographic charting, are described here. The radiographs are viewed and charted in a sequence that is slightly different from the sequence used during a clinical examination. The radiographs are viewed for kinds of changes rather than tooth by tooth (Wuehrmann and Manson-Hing, 1981). For example, first the radiographs are viewed for missing teeth; the clinician scans the radiographs moving from tooth No. 1 to tooth No. 32 and charts missing teeth. Then the radiographs are viewed for the next change, as caries. (Plate 3 and Fig. 11-7 are of the same patient.)

The first radiographic finding to be charted is missing or unerupted teeth. Missing teeth are charted using the previously mentioned line, *X,* or box. Unerupted teeth are circled. Most practitioners differentiate between missing and unerupted

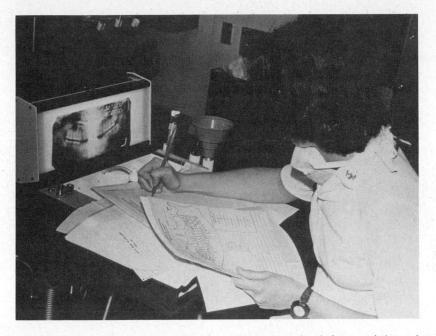

Fig. 11-8. Radiographic chartings should be prepared as a separate procedure before completing an intraoral charting.

teeth; this differentiation is especially important for pedodontic chartings. Notice that all four third molars are missing in Fig. 11-7, but all' other permanent teeth are present.

Existing restorations, including crowns, bridges, and root canal fillings, are charted next. The same symbols used previously are used for the restorations, although it is difficult to distinguish the type of metallic and tooth-colored restorations radiographically. The interproximal extensions of the restorations and pontics can be readily identified from the radiographs; it is important to use the radiographs to detect these findings. Root canal fillings are recorded by darkening the root canal and pulp chamber on the charting and by placing the letters *RC* in the appropriate box. (See tooth No. 9 in Fig. 11-5.)

Note in Fig. 11-7 that there are numerous restorations and two teeth showing endodontic treatment: Nos. 9 and 13. Note the lower right quadrant restorations, as shown in the bitewing films (where the teeth are occluded and the apices are not visible). The knife-edge restoration margins on Nos. 29 and 30 and the mesial aspect of No. 31 indicate that these are cast gold restorations. The restorations appear to provide cuspal coverage, suggesting that these are gold onlays. Compare the shape and the exact margins of the gold onlays with the shape of the restorations on Nos. 5, 6, 11, 12, and 28. The restoration margins on these teeth are less precise, and they appear to be set into the occlusal grooves and pits of the posterior teeth and into the direct distal surfaces of the cuspid teeth.

Tooth-colored restorations usually appear radiolucent on radiographs and can be confused with carious lesions; some of the newer materials have additives to make them radiopaque. Usually a restoration will have well-defined margins, so there will be a well-defined distinction between the radiopaque and radiolucent areas; a carious lesion will not have well-defined margins. Most temporary restorations are also radiolucent and may or may not have well-defined margins.

Tooth No. 8 in Fig. 11-7 shows two tooth-colored restorations, one located either facially or lingually and one on the mesial surface. Tooth No. 23 also shows a tooth-colored restoration, located on the distal surface (see Plate 3, *B* and *C*).

While viewing the radiographs for existing restorations, overhangs can also be recorded. An overhang will appear as an extension of the metallic restorations beyond the tooth. Overhangs are most commonly observed in the gingival third of the tooth (see Chapter 21). It is difficult to detect tooth-colored restoration overhangs radiographically, since the restorations usually appear radiolucent.

Carious lesions can be charted next. Caries appears radiolucent and can be seen as a new lesion or a lesion recurring around a restoration. When detecting caries radiographically, it is important to view each tooth carefully and to check the interproximal areas and around all of the margins of restorations. Lesions can be extremely small or extremely large; some carious lesions will affect the pulp, with this advanced pathology detectable radiographically. (See Fig. 11-9 for interproximal caries.)

After the teeth have been surveyed for carious lesions, the radiographs are surveyed for supernumerary teeth, other developmental disturbances, and retained root tips. These findings are recorded as explained previously.

Next the radiographs are surveyed for *periodontal findings*. The height of the bone level, width of the periodontal ligament space, and continuity of the lamina dura of each tooth are viewed. The *height of the bone* can be drawn on the comprehensive chart or possibly on the periodontal charting (see Chapter 14). The numbers of the teeth with *widened periodontal ligament* spaces and *loss of lamina dura* continuity should be recorded. The letters *PDL* or *LD* can be placed in the boxes corresponding to the teeth.

In Fig. 11-9 the bone between the two molars does not have a defined radiopaque line showing the crest of the bone. That line is the lamina dura, and it is lost or less evident in this area of the dentition. Compare the crest shown here with those depicted in Fig. 11-7, where loss of lamina dura is not evident.

Teeth No. 19 and No. 30 in Fig. 11-7 show evidence of a widened periodontal ligament space on the mesial aspect as seen in the periapical films. Note that this finding is less evident in the bitewing

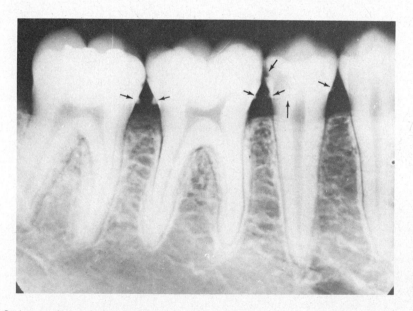

Fig. 11-9. Arrows show calculus extending from proximal surfaces into interdental spaces and ringing the crown of the second premolar. Caries has penetrated proximal surfaces at or below contact points on second premolar and the two molars. Loss of bone height is observable between the two molars and a widened periodontal ligament space is most apparent along distal root of first molar and distal root of first premolar. (From Wuehrmann, A.H., and Manson-Hing, L.R. 1981. Dental radiology, ed. 5. St. Louis: The C.V. Mosby Co.)

films, which is one reason why clinicians prefer having both bitewing and periapical films in order to minimize diagnostic errors due to the differences in the angle of the x-ray beam when the film was exposed.

Calculus can be noted next. Fig. 11-9 shows calculus, loss of bone level, and a widened periodontal ligament space. Calculus will be observed as radiopaque projections from the cervical areas of the teeth. Some clinicians chart calculus according to location by drawing triangles corresponding to the location of the calculus. An equally effective method of noting the calculus is to write a statement such as, ''Radiographic calculus is visible in the maxillary and mandibular posterior areas,'' in the summary of findings.

Periapical disease and other changes in the bone are viewed last. Periapical disease usually appears as a radiolucent area around the apex and can be noted with the letters *PAP* or by drawing a circle around the apex of the affected tooth. While the radiographs are being reviewed for periapical disease, any other abnormalities, radiopaque or radiolucent, should be noted with an asterisk and then described.

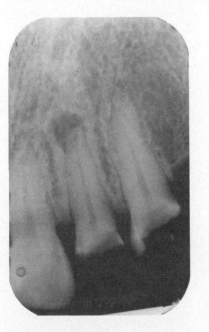

Fig. 11-10. Periapical film of Nos. 10 and 11 showing gross caries and periapical pathology.

In Fig. 11-7 there are radiolucencies near the root tips of Nos. 21, 22, 28, and 29. These are not signs of periapical pathology. These are the shadows caused by a normal anatomic landmark of the mandible: the mental foramen through which the mental nerve and blood vessels pass. Fig. 11-10 shows periapical pathology at the tip of No. 10. The pathology is undoubtedly the result of the extensive caries the crown has suffered. Clinically, only a stub of a tooth would be visible. Such pathology can be seen surrounding root tips of clinically healthy teeth and is often the result of trauma.

The radiographic charting is an involved procedure, but it provides invaluable information to augment other assessment data and help make quality treatment a reality.

• • •

All teeth to which none of these clinical or radiographic characteristics apply are described as *sound*.

Fig. 11-5 describes all the usual charting symbols, with the key to each symbol given in the legend. They are probably never all used for any one patient. However, over the course of charting the dental conditions of a wide variety of patients, each of these charting symbols will probably prove useful.

Describing the charting orally

In some instances the person observing the oral conditions will also be marking the symbols on the charting form, which, of course, does not involve an oral description of the characteristic noted. Far more frequently, an assistant will record what is described aloud. In addition, often the observer or the recorder will need to describe to another person each of the recorded findings for verification.

In order to expedite the charting and/or verification process, an explicit and systematic approach should be used in describing aloud each charted characteristic.

Moving sequentially from 1 to 32 or a to t is the best organizational guideline, with all charted characteristics for each tooth described completely as each tooth is identified. The *tooth number* should be called first. If a restoration is present, the classification, the type of restorative material, and its anatomic location should follow. For example,

"Tooth No. 2 has a Class I occlusal amalgam." In identifying anatomic locations, the basic structure (MOD, DO, MO) should be followed by a description of lingual or buccal extensions and the inclusion of complete cusps. For example, "Tooth No. 2 has a Class II MO amalgam with a buccal extension."

Any defective or carious margins should be described following the description of the restoration in question. For example, "Tooth No. 3 has a Class II MO gold inlay with recurrent caries on the distobuccal margin."

When describing a bridge, it is best to first call the number of units (abutments plus pontics) and then call each involved unit as an abutment or pontic and state the type of restoration present on the unit. For example, "There is a five-unit bridge from tooth No. 17 to tooth No. 21. No. 17 is an abutment with a full gold crown. Nos. 18 and 19 are pontics with gold crowns and a porcelain facing on No. 19. Nos. 20 and 21 are abutments with full gold crowns with porcelain facings."

Caries, decalcification, hypocalcification, attrition, facets, erosion, and abrasion are located anatomically. For example, "Tooth No. 12 has caries in the distal pit. Nos. 13 and 14 have decalcification on the gingival third on the facial surface. No. 27 has a vertical facet on the distal third of the labial surface."

Anomalies are called as the tooth is encountered. For example, "No. 10 is a peg lateral."

Malposed teeth are described by naming the tooth and indicating the direction in which it is inclined. For example, "No. 1 is buccally inclined (or verted)." Rotations are described by stating the proximal surface that is directed facially and describing the rotation. For example, "No. 27—the distal surface is rotated labially."

Proceeding around the mouth in this fashion allows for rapid, precise cross-evaluation of findings.

PEDODONTIC CHARTINGS

For most purposes, the preparatoin of pedodontic chartings is similar to the preparation of adult chartings. Differences include the fact that primary dentition chartings usually use the lower case letters of the alphabet (*a* to *t*). Also, mixed dentition chartings may pose a challenge, since permanent teeth must be differentiated from primary teeth and described with the *1* to *32* system. For instance, a 6-year-old child may have four permanent first mo-

lars (Nos. 3, 14, 19, and 30) and four permanent centrals (Nos. 8, 9, 24, and 25), with all the rest being primary teeth (a, b, c, d, g, h, i, and j on the maxilla and k, l, m, n, q, r, s, and t on the mandible). It should be apparent that assessing present and missing teeth *must* precede the attempt to mark restorations, caries, and other characteristics. A guideline never to be forgotten is that *the first permanent molar appears posterior to the second primary molar; it does not replace a primary molar, and it closely resembles the second primary molar.*

Tooth characteristics that may be encountered in pedodontic chartings include space maintainers and preformed stainless steel crowns. A space maintainer should be identified by drawing the retaining band on the abutment tooth and drawing a bar to show the space being saved. Stainless steel crowns are marked similarly to full gold crowns, except that they are labeled *SSC*.

Practice in reading aloud mixed dentition chartings is particularly helpful, since it is easy to confuse the sequence of teeth to be described and to err in identifying teeth.

In all cases, precision in identifying and recording comprehensive chartings is extremely important, since the chartings serve as legal records and as one basis for treatment planning.

ACTIVITIES

1. Practice reading aloud from a completed anatomic or geometric form a variety of comprehensive chartings to a partner who will record the described findings on a blank form. Compare the chartings for accuracy.
2. Record comprehensive chartings for an advanced student who is assessing his/her patient's oral conditions. Read the findings back to a clinical instructor for verification.
3. In groups of three, take turns (1) observing and describing aloud each tooth's significant characteristics, (2) recording the findings on a charting form, and (3) sitting as a patient observing in a mirror.
4. Translate anatomic or geometric charting symbols to a numerically coded charting form.
5. View a complete series of periapical and bitewing radiographs to practice identifying, recording, and reading aloud the findings.
6. Chart a set of radiographs that has a variety of restorations. Compare the radiographic charting with what you see during an oral examination of the patient. Compare how the restorations look radiographically with their clinical appearance.

7. Compare the radiographic appearance of the teeth and restorations in Fig. 11-7 with the photographs in Plate 3. Some photographs are minor images. Tooth numbering will be backward in those.

REVIEW QUESTIONS

1. Identify at least four basic uses of a comprehensive dental charting.
2. Give one advantage of each of the following charting formats:
   a. Anatomic
   b. Geometric
   c. Numerically coded
3. Following are three columns for the three types of systems used for numbering the teeth and a column for the description of the designated tooth. How would the remaining blanks be filled in so that the designations for a given tooth are identified according to each system and a description of the tooth is included?

	Universal	Palmer's notation	International	Description
a.	—	6⌋	—	—
b.	28	—	—	—
c.	—	—	28	—
d.	—	⌈b	—	—
e.	—	—	—	Maxillary left second premolar

4. Identify each of the following commonly used symbols in charting:
   a. A
   b. T
   c. TC
   d. FGC
   e. GF
   f. C
   g. SSC
   h. DGO
   i. RC
   j. PAP
5. Describe how each of the following findings should be marked:
   a. Tooth anomaly
   b. Pontic
   c. Drifting
   d. Rotation
   e. Attrition
   f. Unerupted teeth
   g. Calculus
   h. Overhang
6. List at least nine conditions that are not readily identified clinically, which can be charted from radiographic surveys.

REFERENCES

Kraus, B.S., et al. 1969. Dental anatomy and occlusion. Baltimore: Williams & Wilkins.

Project ACORDE. 1974. Restoration of cavity preparations with amalgam and tooth-colored materials: instructor's manual. Washington, D.C.: U.S. Department of Health, Education, and Welfare.

Simonsen, R.J. 1980. Preventive resin restorations: three-year results. J. Am. Dent. Assoc. **100**:535.

Simonsen, R.J. 1982. Preventive resin restoration: innovative uses of sealants in restorative dentistry. Clin. Prevent. Dent. **4**(4):27.

Wuehrmann, A.H., and Manson-Hing, L.R. 1981. Dental radiology, ed. 5. St. Louis: The C.V. Mosby Co.

12 CALCULUS DETECTION

OBJECTIVES: *The reader will be able to*

1. Explain the importance of accurate calculus detection.
2. Complete calculus chartings for patients exhibiting various amounts of dental calculus in various locations.
3. Describe the types and locations of calculus usually identified intraorally and radiographically.
4. Describe the role of calculus in the progression of periodontal disease.
5. Identify current theories of calculus formation.

Since removing calculus deposits and planing root surfaces are functions dental hygienists perform regularly in most practice settings, developing basic skills in locating and removing deposits is crucial. In Chapter 5 the beginning manual skills are introduced. This chapter describes the "target" we are seeking when we explore for calculus deposits.

Finding and removing *all* deposits, both above and below the margin of the gingivae, is the ideal toward which clinicians strive. The more closely a clinician approaches accurate detection and complete removal, the more likely it is that the patient will be able to regain and maintain periodontal health. Failure to find calculus, especially when it is several millimeters subgingival or hiding in a root furrow or furcation, can result in persistent, insidious advancement of disease.

TYPES OF DEPOSITS

Calculus deposits are varied in shape, size, and color. The deposits may be chalky and relatively soft, or they may be extremely hard and firmly attached to the root structure (Schroeder, 1969). Calculus is frequently found in children. From 56% to 85% of children examined in a particular study had supragingival deposits; 30% to 67% had subgingival deposits. The occurrence was greater for children 12 to 14 years old than for those 9 to 11 years old. Calculus is more extensive in adults, particularly in those over 30 years old. In children as well as adults, calculus was most commonly found on the lingual aspect of mandibular anterior teeth and on the facial aspect of maxillary molars (Tuersky, 1970).

The most common visible deposits are chalky yellow or white, rough *crustaceous* deposits that are located on the lingual aspect of the mandibular anteriors and on the facial aspect of maxillary molars (Alexander, 1971; Baumhammers et al., 1973). These two sites are adjacent to major salivary ducts. Since many of the elements known to exist in calculus are found in saliva, the flow of saliva over the teeth is believed to influence the deposition of the hard material on the teeth (Alexander, 1971; Listgarten and Ellegaard, 1973; Mandel, 1972; Mislowsky and Mazzella, 1974). Drying the teeth with air and feeling the teeth with the side of the explorer or probe will make it possible to find these deposits. Patients who have not had their teeth cleaned for extended periods of time may have a bridge of calculus covering the lingual surfaces of the mandibular teeth, filling the interdental spaces and literally splinting the teeth from cuspid to cuspid. Similar large deposits are sometimes seen on the facial aspect of the maxillary molars as well (Alexander, 1971). (See Plate 2, *G*, and Plate 4 for clinical examples.)

These visible deposits are referred to as *supragingival*, or *supramarginal*, calculus because they are located coronally to the gingiva. There are many instances in which a deposit that is visible extends subgingivally into the sulcus or pocket and therefore is both supramarginal and submarginal by location.

The visible deposits are usually softer than the

subgingival deposits. They are usually amorphous or follow a pattern on the teeth that is molded by the pressure of the tongue or cheek. Efforts to remove the deposits often cause them to crumble. Therefore complete removal of these types of deposits depends on persistence, good visibility, and frequent use of a stream of air to dry the teeth so that remaining particles are apparent. These fine residual deposits will often be visible only with a disclosant solution. If polishing does not remove the disclosant solution and the surface feels rough, the surface of the tooth should be scaled, since in all probability, the remaining deposit is calculus and not plaque.

Subgingival or submarginal deposits take on a variety of characteristics. They usually are dark brown, green, or black in appearance. They are usually harder than supragingival deposits, and they have a more identifiable form. Their microscopic structure is quite different from that of supragingival calculus (Mislowsky and Mazzella, 1974; Schroeder, 1969).

The calculus deposits can be long *fernlike* or *fingerlike projections* that are relatively flat against the root surface. Or they can be hard spurlike *spicules* that extend outward from the tooth. A deposit can be a ledge or ring of calculus that encircles all or a part of a tooth. Deposits can also be found as hard *nodules* on the tooth surface (Tuersky, 1970) (Fig. 12-1). In most instances the calculus is firmly embedded in the tooth surface (cementum) (Singh, Manhold, and Volpe, 1972) and is removed in chunks rather than in crumblings.

Because the deposits are subgingival, they are rarely visible. It is sometimes possible to direct a stream of air into the sulcus and see the calculus deposits located subgingivally if the tissue is loose around the tooth. If the tissue is relatively tight to the tooth and is not overly fibrous, the shadow of the dark calculus can sometimes be seen through the tissue. This is a particularly useful observation when a patient is being seen for a final evaluation of deposit removal, and the tissue is healing well. The signs of localized continued inflammation and the dark ''shadow'' on the tissue stand out as signals that calculus remains in that particular area.

Veneer, or burnished calculus, is a deposit located subgingivally that has been shaved away rather than fractured away from the tooth in a chunk. If dull instruments or insufficient pressure against

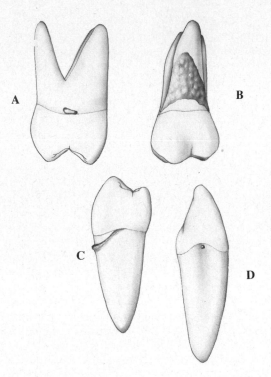

Fig. 12-1. Subgingival calculus can take many forms, including, **A,** small spicule or portion of a ledge of calculus in depression on root, especially at cementoenamel junction; **B,** fingerlike or fernlike projection of calculus down the root; **C,** ledge or ring of calculus surrounding all or part of tooth; and, **D,** small nodules of calculus.

the tooth are used in attempting to remove the deposit, it is possible to simply shave away the rough parts, leaving a very thin sheet of calculus that is still firmly attached to the tooth and now much more difficult to remove, since there is little possibility of engaging the blade of an instrument against it for removal.

CLINICAL SIGNIFICANCE OF CALCULUS

The presence of calculus is a significant aspect of the data to be gathered in assessing a patient's needs. It has long been associated with diseases of the periodontium, although there is still some controversy regarding its role in the initiation and/or the advancement of the disease process (Baer, 1970; Hazen, 1970; Schroeder, 1969; Tuersky, 1970).

It is undisputed that one phase in reducing and eliminating gingivitis and periodontitis includes complete removal of calcareous deposits. These rough deposits harbor volumes of active microorganisms in a covering of dental plaque, which irritate the adjacent soft tissues with their by-products (Baumhammers et al., 1973; Tuersky, 1970). Some researchers believe that the bulk of the deposit limits the free flow of gingival/sulcular fluids and reduces the natural blood circulation to the gingiva, thereby contributing to the advancement of the disease (Schroeder, 1969; Tuersky, 1970). However, in an experiment using rats in which 2% chlorhexidine gluconate, together with brushing and interdental cleaning, was used over a period of time, junctional epithelial cells formed an attachment to the calculus deposits, perhaps because of decreased plaque formation and decreased toxicity of calculus (Listgarten and Ellegaard, 1973). However, until such rinses or combinations of procedures are available and are used by the general public, calculus appears as a significant factor in disease. Therefore, in treatment planning for dental hygiene care, the presence of substantial deposits of calculus would indicate the need for their removal early in treatment and concurrently with an improved routine of daily removal of dental plaque. As long as the hard deposits remain, with plaque adhering to them, reduction in inflammation will be incomplete.

STAGES OF CALCULUS FORMATION

Calculus is composed of an organic matrix of bacterial plaque in which calcium (Ca^{2+}) and phosphate (PO_4^-) ions crystallize to form a hard mass (Armitage, 1974; Goldman and Cohen, 1980; Lustmann, Lewis-Epstein, and Shteyer, 1976; Schroeder, 1969). The formation is not simply a precipitation of ions, but rather an orderly deposition of layers of crystals into the matrix (Armitage, 1974; Goldman and Cohen, 1980; Lustmann, Lewis-Epstein, and Shteyer, 1976; Mislowsky and Mazzella, 1974; Schroeder, 1969). Mineralization occurs with the initiation of crystal growth at nucleation sites in the organic matrix (Lustman, Lewis-Epstein, and Shteyer, 1976; Mislowsky and Mazzella, 1974; Schroeder, 1969). The bacteria themselves may calcify intracellularly. Scanning electron photomicrographs show the patterns of microorganisms, which are both hollow and solid

with the hydroxyapatite and other calcium-phosphate minerals (Lustmann, Lewis-Epstein, and Shteyer, 1976; Schroeder, 1969).

Filamentous organisms are layered over supragingival calculus, whereas subgingival calculus is covered by a mixture of cocci, rods, and filaments. These forms can be seen by examining calculus with a scanning electron microscope. When the filamentous organisms are destroyed with sodium hypochlorite, the calculus shows the patterns of where those microorganisms were attached, which further supports the conclusion that bacteria serve as a matrix for calcification (Friskopp & Hammarström, 1980).

Hydroxyapatite constitutes approximately 55% of the inorganic components, with octacalcium phosphate (31%), whitlockite (25%), and brushite (5%) being the remaining salts (Armitage, 1974). A wide variety of trace elements have been identified in calculus (Retief et al., 1972, 1973), and approximately 6% to 15% of calculus is organic matter (Goldman and Cohen, 1980). Supragingival and subgingival calculus have about the same amounts of calcium, but subgingival calculus has greater zinc and strontium concentrations, and supragingival calculus has higher concentrations of manganese (Knuuttila et al., 1979).

The first stage of calculus formation requires, according to many researchers, the presence of acquired pellicle on the teeth (Canis et al. 1979; Schroeder, 1969). Schroeder (1969) has defined the pellicle as the *exogenous dental cuticle* and describes it as an unstructured, homogenous layer that adheres directly to and penetrates into the crystalline tooth structure, and also to all other firm surfaces in the oral cavity, as well as old dental calculus. It is rapidly formed and renewed constantly. It is presumably formed by microbially altered salivary glycoproteins and is thin (Schroeder, 1969). Bacterial plaque attaches to this exogenous dental cuticle. And given the appropriate conditions, calcification begins. Gram-negative cocci have been seen containing "spherules of amorphous calcium phosphate within the cytoplasm" as they are converted to the hard calculus substance (Sidaway, 1980).

Brushite is formed during the initial stages of calcification. It is slowly transformed into the less porous form of calculus: whitlockite. Thus calculus close to the tooth is harder and less porous, whereas calculus at the outer layers of the deposit that is exposed to saliva is porous (Kani et al., 1983). Calculus close to the cementum often is hardly distinguishable from the tooth structure when viewed microscopically because of its solid structure and its mechanical interlocking with the microscopic topography of the cementum (Canis et al., 1979).

Hard deposits may be detected as early as 2 days after thorough cleansing, although it may require as long as 12 days or more for undisturbed deposits of plaque to calcify and mature (Schroeder, 1969). There is great variability among individuals regarding how rapidly deposits form (Mandel, 1972). Higher levels of calcium ions and urea in the saliva of the submaxillary salivary gland correlate with rapid deposit formation (Mandel, 1972; Schroeder, 1969). One study indicates that smokers are more likely to have calculus deposits than nonsmokers (Kowalski, 1971).

As the calculus matures, the deeper layers of microorganisms calcify. Additional layers of plaque accumulate, and the process continues as the deposit "grows." Subgingival calculus contains fewer microorganisms than supragingival deposits. The current theory, as originally suggested by Black about 1900, is that subgingival calculus draws its calcium phosphate crystals from the exudate of the inflamed tissue that covers it rather than from saliva (Schroeder, 1969). As mentioned earlier, subgingival calculus is extremely hard and is often a dark green or brown in color in contrast to the yellow color of most supragingival calculus.

Microorganisms are directly related to calculus formation. Greater numbers of microorganisms are associated with the presence of calculus (Singh, Manhold, and Volpe, 1972). The role of microorganisms appears to be largely one of providing a matrix for mineralization (Mislowsky and Mazzella, 1974). Devital microorganisms calcify more readily, since acid by-products of microorganisms are antagonistic to crystal nucleation (Schroeder, 1969).

One study suggests that calculus formation is enhanced by the enzymes contained in the layers of dental plaque that cover the forming deposit (Friskopp and Hammarström, 1982).

People who are heavy calculus formers show about 60% more lipid weight in their saliva as compared with light calculus formers. Light calculus formers have much higher levels of free cholesterol and triglycerides in their saliva, whereas the saliva of heavy calculus formers contains more free fatty acids and cholesterol esters. Thus researchers suspect that salivary lipids play a role in calculus formation (Slomiany et al., 1981).

Two distinct types of mineralization centers are seen in calculus: type A, which is initiated by and formed with microorganisms, and adjacent type B centers, which appear unrelated to microorganisms (Lustmann, Lewis-Epstein, and Shteyer, 1976; Schroeder, 1969).

Calculus can form without the presence of any microorganisms, but its nature is quite different. Such sterile calculus is much like mother-of-pearl and does not have the extremely rough surface characteristics of naturally occurring calculus (Theilade et al., 1964).

Calculus deposits penetrate the irregularities of the tooth surface, creating a mechanical lock between the deposit and the tooth (Canis et al., 1979; Selvig, 1970). This is particularly true in areas where a preceding carious process, resorption lacunae, planing grooves, and other defects have created pathways for attachment. One investigator found "minute, atypical crystals within the surface layer of enamel and carious dentin immediately underneath calculus . . . [that] were similar in size to the crystals seen in the adjacent concrement, and characteristically different in size and orientation from the normal crystals of these hard tissues" (Selvig, 1970). When the calculus was chipped off, long needlelike crystals remained. This explains the frequent difficulty encountered in removing mature deposits and points out the importance of planing root structures after calculus removal if the reattachment of future deposits is to be minimized.

Research into the causes and clinical significance of calculus continues. As the many questions about it are finally answered, the clinician's role continues to be, in part, to locate and remove the deposits in combination with helping the patient achieve a high degree of personal control over factors affecting calculus reaccumulation.

PREPARING A CALCULUS CHARTING

A comprehensive charting of oral conditions may include the identification and recording of oral deposits such as calculus and stain. This procedure is particularly useful for beginning students who have had limited experience in detecting calculus and in observing and "feeling" different formations and locations of hard deposits. It also helps the student begin to differentiate calculus deposits from normal anatomic characteristics, such as contact points, the cementoenamel junction, and cementum. It provides an opportunity for students to compare the "feel" of a margin of a restoration with the "feel" of calculus. Finally, comparing the results of the charting with the instructor's findings can help assess how well the student is mastering the art of detection.

As with all other initial assessment procedures, a calculus charting can provide valuable baseline data about the patient's oral conditions, which can then be compared with subsequent evaluations.

In dental hygiene practice, a calculus charting can be a useful tool in developing a dental hygiene treatment plan. A graphic description of the extent of deposits located in the mouth can help the clinician determine the amount of time needed to complete the removal of deposits and can assist in determining which instruments are most appropriate to accomplish the task. A complete calculus charting is probably performed only when a second clinician (hygienist, periodontist, dentist) is likely to perform the deposit removal. In most instances the hygienist who plans and completes the dental hygiene care, including complete scaling, will perform a cursory review of surfaces known to frequently harbor deposits and make an overall assessment based on those findings. This can easily be accomplished during the phase of assessment when pocket depths are assessed. A periodontal probe can readily detect the presence or absence of calculus deposits—particularly those located close to the attachment of the soft tissue to the tooth and those located in furcation areas. Thus, as the probe is used to assess sulcus and/or pocket depth, it can be serving the dual function of assessing the presence or absence of hard deposits.

In most instances heavy subgingival calculus can be seen radiographically, especially those deposits that extend from the proximal surfaces into the interdental spaces. They are seen as radiopaque spicules (spurs) or chunks of calculus, usually at or apical to the cementoenamel junction. Radiographs can be useful adjuncts in preparing a calculus charting and in determining the extent of deposits in the pocket (Fig. 12-2).

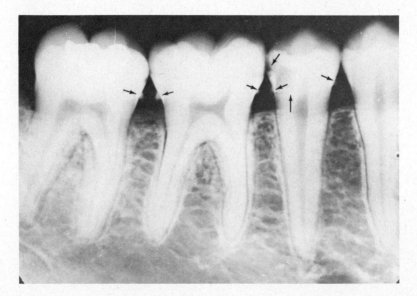

Fig. 12-2. Calculus is observable as spicules extending outward into proximal spaces and as ring around crown of second premolar. Compare radiopacity of calculus with radiolucency of caries on distal aspect of premolar. (From Wuehrmann, A.H., and Manson-Hing, L.R. 1981. Dental radiology, ed. 5. St. Louis: The C.V. Mosby Co.)

Since radiographs can provide such useful information in assessing the presence or absence of calculus, it is wise to review the radiographic survey first, charting the presence of deposits on the standard charting form. Calculus is usually indicated by drawing its shape and size on an anatomic charting form. It can be marked in a color to distinguish it from caries, restorations, and other findings if the calculus charting is to be combined with the comprehensive charting on one form.

In assessing the radiographic survey for calculus, one tooth at a time should be reviewed, focusing on the proximal and cervical areas of the teeth. Observing the most apical aspect of the margins of restorations that extend on the proximal surfaces can often reveal small deposits, otherwise often missed in clinical chartings.

Once the radiographic charting of calculus is complete, the clinician should then begin the clinical charting by exploring each tooth surface, using the basic principles of instrumentation described in Chapter 5, being certain to extend the instrument well across the proximal surfaces from both the facial and lingual aspects, and ensuring that the instrument drops to the base of the sulcus or pocket. Failure to cover all surfaces that are exposed to the oral environment will probably result in an inaccurate charting. It is particularly important to ensure that when the instrument meets resistance in the sulcus, it is because it has reached the elastic resistance of the attachment and not the hard resistance of a piece of ledge calculus. There is a distinct difference in the feeling of the resistance. If the stopping point feels hard, the instrument should be moved out and around the deposit so that it can continue to the bottom of the sulcus or pocket. This is a frequent mistake in calculus detection.

Other frequent mistakes in detecting deposits are:

1. Failure to move the instrument sufficiently across the proximal surface to ensure that the center of the proximal surface is explored from both aspects of the tooth (facial and lingual). Calculus tends to attach in the furrows and other indentations on the teeth, particularly on the mesial and distal aspects. Exploring short of the midpoint of the proximal surface will probably result in undetected deposits (Fig. 12-3).

2. Failure to adequately explore the corners or line angles of the teeth. Frequently a clinician will explore the proximal surfaces thoroughly and then, when turning the instrument to explore the direct facial and lingual surfaces, miss the corner of the root (Fig. 12-4). Spicules of calculus are then left uncharted.

When patients have a low prevalence of plaque and gingivitis, the role of irregular or malposed teeth in the formation of calculus becomes more obvious. There is a positive correlation between malposed teeth and calculus formation (Buckley, 1980, 1981); thus careful exploring for calculus in

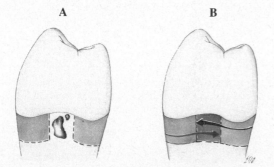

Fig. 12-3. When proximal area is being explored, explorer must cover tooth surface past midpoint of proximal surface. **A,** If exploratory strokes are stopped short of midpoint, calculus that is frequently found in furrows of root and directly below contact area will not be detected. **B,** Exploring past midpoint of tooth from both facial and lingual aspects will ensure that this critical portion of the tooth is thoroughly examined.

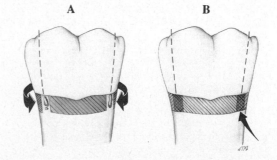

Fig. 12-4. A, Calculus remains undetected on line angles of teeth, **B,** unless exploratory strokes used to cover facial aspect overlap with strokes covering proximal aspects. Undetected calculus at "corners" of teeth is a common error for beginning clinicians.

these areas is important and often challenging because of the limited access caused by the malpositions. Even for patients who practice good oral hygiene, deposits are likely to form in these areas.

As each tooth is explored, it should be examined for the presence of supragingival calculus as well, using air and light and by tracing the tip of the explorer over the visible tooth structure. As deposits are located on each tooth, they should be recorded on the chart form. Being anatomically specific in calling these findings to an assistant will ensure the accuracy of the finished charting. The finished charting should be helpful in planning care and in showing the patient the extent of the deposits present in his/her mouth.

SCORING CALCULUS

It may be necessary in clinical practice to attempt to quantitate the amount of calculus present on teeth. The most widely used indices in epidemiologic studies are the Periodontal Disease Index (PDI) (Ramfjord, 1959) and the Oral Hygiene Index (OHI) (Greene and Vermillion, 1960) or OHI-simplified index (OHIS) (Greene and Vermillion, 1964) in which only six teeth are scored. Calculus is an important component in these indices. In the PDI, presence of calculus is described as *slight*, *moderate*, or *abundant* for grades *1*, *2*, and *3*, respectively. In the OHI indices, both supragingival and subgingival calculus are evaluated, as shown in Table 12-1. Both the PDI and OHI require the use of an explorer to detect the amount and/or location of calculus deposits. These indices are recommended for routine use because of their widespread acceptance and reproducibility (Volpe, 1974).

Table 12-1. Calculus scoring criteria in the OHI or OHIS systems

	Calculus	
Score	Supragingival	Subgingival
0	None	None
1	Less than one third of crown	None
2	Less than two thirds of crown	Single or isolated deposits
3	More than two thirds of crown	Continuous band

These methods have been developed to quantitate calculus on specific tooth surfaces. When these methods were compared with determining the effect of unsupervised toothbrushing on calculus formation after 1 to 2 weeks, all scoring methods showed significant effects; the greatest reduction was scored using the Volpe-Manhold probe method (Tuersky, 1970).

This method measures the extent of a supragingival deposit in three planes (vertical, and diagonally across the deposit from the mesioincisal and distoincisal edges) on the lingual surfaces of the six mandibular anterior teeth with a periodontal probe graduated in millimeters. This technique is most useful in doing clinical surveys but is of limited value in planning care for individual patients, since it assesses only selected teeth, does not address subgingival deposits, and requires that the examiner be highly trained (Volpe, 1974).

ACTIVITIES

1. Examine extracted teeth for the presence of calculus, identifying each type of deposit for its shape, location, consistency, and color.
2. Explore the calculus on extracted teeth, tracing its shape and differentiating it from the cementoenamel junction and margins of restorations. Compare the feel of calculus with the feel of cementum and enamel.
3. Prepare a calculus charting for a more advanced student's patient. Compare findings with those of the advanced student's charting. Observe as heavy deposits are removed by the advanced student.
4. Review Moskow's case description (1978) of a patient with unusual calculus formation. Note the radiographic indications of calculus and bone loss and the shape of the gingivae after calculus was removed.

REVIEW QUESTIONS

1. In what way is a calculus charting a useful assessment tool in clinical practice?
2. Describe the shape and location of the following types of calculus:
   a. Ledge
   b. Veneer
   c. Crustaceous
   d. Fingerlike projections
3. What is the role of calculus in the progression of periodontal disease?
4. True or false
   a. Calculus forms a mechanical lock with the cementum by molding itself to the irregularities of the tooth.

b. Plaque is mineralized to form the hard deposit, calculus.

c. The outer surface of a calculus deposit is less porous than the portion next to the tooth.

d. There is one kind of mineralization center seen in forming calculus, which is initiated by and formed with microorganisms.

e. Hard deposits can form within 2 days of a thorough cleaning.

REFERENCES

Alexander, A.G. 1971. A study of the distribution of supra and subgingival calculus, bacterial plaque and gingival inflammation in the mouths of 400 individuals. J. Periodontol. **42**:21.

Allen, D., and Kerr, D. 1965. Tissue response in the guinea pig to sterile and nonsterile calculus. J. Periodontol. **36**:121.

Armitage, G.C. 1974. Selected lectures in periodontology. San Francisco: University of California.

Baer, P.N. 1970. What is the role of subgingival calculus in the etiology of and progression of periodontal disease? J. Periodontol. **43**:284.

Baumhammers, A., et al. 1973. Scanning electron microscopy of supragingival calculus. J. Periodontol. **44**:92.

Buckley, L.A. 1980. The relationships between irregular teeth, plaque, calculus and gingival disease. Br. Dent. J., **148** (3):67.

Buckley, L.A. 1981. The relationships between malocclusion, gingival inflammation, plaque, and calculus. J. Periodontol. **52**:35.

Canis, M.F., et al. 1979. Calculus attachment. J. Periodontol. **50**:406.

Fischman, S.L., and Picozzi, A. 1969. Review of the literature: the methodology of clinical calculus evaluation. J. Periodontol. **40**:607.

Friskopp, J., an Hammarström, L. 1980. A comparative, scanning electron microscopic study of supragingival and subgingival calculus. J. Periodontol. **51**:553.

Friskopp, J., and Hammarström, L. 1982. An enzyme histochemical study of dental plaque and calculus. Acta. Odontol. Scand. **40**:459.

Goldman, H.M., and Cohen, D.W. 1980. Introduction to periodontics, ed 6. St. Louis: The C.V. Mosby Co.

Greene, J.C., and Vermillion, J.R. 1960. The oral hygiene index: a method for classifying oral hygiene status. J. Am. Dent. Assoc. **61**:171.

Greene, J.C., and Vermillion, J.R. 1964. The simplified oral hygiene index. J. Am. Dent. Assoc. **68**:7.

Hazen, S.P. 1970. What is the role of subgingival calculus in the etiology and progression of periodontal disease? J. Periodontol. **43**:285.

Kani, T., et al. 1983. Microbeam x-ray diffraction analysis of dental calculus. J. Dent. Res. **62**:92.

Knuuttila, M., et al. 1979. Concentrations of Ca, Mg, Mn, Sr, and Zn in supra- and subgingival calculus. Scand. J. Dent. Res. **87**:67.

Kowalski, C.J. 1971. Relationship between smoking and calculus deposition. J. Dent. Res. **50**:101.

Listgarten, M.A., and Ellegaard, B. 1973. Electron microscopic evidence of a cellular attachment between junctional epithelium and dental calculus. J. Periodont. Res. **8**:143.

Lustmann, J., Lewis-Epstein, J., and Shteyer, A. 1976. Scanning electron microscopy of dental calculus. Calcif. Tissue Res. **21**:47.

Mandel, I.D. 1972. Biochemical aspects of calculus formation. J. Periodont. Res. (Suppl.)**10**:7; also **9**:211, 1974.

Mislowsky, W.J., and Mazzella, W.J. 1974. Supragingival and subgingival plaque and calculus formation in humans. J. Periodontol. **45**:823.

Moskow, B.S. 1970. What is the role of subgingival calculus in the etiology and progression of periodontal disease? J. Periodontol. **43**:283.

Moskow, B.S. 1978. A case report of unusual dental calculus formation. J. Periodontol. **49**:326.

Ramfjord, S.P. 1959. Indices for prevalence and incidence of periodontal disease. J. Periodontol. **30**:51.

Retief, D.H., et al. 1972. Quantitative analysis of Mg, Na, Cl, Al, and Ca in human dental calculus by neutron activation analysis and high resolution gamma spectrometry. J. Dent. Res. **51**:807.

Retief, D.H. et al. 1973. The quantitative analysis of Sb, Ag, Zn, Co, and Fe in human dental calculus by neutron activation analysis and high resolution gamma spectrometry. J. Periodont. Res. **8**:263.

Schroeder, H.E. 1969. Formation and inhibition of dental calculus. Berne, Switzerland: Hans Huber Publishers.

Selvig, K.A. 1970. Attachment of plaque and calculus to tooth surfaces. J. Periodont. Res. **5**:8.

Sidaway, D.A. 1980. A microbial study of dental calculus. IV. An electron microscopic study of in vitro calcified microorganisms. J. Periodont. Res. **15**:240.

Singh, S., Manhold, J.H., and Volpe, A.R. 1972. Definitive determination of clinical relationship between dental plaque and calculus. J. Periodontol. **43**:39.

Slomiany, A., et al. 1981. Lipid composition of human parotid saliva from light and heavy dental calculus-formers. Arch. Oral Biol. **26**:151.

Spencer, A.J., et al. 1983. Periodontal disease in five and six year old children. J. Periodontol. **54**:19.

Suomi, J.D., et al. 1971. Oral calculus in children. J. Periodontol. **42**:341.

Theilade, J., Fitzgerald, R.J., and Scott, D.B. 1964. Electron microscopic observation of calculus in germfree and conventional rats. Arch. Oral Biol. **9**:97.

Tuersky, S.S. 1970. What is the role of subgingival calculus in the etiology and progression of periodontal disease? J. Periodontol. **43**:285.

Villa, P. 1968. Degree of calculus inhibition by habitual toothbrushing. Helv. Odontol. Acta **12**:31.

Volpe, A.R. 1974. Indices for the measurement of hard deposits in clinical studies of oral hygiene and periodontal disease. J. Periodont. Res. (Suppl. 14)**9**:31.

13 PLAQUE AND GINGIVAL INDICES

OBJECTIVES: *The reader will be able to*

1. Differentiate among nonmineralized deposits of pellicle, materia alba, debris, and plaque.
2. Describe the nature and formation of plaque and its importance in the etiology of caries, gingivitis, and calculus.
3. Describe the purposes and usefulness of each of the plaque and gingival indices available.
4. Show and describe to patients the differences among the various soft dental deposits and methods for their detection.
5. Select and use one or more of the indices more appropriate for particular dental practice needs as compared with needs for clinical or epidemiologic studies.

SOFT DEPOSITS

Soft, or nonmineralized, dental deposits can occur on all supragingival and subgingival surfaces of the teeth and sometimes on the gingival tissues. They can cause discoloration and fullness of the oral structures. By enhancing the adherence of food particles and bacteria on and around teeth, they initiate the processes associated with caries and periodontal disease. Specific terms have been used by investigators to describe these deposits. Since the clinician should know the differences among the deposits and be able to discuss and demonstrate these differences to the patient, they are defined in this chapter for common understanding. While there have been many in-depth reviews of the non-mineralized dental deposits (Dawes, 1968; Gibbons and Van Houte, 1973; Goldman and Cohen, 1980; Jenkins, 1965; Katz, McDonald, and Stookey, 1979), the general definitions have not significantly changed since the World Health Organization (WHO) report in 1961 on periodontal disease. What has occurred in intervening years has been an increased knowledge of histologic, chemical, microbiologic, and pathogenic information about the effects of these deposits (Armstrong, 1967; Lie, 1978; Osterberg, Sudo, and Folke, 1976; Socransky, 1977). Definitions of deposits according to the guidelines of the WHO report are discussed on p. 205 and are summarized in Table 13-1.

Table 13-1. Silness and Löe Plaque Thickness Index

Index	Description
0	No gingival area plaque. The gingival area of the tooth is literally free of plaque, and no soft matter adheres to the end of a probe passed over the site.
1	A thin film of plaque adhering to the free gingival margin and adjacent area of the tooth. No plaque is observed in situ but is visible on the tip of a probe after it has been moved across the tooth surface.
2	Moderate accumulation of soft deposit at the gingival sulcus, along the gingival margin and/or adjacent tooth surface, seen without disclosing solution. The gingival area is covered with a thin to moderately thick layer of plaque.
3	Abundant soft matter in the gingival pocket and/or at the gingival margin and adjacent tooth surface. The accumulation of soft material obliterates the gingival sulcus between the gingival margin and the tooth surface. Each area of the teeth (facial, mesial, lingual, and distal) is evaluated. Scores for all four areas are totaled and divided by 4 to give a mean score per tooth.

Modified from Silness, J., and Löe, H. 1964. Acta Odontol. Scand. **22:**121.

acquired pellicle An acellular film originating from saliva and gingival fluids. Acquired pellicle cannot be completely removed by vigorous water rinsing or brushing with a dentifrice. It can be removed by professional prophylaxis; however, these acellular deposits will re-form within a few hours. Acquired pellicle will stain with a dental disclosing agent; however, it appears much lighter than disclosed plaque or calculus. Pellicle is a preferred attachment site for bacteria; as such, it is the initial attachment site of organisms that will eventually form the organized matrix defined as plaque. When microorganisms become affixed in pellicle and resolve into plaque, pellicle can no longer be differentiated from the complex plaque.

food debris Particulate matter, mostly of food particles, which can be dislodged by muscular movements, water rinsing, and proper home care. Food debris can become impacted in plaque, between the teeth, or subgingivally and can be broken down by enzymes from plaque or saliva. This type of food debris should be differentiated from fiber strands, which are trapped in areas of food impaction.

plaque A dense coherent mass of microorganisms in an organized intermicrobial matrix, which adheres to tooth or restoration surfaces and remains attached despite muscle action, vigorous water rinsing, or irrigation. The primary sources of microbial plaque are oral microorganisms and salivary components.

materia alba A loosely adherent complex of bacteria and cellular debris that covers plaque deposits. It has no uniform or regular internal pattern as does plaque. Materia alba can be removed by vigorous water rinsing or irrigation. Materia alba is a mixture of living and dead microorganisms.

All of the aforementioned nonmineralized deposits have been defined and described as supragingival deposits. All these deposits, especially plaque, can occur subgingivally. In this chapter only supragingival soft deposits are discussed because these (1) are more abundant, (2) are more easily visualized and demonstrated to the patient, (3) are considered responsible for the initiation of dental disease involving the gingiva, (4) have been studied more extensively for their microbial composition and pathogenic potential, and (5) can be more easily removed (Goldman and Cohen, 1980; Socransky et al., 1977; Tempel, 1975). If supragingival plaque is adequately controlled, no subgingival plaque will form (Waerhaug, 1978).

Of all the soft dental deposits that have been described, *plaque* is considered the most important and has been referred to as the *primary etiologic factor* in the initiation of both caries and periodontal disease. It is the one factor that, if eliminated, will eliminate the cause of the majority of the diseases currently treated in dental practice. With conscientious home care by the patient, all plaque can be removed; with the elimination of plaque, there will be no progression of any dental disease that owes its etiology to that agent.

PLAQUE
Description by location, metabolic activity, and reactions

One convenient way to classify plaque is to describe its location as coronal, gingival, or subgingival (Goldman and Cohen, 1980). *Coronal plaque* is found on the tooth surfaces but not in contact with the gingiva. *Gingival plaque* refers to deposits that are in contact with or at the gingival margin. *Subgingival plaque* then refers to the deposits that are found within the gingival crevice or within the periodontal pocket. Terminology more frequently used defines plaque as being either *supragingival* (i.e., above the gingival margin and in contact with the dentition) or *subgingival* (i.e., below the gingival margin or in the periodontal pocket).

Plaque is also classified by activity. *Metabolizing plaque* is considered the primary etiologic factor in the progression of both caries and periodontal disease. Recently the term *safe-plaque* has been used by several investigators (Yankell, 1984), since clinical studies have been conducted where plaque levels were not reduced by experimental agents; however, gingivitis reductions were observed. In these studies plaque appeared to be neutralized or lacked the ability to produce metabolites that could induce gingival reactions. Additional safety factors that might be ascribed to plaque include its acting as a buffer or a protective barrier, preventing direct food contact with or pH effects on enamel, and as a reservoir for fluoride. Further research is necessary to produce more definitive information about this subject.

Plaque has also been defined by the reactions it produces (Fig. 13-1). When carbohydrate materials, primarily simple sugars such as sucrose and glucose, are metabolized by plaque, an acid situation is produced that can lead to demineralization of enamel, commonly referred to as *caries*. When plaque metabolism develops or results in basic pH, calcification of the microbial content occurs.

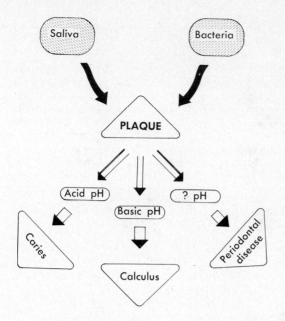

Fig. 13-1. Relationship of plaque to development of oral diseases.

Plaque then becomes mineralized and is referred to or defined as *calculus* or *tartar;* these deposits can no longer be removed by simple home care procedures. These mineralized deposits must be removed by professional scaling. Metabolic changes occuring in plaque can also result in *gingival changes.* However, the relationship of pH to these gingival changes has not been clearly established. If allowed to continue, these metabolic processes within plaque produce continuing changes on or in the gingiva, resulting in both *edematous* (size) and *erythematous* (color) changes. These changes can be accompanied by bleeding pocket formation (separation of the attachment apparatus between the gingiva and the tooth) or can proceed to other signs of periodontal disease (Loë, Theilade, and Jensen, 1965).

Formation

Much of our knowledge regarding the formation and the pathogenic potential of plaque has resulted from two experimental procedures. The first has been to use what are termed *tooth foils* or *strips* (Mandel, 1967).

These foils are attached to the teeth with wire or string ligatures and are removed after various times of deposit formation. The deposits then can be studied for microbial content, weight, and biochemical characteristics. The second procedure, which has resulted in considerable information on the microbiologic components of plaque and its gingival reactions, has been termed *the no-oral-hygiene procedure* (Loë, Theilade, and Jensen, 1965). In this method, subjects refrain from all oral hygiene, including toothbrushing, flossing, the use of mouth rinses, toothpicks, and all other interdental aids. The use of nonantiseptic breath fresheners is often allowed as some reward for the patient during the study. No-oral-hygiene procedures are conducted for various time periods of up to 21 days, or when gingivitis symptoms start to appear.

Early plaque formation occurs in an organized and orderly fashion with distinct differences in microbial succession (Loë, Theilade, and Jensen, 1965; "Periodontal disease," 1961) and is influenced by salivary components (Socransky, 1977). Following a complete dental cleaning, gram-positive cocci are the first organisms to attach to pellicle on days 1 and 2 of the no-oral-hygiene period. On days 3 and 4, gram-positive filamentous organisms begin to appear and eventually grow into the coccal layer and replace these initial organisms. On days 6 to 10, a more mixed bacterial flora begins to appear; the plaque becomes more gram negative and contains anaerobic organisms. From days 10 to 21, initial signs of gingival inflammation can begin. During this time the plaque organisms are spirochetes and vibrios arranged in a densely packed structure (Loë, Theilade, and Jensen, 1965). Plaque weight is essentially maximized from days 8 to 10 (Mandel, 1967).

During no-brushing regimens, several factors become apparent as to the amount of plaque formed in different areas of the mouth. There are no major differences in plaque scores between the maxillary and mandibular arches or among different groups of teeth (incisors, premolars, molars). There are no marked variations in plaque evaluated at the interproximal and buccal areas of the teeth. The lingual tooth areas, however, accumulate less plaque. When gingivitis is evaluated, there are no marked differences in the gingival areas between the teeth of the maxillary and mandibular arches or in any one group of teeth. When the scores from the different gingival areas are compared, the interproximal have higher gingivitis scores than do the buccal surfaces. The lingual surfaces have the lowest index of those evaluated. The interdental areas of the upper molar teeth have the highest gingivitis scores, and the lingual area of the lower molars have the best gingival condition in these experiments (Löe, Theilade, and Jensen, 1965).

It has been proposed that no-oral-hygiene clinical studies for evaluating plaque should be conducted for time periods of 1 to 10 days, and those studies evaluating effects of agents on gingivitis should be conducted for a period of up to 21 days. Since symptoms of gingivitis occur in control groups (i.e., those receiving a placebo or product containing no known active ingredient[s]) after 21 days of no oral hygiene, it is considered that this period should be a maximum. In studies that include toothbrushing, much longer periods are necessary to produce gingivitis. It is difficult to estimate the periods necessary for testing the effectiveness of agents for preventing plaque or gingivitis when toothbrushing regimens are included (Mandel, 1974).

Prevention and control

Several review articles have described the rationale for preventing plaque and chemotherapeutic approaches for preventing plaque (Lobene, 1976; Loesche, 1976). Several categories of these test agents are briefly reviewed as follows:

Enzymes. The rationale behind this category of agents is the attempt to dissolve the intermatrix substance that binds the bacteria together within plaque.

Surface-active agents. The rationale for testing this category of agents is that they are similar to cleaning detergents, which lower the ability to adhere. Theoretically, in plaque, the ability of bacteria to adhere to enamel or pellicle would be decreased. Similarly, agents in this category would attempt to dissolve or lift off the bacteria by reducing surface tension.

Antibiotics. These agents have potent antibacterial properties. When applied topically, several broad-spectrum antibiotic agents are highly effective in controlling plaque. A major problem associated with these agents is that long-term use may result in overgrowth of microorganisms, either by bacteria-resistant strains developing or by opportunistic organisms being favored, such as yeast or molds that cause "black hairy tongue," staining, and other undesirable side effects. The primary difficulty with agents in this category is that they are used for life-threatening diseases and should not be used for a "minor problem" such as plaque control.

Antibacterial agents. These are agents with less potent antibacterial effects than antibiotics. Many have been tested for prevention of plaque and gingivitis. Several have shown excellent results in short-term studies; however, none have yielded significant activity when tested in clinical studies of 1 to 2 year's duration.

Flavor oils. Various individual and combinations of flavor oils (e.g., thymol, menthol, eucalyptol) have shown antibacterial properties in laboratory studies. In short-term clinical studies antiplaque activity has also been demonstrated.

To date, there are no agents or product formulations that have been classified by the Food and Drug Administration as safe and effective (Loesche, 1976), or that the American Dental Association has granted acceptance to, with regard to plaque claims.

INDICES

Several methods are used to attempt to quantify the accumulation of soft materials on tooth surfaces. Most of these procedures have been developed to evaluate plaque in epidemiologic surveys or clinical studies. Little attention has been paid to developing procedures for use in clinical practice, which would be meaningful to both the clinician and the patient. The purpose of this section is to describe the rationale behind what we consider the more practical plaque scoring methods available and attempt to give the dental professional some ideas that might be used when treating patients.

In epidemiologic and community programs

Before describing particular indices, it might be useful to describe the rationale for developing dental indices in general and their use in various populations. The first use of indices was in epidemiologic studies where the incidence and prevalence of dental disease in large populations had to be determined. An epidemiologic study is a cross-sectional evaluation or survey of large groups of people to evaluate such factors as age, sex, nutritional differences, income, etc. (Biswas, Duperon, and Chebib, 1977). Indices used in epidemiologic studies are also useful in evaluating the success of community health planning and public health programs and in indicating the need for changes.

In research

With the development of agents that prevented dental disease in laboratory and animal models, more critical indices had to be developed to evaluate the success of these materials in the clinic. By necessity, this also involved training and standardization among investigators. The basic principles that should be adhered to by the investigator when using particular clinical quantitating procedures have been described in detail (Volpe, 1974). Briefly, these include (1) thorough familiarization with an index; (2) the use of specific and appropriate equipment; (3) having an assistant record the findings using a standard examination form; and, perhaps most important, (4) resisting the temptation to modify the procedure or equipment for the investigator's particular needs.

In clinical practice

Plaque scoring can be done for all teeth present in the mouth or for selected teeth. The concept of using specific teeth instead of the whole mouth score was introduced by Ramfjord (1956). Six teeth are measured; these are the maxillary right first molar, maxillary left central incisor, maxillary left first premolar, mandibular left first molar, mandibular right central incisor, and mandibular right first premolar. The use of a six-tooth index has been shown by other investigators to be a valid representation of plaque scores for the entire dentition (Jamison, 1960; Shick and Ash, 1961). This approach is most useful in epidemiologic studies or, with more critical indices, in clinical efficacy investigations. Plaque scoring only selected teeth may be useful in the dental office when it is desirable to chart the progress of specific teeth or particular problematic areas.

Plaque scoring methods

Plaque scoring has been divided into three methods used to quantitate supragingival plaque occurrence on teeth. These are plaque *thickness, area,* and *weight.*

Thickness. The method developed by Silness and Löe (1964) has been referred to as the *Plaque Thickness Index (PTI).* This index focuses on the gingival area of the tooth and attempts to characterize the thickness of the accumulations. Because plaque thickness varies on different parts of the tooth, measurements are taken at the buccal, lin-gual, mesial, and distal aspects. Scores from these areas are added, and the total is divided by 4 to give the plaque thickness for the individual tooth. Scores for all of the teeth are then added and divided by the number of teeth examined to give the mean plaque thickness score for the patient. The criteria for evaluating thickness are described in Table 13-1. Scoring according to the PTI requires the use of a probe to evaluate the lower, or 0 to 1, scores. A probe is traced across the defined tooth surface area at the level of the gingival margin to determine if plaque is present. If a "globule" of plaque is present on the probe, a score of 1 is assigned to this area. When a score of 2 or more is evaluated in this system, plaque is visible to the naked eye. Disclosing solutions are not used in the plaque thickness scoring system.

Area. In scoring plaque thickness, only differences in thickness of the deposit in the gingival area of the tooth are scored; no attention is paid to the coronal or surface extension of plaque. Indices that evaluate this factor (i.e., plaque extension) are referred to as plaque area scoring systems. All plaque area scoring systems require the use of plaque disclosing agents. Many of the early plaque area systems evaluated the tooth surface by arbitrarily dividing the tooth into thirds or quarters. Since the periodontal pathogenic potential of plaque leading to gingivitis is considered to be at the gingival margin, recent scoring procedures have paid more attention to, or have arbitrarily given higher scores to, plaque that occurs in the gingival third of the tooth (Mandel, 1974). One of these procedures is Turesky, Gilmore, and Glickman's modification (1970) of the Quigley and Hein index. While the areas evaluated by both indices are the same, the criteria for this scoring system have been better defined, as shown in Fig. 13-2. Two other area scoring indices that have placed emphasis not only on the gingival margin but also on the interproximal areas are the *Modified Navy Plaque Index* (Elliott et al., 1972) (Fig. 13-3, *A*) and the Martens and Meskin (1972) adaptation of the Podshadley and Haley index (Fig. 13-3, *B*). In these modified indices, the tooth is divided into four or five segments respectively, and each segment is assigned a letter and a score of 0 or 1.

The *O'Leary Plaque Control Record* (O'Leary, Drake, and Naylor, 1972) was designed as a simple method for the dental professional to use in scoring

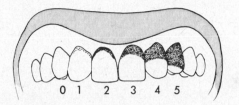

CROWN AREA COVERED BY PLAQUE

Fig. 13-2. Turesky, Gilmore, and Glickman's plaque area scoring method.

0 — None

1 — Separate flecks

2 — Continuous band to 1 mm

3 — >1 mm and < 1/3

4 — > 1/3 and < 2/3

5 — > 2/3

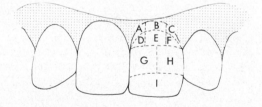

A

CROWN AREA COVERED BY PLAQUE

A,B,C — Continuous band to 1 mm

D,E,F — >1 mm and < 1/3

G,H — > 1/3 and < 2/3

I — > 2/3

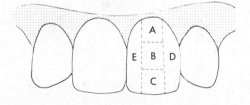

B

CROWN AREA COVERED BY PLAQUE

Middle area:

    A — Gingival 1/3

    B — Middle 1/3

    C — Incisal 1/3

D — Distal area

E — Mesial area

Fig. 13-3. **A,** Modified Navy Plaque Index. **B,** Martens and Meskin adaptation of Podshadley and Haley index.

areas of plaque accumulation for individual patients. An oval symbol, representing each permanent tooth, has been divided into four segments to represent the mesial, distal, facial, and lingual surfaces. The use of this form to record baseline and recall plaque scores allows both the patient and the professional to visualize exactly where plaque remains. This visualization is valuable during plaque control instruction, since specific problem areas can be pointed out and discussed with the patient along with possible solutions. In addition, both the professional and the patient can see visual evidence of progress at recall appointments when improved plaque records are compared with the initial record. This objective measure of patient progress can provide a sense of accomplishment and motivation for the patient.

The record is scored by disclosing the patient's teeth and then examining each tooth surface, using an explorer or the tip of a probe, for the presence of soft stained accumulations on the cervical third of the tooth at the dentogingival junction. If a soft deposit is visible, the corresponding surface is marked on the plaque control record by shading it or placing a dash in the area. Only plaque accumulation that occurs at the dentogingival junction is recorded on the form. Those surfaces that have soft accumulations that are not at the distogingival

junction are not recorded. No attempt is made to differentiate between varying amounts of plaque on the tooth surfaces. Teeth that are not present in the mouth should be crossed out on the recording form (Fig. 13-4).

After all teeth have been examined, an index can be calculated by dividing the number of plaque-containing surfaces by the total number of available surfaces (total number of teeth × 4 surfaces). This procedure is repeated at each appointment and the percentages of plaque-covered surfaces are compared to evaluate the patient's progress.

Plaque area measurements require that plaque be visualized by the use of disclosing agents (Yankell and Emling, 1978). There are several commercially available plaque disclosing preparations that have been accepted by the American Dental Association. Following is a brief description of several available materials.

The most widely used disclosing agent has been erythrosine, or FD & C (Food, Drug, and Cosmetic) red No. 3 (Arnim, 1963). The primary problem with this material is that because of its red color it can be difficult to distinguish between stained deposits and stained gingiva. This agent stains the gingiva and other oral soft tissues, including the lips; it also has a potential for staining silicate fillings, clothing, and sink materials.

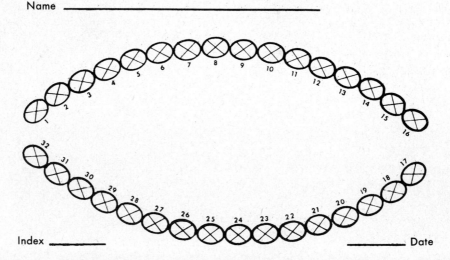

Name _____

Index _____   _____ Date

Fig. 13-4. O'Leary Plaque Control Record. (From O'Leary, T.J., Drake, R.B., and Naylor, J.E. 1972. J. Periodontol. **43**:38.)

Another visible colorant used is FD & C green No. 3 (Mandel, 1974). This agent readily distinguishes plaque from the gingiva; however, it has the same staining drawbacks as erythrosine. There are no commercially available products containing this colorant, and 2% to 5% solutions must be prepared by the researcher.

A commercially available combination of FD & C red No. 3 and FD & C blue No. 1 differentiates between old and newly formed plaque (Block, Lobene, and Derdivanis, 1972; Gallagher, Fussell, and Cutress, 1977). This differentiation is due to differences in plaque penetration or permeability of these two different colorants. Again, this combination of food colors has the disadvantages of discoloring soft tissues and undesirable staining.

A different type of plaque disclosing system is Plak-Lite.* This system uses sodium fluorescein, which is not visible under normal light. Plaque stained with sodium fluorescein becomes visible only under a properly filtered light source (Lang, Ostergaard, and Löe, 1972). In laboratory studies, uptake of sodium fluorescein by plaque bacteria has been shown to be more specific than uptake of erythrosine (Landay et al., 1974).

Weight. A third method used in clinical studies for determining plaque is plaque weight (Lobene, 1970). With this procedure, after a disclosing agent is used, all plaque is removed from specified teeth and evaluated by determining wet and/or dry weight. This procedure involves the use of excellent research facilities and probably cannot be done in the general dental office.

Miscellaneous. Other methods to quantitate plaque include evaluating the chemical content, such as calcium, phosphorus, protein, etc., or attempting to determine the percent of the tooth surface covered by stained plaque by planimetry (Mandel, 1974). These parameters are too sophisticated for routine use in clinical practice.

Measurement of gingival inflammation

Gingivitis. Following are descriptions of several methods for measuring gingival inflammation. Criteria used for specific research studies have been compared with those that are practical for use in the dental office.

In 1950 Massler, Schour, and Chopra introduced the concept of measuring gingivitis at the *P (papillary)*, *M (marginal)*, and *A (attached)* gingival units. The Massler PMA Index is then used in an all-or-none type of description to indicate whether reddening or gingivitis is present. This index has served as the basis for many epidemiologic studies; however, it is not sensitive enough to detect differences among individuals with regard to either gingivitis incidence or increases or decreases in gingivitis (Hazen, 1974).

There is considerable controversy concerning when bleeding occurs in the process of progressing from normal to diseased gingivae. Although no conclusions have been reached, an excellent discussion of this subject is available (Mandel, 1974).

Two primary procedures have been to emphasize gingival bleeding as being more important in evaluating the gingival condition. The first of these indices scores the papillary and marginal areas of the gingiva, after a probe is gently passed around the gingival margin. The criteria for this index are shown in Table 13-2. The primary emphasis of this index, the *Sulcular Bleeding Index (SBI)* (Muhlemann and Mazor, 1958), is that bleeding occurs very early in the inflammatory process of gingivitis before gingival changes in color or size are apparent, and this is emphasized in the score of 1. In the *Gingival Bleeding Index (GBI)* (Carter and Barnes, 1974), unwaxed dental floss is passed first on one side of the papilla and then on the other. Bleeding is evaluated as an all-or-none reaction on either the floss or the interproximal area.

Another approach is the Löe and Silness (1963) *Gingival Index (GI)*. Each gingival unit (i.e., the buccal, lingual, mesial, and distal aspects) of the individual tooth is scored after gentle probing. As

*Plak-Lite, Brilliant International, Bala Cynwyd, Pa.

Table 13-2. Sulcular Bleeding Index (SBI)

Index	Description
0	No inflammation.
1	Bleeding from the gingival sulcus on gentle probing. Tissues otherwise appear normal.
2	Bleeding on probing plus a color change due to inflammation. No swelling or edema.
3	Bleeding, color change, and edematous swelling.
4	Ulceration or additional symptoms.

Modified from Muhlemann, H.R., and Mazor, Z.S. 1958. Helv. Odontol. Acta **2:**3.

Table 13-3. Löe and Silness Gingival
Index (GI)

Index	Description
0	Normal gingivae. Gingivae are pink or pale color. On palpation, the gingivae should be firm.
1	Mild inflammation. Gingival margin is slightly more reddish or bluish than normal. Bleeding is not provoked when tissues are probed by running a probe along the soft tissue wall of the sulcular orifice.
2	Moderate inflammation. The gingivae exhibit redness, edema, and glazing. There is enlargement of the margin due to edema. Bleeding is provoked by probing in the presence of either mild or moderate inflammation.
3	Severe inflammation. The gingiva is markedly red or reddish blue and enlarged. Ulceration or a tendency to spontaneous bleeding (e.g., after the use of air).

Modified from Löe, H., and Silness, J. 1963. Acta Odontol. Scand. **21**:533.

Table 13-4. Suomi and Barbano
Gingivitis Index

Index	Description
0	Absence of inflammation. Stippling usually noted.
1	Inflammation, evidenced primarily by distinct color change.
2	Severe inflammation. A distinct color change coupled with swelling, loss of stippling, a spongy consistency, and bleeding on probing; or inflammation has spread to the attached gingiva.

Modified from Suomi, J.D., and Barbano, J.D. 1968. J. Periodontol. **39**:71.

with the Silness and Löe PTI (1964), the individual tooth score is divided by 4 to obtain the gingival index for the particular tooth. The criteria for this index are presented in Table 13-3. With this index, the initial score for the occurrence of bleeding is 2, and this occurs only after or in combination with visual changes in the gingival condition.

Several scoring systems are also available in which the gingival area around each tooth is considered as a distinct unit. An example of a generalized descriptive scoring approach is presented in Table 13-4.

Photographic methods have been used to keep a permanent record and to assess gingival conditions. Difficulties occur with this procedure because films vary from batch to batch, and color is often not replicative if film is developed at different times (Dunne, Day, and Alexander, 1979; Gjermo, 1974; Jones and McFall, 1977).

Gingival health has also been assessed by monitoring *gingival crevicular fluid (GCF) flow.* Flow of GCF begins before clinical signs of gingivitis can be ascertained (Borden, Golub, and Kleinberg, 1977; Löe and Holm-Pedersen, 1965; Pashley, 1976). Although GCF may not be related to preexisting gingival conditions, such as single measurements in the dental office, GCF flow can be used to monitor progress or control of gingival inflam-

mation (Cimasoni, 1974; Golub and Kleinberg, 1976). A commercial digital unit to monitor GCF (Periotron*) is available. Following is a description of the procedure for taking samples of GCF:

Procedure†

Isolate with cotton rolls and dry with gauze the region of the mouth under examination.

Place a dry paper strip in the facial crevice of the tooth to be monitored for 3 seconds to empty the crevicular pool of fluid; remove with tweezers and discard this strip.

Wait 27 seconds, and insert a dry paper strip in the crevice; wait for 3 seconds.

Remove the paper strip and immediately place in the Periotron for recording the crevicular fluid in this strip.

This procedure could be of value to the clinician monitoring treatment procedures or provide an incentive to the patient to improve home care of critical gingival areas.

Because of the difficulties involved in using gingival indices, investigators should be trained in following standardized procedures before conducting clinical studies. Unfortunately, training of the dental professional today does not always include the learning of gingival indices. These indices are valuable to demonstrate to the patient those areas that require more attention during home care procedures. Even if only an all-or-none type of index is recorded, it is strongly recommended that the practitioner maintain a record of location

*Periotron, Harco Electronics, Winnipeg, Canada.
†Modified from Borden, A.M., Golub, L.M., and Kleinberg, I. 1974. IADR Abstract No. 482.

of gingival problems, since it is this parameter that often forecasts major periodontal disease problems.

Patient motivational index focusing on gingival bleeding

Since patients associate gingival bleeding with dental disease, Muhlemann (1977) has developed the *Papillary Bleeding Index (PBI)* for use in daily clinical practice. This index differs from other gingivitis scoring methods focusing on bleeding, since attempts are made to classify the intensity of bleeding from the sulcus rather than recording bleeding as an all-or-none condition (Carter and Barnes, 1974; Muhlemann and Mazor, 1958). Briefly, the procedure for conducting the PBI is as follows. Start lingually at the upper right quadrant, at the distal aspect of tooth No. 2 (the papilla between Nos. 1 and 2). Draw an imaginary line across the base of the papilla to form an isosceles triangle (three equal sides). Insert a periodontal probe at the gingival margin, and with a light sweeping movement bring the end of the probe toward the tip of the papilla. Probe gently, using a probing depth of 1 to 3 mm. First probe the mesial aspect of No. 1, then the distal aspect of No. 2. Go to the papilla between Nos. 2 and 3 and probe the mesial aspect of No. 2 and the distal aspect of No. 3 as above. Continue to the papilla around the distal aspect of No. 8. Repeat this procedure on the buccal left maxillary, the left lingual of the mandible, and the lower right buccal. After probing each quadrant, which takes about 20 to 25 seconds, evaluate the bleeding scores of the probed sulci beginning from the last papilla. If no bleeding occurs within 10 to 15 seconds, repeat the probing on individual papillae. Assessment of bleeding intensity is based on the criteria shown in Table 13-5 and depicted in Plate 1.

Bleeding scores as they are evaluated at each visit are filled in on the PBI form (Fig. 13-5). When all teeth are present, 28 papillae can be scored. All papillae in the mouth are scored except between Nos. 8 and 9 and 24 and 25 and the distal aspects of third molars if present. If a tooth is missing, its corresponding papilla is crossed out on the form. After the individual scores are recorded, the scores for the four quadrants are added together and a total value is recorded for that session and entered to the right of the form. The Roman numerals I to V are intended for use during visits when the patient

Table 13-5. Scoring the PBI

Assigned score	Description
0	No bleeding.
1	Appearance of isolated dots of blood and/or a thin line of bleeding less than one half of area probed.
2	Appearance of a thin line of bleeding more than one half of probed area or a discrete speck of blood interdentally.
3	Interdental triangle filled with blood. Blood flows slowly toward the marginal gingiva.
4	Profuse bleeding immediately on probing. Interdental triangle filled with blood. In the mandible blood flows immediately into the marginal area; in the maxilla it flows toward the incisal or occlusal surfaces.

is developing improved oral hygiene procedures. The use of Roman numerals plus *R* is for recall appointments.

The patient should follow the probing with a hand mirror. The procedure should be explained, and the patient should participate in the evaluation of the number of bleeding sites and the intensity of the bleeding at each site. At the end of each session, the patient is told the total PBI score. Total scores are used rather than an average, since it is more impressive for a patient to witness a reduction from 83 to 53 instead of a mean index of 3.46 to 2.21. The goal for all patients is to reduce the index to a score of lower than 10.

The use of this index, from a hygienist's point of view, has recently been reported (Craig and Duhamel, 1981). In addition to its usefulness in the dental office, the PBI scoring method has been demonstrated to be effective in both school-based and public health programs (Saxer, Turconi, and Elsasser, 1977).

INVOLVING THE PATIENT IN DETERMINING PLAQUE LEVELS

Perhaps the best way to demonstrate plaque to patients would be to use the following method. When the patient arrives in the office, he/she is questioned as to when, prior to the visit, he/she had brushed and/or flossed or performed any other dental home care. At this point a disclosing agent

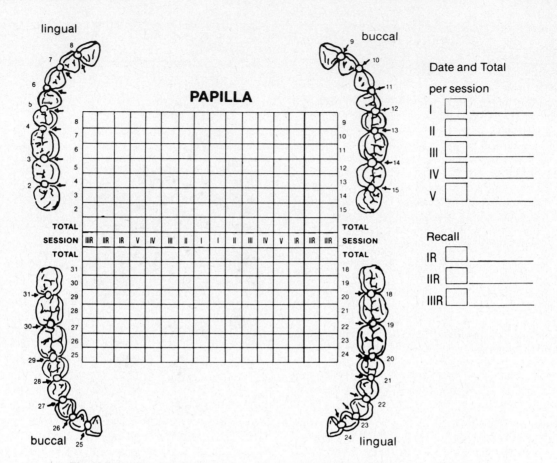

Fig. 13-5. Papillary Bleeding Index form. (Courtesy University of Pennsylvania, Philadelphia.)

is used, and the patient is examined before the mouth is rinsed with water.

The patient is shown the results, and the terms *plaque, materia alba,* and *food debris* are explained. At this point vigorous rinsing of the mouth is conducted, the patient's teeth are redisclosed, and the difference in appearance of deposits is observed and explained. The professional indicates that the materials removed were materia alba and food debris; plaque remains. Next the patient is instructed in and performs toothbrushing and flossing. After these procedures the patient again uses a disclosing agent. If toothbrushing and flossing were done properly, all nonmineralized deposits should have been removed. With a probe or ex-

plorer any stained deposits remaining are demonstrated to the patient, and at this point calculus is described and defined. After calculus deposits have been removed by the dental professional, reuse of a disclosing agent is performed; now the patient should observe no staining on any dental surfaces. At this point the patient's ability to prevent further deposits from forming and the suggested at-home use of disclosants are discussed.

SUMMARY

The use of soft deposit and gingival indices in the dental office is important for several reasons. Initially, they are used as the basis for the patient's permanent record. From information obtained, the professional will be better able to establish a diagnosis and design the treatment plan. Indices also should be used to educate and motivate the patient. Scoring criteria where the characteristic being examined can be clearly stated by the professional and understood by the patient should be used. Indices properly used can evaluate the success of treatment and preventive home care programs and the long-term benefits of disease control.

ACTIVITIES

1. Examine plaque microscopically, identifying the kinds of microorganisms present.
2. Conduct a 3- to 5-day no-oral-hygiene study in the class, observing changes in the mouth. After using a plaque disclosant, document changes with intraoral photographs or by exposing several frames of 8 mm movie film each day to record and condense the progression of disease. Reverse the process by instituting brushing and flossing; record with photographs or daily exposure of movie film.
3. Use each of the described plaque and gingival indices on a student partner. Determine which methods are most easily incorporated in clinical practice for purposes of documentation and patient instruction.
4. Use a variety of disclosing solutions and evaluate each for its effectiveness, acceptability to the patient, and ease of use.

REVIEW QUESTIONS

1. Match the following terms with the appropriate descriptions. More than one answer may be correct.
   _____ Acquired pellicle
   _____ Materia alba
   _____ Food debris
   _____ Plaque
   a. Cannot be dislodged from the teeth with muscle action and vigorous water rinsing or irrigation.
   b. A dense coherent mass of microorganisms in an intermicrobial matrix.
   c. Primary source is oral microorganisms and salivary components.
   d. Can become impacted interdentally or mechanically in the plaque.
   e. A loosely adherent complex of bacteria and cellular debris that covers plaque.
   f. Will stain with a disclosant but appears lighter than disclosed plaque or calculus.
   g. Can be dislodged with muscular movements and water rinsing or irrigation.
   h. Re-forms in a few hours after professional prophylaxis; cannot be brushed away.
   i. Major etiologic factor in dental caries and gingivitis.

2. When plaque metabolizes or develops a basic pH, _____ of the microbial content occurs.
3. When plaque metabolizes carbohydrates, a(n) _____ pH occurs that leads to _____.
4. In no-oral-hygiene procedures, describe the plaque formation that occurs in the following organized and orderly fashion:
   a. Days 1 to 2
   b. Days 3 to 4
   c. Days 6 to 10
   d. Days 8 to 10
   e. Days 10 to 21
5. Identify five categories of agents that are currently being evaluated for the prevention of plaque formation.
6. Identify the three essential types of methods used for scoring plaque.
7. In gingival indices, the primary determinant in scoring is usually _____ and/or _____ in several aspects of each tooth or considering each tooth as a unit.
8. Why should plaque and gingival indices be incorporated routinely into clinical practice?

REFERENCES

Armstrong, W.G. 1967. The composition of organic films formed on teeth. Caries Res. **1**:89.

Arnim, S.S. 1963. The use of disclosing agents for measuring tooth cleanliness. J. Periodontol. **34**:227.

Biswas, S., Duperon, D.F., and Chebib, F.S. 1977. Study of periodontal disease in children and young adolescents. J. Periodont. Res. **12**:250.

Block, P.L., Lobene, R.R., and Derdivanis, J.P. 1972. A two-tone dye test for dental plaque. J. Periodontol. **43**:423.

Borden, A.M., Golub, L.M., and Kleinberg, I. 1974. An intra-crevicular technique for monitoring gingival crevicular fluid. IADR Abstract No. 482.

Borden, S.M., Golub, L.M., and Kleinberg, I. 1977. The effect of age and sex on the relationship between crevicular fluid flow and gingivitis index in humans. J. Periodont. Res. **12**:160.

Carter, H.G., and Barnes, G.P. 1974. The gingival bleeding index. J. Periodontol. **45**:801.

Cimasoni, G. 1974. The crevicular fluid, ed. 3. Basel, Switzerland: S. Karger AG.

Craig, D., and Duhamel, L. 1981. The papillary bleeding index: a new aspect in motivation. Eighth International Symposium on Dental Hygiene. Brighton, England.

Darwish, S., Hyppa, T., and Socransky, S. 1978. Studies on predominant cultivable microbiota of early peridontitis. J. Periodont. Res. **13**:1.

Dawes, E. 1968. The nature of dental plaque, films, and calcareous deposits. Ann. N.Y. Acad. Sci. **153**:102.

Dunne, S.M., Day, C.R., and Alexander, A.G. 1979. An evaluation of the use of color transparencies for scoring gingivitis. J. Dent. Res. **58C**:1237.

Elliott, J.R., et al. 1972. Evaluation of an oral physiotherapy center in the reduction of bacterial plaque and periodontal disease. J. Periodontol. **43**:221.

Gallagher, I.H.C., Fussell, S.J., and Cutress, T.W. 1977. Mechanism of action of a two-tone plaque disclosing agent. J. Periodontol. **48**:395.

Gibbons, R.J., and Van Houte, J. 1973. On the formation of dental plaques. J. Periodontol. **44**:347.

Gjermo, P. 1974. Formal and informal discussions: indices for the measurement of gingival inflammation in clinical studies of oral hygiene and periodontal disease. J. Periodont. Res. **9**:70.

Goldman, H.M., and Cohen, D.W. 1980. Periodontal therapy, ed. 6. St. Louis: The C.V. Mosby Co.

Golub, L.M., and Kleinberg, I. 1976. Gingival crevicular fluid: a new diagnostic aid in managing the periodontal patient. Oral Sci. Rev. **8**:49.

Hazen, S.P. 1974. Indices for the measurement of gingival inflammation in clinical studies of oral hygiene and periodontal disease. J. Periodont. Res. **9**:61.

Jamison, H.D. 1960. Prevalence and severity of periodontal disease in a sample of a population. Thesis. Ann Arbor: University of Michigan, School of Public Health.

Jenkins, G.N. 1965. The chemistry of plaque. Ann. N.Y. Acad. Sci. **131**:786.

Jones, J., and McFall, W.T., Jr. 1977. A photometric study of the color of healthy gingiva. J. Periodontol. **48**:21.

Katz, S., McDonald, J.L., and Stookey, G.K. 1979. Preventive dentistry in action, ed. 3. Upper Montclair, N.J.: D.C.P. Publishing.

Landay, M.A. et al. 1974. A fluorescent microscopic study of human bacterial plaque smears stained with the plaklite fluorochrome. Calif. Dent. Assoc. J. **2**:60.

Lang, N.P., Ostergaard, E., and Löe, H. 1972. A fluorescent plaque disclosing agent. J. Periodont. Res. **7**:59.

Lie, T. 1978. Ultrastructural study of early dental plaque formation. J. Periodontol. Res. **13**:391.

Lobene, R.R. 1970. A clinical study of the effect of dextranase on human dental plaque. J. Am. Dent. Assoc. **82**:132.

Lobene, R.R. 1976. Chemotherapeutics for the prevention of dental plaque. J. Prevent. Dent. **3**:32.

Löe, H., and Holm-Pedersen, P. 1965. Absence and presence of fluid from normal and inflamed gingivae. Periodontics **3**:171.

Löe, H., and Silness, J. 1963. Periodontal disease in pregnancy. I. Prevalence and severity. Acta Odontol. Scand. **21**:533.

Löe, H., Theilade, E., and Jensen, S.B. 1965. Experimental gingivitis in man. J. Periodontol. **36**:177.

Loesche, W.J. 1976. Chemotherapy of dental plaque infections. Oral Sci. Rev. **9**:65.

Mandel, I.D. 1967. Plaque and calculus measurements—rate of formation and pathologic potential. J. Periodontol. **38**:721.

Mandel, I.D. 1974. Indices for measurement of soft accumulations in clinical studies of oral hygiene and periodontal disease. J. Periodont. Res. **9**:7.

Martens, L.V., and Meskin, L.H. 1972. An innovative technique for assessing oral hygiene. J. Dent. Child. **39**:12.

Massier, M., Schour, I., and Chopra, B. 1950. Occurrence of gingivitis in suburban Chicago school children. J. Periodontol. **21**:146.

Muhlemann, H.R. 1977. Psychological and chemical mediators of gingival health. J. Prevent. Dent. **4**:6.

Muhlemann, H.R., and Mazor, Z.S. 1958. Gingivitis in Zurich school children. Helv. Odontol. Acta **2**:3.

O'Leary, T.J., Drake, R.B., and Naylor, J.E. 1972. The plaque control record. J. Periodontol. **43**:38.

Osterberg, S.K.-A., Sudo, S.Z., and Folke, L.E.A. 1976. Microbial succession in supragingival plaque of man. J. Periodont. Res. **11**:243.

Pashley, D.H. 1976. A mechanistic analysis of gingival fluid production. J. Periodont. Res. **11**:121.

Periodontal disease. Report of an expert committee on dental health. 1961. Technical Report Series, No. 207. Geneva: World Health Organization.

Ramfjord, S. 1956. Indices for prevalence and incidence of periodontal disease. J. Periodontol. **30**:51.

Saxer, U.P., Turconi, B., and Elsasser, C.H. 1977. Patient motivation with the papillary bleeding index. J. Prevent. Dent. **4**:20.

Shick, R.A., and Ash, M.M., Jr. 1961. Evaluation of the vertical method of tooth brushing. J. Periodontol. **32**:353.

Silness, J., and Löe, H. 1964. Periodontal disease in pregnancy. II. Correlation between oral hygiene and periodontal condition. Acta. Odontol. Scand. **22**:121.

Socransky, S.S. 1977. Microbiology of periodontal disease—present status and further considerations. J. Periodontol. **48**:497.

Socransky, S.S., et al. 1977. Bacteriological studies of developing supragingival dental plaque. J. Periodont. Res. **12**:90.

Suomi, J.D., and Barbano, J.P. 1968. Patterns of gingivitis. J. Periodontol. **39**:71.

Tempel, T.R., Mareil, J.F.A., and Seibert, J.S. 1975. Comparison of water irrigation and oral rinsing on clearance of soluble and particulate materials from the oral cavity. J. Periodontol. **46**:391.

Turesky, S., Gilmore, N.D., and Glickman, I. 1970. Reduced plaque formation by the chloromethyl analogue of victamine C. J. Periodontol. **41**:41.

Volpe, A.R. 1974. Indices for the measurement of hard deposits in clinical studies of oral hygiene and periodontal disease. J. Periodont. Res. **9**:31.

Waerhaug, J. 1978. Healing of the dentoepithelial junction following subgingival plaque control. J. Periodontol. **49**:1.

Yankell, S.L. 1976-1984. Personal communications with Dr. R.R. Lobene, Dr. I.D. Mandel, and Dr. H.R. Muhlemann.

Yankell, S.L., and Emling, R.C. 1978. Understanding dental products: what you should know and what your patient should know. Continuing Dental Education, University of Pennsylvania School of Dental Medicine **1**(7):1.

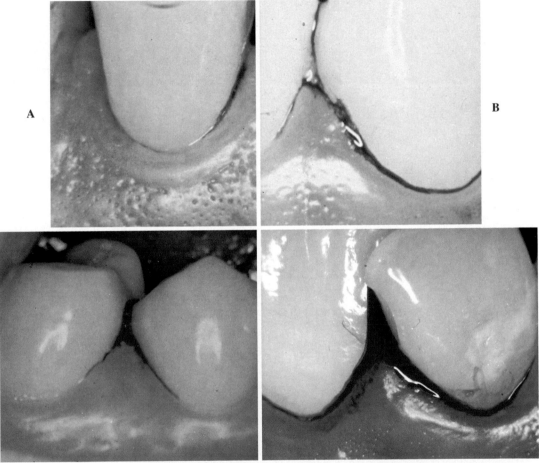

Plate 1. Photographs of PBI scores of 1 to 4 (see Table 13-5 for description of assigned scores) on mandibular papillae. **A,** Score of 1. **B,** Score of 2. **C,** Score of 3. **D,** Score of 4. (Courtesy Elida Cosmetic AG, Zurich, Switzerland.)

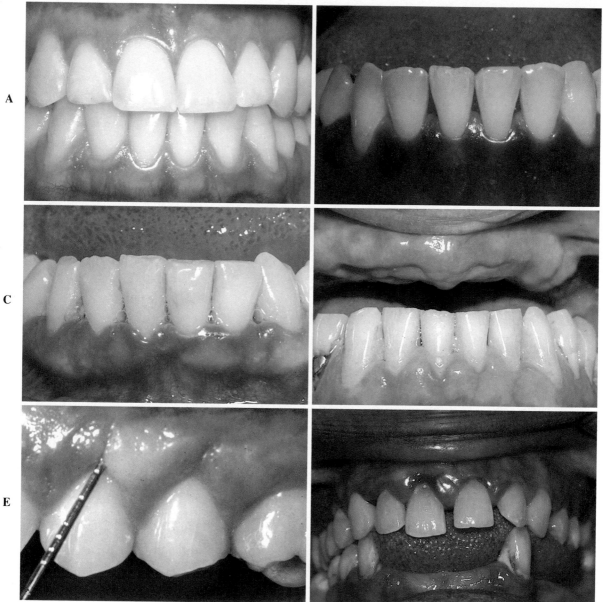

Plate 2. **A,** Clinically healthy gingiva. **B,** Normal melanin pigmentation is visible on free and attached gingiva of this patient. **C,** Signs of marginal inflammation are visible, including redness, rolled margins, and loss of contour. Papillae appear blunted and swollen. Note differences in appearance between attached gingiva and alveolar mucosa. **D,** Fibrotic (hyperplastic) tissue, as seen in mandibular arch of this patient, may appear normal or near normal in color and has a very firm, hard consistency. **E,** Gingival clefting is evident on facial surfaces of premolars. **F,** Marginal gingivitis and periodontitis. Clinical signs of inflammation are visible, especially around Nos. 6 to 10. Note open contacts between teeth and extrusion of maxillary right central incisor, indicating loss of periodontal support. Melanin pigmentation can also be seen in this patient's gingiva.

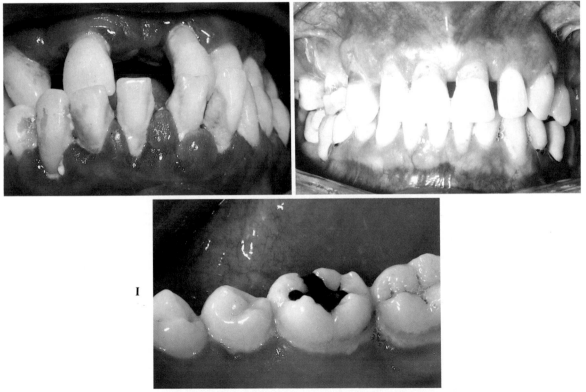

Plate 2, cont'd. **G,** Severe periodontal disease. Presence of heavy hard and soft deposits can be seen. Gingiva exhibits signs of both acute (redness, edema) and chronic inflammation (hyperplasia). Note presence of extruded and shifted teeth and recession due to periodontal destruction. Anterior teeth are clinically mobile. **H,** Generalized recession of maxillary gingivae due to periodontal disease. **I,** Clinical signs of acute necrotizing ulcerative gingivitis can be seen. Tissues are red, swollen, and extremely painful. Necrotic ulceration, which began in interdental papillae, now includes marginal gingiva in this patient. Yellowish ''pseudomembrane'' is actually a collected mass of bacteria, dead inflammatory cells, and necrotic tissue. (Courtesy Catherine Schifter, R.D.H., M.Ed.)

14 PERIODONTAL EXAMINATION AND CHARTING

OBJECTIVES: *The reader will be able to*

1. Discuss seven uses of the periodontal examination and charting.
2. Identify the significance of the following factors to the periodontal examination: missing teeth; unerupted, impacted, or supernumerary teeth; malpositioned teeth; open contacts; poorly contoured restorations and crowns; prosthetic devices, and carious lesions.
3. Discuss the procedure for examining and charting each of the following:
   a. Pocket depths
   b. Gingival height/recession
   c. Masticatory mucosa
   d. Attached gingiva
   e. Mobility
   f. Furcations
4. Describe four complications of periodontal probing and explain how to handle them.
5. Discuss the characteristics of effective probing in terms of adaptation and angulation of the tip, amount of pressure needed, and number and location of probe readings on each tooth.

PERIODONTAL DISEASE

The major purpose of the periodontal examination is to correlate those clinical signs and patient symptoms that point to either the presence of or the potential for periodontal disease. Periodontal disease may be inflammatory in nature, such as in gingivitis and periodontitis, or it may be noninflammatory, as in occlusal trauma. A basic understanding of these conditions is necessary to distinguish among their clinical signs and to understand the significance of collecting data for periodontal examination.

Gingivitis is an inflammation of the gingival soft tissues. It may occur in an acute stage of short duration, which is characterized by a sudden onset and the severe symptoms of pain, bleeding, swelling, and tissue destruction. An example of this type of gingivitis is the condition known as *acute necrotizing ulcerative gingivitis (ANUG)*. This acute gingival inflammation is also known as trench mouth, Vincent's gingivitis, Vincent's gingivostomatitis, and necrotizing gingivitis. It is most prevalent in young adults between the ages of 18 and 30 and is associated with factors other than those that cause chronic gingivitis. Three specific factors seem to be most frequently implicated in the occurrence of this condition: (1) poor oral hygiene in the presence of an existing chronic gingivitis; (2) smoking (Goldhaber and Giddon, 1964); and (3) emotional stress (Giddon et al., 1964).

The most obvious clinical sign of ANUG is ulceration of the marginal gingiva and interdental papilla. This destruction begins with the appearance of a necrotic ulcer on the papilla that rapidly progresses until the entire papilla is destroyed, leaving a central depression or crater where the intact papilla once stood. The necrosis spreads to the adjacent marginal gingiva and other papillae. The affected gingiva is often covered with a greyish or yellowish "pseudomembrane," composed of necrotic tissue, bacteria, and destroyed blood cells, which forms over the red, raw, exposed connective tissues. This lesion is extremely painful to the patient, so that the situation is exacerbated by a continued lack of plaque control. Spontaneous bleeding and a characteristic foul odor are also common findings. In advanced cases swelling of the regional lymph nodes (regional lymphadenitis) may also be present.

The initial treatment of ANUG involves relief of the acute symptoms by removing local etiologic factors. Gross scaling, preferably accomplished with an ultrasonic scaler, will help relieve the acute symptoms. This initial debridement can be followed at a later appointment by fine scaling and curettage, once the pain and discomfort have been reduced. Patients should be instructed to perform gentle but thorough plaque control in all areas. Since it is painful to touch the inflamed tissues, brushing and frequent rinsing should be instituted first, to be followed by flossing after some healing has occurred. The patient should rinse the mouth frequently with equal parts of hydrogen peroxide and warm water as a supplement to plaque control.

Following removal of all local etiologic factors, the other cause-related factors (e.g., poor oral hygiene habits, smoking, stress), must be addressed to avoid recurrence. After initial therapy has been completed, periodontal surgery may be indicated to restore a normal contour to the gingiva, which will support the patient's plaque removal efforts (Goldman and Cohen, 1980; Lindhe, 1983).

The most common type of gingivitis is *chronic* in nature. A chronic condition is one that has the same inflammatory symptoms and signs as the acute stage but is less severe in nature and persists over a longer period of time. The clinical signs of chronic gingivitis are described in more detail in Table 14-1.

Table 14-1. Gingival assessment: clinical characteristics

Clinical characteristic	Normal	Abnormal
Color	Uniformly coral pink Variations may occur depending on patient's complexion and race	Acute—bright red Chronic—red, bluish red, dark pink Color changes may be restricted to papilla or extend to marginal and attached gingiva
Contour	Margins are knifelike Contour of free margin forms regular parabolic curve as it goes around teeth Papillae are pointed and fill embrasure space	Margins become rolled, bulbous, enlarged; irregular contour may be noted; clefting, festooning Papillae may be flattened, bulbous, blunted, or cratered
Size	Free margin is at cementoenamel junction (CEJ) Margin adheres closely to tooth	Enlarged because of excess fluid in tissues (edematous) or buildup of collagen fibers (fibrotic) Margin may be retracted away from tooth with air or instrument
Consistency	Firm	Edematous, soft, spongy; pressure on tissues with an instrument will leave a dent Fibrotic, firm, hard tissue
Surface texture	Smooth free gingiva Stippled attached gingiva	Acute—loss of stippling; smooth, shiny Chronic—stippling present; may increase in occurrence
Position of gingival margin	1 to 2 mm above CEJ in fully erupted teeth	May be enlarged so that margin is more coronal than CEJ May show apical recession so that root surface is exposed
Position of junctional epithelium	At CEJ in fully erupted teeth	Apical migration onto root surface
Mucogingival junction	Clear distinction between appearance of attached gingiva (pink, stippled, immobile, firm) and alveolar mucosa (red, shiny, smooth, mobile)	Lack of attached gingiva determined by 1. Loss of junctional line 2. Mobility of all existing tissues 3. Probing extends beyond mucogingival junction
Bleeding	No bleeding detectable with palpation or probing	Spontaneous bleeding Bleeding resulting from probing
Exudate	No exudate with palpation or probing	Increase in amount of clear crevicular fluid Presence of white fluid (pus) with palpation

Data from "Examination and Diagnosis," 1975; Goldman and Cohen, 1980; Wilkins, 1983.

Periodontitis is an inflammation that involves not only the gingival tissues, but also the attachment apparatus of the tooth. The attachment apparatus consists of alveolar bone, cementum, and periodontal ligament. Although an inflammation may begin as gingivitis, as it continues to spread into the deeper tissues it affects the supporting structures and then becomes the condition known as periodontitis. Periodontitis is characterized by gingival inflammation, formation of periodontal pockets, recession of the gingiva, resorption of alveolar bone, destruction of periodontal ligament fibers, and tooth mobility (Goldman and Cohen, 1980).

Chronic gingivitis and periodontitis are associated with the presence of microbial plaque. The microorganisms that form dental plaque contain or release substances that cause inflammatory responses in the gingiva (Lindhe, 1983). Even in a healthy gingival crevice, there may be a small number of bacteria and a slight inflammatory response (connective tissue infiltrate) at all times (Page and Schroeder, 1976), but the body response and the quantity of the microorganisms balance each other, so that there are no clinical signs of disease from this relationship. This equilibrium can be maintained over an indefinite length of time as long as both the host tissue and the bacteria remain balanced. If the quantity of microorganisms increases (i.e., plaque accumulation), however, this balance is upset and the body initiates an increased inflammatory response to remove the toxic substances. Clinical changes include the signs of redness, swelling, and bleeding on probing. Histologically, the signs of inflammation begin in the coronal part of the junctional epithelium and the adjacent connective tissues, resulting in an increase in inflammatory cells and destruction of the collagen fibers that provide the supporting framework of the gingiva. The collagen content is reduced by 60% to 70% in the inflamed areas of the connective tissue (Lindhe, 1983). The junctional epithelium loses its attachment to the tooth surface and no longer can provide an effective barrier against the advancing plaque front. The loss of epithelial attachment also creates a deeper sulcus where more submarginal plaque can form. As the plaque moves apically, it continues to excite an inflammatory response. The result is destruction of the connective tissues including the principal fiber groups that attach to the root surface. Loss of these fibers is followed by

loss of alveolar bone. And so the process continues as the pocket becomes pathologically deepened.

Periodontal disease is a chronic condition that is progressive and destructive. Loss of connective tissue attachment has been estimated to occur at a rate of 0.1 to 0.2 mm per tooth surface per year (Waerhaug, 1977). The condition increases in severity with age. It develops and progresses at different rates in different parts and surfaces of the dentition. Periodontal disease is site specific, meaning that the onset of the disease can occur in some areas of the mouth without affecting others (Haffajee et al., 1983; Socransky et al., 1984). Periodontal disease is cyclical in nature. It does not demonstrate a constant linear progression over time. Instead, it occurs as bursts of activity that last for a short time and are followed by periods of quiescence or inactivity (Lindhe, 1983).

One explanation for the cyclical nature of the disease is that the host tissue and the oral microbiota enjoy an equilibrium until large numbers of microorganisms are allowed to colonize a specific site, upsetting the balance. The tissues respond by setting up an inflammatory response that will result in tissue destruction and apical migration of the microbial plaque. The body's immune response also participates in the defense. After a few weeks of exaggerated host response (acute inflammation), the equilibrium between microbes and the tissues is again established, resulting in a chronic gingivitis. This balance could be maintained for months, years, or decades without any additional destruction, so that the patient would have a chronic gingivitis, but there would be no progression of the condition to periodontitis. If, however, these inflammatory bursts occur with frequency and result in significant tissue destruction beyond the cementoenamel junction (CEJ), there could be eventual loss of connective tissue attachment and the chronic gingivitis would become chronic periodontitis (Lindhe, 1983).

In summary, an inflammatory process that affects only gingival soft tissues is called *gingivitis*. If this condition persists and spreads into the supporting tissues so that destruction of bone occurs, it is called *periodontitis*.

The prognoses for these two forms of periodontal disease are quite different. The damaged epithelium and connective tissues that form the gingival unit can regenerate if the cause of the inflammation, called the *etiologic agent*, is removed from the soft tissue environment. Therefore a simple gingivitis can often be treated quite successfully and the tissues brought back to normal form and function. This is not the case with periodontitis, because supporting bone does not have this same ability to completely repair and restore the bone that has been destroyed by the inflammatory process. Another result of this disease is the apical migration of the junctional epithelium, which results in the formation of deep periodontal pockets that are difficult, if not impossible, for the patient to maintain free of plaque. Once the disease process has spread to involve the supporting structures, there is permanent loss of tissues and an increased potential for the condition to persist or recur. This makes it painfully clear that the only effective method of curbing this disease and restoring the tissues to complete health is to recognize early signs of gingival inflammation and eliminate the etiologic factors that cause it to occur. This especially includes teaching the patient to control etiologic factors, mainly dental plaque, before the condition develops into periodontitis.

The third form of periodontal disease is not inflammatory but rather is degenerative in nature. This condition, known as *occlusal trauma*, is one in which the supporting structures of affected teeth are damaged because they cannot withstand the occlusal forces that act on them. The result is a breakdown of the periodontal ligament fibers, loss of supporting bone, widening of the periodontal ligament space, and tooth mobility. When this destruction is caused by excessive occlusal forces acting on an otherwise normal periodontium, the condition is referred to as *primary occlusal trauma*. The sources of the pressure may include bruxism, night grinding, malocclusion, or poorly constructed dental restorations. These factors can produce more stress than the supporting structures were designed to withstand, and the result is that they are slowly destroyed. *Secondary occlusal trauma* is the result of normal occlusal forces on an attachment apparatus that has already been damaged and weakened by periodontitis. Some of the clinical signs of occlusal trauma include a widened periodontal ligament space, root fractures, loss of lamina dura, mobility, and signs of attrition or facets on the crowns of teeth (Goldman and Cohen, 1980).

It is not our purpose to provide detailed descrip-

tions of these three forms of periodontal disease; a periodontal text will best serve that need. However, a basic understanding of their similarities and differences will help the beginning student understand the purpose for gathering as much data describing the periodontal condition of each patient as possible to ensure that accurate diagnosis and effective treatment planning will follow.

PURPOSE OF THE PERIODONTAL EXAMINATION

In this chapter the complete periodontal examination is described, and suggestions as to how it may be recorded on the periodontal charting form are given. The information gathered and recorded during the periodontal examination will assist the clinician in correlating all factors that might aid in assessing and describing the level of periodontal health or disease present in each patient. Without the information from a complete periodontal examination, diagnosis and treatment planning could be a hit-and-miss proposition, based on conjecture and not on reliable observed data.

In addition to the periodontal charting, there are many other diagnostic aids that contribute vital information to the clinician. These aids include medical and dental histories, a head and neck examination, dental chartings, radiographs, study models, bite registration, photographs, and plaque and gingival indices. All of these assessment tools together provide a total picture of the patient's periodontal condition and permit comprehensive treatment planning. Exact descriptions of these other components are contained elsewhere in this text. The information they provide is supplemental to the periodontal examination, and specific situations in which they may be used are mentioned as the periodontal examination is described.

USES OF PERIODONTAL CHARTING

The data that are collected and recorded in a periodontal charting serve a number of purposes for both the patient and the clinician. As part of an initial examination, periodontal charting provides a record of *baseline data* that describes the patient's periodontal condition before initial therapy is instituted. This data base will later serve as a means for evaluating the success of treatment and preventive practices. Over a period of time, changes in the patient's periodontal status can be noted to trace the control of disease and restoration of health. The periodontal charting provides *information that is necessary to establish a diagnosis* of the patient's condition. It consolidates a comprehensive collection of clinical data, which, along with the other components of the periodontal examination, allows for a careful analysis of all observable conditions so that an accurate diagnosis can be made. Since the periodontal charting represents the clinical conditions in written form, this analysis can occur without the patient's presence. The accumulation of all available clinical signs and symptoms will help the dental professional identify early signs of inflammatory disease while it may still be reversible.

After a diagnosis is made and confirmed, the periodontal charting continues to serve as a *resource for treatment planning*. Its information assists in establishing treatment priorities and in answering the following questions:

1. What areas show the most acute signs of disease and appear to have the highest potential for causing pain and/or destruction?
2. Which conditions demand additional examination or testing?
3. What types of treatment might be most effective?
4. What etiologic factors are present?
5. What combination of patient and professional efforts will be necessary to restore the tissues to health?

Data that have been recorded as part of a complete periodontal charting can be used to formulate treatment plans for restorative, periodontal, and preventive therapy. During the presentation of the treatment plan, the periodontal charting and other diagnostic aids provide visual evidence of the clinical findings to the patient, so that the diagnosis and its treatment can be understood.

The periodontal chart also serves as a valuable aid for the clinician during *implementation of the treatment plan*. During probing, scaling, root planing, and curettage, the chart can be used as a road map for instrumentation. Information such as the depth of pockets, root morphology, exposure of furcation areas, and mobility will affect the clinician's choice of instruments and the approach to scaling and root planing. When it is known from the chart that deep and complex pocket morphologies are present, the clinician can be more alert to tactile clues during exploring and probing and can plan effective approaches to areas in which access may prove challenging. Information recorded during the periodontal charting will help identify the need for special treatment procedures, such as temporary ligation of mobile teeth to facilitate scaling and root planing. It may also identify a need to recontour restorations so that their plaque-retentive characteristics are eliminated or at least reduced. The description of the pocket morphology and degree of destruction incurred by the soft and hard tissues will assist the clinician in determining indications for subsequent root planing and soft tissue curettage.

After treatment is completed, the periodontal chart serves as a valuable *reference for evaluating treatment success*. A posttreatment charting when compared with pretreatment records will indicate in which areas the soft tissues have been restored to some degree of normal form and function. It will also serve as a point from which referrals for more advanced treatment, such as periodontal surgery, may be made. The periodontal chart should be updated during recall appointments to document the patient's periodontal status over a period of time. If the gingiva remains healthy and shallow probing depths are maintained, it is an indication that home care, professional treatment, and recall intervals have been effective in health maintenance. If, on the other hand, subsequent chartings show that periodontal destruction is continuing, this is a flagrant signal that one or all of these criteria need additional assessment and modification.

This permanent record of peridontal status is valuable not only for the clinician, but also for the patient who is receiving verification of the success of treatment at the same time. Periodontal charting can be useful as *legal evidence* to support a diagnosis and to justify subsequent treatment. In addition, a periodontal chart can provide information about the rationale for proposed or actual treatment in cases involving a third-party payer such as an insurance carrier. A less familiar use of dental records, including periodontal charts, is their application in *forensic dentistry*. A periodontal chart may be used to identify deceased individuals. Their dental and periodontal conditions are as specific to them as their fingerprints; thus dental records are invaluable for making or confirming positive identification.

In summary, periodontal charting is an important tool to the dental professional and well worth the time it takes to collect and record the data. This information is a necessary element of diagnosis and treatment planning.

PREAPPOINTMENT CHARTING

Before the actual clinical examination of a patient there are many factors relevant to the periodontal diagnosis that may be assessed and charted from study models and radiographs. The advantage of studying these records is twofold. First, they provide information that can be reviewed when the patient is not present. This allows the clinician to take the time needed to examine both the study models and radiographs carefully and in detail for possible etiologic factors that might affect the periodontal diagnosis and final treatment plan. Second, information from the study models and radiographs alerts the dental professional to search for particular clinical signs and symptoms that might be overlooked otherwise. This preparation can save time during the appointment and can reduce the time required to reach a diagnosis. In the following paragraphs those factors of the periodontal charting and examination that can be assessed in advance with the aid of radiographs and study models are identified. The significance of each factor to the periodontal examination is described. Many of these factors have already been identified as components of a comprehensive charting (see Chapter 11).

Missing teeth should be noted, whether they are congenitally missing, extracted, or unerupted. This factor can be assessed from both the radiographs and the study models. Radiographs can help the professional determine whether the teeth are actually missing or simply unerupted. Radiographs will also provide the clinician with a view of root morphology and will assist in tooth identification. Study models assist in the identification of missing teeth by providing the clinician with the coronal anatomy of all erupted teeth. Missing teeth are significant in a periodontal examination because they may indicate a past history of periodontal disease. Areas left vacant by missing teeth also affect the distribution of occlusal forces on remaining teeth. The imbalanced forces can result in periodontal breakdown and occlusal trauma (Goldman and Cohen, 1980).

Malpositioned teeth should be noted during the periodontal examination. Malpositioned teeth are not only susceptible to occlusal trauma, but may also point to previous destructive disease since the shifting may have been caused by breakdown of periodontal support (see Plate 2, *F* and *G*). Other signs of abnormal occlusal stresses or wear can be detected in radiographs and study models. The radiographs will reveal signs of occlusal trauma such as periodontal ligament spaces, which may appear to be abnormally wide because of increased pressures on the teeth. There may be signs of root fracture or loss of lamina dura. Attrition patterns on occlusal or incisal surfaces (wear facets) may be detectable on the radiographs but can be seen more clearly on the study models as flattened areas on the cusp tips or occlusal surfaces that result from constant wear of opposing teeth. Wear facets are charted by shading that portion of the tooth that has undergone the wear on either the facial or occlusal views of the teeth.

Teeth that are *impacted or supernumerary* can also be detected in radiographs. An unerupted tooth is one that is incomplete in its formation or not yet visible in the mouth. An impacted tooth is one that may be completely formed but is obstructed from normal eruption by an adjacent tooth or because of its position in the dental arch. A supernumerary tooth is an "extra" tooth. These teeth are usually formed after the permanent dentition, and they remain apical to the erupted teeth in the alveolus. A common area for supernumerary teeth is apical to the maxillary central incisors. The significance of these conditions is that unerupted teeth can develop infections that affect the surrounding tissues. The constant pressure of an unerupted or impacted tooth against other hard tissues, such as an adjacent tooth or bone, can cause resorption or permanent destruction of these tissues. *Partially erupted teeth* should also be noted on the charting form. If, for some reason, full eruption is not completed (e.g., impaction), it becomes difficult for the patient to keep these teeth clean and to keep the surrounding soft tissues healthy. These areas become prime sites for food impaction and gingival inflammation. *Pericoronitis* is an acute localized inflammation that commonly occurs in the soft tissues surrounding a partially erupted molar (Goldman and Cohen, 1980).

An *open contact,* called a *diastema,* can be detected on radiographs and study models. A good-quality radiograph will show the space between the adjacent teeth, and this can be confirmed by the study models. Clinically, the presence of a diastema can be determined visually if the diastema is wide (see Plate 2, *F* and *G*). Open or deficient contacts can also be detected by passing a piece of dental floss between the teeth. When the contact areas do not offer sufficient resistance to the floss, a deficient contact should be charted. Open or deficient contacts may be significant because of the potential for food impaction in these areas. They may also indicate tooth movement from periodontal destruction if the patient indicates that they have not always been present. The presence of *plunger cusps* should also be noted during the periodontal examination. These are cusps of teeth in one arch that fit directly into the area between two teeth in the opposing arch. The significance of this phenomenon is that the plunger cusps can push food directly into the space between the opposing teeth; this may cause trauma to the soft tissues in the area (Pennel and Keagle, 1977). A plunger cusp should be detectable in the study models if the occlusal relationships have been properly reproduced in the wax bite (see Chapter 15).

Abnormal crown and root morphologies may be detected radiographically or on the study models and should be charted by drawing the existing anatomic shape over the symbol of the affected tooth so that the drawing represents reality as closely as possible. Examples of these deviations are teeth that are exceptionally large or small in relationship to other teeth in the dentition, teeth with dilacerated roots, abnormal distances from the CEJ to furcations, and teeth with roots that are spread abnormally or with more or fewer roots than normal. The discovery of any of these deviations is significant for the determination of a tooth's susceptibility to disease, its roots' "anchoring" ability, and how its roots should be treated during root planing or surgical procedures.

Two anomalies that may affect a tooth's susceptibility to disease are the *distopalatal groove* and *cervical-enamel projections*. The former is a groove that extends apically along the root on some maxillary incisors. Most distopalatal grooves are found on maxillary lateral incisors (Withers et al., 1981). Its presence as a plaque-retentive area increases the chances of periodontal destruction. Enamel projections occur in mandibular furcation areas, causing a lack of normal attachment and a predisposition for the buildup of plaque in those locations (Pennel, 1977). Areas affected by *abrasion* or *erosion* are also significant in the periodontal examination because of their potential as etiologic factors in the harboring of plaque. This loss of tooth structure affects the normal self-cleansing abilities of the dentition.

Other conditions that are plaque retentive and serve as etiologic factors include *poorly contoured crowns and restorations, prosthetic devices,* and *carious lesions*. Until these problems are either removed, replaced, or restored, the patient will find it difficult to practice optimal plaque control and periodontal disease will persist (Rodriguez-Ferrer et al., 1980). *Periapical conditions* should be carefully examined on the radiographs and charted in the location where they appear. Any radiopacities or radiolucencies in the periapical regions or supporting bone should be noted, and a tentative diagnosis should be made. In order to reach a final diagnosis, however, the dentist may require that additional tests and questioning of the patient be performed during the clinical examination.

Bone levels and the appearance of *boney defects* should be carefully examined on the radiographs. The topography of the bone should be scrutinized for the presence of vertical or horizontal defects. The extent of these defects should be estimated to guide periodontal probing during the clinical appointment. At that time the clinical readings and the appearance of bone levels on the radiographs should be correlated to ensure that deep boney defects have not been overlooked. The crestal bone patterns should be examined for loss of definition or loss of lamina dura to determine the level of bone destruction. The presence of boney craters can also be observed on the radiographs (Newman and Moran, 1980).

Many of the aforementioned conditions may have already been charted as part of the comprehensive charting. If so, they need not be included on the periodontal chart, since the time and effort of duplication are unnecessary as long as the other chart is available for consultation when the periodontal treatment plan is being considered. The dental professional may also consider combining the periodontal and restorative charts into one form rather than having two separate ones. The purpose of identifying these elements as part of a periodontal examination is that they are pertinent not only in ascertaining a restorative treatment plan, but also in determining the etiologies of periodontal conditions and in selecting the best sequence of priorities to meet patient needs during comprehensive treatment planning.

After a close examination of the radiographs and study models and after all pertinent findings have been reviewed from the restorative chart and/or charted on the periodontal charting form, the dental professional who will be conducting the clinical periodontal examination should make notes to indicate any special evaluations or tests that might be helpful in verifying diagnoses suggested by this initial assessment of data. When the patient is seated, the clinical examination should assess all characteristics of the soft and hard tissues that could not be evaluated from the radiographs, study models, or restorative charting and confirm clinically any details that are in question.

CLINICAL EXAMINATION

Before beginning the periodontal examination, the patient's medical history should be reviewed and confirmed with the patient so that any potential complications in treatment can be detected. Information gathered from the medical history of the patient can assist the clinician in identifying medical reasons for certain gingival and periodontal conditions. Systemic diseases such as diabetes, blood dyscrasias, and hormonal imbalances can affect the ability of the body to resist and repair damage that occurs as the result of inflammatory conditions. These patients may be more susceptible to periodontal destruction. Medications may also affect the periodontal tissues. Patients who take sodium dilantin for control of seizures often exhibit hyperplasia or fibrotic overgrowth of gingival tissues. Patients who use oral contraceptives may exhibit gingival changes similar to those seen during pregnancy. Corticosteroids are antiinflammatory drugs, and their use can mask the usual signs of inflammation in the gingival soft tissues even though the inflammatory process is active. Poor nutrition and emotional stress can also exacerbate the inflammatory response in the gingival and periodontal tissues.

Patients who require premedication for scaling procedures should be premedicated for all periodontal procedures. Periodontal probing can cause a bacteremia in a susceptible patient, as can any other periodontal or dental procedure. As soon as all necessary medical precautions have been taken, the procedure can be performed. Information from the dental history will indicate past dental or periodontal treatment that might affect the present periodontal examination, such as surgical treatment or explanations regarding tooth loss. The dental history will also reveal information about the patient's attitudes regarding periodontal and preventive therapy, which will aid in treatment planning.

The purpose of the periodontal examination and charting should be discussed with the patient, and the procedure should be explained to answer any questions that the patient might have. The patient must understand that this is an exacting procedure that must be done carefully. The patient may experience some discomfort, depending on the severity of the inflammation. The need for pain control (either topical, local, or nitrous oxide) should be considered. After the purpose of the clinical periodontal examination has been explained to the patient and consent for treatment has been obtained, the procedure can begin.

Gingival assessment

The first areas to be studied during the clinical examination are the free and attached gingiva. Fig. 14-1 and Plate 2, *A,* show the normal structures of the gingiva and alveolar mucosa. The clinical appearance of the gingiva in all parts of the mouth should be closely examined for signs of inflammation. Table 14-1 contrasts the appearance of normal gingiva and inflamed gingiva. A careful examination is necessary to determine subtle changes in the gingiva because the patient's prognosis for treatment is much improved if gingivitis is recognized and treated in its earliest stages. Deviations from normal gingival characteristics should be noted and described as part of the periodontal examination. This description should include not only the appearance of the gingiva, but also the location and extent of the condition so that later comparisons and evaluation of the success or failure of professional treatment or home care procedures can be made.

The clinician should assess the condition of the gingiva by examining it for each of the following characteristics: color, contour, consistency, and texture. Normal characteristics and changes that

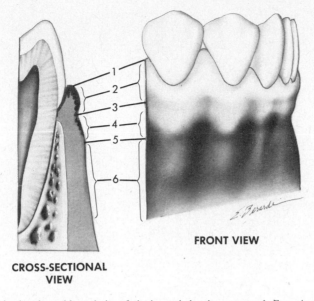

CROSS-SECTIONAL VIEW

FRONT VIEW

Fig. 14-1. Normal landmarks and boundaries of gingiva and alveolar mucosa. *1*, Free gingival margin; *2*, free gingiva; *3*, free gingival groove; *4*, attached gingiva, *5*, mucogingival junction; *6*, alveolar mucosa. Clinician should be able to relate these landmarks to their appearance in patient's mouth.

may be visible as a result of inflammation should be well-known to the clinician so that exact descriptions of the character of the gingiva can be recorded. The extent of gingival changes due to inflammation can vary. Signs of inflammation may extend into all attached and free gingiva, or they may be restricted to only the marginal gingiva or interdental papillae. Specific changes may also be localized around one or several teeth, or generalized to an entire arch. The clinician must evaluate the degree of inflammation and extent of tissue involvement to determine if the inflammation can be considered as slight, moderate, or severe in quality.

The *color* of normal gingiva is usually a uniform, coral-pink shade. The light pink color should extend all the way from the mucogingival attachment to the gingival margin (see Plate 2, *A*). Shade variations will occur among different individuals, much the same as facial complexions differ. The amounts of normal melanin pigmentation present in the gingiva will also vary. This pigmentation may be visible as brown patches of color distributed in varying degrees throughout the tissue. This type of pigmentation is prevalent in black individuals.

An example of melanin pigmentation is shown in Plate 2, *B* and *F*.

The earliest color change associated with gingival inflammation often begins as a subtle change in the interdental papilla from light pink to a darker pink or red. This color change will extend to the marginal gingiva and into the rest of the free and attached gingiva as the inflammation becomes more severe. Acutely inflamed gingiva will have a red color (see Plate 2, *G*), whereas chronically inflamed gingiva may take on a bluish or cyanotic cast. This blue color change may be discernible around the margins of poorly contoured crowns (see Plate 3, *D*, No. 8). In many cases the color of fibrotic, chronically inflamed gingiva may be close to normal in appearance. Both chronic and acute signs of gingival inflammation may exist simultaneously within the same patient.

The *contour* of normal gingival tissues also can be seen in Plate 2, *A*. The interdental papillae fill the embrasure spaces and come to a sharp point at the contact area. The free gingival margins are knifelike and hug the coronal surface of the tooth. The margins also create a regular series of parabolic curves as the eye moves from tooth to tooth. The level of the free gingival margin should be at or slightly coronal to the CEJ of the tooth.

A number of changes occur in the contour of the gingiva as a result of inflammation. The interdental papillae become swollen and edematous. In later stages of the disease, they may become flattened, blunted, or cratered. This ''punched-out'' appearance caused by loss of the papilla is characteristic in patients who have had ANUG. The marginal gingiva may also appear bulbous and swollen with rolled margins. As the edema increases, other gingival changes may occur such as clefting (see Plate 2, *E*) or festooning. The inflamed marginal gingiva also loses its elastic ability to adhere closely to the contour of the tooth. The inflamed tissues may stand away from the tooth, or they can be easily displaced with air or instrument retraction (see Plate 2, *G*). When gingival tissues undergo a change in the inflammatory response from acute to chronic inflammation, the constant destruction of the tissues results in the appearance of scar tissue or fibrotic tissue that is extremely firm and often enlarged and irregular in contour (see Plate 2, *D*).

Normal gingival tissues have a *consistency* that is firm and resilient. With the onset of inflammation, the consistency becomes edematous, soft, and spongy. This can be detected by applying slight pressure on the dried tissues with the tip or side of a probe or other blunt instrument. A ''dent'' will remain visible in the edematous tissues. The consistency of chronically inflamed, fibrotic tissues is very firm, hard, and unyielding because of the buildup of excessive amounts of repair or scar tissue.

The *surface texture* of normal free gingiva is smooth. The attached gingiva may exhibit a smooth or stippled appearance. Stippling will appear as tiny indentations in the surface of the attached gingiva similar to the appearance of an orange peel (see Plate 2, *A* and *B*). Although many individuals display this normal characteristic, its absence is not necessarily an indication of disease (Goldman and Cohen, 1980). Stippling may be easily detected if the tissues are dried with a stream of air.

Acute inflammation usually results in the loss of stippling because of the increase in tissue edema. The surface texture becomes very smooth and glossy (see Plate 2, *C* and *F*). During chronic inflammation, stippling will often be present and may actually increase in prevalence.

Evaluation of the external appearance of the gingiva is useful as an assessment tool for describing the presence of gingival inflammation. It can be less reliable as a means of assessing inflammation within the sulcus or pocket area. Waerhaug (1978a, 1978b) demonstrated that inflammatory changes that affect the marginal gingiva may occur independently of inflammatory changes in the sulcular areas. Patients who performed effective supramarginal plaque control displayed normal-appearing gingiva in spite of the presence of submarginal plaque and sulcular inflammation. Waerhaug warned clinicians not to be misled by the overt appearance of the gingival tissues, especially when the patient has been effective in plaque control removal. Other methods of clinical assessment, such as the presence of bleeding or exudate from the sulcus or pocket, should complement the gingival evaluation to provide a more accurate clinical evaluation.

The presence of sulcular bleeding can be detected during periodontal probing. One of the first signs of gingival inflammation is bleeding during gentle probing of the sulcus area (Meitner et al., 1979; Muhlemann and Son, 1971), and this is an immediate indicator of the need for improved home care and possibly for professional treatment. Bleeding is the result of an ulcerated epithelial lining in the sulcus or pocket and may occur to varying degrees. An acutely inflamed sulcus will bleed spontaneously from finger pressure against the tissue or from probing. Bleeding from incipient gingival inflammation may not be apparent at the surface of the free margin of the gingiva for as long as 30 seconds after complete probing of the entire sulcus depth (Carter and Barnes, 1974). Fibrotic tissues, because of a long-standing inflammation, may bleed little or not at all. All areas of gingival bleeding should be charted according to where they occur in the mouth as a method of assessing the extent and location of the inflammation. In Fig. 14-2 a check mark indicates the presence of bleeding when each area is probed. The amount of gingival bleeding may also be translated into a bleeding index by assigning a numeric value to its occurrence (see Chapter 12).

The presence of inflammatory exudate should be charted during the periodontal examination. The amount of gingival crevicular fluid (GCF) is an indicator of the amount of gingival inflammation

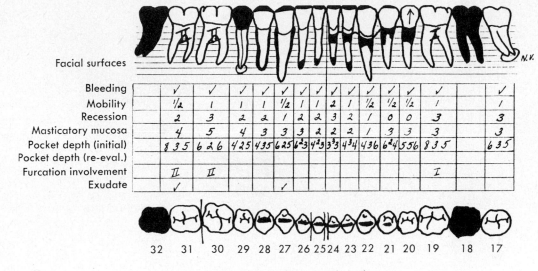

																N.V.
Facial surfaces																
Bleeding	✓	✓	✓	✓	✓	✓	✓	✓	✓	✓	✓	✓	✓			✓
Mobility	½	1	1	1	½	1	1	2	1	½	½	½	1			1
Recession	2	3	2	2	1	2	2	3	2	1	0	0	3			3
Masticatory mucosa	4	5	4	3	3	3	2	2	2	1	3	3	3			3
Pocket depth (initial)	8 3 5	6 2 6	4 2 5	4 3 5	6 2 5	6²3	4²3	3³3	4³4	4 3 6	6²4	5 5 6	8 3 5			6 3 5
Pocket depth (re-eval.)																
Furcation involvement	II	II										I				
Exudate	✓			✓												

32 31 30 29 28 27 26 25 24 23 22 21 20 19 18 17

Fig. 14-2. Periodontal charting—sample section.

present in the area. Although this fluid is present in small amounts under normal conditions, it increases when gingival inflammation is present (Muhlemann and Son, 1971). A more obvious sign of acute inflammation and infection is the presence of pus, an inflammatory exudate composed of white blood cells and other debris. This exudate can be expelled from affected pockets by applying gentle finger pressure to the gingiva. The expulsion of exudate from pockets may have been noted previously when the alveolar ridges and gingiva were palpated during the intraoral examination. The presence of exudate has been charted with a check mark in the affected area in Fig. 14-2.

The soft tissue that covers the supporting bone should be examined for signs of swellings, such as those that might be caused by periapical or periodontal abscesses, granulomas, or cysts. Initial signs of bone destruction caused by these lesions might have been detected during the radiographic examination, and the clinical examination can confirm the tentative diagnosis. The clinician should never rely solely on the use of radiographs to diagnose these lesions, since they are not always detectable radiographically. Signs of openings or breaks in the gingiva or mucosa (e.g., draining fistulas) should be carefully examined and noted.

Periodontal probing

Periodontal charting is the culmination of a variety of characteristics of the dentition and attachment apparatus, which are either measured or observed and then recorded with symbols on paper. Those aspects of the periodontium that are commonly measured are sulcus or pocket depth, masticatory mucosa, gingival recession, and mobility. The first three are measured with a periodontal probe. As explained in Chapter 5, the probe is an instrument whose working end is calibrated in millimeters to facilitate clinical measurements. There are a wide variety of probe designs, and the choice of a particular design is based mainly on individual preferences. The diameter of the working end is important for detection during insertion into tight pockets. It should be long enough and narrow enough so that it can be easily inserted without causing undue distension of the soft tissue side of the sulcus. The tip, however, should be blunt so as not to puncture or damage the soft tissues of the sulcus base.

Calibrations of probes vary; some are calibrated at each millimeter up to 10, and others are calibrated in millimeter increments, with the markings at 4 and 6 left off for ease of reading. A probe that is even less complex has calibrations only at 3, 6, and 8 mm. Some clinicians prefer color-coded probes to assist reading. Examples of several different probe designs are shown in Fig. 5-3. No matter what type of probe is chosen, the accuracy of probing pocket depths depends on the skill and clinical judgment of the dental professional.

Other instruments that are necessary for periodontal charting include a mouth mirror, a writing implement, and a form on which the charting will be recorded. In addition, it is helpful for an assistant to record the findings as they are detected clinically. This enables the clinician to work more efficiently and makes it easier to prevent cross-contamination, since it is no longer necessary to go constantly from the mouth to the chart and back again. If an assistant is not available, the hygienist should minimize cross-contamination by disinfecting the writing implement before and after each patient.

For some patients periodontal probing may be painful, especially in the presence of advanced periodontal disease and acute inflammatory responses. In these situations a local anesthesia setup may be required to make the patient more comfortable. A saliva ejector and tri-syringe (air-water syringe) should be used during the procedure to keep the field clear of saliva and blood. Two other instruments that are helpful in special situations are a shepherd's hook explorer for detecting exposed furcation areas that are not accessible to the straight design of the periodontal probe and a curette for gross removal of heavy calculus pieces that might interfere with probing.

It is important to establish an effective and efficient order of instrumentation as in any dental procedure involving more than one tooth. This order is helpful to the hygienist working with an assistant because recording the location where the hygienist is working is then unnecessary because of the pattern's predictability. It is also helpful for the clinician who is personally recording results because it is easier to recall which segments of the mouth have been done and which have not. The order of instrumentation prevents unnecessary motion and time spent moving back and forth from one position to another. A recommended order of instrumentation is described in Chapter 5.

The actual adaptation and activation of the periodontal probe within the sulcus is described in Chapter 5. It is important to remember, however,

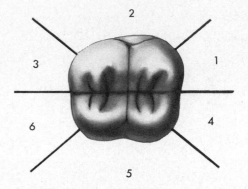

Fig. 14-3. Occlusal view of this molar shows areas where periodontal pocket depth readings are usually taken. Highest reading within each area is the one that should be recorded on charting form.

that only six probe readings will be taken for the periodontal charting. These are in the areas shown on the molar tooth in Fig. 14-3. Although only six readings are recorded, the pockets are not probed at only six points around the tooth. The technique for probing involves carefully "walking" the probe around the entire circumference of the tooth and recording the greatest depth reading for each of the areas defined. If, for instance, the pocket reading is deeper near the distobuccal line angle on the buccal surface of the tooth than it is on the exact center of the buccal surface, the correct record for this area would be the deeper of the two readings. The technique of "walking" the probe tip around the tooth allows the examiner to explore carefully the morphology of the entire pocket so that all defects are noted (Hassell et al., 1973; Tibbetts, 1969) (see Fig. 5-39).

For the most part, the probe's working end is kept as closely parallel to the long axis of the tooth as possible with the tip in close contact with the tooth surface at all times. The tip must always be kept snug against the tooth to prevent damage to soft tissues. As the mesial and distal surfaces are approached, the probe should be moved proximally until it touches the contact and then should be angled slightly into the proximal area so that the tip is measuring directly beneath the contact. This position is shown in Fig. 14-4, *A*. A common error is keeping the working end of the probe too straight with the long axis of the tooth when the interprox-

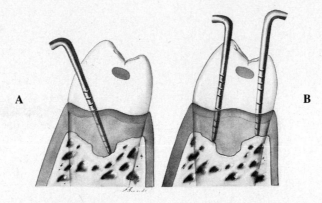

A

B

*Fig. 14-4. **A***, Correct interproximal adaptation of probe. Both facial and lingual readings should detect this crater if probe is angled in this manner. **B**, Deep interproximal bony defects are missed if probe is not angled below contact area interproximally. No matter how hard this clinician tries, neither facial nor lingual reading will be accurate representation of disease present in this area.

imal area is reached and, therefore, failing to measure adequately the entire proximal surface. This error is shown in Fig. 14-4, *B*. (To review correct adaptation of the probe to the tooth, see Fig. 5-39.) Success with this adaptation depends on the tactile sense of the clinician in keeping the tip against the tooth. The *col* area, which is apical to the contact, is a frequent site for periodontal breakdown and destruction (Goldman and Cohen, 1980), and it is important to probe it carefully from both facial and lingual aspects. When the procedure is done correctly, there will be a slight overlap between the area probed for the mesiofacial and the area probed for the mesiolingual. In Fig. 14-4, *A*, the probe has gone slightly beyond the midline of the tooth to obtain its reading. If a choice must be made, it is better for the probe to be slightly overangled than underangled. With the former there is a slight risk of getting a deeper pocket reading than is accurate, but with the latter there is the possibility of missing a deep vertical defect altogether. With some clinical judgment and practice the clinician will be able to visualize the distance and angle that will ensure that this vital area has been thoroughly explored and accurately measured.

When the probe is being maneuvered around the tooth and a reading is taken, it is easiest to read the correct pocket or sulcus depth from the top of the probe down to the free gingival margin. The deepest reading for each of the six probed areas of the tooth should be recorded on the periodontal charting form. Fig. 14-2 shows pocket depths recorded for the buccal surfaces of the mandibular teeth; there is one box for all three buccal readings. It should be noted that the three readings for tooth No. 31 are: distobuccal = 8 mm; buccal = 3 mm; and mesiobuccal = 5 mm. The readings are taken for each tooth in the mouth. When a pocket depth falls between two millimeter marks, it should be rounded off to the higher of the two numbers and recorded only as whole millimeters. In most situations it is not necessary to spend the time and effort required to estimate within less than a millimeter. A more graphic method of charting periodontal depths is shown for teeth No. 20 to No. 24 in Fig. 14-2. Here the recorded depths have been shaded onto the picture of the tooth so that pocket morphology can be clearly visualized.

Significance of pocket depth measurements. The periodontal probe is a valuable clinical tool for exploring and measuring the extent of the healthy gingival sulcus and its pathologic counterpart, the periodontal pocket. For years it has been assumed that this measurement of a clinical sulcus or pocket was an accurate representation of the actual histologic attachment of soft tissues to the tooth surface at the dentogingival junction. Based on this assumption, clinicians measured the depths of inflamed pockets prior to their treatment and compared these measurements with those obtained following treatment. The resultant decrease in pocket depth was interpreted and described as a gain in attachment level.

More recent reports, however, have demonstrated that the probe does not measure the exact extent of the dentogingival junction in either health or disease (Listgarten, 1980). A number of factors contribute to this discrepancy, including the degree of inflammation present in the tissues, the amount of pressure used during probing, and the diameter of the probe.

As the inflammatory lesion of chronic periodontitis advances from early to established to advanced stages, there is a progressive disruption in the soft tissues of the dentogingival attachment. The junctional epithelium becomes more permeable to inflammatory cells and eventually loses its attachment to the tooth surface. The underlying and adjacent connective tissue fibers undergo destruction of the dense collagen network of supportive tissues that were present in health. These inflamed tissues cannot resist the normal forces of probing, so that the probe tip will usually penetrate past the junctional epithelium and not come to rest until the increased resiliency of healthy connective tissue fibers is detected. The probe tip penetrates through the partially destroyed fibers and comes to rest approximately 0.25 to 0.4 mm apical to the termination of the junctional epithelium according to a number of investigators (Listgarten et al., 1976; Powell and Garnick, 1978; Saglie et al., 1975; Sivertson and Burgett, 1976; Spray et al., 1978). Since the clinician cannot feel the presence of the inflamed tissues that are being penetrated, the resulting measurement of the pocket depth might be overestimated by as much as several millimeters (Listgarten, 1980).

Armitage et al. (1977) studied the penetration of the probe tip in the gingival tissues of beagle dogs. They found that in healthy gingiva the probe tip stopped before reaching the apical termination of the junctional epithelium. When areas of gingival inflammation were probed, the probe came near, but not to, the apical termination of the junctional epithelium, and when areas displaying periodontitis were probed, the probe tip consistently went past the most apical junctional epithelial cells and into the underlying connective tissue. This study demonstrated that there is a relationship between the amount of inflammation present in the tissues and the level of probe penetration. Other investigators have studied the extent of probe tip penetration in healthy tissues and have reported that the probe usually comes to rest within the junctional epithelium (Hancock et al., 1978) or coronal to the junctional epithelium (Hancock and Wirthlin, 1979). The results of these studies demonstrate that clinical probing measurements seldom are reliable in predicting the actual histologic or anatomic sulcus or pocket depth, although they are closer to that prediction when a healthy, shallow sulcus is being measured than when an inflamed sulcus or pocket is being measured.

When pockets are treated with scaling, root planing, curettage, and daily plaque removal, the inflammatory conditions subside and the soft tissues of the dentogingival junction undergo repair. The clinical result, when measured by the periodontal probe, may be reported as a decrease in probing depth caused by an apparent gain in the level of the attachment and tissue shrinkage. Investigators have taken a closer look at the reported "gain" of attachment and have found that a decrease in pocket depth does not necessarily represent a gain of new attachment. Instead, the healed periodontal tissues can regain their dense collagen network and provide resistance to the penetration of the probe tip so that it can no longer extend as far apically into the soft tissues (Fowler et al., 1982; Magnusson and Listgarten, 1980). In these cases there has been no actual change in the level of connective tissue attachment, as determined histologically. The only change is that the healthy dentogingival fibers are able to resist penetration by the probe, which they were unable to do when they were inflamed. The actual levels of attachment, however, have not been altered as a result of treatment. In addition, a common healing response to initial therapy (scaling, root planing, curettage, etc.) is the formation of a long junctional epithelium that forms a new biologic attachment to the tooth. The length of the new junctional epithelium has been estimated in one study to range from 1.0 to 4.5 mm (Listgarten and Rosenberg, 1979). The long junctional epithelium will resist penetration by the probe in a healthy sulcus or pocket. Clinical pocket measurements following initial therapy are more likely to estimate the actual anatomic or histologic pocket depths than were the initial pocket measurements in the presence of inflammation.

In summary, then, clinical probing measurements seldom represent the actual anatomic sulcus or pocket depths. When baseline periodontal examinations are performed on new patients who demonstrate signs of inflammation, the pocket measurements may overestimate the actual pocket depths by 1 to 2 mm (Listgarten, 1980). Following treatment, resolution of the inflammation may result in a decrease in the pocket measurement, but the clinician has no way of knowing whether the decrease is due to new connective tissue attachments, decreased penetrability of repaired connective tissue fibers, or the presence of a new long junctional epithelium on the basis of pocket measurements alone. Listgarten (1980), in his review of this topic, suggests that clinicians would be more accurate in referring to pocket measurements as "clinical pocket depths" rather than simply as "pocket depths."

The amount of pressure that is applied to the tip of the probe may also affect the accuracy of the clinical pocket depth measurements. Only a light pressure is necessary to determine these measurements. Additional error is introduced into the procedure when differing amounts of pressure are used in different areas of the mouth, usually because of access problems, or at different examination times. For research purposes, a special pressure-sensitive probe has been developed so that the pressure that is delivered can be standardized (Gabathuler and Hassell, 1971; van der Velden and de Vries, 1978). Since this equipment is not available or practical for general clinical practice at this time, the problem of obtaining reliable probing measurements remains unsolved.

The size of the tip of the probe will also affect the pocket measurements. Probes that are extremely thin can gain easier access into narrow or tight pocket areas but can also penetrate the soft tissues more readily. Less pressure is required to direct a thin tip into soft tissue, so that the clinician should evaluate and control the amount of probing force that is applied to thin probes. In contrast, a very thick probe can become wedged between healthy dense tissues and the tooth before it has reached the base of the sulcus. The use of these thick probes can also be painful for the patient if they are forced into tight, healthy sulci.

Complications of probing. Some of the complications that may interfere with periodontal probing include bleeding, sensitivity, saliva, and cal-

culus. A patient with any degree of inflammation in the soft tissues is likely to exhibit bleeding with probing. If the principles of adaptation are being followed and probing is accomplished with only gentle pressure, the clinician can be assured that signs of bleeding represent an inflammatory response rather than poor probing technique. Bleeding areas should be noted carefully because they are one of the first signs of inflammation and appear before other clinical changes in the gingiva can be detected. If a bleeding index is to be taken, it is wise to incorporate it with the periodontal probing and to record signs of gingival bleeding as they occur. It is also important to use this opportunity to explain the cause and significance of bleeding to the patient so that it is not associated with the probing technique but rather with the inflammatory state of the soft tissues. This method of assessment is one that the patient should be encouraged to use at home to detect areas where home care may not be optimal. Many patients have experienced bleeding from toothbrushing or flossing and may regard this sign as a normal occurrence rather than as a sign of inflammatory disease. This is an excellent opportunity to educate patients by showing them which areas need special attention during their home care practices.

Sensitivity from the probing procedure may result from two sources. If the clinican uses an excessive amount of pressure against the soft tissues at the base of the sulcus or pocket, the patient is likely to experience unnecessary sensitivity. Studies have shown that even gentle probing by an experienced clinician can send the tip of the probe through the junctional epithelium and down to the connective tissue attachment below it. This phenomenon is even more likely to occur when the sulcular and junctional epithelium is inflamed and lacks its usual resiliency and tissue firmness.

Another source of sensitivity may be entirely unrelated to poor technique but may simply be the normal response of acutely inflamed tissues to any type of contact by the probe. Inflamed tissues are ulcerated and bleeding, and they have an exaggerated response to any kind of instrumentation, whether it be probing or scaling. In situations like these, the clinician should be prepared to give an anesthetic for patient comfort to complete this procedure. Another alternative is to postpone probing and give home care instructions that may lead to healing of the acutely inflamed tissues. A reduction of inflammation will serve to decrease the pain response to probing at a later appointment.

Visibility of the sulcus area is important during probing to ensure that the probe can be seen and read accurately. Excessive saliva in the area can make reading the probe difficult, and thus, patients may require the use of a saliva ejector during the procedure if they are salivating excessively. The use of the tri-syringe can also help clear the area of blood and saliva and dry the teeth and tissues that are being examined.

Another factor that can inhibit periodontal probing of pockets is calculus. If the deposits are small and scattered throughout the mouth, it is usually possible simply to move the probe away from the deposit and then continue apically into the pocket. One of the traps into which an inexperienced clinician might fall is that of mistaking a calculus deposit for the base of the sulcus or pocket (Fig. 14-5). A good tactile sense will help the clinician determine the difference between the hard resistance of the calculus and the more elastic resiliency of the pocket or sulcus base. If the calculus deposits that are encountered are large and prohibit convenient access to the probe, these gross deposits should be removed by means of ultrasonic or hand scaling to facilitate the probing procedure. There is no need to put the patient through the discomfort of a time-consuming probing procedure if the accuracy of the readings might be questionable. Instead, periodontal probing should be postponed until after these gross deposits have been removed.

Gingival enlargement or recession. Another measurement that must be made and recorded on the periodontal charting form is the height of the gingival margin on each tooth. The gingival height is measured as the distance of the free gingival margin from the CEJ. If the height of the gingival margin is above the CEJ, it is measured by placing the tip of the probe at the CEJ and measuring in millimeters to the free margin of the gingiva. If the free gingival margin has receded apically from the CEJ, the amount of recession is measured by placing the probe tip on the level of the free gingival margin and measuring to the level of the CEJ. Areas of gingival enlargement are recorded by noting a plus sign (+) in front of the number; areas of apical recession are recorded by placing a minus sign (−) before the number; areas where the free gingival margin lies at the level of the CEJ are noted as zero (0) recession. Usually only one reading is taken on the buccal surface of each tooth, and another one is taken on the lingual surface. The highest readings obtained for each of these two areas are then recorded in the appropriate box on the charting form (Fig. 14-2).

Another method of depicting gingival height is to draw a line representing the height of the gingival margin on the pictures of the teeth. This provides visual information for those reading the chart, which is much easier to interpret than numeric millimeter readings alone. This method of charting gingival height is shown for teeth No. 20 to No. 24 in Fig. 14-2.

It is important that the clinician realize that pocket depth readings alone have little or no significance unless they can be compared with the level of the free gingival margin. For instance, a pocket reading of 3 mm on the buccal surface of a mandibular first molar may not sound significant by itself, but when the same area has 4 mm of apical recession, the situation is one of exposed root surfaces, possible furcation involvement, and bone destruction. If the periodontal charting is to be used for diagnosis and

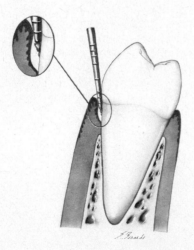

Fig. 14-5. Often calculus ledges prohibit tip of probe from reaching base of pocket. An inexperienced clinician may mistake hard unyielding pressure offered by calculus as the pocket base. If piece is small enough, it may be possible to navigate probe out and around it and continue on down to more resilient texture of pocket base. If calculus piece is too large, it must be removed before accurate probing can be done.

treatment planning, the total picture must be represented. Simply recording pocket depths alone reveals insufficient information about the true status of the periodontal structure.

Amount of masticatory mucosa. The third measurement of soft tissue that is necessary for a complete periodontal charting is the amount of masticatory mucosa on each tooth. This is measured by placing the tip of the probe at the mucogingival junction and measuring the width of the masticatory mucosa, including all attached and free gingiva up to the free gingival margin. This measurement is being shown by probe *A* in Fig. 14-6. Usually this measurement can be made by simply identifying the difference in the appearance of the darker, shinier alveolar mucosa and the light pink, stippled attached gingiva (see Plate 2, *C* and *H*). If this line is not clearly demarcated because of lack of attached gingiva or color changes due to inflammation, it may be helpful to retract the lip or cheek and move it coronally to determine where the junction lies. Tissue that is freely movable is alveolar mucosa, and tissue that is fixed is attached gingiva (Kopczyk and Saxe, 1974; Vincent et al., 1976). This test is also valuable for determining whether or not frena or muscle attachments are pulling on attached gingiva and causing recession. Once the junction has been identified, one measurement can be taken for the buccal surface of each tooth and another for the lingual surface. The

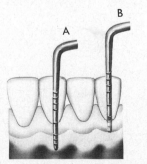

Fig. 14-6. The two measurements necessary to estimate amount of attached gingiva present. Probe *A* is measuring from mucogingival junction to free gingival margin on facial aspect of tooth. Probe *B* is measuring pocket depth. A comparison of the two readings, both taken on facial aspect of same tooth, will indicate amount of attached gingiva that is present.

measurement representing the smallest amount of masticatory mucosa for any one tooth surface should be recorded on the charting form (Fig. 14-2). This measurement is not necessary on the palatal surfaces of maxillary teeth, since the attached gingiva is continuous with the masticatory mucosa of the hard palate.

From the information recorded for pocket depths and masticatory mucosa, the amount of attached gingiva can be calculated. If the buccal pocket depth for a given tooth is subtracted from the masticatory mucosa measurement, the result is the amount of attached gingiva. These two measurements are depicted in Fig. 14-6 as they are being taken on two different teeth. This information is important for determining the periodontal prognosis of a given tooth. To be maintained in a healthy state, a tooth must have an adequate amount of attached gingiva. Experts disagree on exactly how much is "adequate," but studies have shown that as little as 1 mm may be sufficient to maintain gingival health. Less than that may be a significant factor in the etiology of periodontal destruction. The delicate, movable, elastic alveolar mucosa cannot withstand the rigors of mastication and the trauma of brushing as well as the tougher masticatory mucosa. If forced to do so, the result will be loss of gingival height and destruction of periodontal tissues (Bowers, 1963; Lang and Loe, 1972; Hall, 1977, 1981).

The amount of attached gingiva on each tooth is also an important consideration when considering root planing, curettage, and periodontal surgery. Often the treatment of choice will vary, depending on the amount of attached gingiva that is present. Root planing and curettage are frequently contraindicated for areas where there is inadequate or no attached gingiva. Surgical techniques are necessary for successful treatment of these areas.

Mobility

After completing the periodontal probing and soft tissue measurements, the clinician should continue to document the degree of bone destruction and loss of periodontal support by checking the mobility of all teeth. This can be accomplished by using two single-ended instruments, placing the flat end of the handle of each instrument against opposite sides of the tooth, and attempting to move them alternately in a buccolingual direction and then in a mesiodistal direction. Any mobility that is more than the normal amount should be noted on the charting in the following manner ("Periodontal Syllabus," 1975):

1 = Slight mobility
2 = Mobility of up to 1 mm in any direction
3 = Mobility of greater than 1 mm in any direction; tooth may be depressed in the socket

The amount of mobility should be noted in the box for each tooth on the charting form (Fig. 14-2). This box should be left empty if no pathologic mobility has been detected.

Furcation involvement

Areas where loss of bone has caused detectable furcations should be charted. As suggested earlier, it may be helpful to use a curved instrument such as a curette or a shepherd's hook explorer to enter these areas because of the difficulty of access with a straight periodontal probe. A specially designed curved probe, called the *Naber's probe,* is also available for this purpose (Fig. 14-7). Once the furcation is explored, the extent of destruction should be classified as follows:

Class 1. The explorer or probe can detect the concavity of the furcation but cannot enter it. This amount of involvement cannot be detected radiographically.
Class II. The explorer or probe can enter the furcation area but not extend through to the opposite side. A slight radiolucency in the furcation area may be detected with this amount of involvement.
Class III. The explorer or probe can pass all the way through the furcation to the opposite side. An obvious radiolucency should be visible, showing the total destruction of bone in the furcation area.

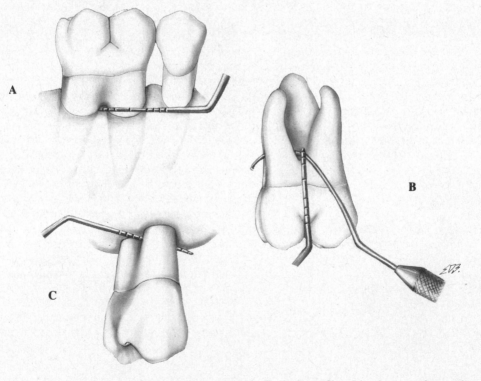

Fig. 14-7. Three teeth with furcation involvements. **A,** Tooth shows Class I involvement where probe can barely detect entrance to furcation. **B,** Tooth shows advantage of having a curved instrument, such as Naber's probe, for detection of furcations. **C,** Tooth has Class III involvement going all the way through to other side. (From Matarazzo, F., and Casullo, D. 1978. Continuing Dental Education, University of Pennsylvania School of Dental Medicine **1:** No. 7.)

The classification Roman numeral I, II, or III should be placed over the picture of the affected tooth in the area of the furcation. This can be seen on teeth No. 31, No. 30, and No. 19 in Fig. 14-2.

USE OF DARK-FIELD MICROSCOPY TO EVALUATE PERIODONTAL STATUS

Clinical signs of inflammation and periodontal destruction such as those described in this chapter (i.e., changes in gingival color, contour, consistency, texture, recession, pocket depths, etc.) can describe existing gingival inflammation or past periodontal disease, but they cannot determine which patients or which sites are currently undergoing active periodontal destruction, or predict which areas of the mouth are more susceptible to the disease process than others. Haffajee et al. (1983) studied the predictive abilities of clinical parameters, including gingival redness, plaque accumulation, bleeding, suppuration, and pocket depth, and found that they could not be used to predict destructive periodontal disease activity in individual sites of the mouth. Hancock (1981), in a review of different methods used to predict disease activity, notes that the traditional methods of evaluating disease activity (i.e., bleeding, signs of gingival inflammation, radiographs, pocket depth measurements) cannot determine the rate of connective tissue or bone loss in periodontal disease until significant destruction has occurred. Although these signs can indicate the presence of gingival inflammation, they do not allow the clinician to determine when the course of the disease has changed into actively progressing periodontal disease.

Listgarten and Hellden (1978) investigated the use of dark-field microscopy to examine the bacterial composition of submarginal plaque in both healthy and diseased periodontal pockets. They found that the distribution of bacteria in the healthy sites was primarily coccoid (90%) and straight rods, with a small percentage of the bacteria being spirochetes (1.8%). In addition, most of the bacteria at these healthy sites were nonmotile rather than motile. When periodontally diseased sites were examined, the distribution of bacteria was very different. In these sites spirochetes made up 37.7% of the total bacterial flora of the pocket, and coccoid and rod types made up only 40% of the bacterial flora. There were also equal numbers of motile and nonmotile bacteria. These investigators proposed that the simple technique of collecting bacterial samples from the pocket areas, examining them under the dark-field microscope, and counting the relative distribution of different types of bacterial cells would allow clinicians to determine exactly which sites were undergoing periodontal disease activity at any given point in time.

Listgarten et al. (1978) found that the numbers of spirochetes were reduced in pockets following treatment by tetracycline and/or scaling, as were other clinical parameters of disease, demonstrating that identification of the proportion of spirochetes and motile rods by dark-field microscopy could be used as a means of evaluating treatment effectiveness. Singletary et al. (1982) confirmed that microscopic evaluation of the subgingival flora was both accurate and convenient as a means of evaluating periodontal disease activity and to monitor the progress of treatment.

Listgarten and Levin (1981) continued to expand the usefulness of this method of periodontal evaluation by testing the reliability of dark-field bacterial analysis in predicting which patients were more likely to experience periodontal breakdown. They concluded that this method provided the clinician with a practical test to determine the susceptibility of patients to periodontal destruction as a result of chronic periodontitis.

Listgarten and Schifter (1982) demonstrated that differential dark-field microscopy could be used as a method for determining the length of the recall interval for an adult population. Patients were assigned "customized" recall intervals based on the relative proportion of spirochetes and motile rods in pooled samples of their subgingival pocket flora. Many patients in the experimental group did not receive a regular prophylaxis for as long as 15 to 18 months, and yet the periodontal health of these patients was found to be no different than that of those who were seen at regular 6-month intervals.

These results indicate that dark-field microscopy may be valuable as a method for assessing periodontal disease activity, for evaluating the success of initial therapy, and for predicting which patients and which intraoral sites are most likely to suffer periodontal destruction. Access to this information would be valuable to the clinician in all aspects of periodontal treatment. In addition, it may offer a more scientific and effective way to determine how frequently patients should receive professional maintenance care, rather than basing this decision on the subjective judgment of the clinician, as has been done in the past. This new method of periodontal evaluation should continue to be evaluated as an adjunct in performing a complete periodontal examination.

SUMMARY

A method of periodontal examination and charting has been presented to aid the clinician in performing and recording this assessment data. Although only one method of charting has been illustrated and described in detail, there are certainly other symbols, figures, and criteria that may be used to achieve the same goals. It is important for the student to realize that the emphasis in periodontal examination and charting is more on the criteria of comprehensiveness, accuracy, and clarity than on the exact way the information is represented on paper. These data, as well as all the other patient assessments discussed in this chapter, must be as complete and easy to interpret as possible, so that those responsible for diagnosis and implementation of treatment can optimally perform their responsibilities to meet the patient's needs.

ACTIVITIES

1. View slides of actual clinical cases and describe and record the most accurate and specific gingival assessments possible of what is seen. Discuss descriptions in small groups and resolve discrepancies by reviewing the slides and discussing the most appropriate descriptions.
2. Watch slides depicting various factors that should be included on the periodontal charting form, such as the clinical appearance of tissues, radiographic findings, and study model records. (Study models could also be available for inspection.) Chart what is seen individually while the faculty member charts findings on an overhead transparency. When the faculty member projects the transparency and slides together, check the accuracy and consistency of your chartings.
3. Research the literature and private offices for charting forms and compare samples for similarities and differences. Review the Computerized Periogram* charting method for accurate graphic data depiction.
4. In small groups discuss the many different ways in which periodontal findings can be recorded. For example, in how many different ways can the periodontal pocket depths be depicted? Use the same approach for gingival height, mobility, masticatory

*Rhelco, Inc., P.O. Box 325, Easton, Conn. 06612.

mucosa, and furcations. After the discussion, analyze these alternative methods in terms of *clarity* (Could anyone understand what was being depicted?), *simplicity* (How complicated is it to reproduce?), and *efficiency* (Can it be charted quickly?).

REVIEW QUESTIONS

1. Identify seven uses of the periodontal examination and charting.
2. How is the amount of attached gingiva on a given tooth surface measured?
3. Is it better to overangulate or underangulate the probe in interproximal areas?
4. On a charting, are pocket depths alone sufficient to describe the presence or absence of disease?
5. True or false
   a. The calibrated end of the probe is adapted exactly parallel to the long axis of the tooth in all areas of the mouth.
   b. Periodontal charting will always be completed before any scaling is performed.
   c. Periodontal pocket readings are taken at the same points on every tooth.

REFERENCES

Armitage, G.C., et al. 1977. Microscopic evaluation of clinical measurements of connective tissue attachment levels. J. Clin. Periodontol. **4:**173.

Armitage, G.C., et al. 1982. Relationship between the percentage of subgingival spirochetes and the severity of periodontal disease. J. Periondontol. **53:**550.

Bowers, G.M. 1963. A study of the width of attached gingiva. J. Periodontol. **34:**201.

Carter, H.G., and Barnes, G.P. 1974. The gingival bleeding index. J. Periodontol. **45:**801.

Examination and diagnosis of periodontal disease. 1975. Bethesda, Md.: U.S. Department of Health, Education, and Welfare.

Fowler, C., et al. 1982. Histologic probe position in treated and untreated human periodontal tissues. J. Clin. Periodontol. **9:**373.

Gabathuler, H., and Hassell, T. 1971. A pressure-sensitive periodontal probe. Helv. Odontol. Acta **15:**114.

Giddon, D.B., et al. 1964. Acute necrotizing ulcerative gingivitis in college students. J. Am. Dent. Assoc. **68:**381.

Goldhaber, P., and Giddon, D.B. 1964. Present concepts concerning the etiology and treatment of acute necrotizing ulcerative gingivitis. Int. Dent. J. **14:**468.

Goldman, H.M., and Cohen, D.W. 1980. Periodontal therapy, ed. 6. St. Louis: The C.V. Mosby Co.

Haffajee, A.D., et al. 1983. Comparison of different data analyses for detecting changes in attachment level. J. Clin. Periodontol. **10:**298.

Hall, W.B. 1977. Present status of soft tissue grafting. J. Periodontol. **48:**587.

Hall, W.B. 1981. The current status of mucogingival problems and their therapy. J. Periodontol. **52:**569.

Hancock, E.B. 1981. Determination of periodontal disease activity. J. Periodontol. **52:**492.

Hancock, E.B., and Wirthlin, M.R. 1979. Histologic assessment of probing in the presence of gingivitis. J. Dent. Res. (Special Issue A)**58**:239.

Hancock, E.B., et al. 1978. Histologic assessment of periodontal probes in normal gingiva. J. Dent. Res. (Special Issue A)**57**:309.

Hangorsky, U. 1980. Early detection of periodontal disease by the general practitioner. Compend. Contin. Dent. Educ. **1**:409.

Hassell, T.M., et al. 1973. Periodontal probing: interinvestigator discrepancies and correlation between probing force and recorded depth, Helv. Odontol. Acta **17**:38.

Kopczyk, R.A., and Saxe, S.R. 1974. Clinical signs of gingival inadequacy: the tension test. J. Dent. Child. **41**:22.

Lang, N., and Hill, R.W. 1977. Radiographs in periodontics. J. Clin. Periodontol. **4**:16.

Lang, N.P., and Loe, H. 1972. The relationship between the width of keratinized gingiva and gingival health. J. Periodontol. **43**:623.

Lindhe, J. 1983. Textbook of clinical periodontology. Copenhagen: Munksgaard.

Lindhe, J., et al. 1982. Critical probing depths in periodontal therapy. Compend. Contin. Educ. **3**:421.

Listgarten, M.A. 1980. Periodontal probing: what does it mean? J. Clin. Periodontol. **7**:165.

Listgarten, M.A., and Hellden, L. 1978. Relative distribution of bacteria at clinically healthy and periodontally diseased sites in humans. J. Clin. Periodontol. **5**:115.

Listgarten, M.A., and Levin, S. 1981. Positive correlation between the proportions of subgingival spirochetes and motile bacteria and susceptibility of human subjects to periodontal deterioration. J. Clin. Periodontol. **8**:122.

Listgarten, M.A., and Rosenberg, M. 1979. Histological study of repair following new attachment procedures in human periodontal lesions. J. Periodontol. **50**:333.

Listgarten, M.A., and Schifter, C. 1982. Differential dark field microscopy of subgingival bacteria as an aid in selecting recall intervals: results after 18 months. J. Clin. Periodontol. **9**:305.

Listgarten, M.A., et al. 1976. Periodontal probing and the relationship of the probe tip to periodontal tissues. J. Periodontol. **47**:511.

Listgarten, M.A., et al. 1978. Effect of tetracycline and/or scaling on human periodontal disease. J. Clin. Periodontol. **5**:246.

Magnusson, I., and Listgarten, M.A. 1980. Histologic evaluation of probing depth following periodontal treatment. J. Clin. Periodontol. **7**:26.

Meitner, S.W., et al. 1979. Identification of inflamed gingival surfaces. J. Clin. Periodontol. **6**:93.

Muhlemann, H.R., and Son, S. 1971. Gingival sulcus bleeding—a leading symptom in initial gingivitis. Helv. Odontol. Acta **15**:107.

Newell, D.H. 1981. Current status of the management of teeth with furcation invasions. J. Periodontol. **52**:559.

Newman, P.S., and Moran, J.M. 1980. Aspects of bone in periodontal disease. Dent. Update **7**:453.

Page, R.C., and Schroeder, H.E. 1976. Pathogenesis of inflammatory periodontal disease: a summary of current work. Lab. Invest. **33**:235.

Parr, R.W. 1975. Examination and diagnosis of periodontal disease. DHEW Pub. No. (HRA) 74-36. Washington, D.C.: U.S. Government Printing Office.

Pennel, B.M., and Keagle, J.G. 1977. Predisposing factors in the etiology and treatment of chronic inflammatory periodontal disease. J. Periodontol. **48**:517.

Periodontal syllabus. 1975. Bethesda, Md.: Naval Graduate Dental School, U.S. Navy Dental Corps.

Powell, B., and Garnick, J.J. 1978. The use of extracted teeth to evaluate clinical measurements of periodontal disease. J. Periodontol. **49**:621.

Ramfjord, S.P., and Ash, M. 1981. Significance of occlusion in the etiology and treatment of early, moderate and advanced periodontitis. J. Periodontol. **52**:511.

Repine, K.D. 1983. Periodontal procedures for the general practitioner. I. Periodontal diagnosis, patient education, and referral procedures. Compend. Contin. Dent. Ed. **4**:125.

Rodriguez-Ferrer, H.J., et al. 1980. Effect on gingival health of removing overhanging margins of interproximal subgingival amalgam restorations. J. Clin. Periodontol. **7**:457.

Saglie, R., et al. 1975. The zone of completely and partially destructed periodontal fibres in pathological pockets. J. Clin. Periodontol. **2**:198.

Schifter, C.C., and Levin, S.I. 1984. Dark field microscopy: adjunct in assessment. RDH **4**:52.

Setchell, D.J., and Shaw, M.J. 1980. The graduated periodontal probe. Dent. Update **7**:431.

Singletary, M.M., et al. 1982. Dark-field microscopic monitoring of subgingival bacteria during periodontal therapy. J. Periodontol. **53**:671.

Sivertson, J.F., and Burgett, F.G. 1976. Probing of pockets related to the attachment level. J. Periodontol. **47**:281.

Socransky, S.S., et al. 1984. Changing concepts of destructive periodontal disease. J. Clin. Periodontol. **11**:21.

Spray, J.R., et al. 1978. Microscopic demonstration of the position of periodontal probes. J. Periodontol. **49**:148.

Theilade, J. 1960. An evaluation of the reliability of radiographs in the measurement of bone loss in periodontal disease. J. Periodontol. **31**:143.

Tibbetts, L.S. 1969. Use of diagnostic probes for detection of periodontal disease. J. Am. Dent. Assoc. **78**:549.

van der Velden, U., and de Vries, J.H. 1978. Introduction of a new periodontal probe: the pressure probe. J. Clin. Periodontol. **5**:188.

Vincent, J.W., et al. 1976. Assessment of attached gingiva using the tension test and clinical measurements. J. Periodontol. **47**:412.

Waerhaug, J. 1977. Subgingival plaque and loss of attachment in periodontosis as evaluated on extracted teeth. J. Periodontol. **48**:125.

Waerhaug, J. 1978. Healing of the dento-epithelial junction following subgingival plaque control. I. As observed in human biopsy material. J. Periodontol. **49**:1. (a)

Waerhaug, J. 1978. Healing of the dento-epithelial junction following subgingival plaque control. II. As observed on extracted teeth. J. Periodontol. **49**:119. (b)

Wilkins, E. 1983. Clinical practice of the dental hygienist, ed. 5. Philadelphia: Lea & Febiger.

Withers, J.A., et al. 1981. The relationship of palato-gingival grooves to localized periodontal disease. J. Periodontol. **52**:41.

15 PREPARATION OF STUDY MODELS

OBJECTIVES: *The reader will be able to*

1. List and describe the four uses of study models
2. Identify the armamentarium used for pouring alginate impressions and for pouring the models.
3. Discuss the health hazards associated with alginate, alginate impressions, and gypsum casts.
4. Briefly describe the significance of each of the following factors for alginate and for gypsum:
   a. Water-to-powder ratio
   b. Water temperature
   c. Method of manipulation
5. Justify the use of beading wax.
6. Describe how to prepare a patient who is to have an alginate impression.
7. List and evaluate the possible approaches to assist a patient with a gagging problem.
8. Describe how to determine if a tray is the proper size.
9. List and describe the steps for taking maxillary and mandibular impressions.
10. Define the term *muscle molding*.
11. Explain why an alginate impression should be removed from a patient's mouth with a quick, steady motion.
12. State the rationale for taking an interocclusal record, and describe the technique.
13. Identify three methods for producing an art base.
14. List the steps for pouring an alginate impression with plaster or stone.
15. Describe the effects of separating the impression too soon or too late from the cast.
16. List and describe the steps for trimming maxillary and mandibular casts.
17. Perform the following procedures for a partner:
    a. Assemble the armamentarium.
    b. Prepare the patient.
    c. Prepare the alginate impressions.
    d. Prepare the interocclusal record.
    e. Pour the models.
    f. Trim the models.

STUDY MODELS

Study models, or diagnostic casts, are exact plaster or stone replicas of the patient's mouth. The models are constructed from impressions taken of the patient's mouth, which are then filled with plaster material. When the impression and plaster are separated, the resulting model is referred to as the study model (Fig. 15-1). Before the models can be used, they must be trimmed and finished. The finished study models can be used as permanent records, diagnostic aids, educational aids, and for the fabrication of temporary appliances (Craig, O'Brien, and Powers, 1983; Goldman and Cohen, 1980; Hirshfeld, 1933; Rudd, 1968).

Permanent records

Study models may be included in the initial records collected to document the conditions existing in a patient's mouth at the beginning of treatment. Since the models are a three-dimensional record of the patient's mouth, they are a helpful addition to the two-dimensional charts and radiographs nor-

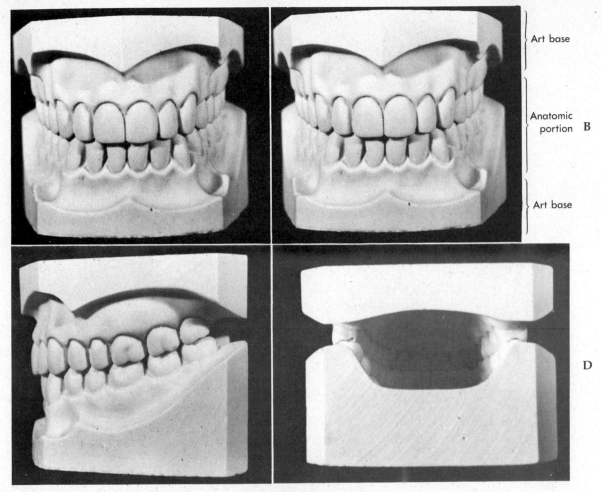

Art base

Anatomic portion

Art base

A

B

C

D

Fig. 15-1. Trimmed study models. **A,** Anterior view. **B,** Anterior view with anatomic portion and art bases indicated. **C,** Side view. **D,** Posterior view.

mally included in an initial set of records. Some dentists may use study models to document the progress of involved or long-term treatment. In these instances study models are taken periodically during treatment as well as at the end of the treatment. Several of the dental specialties (i.e., orthodontics, prosthodontics, periodontics, oral surgery) and some general dentists routinely include study models in records gathered for each patient.

Diagnostic aid

Study models permit the clinician to examine the conditions in the patient's mouth from all views,

including some views that are impossible during a clinical examination (i.e., from the lingual or the direct distal aspects) (Fig. 15-1). The relationships between adjacent teeth and opposing teeth can be examined, measured, and analyzed for as long as is necessary without causing discomfort to the patient. The clinician can draw or perform proposed treatments on the study models. Occlusal relationships can also be examined on the models; if the clinician wants to examine the precise movements of the mandible, the models can be mounted on an articulator (Rudd, 1968) (Fig. 15-2). When the models are mounted on an articulator, some of the

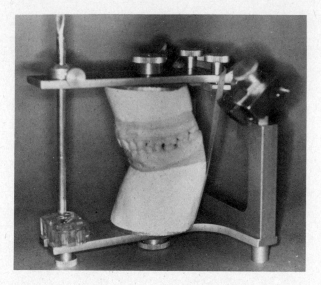

Fig. 15-2. Models mounted on an articulator. (From Gilmore, H.W., et al. 1982. Operative dentistry, ed. 4. St. Louis: The C.V. Mosby Co.)

patient's mandibular movements can be replicated so that the dentist can consider those movements when designing appliances and restorations for the patient.

Study models are also useful during charting procedures, particularly periodontal chartings (Goldman and Cohen, 1980; Hirshfeld, 1933). Wear facets, open contacts, rotated teeth, recession, and other such findings may be viewed on the models and recorded on the chart. The use of study models for recording these findings can save valuable chairside time.

Educational aid

Study models can be used as an educational tool during case presentations and patient education sessions. The clinician can use the models to explain the patient's existing conditions and to illustrate the various possible treatments. The patient can become an active partner during these sessions because she/he is able to view the mouth in the same way the clinician does. Many clinicians have discovered that study models are an excellent tool for describing and demonstrating individualized home care procedures to patients (Hirshfeld, 1933). Patients can practice the techniques on the models before performing the techniques in their mouths.

Fabrication of temporary appliances

Mounted and/or unmounted study models can be used to make temporary appliances such as mouth guards or some orthodontic appliances (Craig, O'Brien, and Powers, 1983; Rudd, 1968). Study models being used for this purpose, sometimes referred to as *working models*, are constructed of a more durable material than are regular study models (Fig. 15-3).

An increasing number of states' dental practices acts permit dental hygienists, and in some states dental assistants, to take alginate impressions and construct study models (see Table 1-1). The purpose of this chapter is to describe the procedures for taking alginate impressions and constructing study models. Brief descriptions of each of the materials used are presented; however, the reader should consult a dental materials textbook for more in-depth discussions of each of the materials.

OVERVIEW OF THE PROCEDURES

Study models are the final product, but several procedures must be performed to obtain the final product: assembling the armamentarium, preparing the patient, taking the alginate impressions, taking the interocclusal record, pouring the models, and trimming and finishing the models. Obtaining study

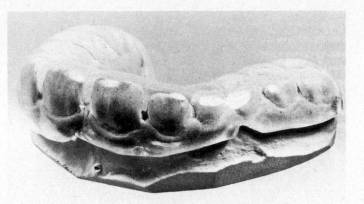

Fig. 15-3. Working model with clear plastic mouth protector in place. (From Craig, R.G., O'Brien, W.J., and Powers, J.M. 1983. Dental materials: properties and manipulation, ed. 3. St. Louis: The C.V. Mosby Co.)

models is an involved process that can be mastered in stages.

Assembling the armamentarium

The armamentarium needed to take alginate impressions and to pour the study models is as follows.

Taking the impression	*Pouring the model*
Bowl and spatula	Bowl and spatula
Alginate with powder and water measures	Plaster or stone
	Vibrator
Impression trays	Buffalo knife
Beading wax	Model base formers or boxing wax, glass slab, or other materials(s) to form the base
Baseplate wax	
Buffalo knife	
Mouthwash	
	Model trimmer (in the laboratory)

Alginate is a flexible irreversible hydrocolloid impression material. Alginate is composed of sodium alginate salt (derived from marine kelp); calcium sulfate; potassium sulfate, zinc fluoride, silicates, or borates; sodium phosphate, diatomaceous earth or silicate powder; and flavoring and coloring agents (ADA Council, 1981; Craig, 1980). The material is supplied as a powder in either premeasured pouches or in a bulk-pack can to be measured as used. If the bulk-pack can is used, the manufacturer supplies a scoop and vial to measure the water and powder in the proper proportions.

When the powder is mixed with water, it forms a gel that flows around the oral structures and hardens in the mouth. When the alginate is removed from the mouth, it stretches slightly (this permits the alginate to be pulled over the rounded oral structures) and then springs back to the form it held in the mouth. Alginate is relatively pleasant tasting, easily mixed, inexpensive, and relatively accurate, making it the material of choice for study model impressions (Craig, O'Brien, and Powers, 1983).

There are a few important factors to keep in mind when manipulating alginate: the water-to-powder ratio, the water temperature, and the mixing method (Craig, O'Brien, and Powers, 1983; Roswick and Simon, 1974a). The manufacturer's directions should be followed for each of these factors. Too much water will result in a runny, slow-setting, weakened mix; too little water will produce a stiff, fast-setting, and hard-to-manipulate mix. The water temperature will also affect the setting time of the alginate mix. Ideally, the water should be 70° F (21° C); warmer water will decrease the setting time, and colder water will increase the setting time. The method used to mix the alginate should minimize the amount of air incorporated into the mix. The alginate powder is added to the water and wetted; a wiping motion is used to mix the alginate. The spatula is wiped against the side of the bowl while the bowl is rotated (Fig. 15-4). At the completion of the mixing, the alginate should be homogeneous, smooth, and creamy (Fig. 15-5).

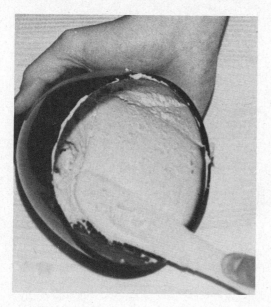

Fig. 15-4. Spatula is wiped against side of bowl to minimize air bubbles during mixing.

Fig. 15-5. Proper consistency of mixed alginate. (From Craig, R.G., O'Brien, W.J., and Powers, J.M. 1983. Dental materials: properties and manipulation, ed. 3. St. Louis: The C.V. Mosby Co.)

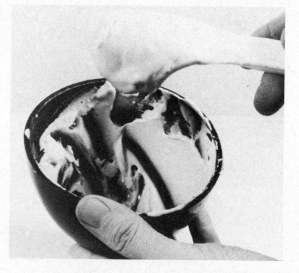

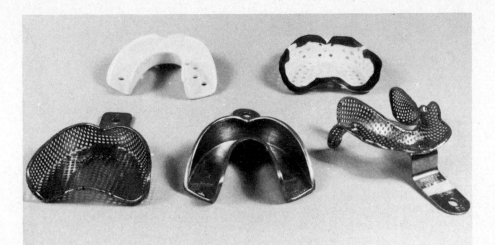

Fig. 15-6. Examples of impression trays: disposable and Styrofoam trays are also available. Note beading wax applied to upper right plastic tray. (From Craig, R.G., O'Brien, W.J., and Powers, J.M. 1983. Dental materials: properties and manipulation, ed. 3. St. Louis: The C.V. Mosby Co.)

Alginate is available in fast-set or normal-set formulas. Fast-set alginate gels in 1 to 2 minutes from the beginning of the mix; normal-set alginate gels in 2 to 4½ minutes (ADA Council, 1981). Fast-set alginate is ideal for use with patients who have a tendency toward gagging and with children. The clinician must be able to work quickly to obtain satisfactory results. It is recommended that both fast-set and regular-set alginate remain in the mouth for 2 minutes, whenever possible, to allow sufficient flowing of the material around the structures and then gelling (ADA Council, 1981).

Alginate impressions lose water when exposed to air. The loss of water will cause the impression to dry out, shrink, and eventually become very brittle. If the impression is not going to be poured immediately, it should be wrapped in a wet paper towel until it is poured (ADA Council, 1981; Craig, O'Brien, and Powers, 1983).

Impression trays. Various types of metal, plastic, and Styrofoam trays are available to use with alginate (Fig. 15-6). The type of tray used depends on the clinician's preference and convenience. The metal trays can be sterilized and reused; the plastic trays can be reused after disinfection but cannot be sterilized with heat. With increasing knowledge of disease transmission and asepsis, it seems highly inappropriate to use a tray that cannot be sterilized

(Greenlee, 1983). The Styrofoam trays are used once and then discarded. The trays can be solid or perforated as long as there is some means of mechanically locking the alginate into the tray so that the alginate remains in the tray when the impression is removed from the mouth. An adhesive may have to be used with some Styrofoam trays. All of the trays are available in several sizes to accommodate any size mouth.

Beading wax. Beading wax is a soft wax available in strips, which are placed around the edges of metal and plastic trays (Fig. 15-6). The wax extends the trays to include the vestibule and posterior areas in the impression. The wax also makes the trays more comfortable for the patient (Craig, O'Brien, and Powers, 1983).

Plaster and/or stone. Plaster and stone are two types of gypsum products that can be used to construct study models. Dental plaster and stone are derived from the mineral gypsum. Chemically, gypsum is the dihydrate form of calcium sulfate (Craig, O'Brien, and Powers, 1983). Plaster is usually used for study models because it is less dense and easier to trim and finish. Some practitioners prefer to use stone because it is a stronger material and is less likely to fracture. As with alginate, it is important to remember several factors when working with plaster and/or stone: water-to-powder ratio, water temperature, and mixing technique. (Craig, O'Brien, and Powers, 1983; Roswick and Simon, 1974b) The manufacturer's recommendations should be followed for the water-to-powder ratio. The recommended ratio for plaster ranges from 40 to 50 ml of water for each 100 g. of plaster; the range for stone is from 30 to 40 ml of water for each 100 g of stone (ADA Council, 1981). Some laboratories provide scales and vials to measure the proper amount of each component; many do not. If these are not provided, the clinician will learn to recognize the proper consistency through experience. Too much water will increase the setting time and produce a weak final product. Too little water will decrease the setting time and produce a stronger final product; however, the mix will be extremely difficult to manipulate, and it will not flow into the impression readily. The water temperature should be 21° C (70° F); cold water will increase the setting time. Water above 21° C and below 37° C (98.6° F) will decrease the setting time, but if the water is above 37° C, no reaction will occur. As can be seen, the water temperature and water-to-powder ratio are very important when trying to mix plaster and/or stone (Craig, O'Brien and Powers, 1983; Roswick and Simon, 1974b).

The gypsum product is mixed by placing the water in the rubber bowl and adding the powder. Craig, O'Brien, and Powers (1983) recommend that the powder be allowed to sit in the water, undisturbed, for about 30 seconds prior to mixing to decrease the amount of air incorporated into the gypsum. The mixing technique is similar to the one used with the alginate: rotary and wiping strokes are used. Once the gypsum is mixed, the bowl can be placed on the activated vibrator so that the air bubbles will rise to the surface and burst. Eliminating air from the gypsum at this stage will lessen the chance of having air bubbles, which cause voids in the final study models. At the completion of the mixing, the material should be homogeneous, smooth, and about the consistency of sour cream (see Fig. 15-17).

Vibrator. The vibrator is used to flow the gypsum into the impression and spread it evenly throughout the impression. The vibrator is especially useful to eliminate air bubbles. The use of the vibrator is discussed further in the section pertaining to pouring the model.

Model trimmer. The model trimmer is used to shape the hardened gypsum into the proper form.

Only the base and borders of the model are trimmed; none of the anatomic structures recorded on the model are trimmed.

Considering health hazards

Health hazards in the work place are, rightly, of great concern to all working persons. The dental work place, including the operatories, laboratory, and radiograph exposure and development rooms, is filled with materials and devices that are of potential harm to the patient and the clinician (ADA Council, 1981). Within dentistry, concern for the safety and welfare of the patient has become tantamount. This is as it should be, since patients entrust themselves into the care of the dental health care providers. Yet, the safety and welfare of the health care providers has sometimes been overlooked. Health care providers must accept responsibility to gain knowledge about materials and devices with which they are working, particularly about the health hazards. Such responsibility has been accepted and acted on in regard to radiation safety. But, even seemingly harmless materials such as alginate, the impressions, and gypsum models have health risks that must be considered and guarded against. The purpose of this section is to discuss the health hazards associated with alginate and gypsum models. The health hazards fall into three categories: those associated with cross-contamination from gypsum models, release of fluoride from alginate, and airborne particles from alginate.

Cross-contamination can occur between patients and dental personnel via gypsum models. Microorganisms have been recovered from stone casts, showing that the casts may be a medium for transmitting disease from patients to dental personnel, especially personnel working with the casts in a laboratory (Leung and Schonfeld, 1983). If a patient with known viral hepatitis were being treated, the clinician would wear gloves and a mask during the alginate impression procedure and thus be protected. However, the impression, carrying the microorganisms, would be poured and trimmed by personnel who in most instances would not be wearing gloves and a mask; thus this person would be exposed to the virus. In addition, anyone handling the model would also be exposed to the virus. Thus far, no cases of viral hepatitis or any disease has been reported to have been transmitted in this way. Yet, the dental personnel are at risk.

Presently investigations are being conducted to determine the feasibility of sterilizing impressions before they are poured to eliminate the chance of cross-contamination. A few studies have been conducted. Leung and Schonfeld (1983) recommend that personnel wear gloves and masks when handling casts from patients with known viral hepatitis. In addition, they recommend that the casts be sterilized. One of the problems with sterilizing either the casts or the impressions is the likelihood of the sterilization procedure causing dimensional change to the impression or the cast. Storer et al. (1981) investigated several methods of sterilizing an impression to eliminate hepatitis B and found that many solutions caused severe damage to alginate impression materials. Their recommendation is to soak the impression overnight in a hypochlorite solution containing 1% available chlorine. Other researchers (Rowe et al., 1978) have suggested spraying or soaking impressions for 1 minute with a solution of chlorhexidine. This method will reduce the level of bacterial contamination but will not eliminate hepatitis virus. Additional information about the sterilization of impressions and models should be sought in the future.

The *release of fluoride* that is present in alginate has been researched recently. High blood levels of fluoride can be toxic. Fluoride is one of the components in alginate, and it is released and absorbed by patients (Hettab, 1981; Hattab et al., 1978). Hattab has indicated that the amount of fluoride absorbed does not cause a significant increase in the blood plasma level of fluoride, except in one instance. If alginate is swallowed, there is a significant increase in the fluoride level. This is particularly important if the patient is a child; therefore, the patient should be cautioned not to swallow alginate material. Hattab (1981) also measured the amount of fluoride absorbed by personnel through routine exposure to alginate during mixing and found it to be negligible.

The final health hazard to be considered is exposure to *airborne particles* from alginate. Most manufacturers recommend that the alginate be shaken before it is measured; this shaking introduces particles of the alginate into the air when the can or pouch is opened. Dental personnel are exposed to powders, lead, and silicone particles (Brune et al., 1978) while measuring and mixing the alginate. It has been found that masks do not filter out the particles and that there is no adequate protection. The concentrations of the airborne particles is greatly reduced after 10 minutes. The precise effect of breathing these particles is uncertain, but working in a well-ventilated area is recommended (de Freitas, 1980).

Preparing the patient

One of the most important keys to obtaining acceptable impressions and, ultimately, acceptable study models is proper patient management. Explaining the procedure and reassuring the patient usually help put the patient at ease and help increase the patient's confidence in the clinician. The armamentarium should be ready before the procedure is begun, and then a brief explanation of what will be done and how the patient can help is appropriate. Having the procedure explained to them and being prepared are important for both adult and pedodontic patients. Children want to know what is to be done and how they should help; it is helpful to liken the materials to be used to objects with which the child is familiar (i.e., the tray is like a big spoon) (Hill and Gellin, 1970). However, it should be pointed out that unlike with a spoon, the material in the tray *should not* be swallowed. As with any procedure, the patient will have confidence in a clinician whose work is thorough, efficient, and done with confidence.

The patient may be seated in either an upright or a supine position for the alginate impression procedure. When working without an assistant, many practitioners seat the patient in an upright position to prevent patient gagging (Chasteen, 1978). An increasing number of practitioners place the patient in a supine position and use four-handed dentistry procedures to take the alginate impressions. These practitioners believe that gagging is less of a problem when the patient is in a supine position because the tongue is in a relaxed position, resting against the soft palate and closing off the oropharynx, thus lessening the chance of gagging (Hill and Gellin, 1970). Regardless of the patient's position, gagging can be a problem for some patients during the impression-taking procedure. Several approaches can be used to minimize patients' gagging.

One approach is to encourage the patient to breathe through the nose rather than through the mouth when the tray is in place. The patient can practice breathing through the nose before the tray is placed; this may help the patient feel less panicky if gagging occurs. If the patient is a known gagger, the patient can hold an ice cube in the mouth or rinse with an anesthetic mouthwash before the tray is placed. Both of these procedures will have a slight numbing effect on the patient's mouth. Some clinicians use topical anesthetic ointment or spray to avert gagging. The use of a topical anesthetic spray is not recommended (see Chapter 32), because the clinician has little control over its application, and the use of ointment in the case of gagging does not always make sense. The topical anesthetic is applied to the soft palate, and the patient will experience a numbing sensation in that area; having a numb soft palate may stimulate a gagging sensation. In addition, gagging is a reflex to prevent aspiration of a foreign object; eliminating the reflex can be dangerous. In a few instances a patient may have such a severe gagging problem that the dentist may decide to prescribe an agent such as nitrous oxide and oxygen sedation for the procedure. (Chasteen, 1978).

Most patients will not have a gagging problem during the procedure. If a patient gags, the clinician can ask the patient to breathe through the nose, as mentioned previously. Sometimes having the patient concentrate on something other than the gagging sensation, such as looking at a spot on the wall or holding one leg up, will help. It is very important for the clinician to remain calm and to reassure the patient. The alginate should not be removed until it has set; removing it too soon would worsen the situation, since the material would be very gooey.

Taking the impression

After explaining the procedure to the patient, the clinician can select and fit the trays. The trays should be large enough to permit ¼ inch (6 mm) of alginate to flow between the tray and the oral structures (Fig. 15-7); however, the tray should not be so large that it impinges on the soft tissues or causes the patient pain (Fig. 15-8). Once the proper trays have been selected and beaded with wax, the alginate material can be mixed for the lower impression. While the material is being mixed or before it is mixed, the patient can rinse with the diluted mouthwash. The tray should be filled up to the level of the beading wax and smoothed with damp fingers (Fig. 15-9). Smoothing the material with damp fingers has been shown to produce better

gypsum models (Morris et al., 1983). Filling the tray above the level of the beading wax will cause an excessive amount of material to flow out of the tray and into the patient's mouth; however, underfilling the tray may cause voids in the impression. When the tray is properly filled, the clinician can invert the tray, retract one of the cheeks with the side of the tray, and rotate the tray into the mouth while retracting the other cheek with a finger (Fig. 15-10). Once the tray is in the mouth and centered, the posterior borders can be seated, the patient can be asked to raise the tongue, and the rest of the tray can be seated (Fig. 15-11). The tray is held in position with a light pressure, and the lip is pulled up to ensure the inclusion of the frenum and the muscle attachments. This procedure of pulling the patient's lip is called *muscle molding* or *muscle trimming* and is performed to record the patient's muscle attachment and mucobuccal fold in the impression (Roswick and Simon, 1974a). When the alginate is set, the tray, with the impression, is removed from the mouth with a quick, steady, upward motion. This can be accomplished by placing the thumbs on the occlusal portion of the tray to insulate the opposing teeth from the tray and by placing the index fingers in the vestibule to break the seal around the tray and lifting the tray upward (Fig. 15-12). An alternative method of removing the tray is to use the handle to pull the tray upward and the fingers from the other hand to insulate the opposing teeth (Fig. 15-13, *H*). It is important to use a quick motion when removing an alginate impression to reduce distortion of the material. If the alginate impression is rocked during removal, this will cause permanent distortion of the material (Craig, O'Brien, and Powers, 1983; Roswick and Simon, 1974a).

A similar technique (Fig. 15-13) is employed to take and to remove the maxillary and mandibular impressions, but the possibility of a gagging problem is greater during the maxillary impression procedure, so it is important to employ methods to reduce gagging. Loading excess alginate in the posterior region should be avoided to lessen chances of gagging.

An acceptable impression is shown in Fig. 15-14.

The alginate impressions should be poured as soon as possible to prevent distortion, but they can be wrapped in damp paper towels for brief storage.

Text continued on p. 252.

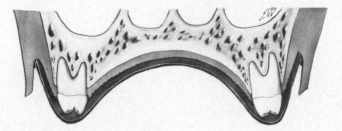

Fig. 15-7. Alginate flows between tray and oral structures. Note that there is about ¼ inch (6 mm) of material between tray and structures. Some of the alginate extends into mucobuccal fold area.

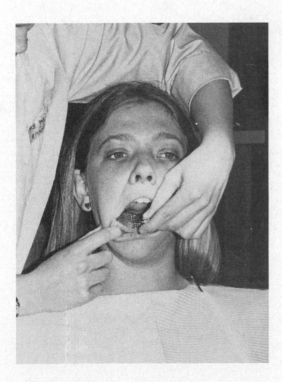

Fig. 15-8. After initial fitting of tray, beading wax has been applied to lower tray, and tray is fitted once more.

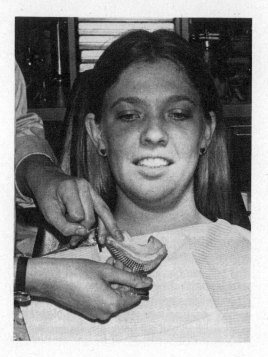

Fig. 15-9. Tray is filled to level of beading wax with alginate and smoothed with a damp finger.

Fig. 15-10. Tray is inverted; one side is used to retract patient's right cheek while clinician retracts left cheek with a finger and rotates tray into mouth. Note that clinician is between 10 and 12 o'clock positions.

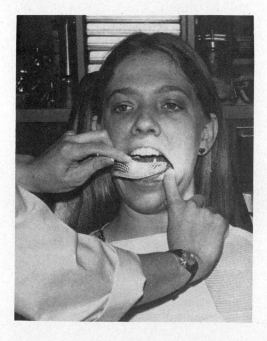

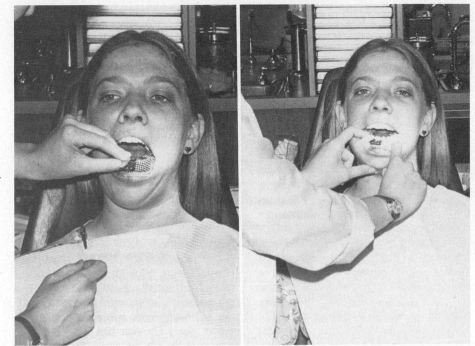

Fig. 15-11. A, Tray is centered, and posterior border is seated. **B,** Remainder of tray is seated and then stabilized until alginate sets.

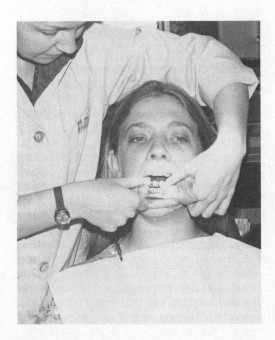

Fig. 15-12. Seal is broken with index fingers, and tray is removed with thumbs protecting upper teeth from impact with tray.

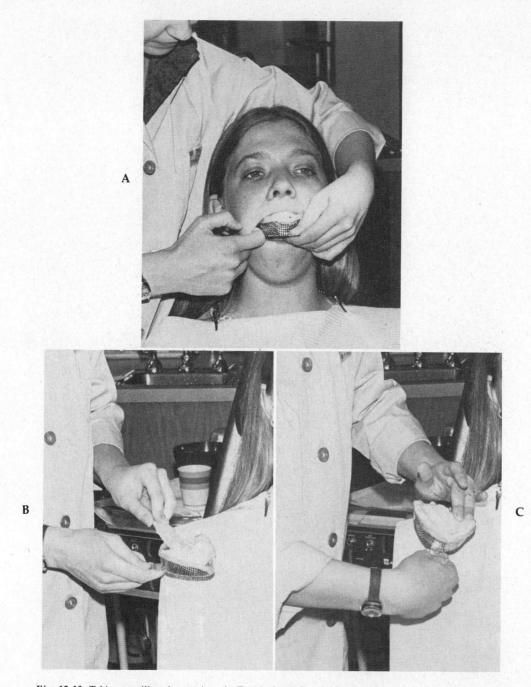

Fig. 15-13. Taking maxillary impression. **A,** Tray is fitted. **B,** Alginate is wiped into tray and, **C,** smoothed with damp fingers. **D,** Patient's left cheek is retracted with side of tray and right cheek with clinician's finger. **E,** Tray is rotated into mouth. **F,** Posterior border is seated; then remainder of tray is seated. **G,** Clinician muscle molds by pulling lip downward. **H,** Teeth in opposite arch are protected while tray is removed. **I,** Tray is removed completely.

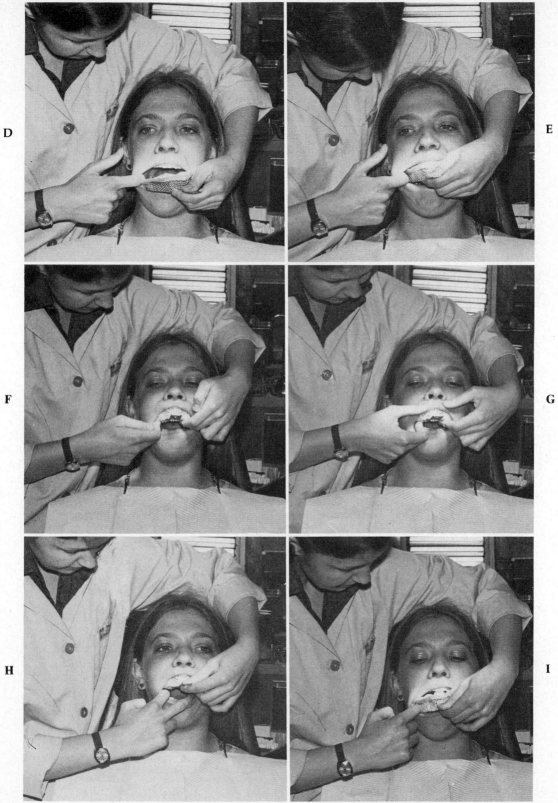

D

E

F

G

H

I

Fig. 15-13, cont'd. For legend see opposite page.

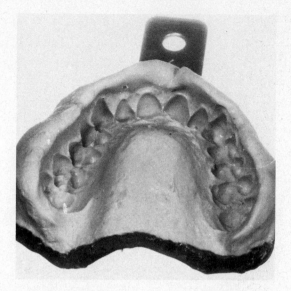

Fig. 15-14. Acceptable alginate impression. (From Craig, R.G., O'Brien, W.J., and Powers, J.M. 1983. Dental materials: properties and manipulation, ed. 3. St. Louis: The C.V. Mosby Co.)

Taking the interocclusal record

An interocclusal bite record is needed to correctly relate the mandibular model to the maxillary model during the trimming. A soft moldable wax is used to take the interocclusal record. One method of taking the interocclusal record uses pink baseplate wax folded in half. The wax is trimmed into the shape of the patient's dental arch with a Buffalo knife and is softened in warm water. The softened sheet of wax is held against the maxillary arch, and the patient is guided into occlusion (Fig. 15-15). The patient's physiologic bite is to be recorded; it sometimes helps to tell the patient to bite on the back teeth (checking to be sure the patient is biting "as usual"). The wax is carefully removed from the patient's mouth to avoid distortion and is hardened in cold water (Graber, 1972).

At the completion of the alginate impression and interocclusal record procedures, the clinician can reassure and thank the patient for being cooperative. It is also a good idea to wipe the patient's face and chin with a damp paper towel to remove any excess alginate.

Pouring the study models

The maxillary and mandibular models are each composed of an art base and an anatomic portion. The anatomic portion is formed by the impression—the teeth and the soft tissues recorded in the impression. The art base can be formed by several methods: base formers, boxing wax, and single-pour and double-pour techniques. Base formers, boxing wax, and the single-pour technique are described in this section. Whichever method is used to form the base, it should be large enough to allow the trimmed models to have a ½ inch (12.5 mm) base and borders that extend about ¼ inch (6 mm) beyond the recorded vestibule.

Prior to pouring, the impression can be gently rinsed with plain or soapy water to remove debris and saliva from it. A gentle stream of air can be used to dry the impression to reduce the amount of excess moisture in it. Excess water or saliva pooled in the impression can cause air bubbles and/or voids in the final study model.

That part of the mandibular tray that is open for the tongue must be filled in with alginate before the model is poured (Fig. 15-16). The tray is placed on a flat surface, and a damp paper towel is folded and placed in the opening; the towel should be about one half the height of the tray. One measure of alginate is mixed and is placed in the opening over the paper towel. The clinician must be careful not to allow the alginate to flow into any of the teeth. Once the alginate has hardened, the impression is ready to be poured.

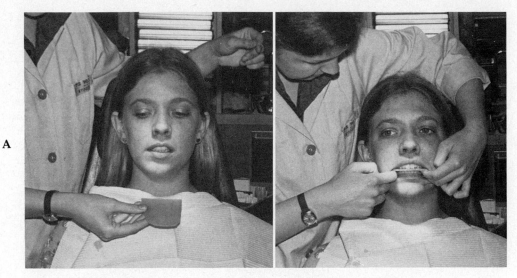

Fig. 15-15. Taking interocclusal record. **A,** Trimmed baseplate wax. **B,** Softened wax is held against upper arch as patient bites.

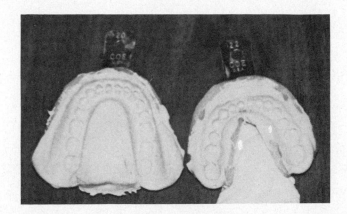

Fig. 15-16. Mandibular impression on left has had tongue area filled in with alginate; impression on right is ready for alginate to be smoothed into tongue area. This procedure eliminates void area in mandibular impression and prepares it for accepting stone or plaster during the pouring process.

The plaster or stone is mixed, and a small increment is flowed from one end of the impression to the other by rolling the impression and tray on the vibrator (Roswick and Simon, 1974b) (Fig. 15-17). Increments of the gypsum are added and manipulated, as described previously, until all of the teeth are filled. A downward pressure can be applied to the tray while it is on the vibrator to eliminate air bubbles in the gypsum (Fig. 15-18). Throughout mixing and pouring, the clinician should try to prevent and/or eliminate air from the mix. Once all of the teeth are filled, larger increments can be added, and the base can be formed by one of the methods described here (Fig. 15-19).

The use of *base former* is a simple way to obtain

an acceptable shape and size base for the model. The base former is filled with the gypsum and placed on the vibrator for a few seconds to remove any air bubbles (Fig. 15-20). The base former is then moved to a flat surface away from the vibrator. The impression filled with gypsum is inverted, centered, and gently pressed into the gypsum in the base former (Fig. 15-21). The tray should be placed into the gypsum so that the occlusal plane of the impression is parallel to the table; this must be estimated. The impression tray and base former should be inspected to be sure that the gypsum in the tray has joined the gypsum in the former; however, the gypsum should not extend up and around the sides or top of the impression tray. If the gypsum does extend onto the tray, the tray will be "locked into" the gypsum, and it will be extremely difficult to separate the tray and impression from the hardened model.

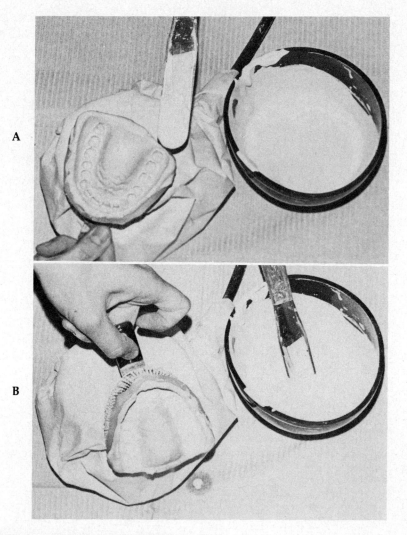

Fig. 15-17. A, A small increment is flowed into maxillary impression. **B,** Gypsum has been flowed around tray to fill all teeth. Note sour cream consistency of gypsum.

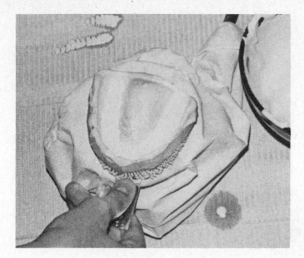

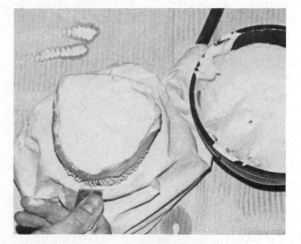

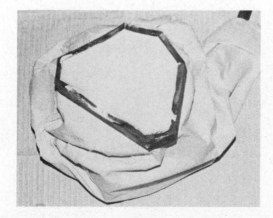

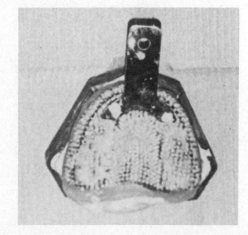

Fig. 15-18. Gypsum is added, and downward pressure is applied to tray on vibrator.

Fig. 15-19. Larger increments are added to fill tray.

Fig. 15-20. Base former is filled with gypsum and vibrated to remove bubbles.

Fig. 15-21. Impression is inverted and joined with gypsum in base former.

Another way to form the art base is with the *single-pour* method, which is probably the most commonly used one. After the tray is filled with gypsum, the remaining material is formed into a shape approximating the tray, about ¾ inch thick, on a glass slab that is away from the vibrator. Once the gypsum is formed, the tray is inverted and joined to the base. The tray should be adjusted so that the occlusal plane of the teeth is parallel to the glass slab; this will have to be estimated, since the clinician will not be able to see the occlusal plane (Figs. 15-22 to 15-24).

The third way to form the art base is with *boxing wax*. This method is popular in prosthodontics, particularly for working casts to be used to construct dentures or pemanent restorations such as bridges. Before the tray is filled with gypsum, a row of beading wax is attached to the outside of the tray. Sometimes the posterior portion of the alginate must be trimmed with a Buffalo knife; this must be done with care so that no anatomic features are removed. Once the beading wax is applied,

boxing wax is molded around the tray, extending above the tray to hold the gypsum and form the art base (Figs. 15-25 to 15-27). The gypsum is then flowed into the tray with the boxing wax attached. This method decreases the amount of trimming but increases the chances of incorporating air, since the excess gypsum cannot flow out.

A fourth way of forming the art base is with the double-pour method. The double-pour method is more involved than any of the other methods described; for a thorough description, consult Roswick and Simon, (1974b).

Once the art base is formed, the model should be left undisturbed for approximately 45 minutes while the gypsum hardens and sets. When the gypsum is cool and no longer hot or warm (gypsum gives off heat while it is setting) to the touch, the impression can be separated from the cast. If the impression is removed from the cast too soon, the model may fracture; if the impression remains on the cast too long, the surface of the model will become extremely rough (Craig, O'Brien, and Powers, 1983; Phillips, 1982).

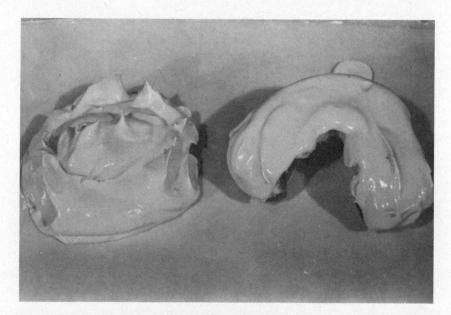

Fig. 15-22. Single-pour method. A mound of gypsum approximating shape of tray has been formed. Filled tray on right is ready to be inverted and joined to base.

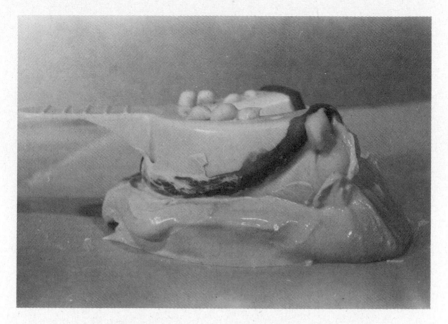

Fig. 15-23. Filled tray is joined to base so that tray and occlusal plane are parallel to table.

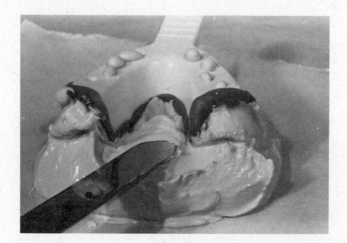

Fig. 15-24. Since tongue area was not filled in with alginate, gypsum from that area is cleared with spatula.

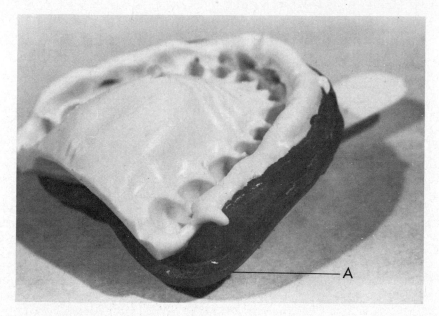

Fig. 15-25. Boxing wax method: an extra row of beading wax *(A)* has been applied to tray.

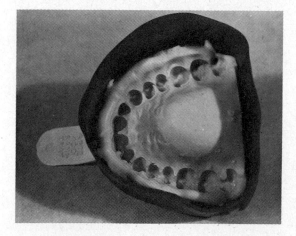

Fig. 15-26. Boxing wax is molded around tray and joined to beading wax.

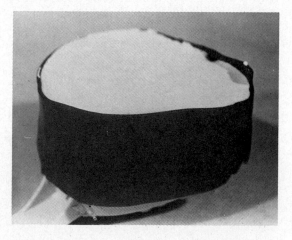

Fig. 15-27. Tray with boxing wax is filled with gypsum.

Trimming and finishing the study models

If no art base former is used, the base and borders of the models are trimmed to form the art base shapes illustrated in Fig. 15-28. The following guidelines should be followed when trimming models. Some practitioners recommend very specific guidelines for trimming models, such as those presented by Robson (1973) or by Roswick and Simon (1974b). The generally accepted guides recommended by Thurow (1977) are presented and described in the accompanying illustrations.

The models should be soaked in water before trimming (Fig. 15-29). The maxillary cast is trimmed first; then the mandibular cast is trimmed to match the maxillary cast. As mentioned previously, only the art base is trimmed; the anatomic portions are not trimmed. The posterior border of the maxillary cast is trimmed first so that it is flat and perpendicular to the midline of the palate (Fig. 15-30). Ultimately, the models will be able to stand on end without wobbling or moving out of occlusion (Fig. 15-31). The top of the maxillary cast is trimmed next so that it is parallel with the occlusal plane (Fig. 15-32). Then the sides of the cast are trimmed to remove the gross excess and to begin the shape of the art base (Fig. 15-33). The shapes of the art bases of the maxillary and mandibular casts are shown in Figs. 15-1 and 15-28. Note that the posterior borders and the sides of both casts are the same shape—the posterior borders are perpendicular to the midlines; the posterior angles are trimmed to be parallel with the opposite cuspids;

and the sides are parallel to a line through the cusps of the cuspids and the central grooves of the posterior teeth. On the maxillary cast the anterior border forms a point over the midline; each side is parallel to a line through the incisal edges of the anterior teeth. The anterior border of the mandibular cast is rounded from cusp to cusp of the cuspids. After the rough shape of the maxillary cast is formed, the mandibular cast is trimmed to form the rough outline. The first step is to trim off the excess width of the mandibular cast (Fig. 15-34). Then the posterior border of the mandibular cast is trimmed to be even with the posterior border of the maxillary cast (Fig. 15-35). It is a good idea to keep the interocclusal record between the teeth during this step to prevent damage to the teeth. The wax should be cut back so that it is not touching the spinning trimmer. Next, the bottom of the model is trimmed to be parallel with the top of the maxillary cast (Fig. 15-36). Since the top of the maxillary cast is parallel to the occlusal plane, the bottom of the mandibular cast also should be parallel to the occlusal plane. The finished product should be able to sit on a flat surface so that the bottom of the mandibular cast, the occlusal plane, and the top of the maxillary cast are all parallel to the flat surface (Fig. 15-1). The sides of the mandibular cast are trimmed (Fig. 15-37). After the approximate shapes of both casts are formed, each is gradually trimmed to form the final shape (Fig. 15-38). Fig. 15-39 shows casts being trimmed with a model trimmer.

Text continued on p. 266.

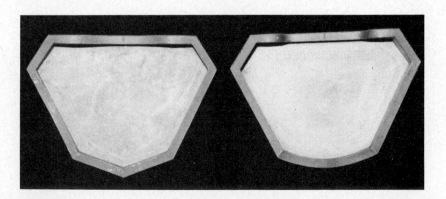

Fig. 15-28. These base formers show outline shapes of properly trimmed models. Pointed former on left is shape of maxillary model. Rounded former on right is shape of mandibular model.

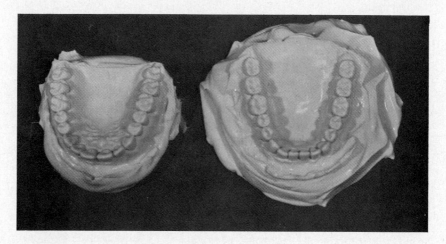

Fig. 15-29. Models removed from alginate impressions and ready to be soaked in water prior to being trimmed.

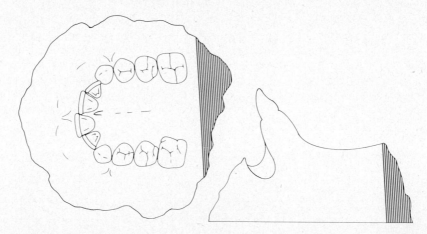

Fig. 15-30. Back surface of maxillary model is trimmed flat. (From Thurow, R.C. 1977. Atlas of orthodontic principles, ed. 2. St. Louis: The C.V. Mosby Co.)

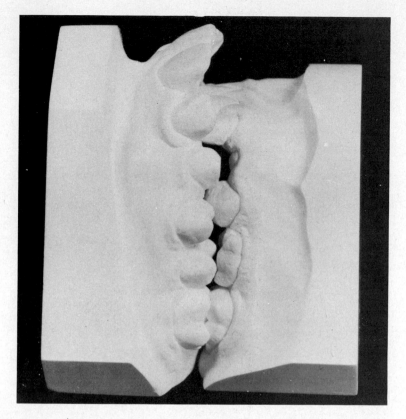

Fig. 15-31. Casts are trimmed so that they will occlude correctly when resting on posterior surfaces. (From Thurow, R.C. 1977. Atlas of orthodontic principles, ed. 2. St. Louis: The C.V. Mosby Co.)

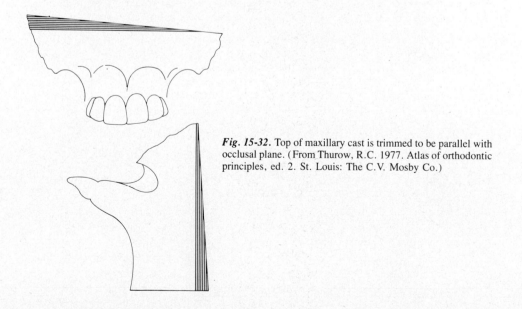

Fig. 15-32. Top of maxillary cast is trimmed to be parallel with occlusal plane. (From Thurow, R.C. 1977. Atlas of orthodontic principles, ed. 2. St. Louis: The C.V. Mosby Co.)

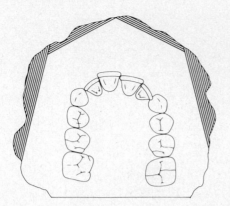

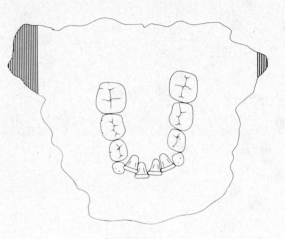

Fig. 15-33. Sides of maxillary cast are trimmed. (From Thurow, R.C. 1977. Atlas of orthodontic principles, ed. 2. St. Louis: The C.V. Mosby Co.)

Fig. 15-34. Gross excess is trimmed from mandibular model. (From Thurow, R.C. 1977. Atlas of orthodontic principles, ed. 2. St. Louis: The C.V. Mosby Co.)

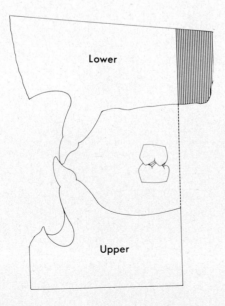

Fig. 15-35. Posterior border of mandibular model is trimmed to match maxillary model. (From Thurow, R.C. 1977. Atlas of orthodontic principles, ed. 2. St. Louis: The C.V. Mosby Co.)

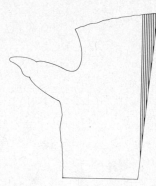

Fig. 15-36. Bottom of mandibular model is trimmed. (From Thurow, R.C. 1977. Atlas of orthodontic principles, ed. 2. St. Louis: The C.V. Mosby Co.)

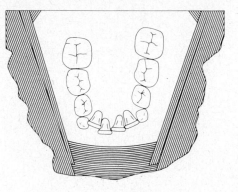

Fig. 15-37. Sides of mandibular cast are trimmed. (From Thurow, R.C. 1977. Atlas of orthodontic principles, ed. 2. St. Louis: The C.V. Mosby Co.)

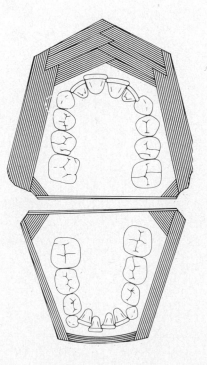

Fig. 15-38. Final shapes of both casts are achieved. (From Thurow, R.C. 1977. Atlas of orthodontic principles, ed. 2. St. Louis: The C.V. Mosby Co.)

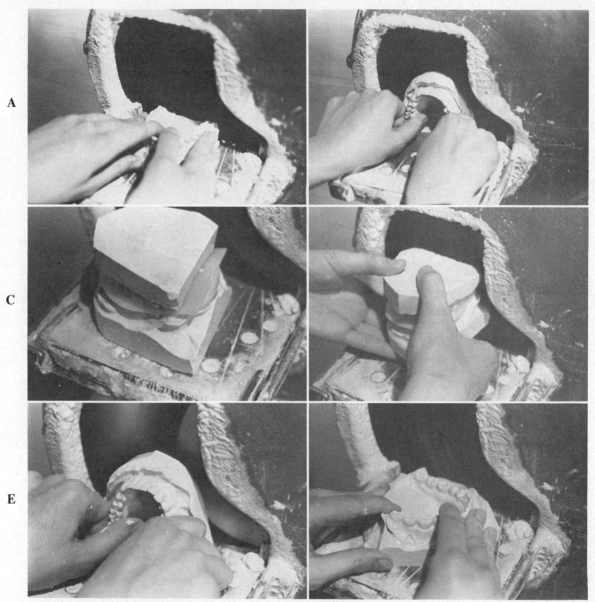

Fig. 15-39. Trimming casts with model's trimmer; note firm grip used to hold cast against blade. **A,** Back surface of maxillary cast is trimmed flat. **B,** Top of maxillary cast is trimmed. **C,** Maxillary and mandibular casts are related with interocclusal record. **D,** After posterior border of wax is removed, casts are trimmed together. **E,** Bottom of mandibular cast is trimmed. **F,** Sides of mandibular cast are trimmed.

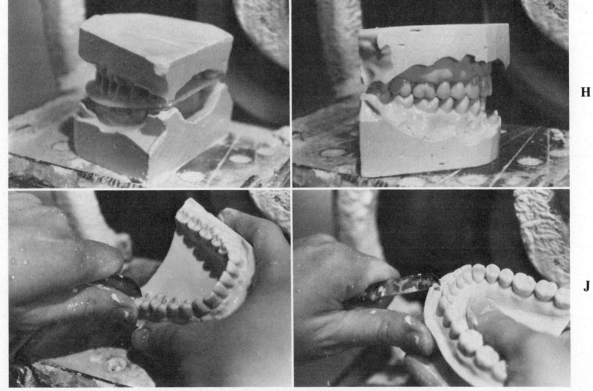

Fig. 15-39, cont'd. **G,** Mandibular casts are related to each other to see if further trimming is needed. **H,** Basic outline is achieved; top, occlusal plane, and bottom are parallel. **I,** Occlusal blebs are removed with Buffalo knife. **J,** Extensions of gypsum are removed.

Study models can be smoothed and polished with fine sandpaper and then soaked in a soap solution and buffed to make smooth models worthy of display. Most practitioners trim the models but do not finish them unless they are to be used for a professional presentation. Most practitioners mark each model with an identifying number or the patient's name in case the models become separated. Models can be stored in a model box labeled with the patient's name and chart number.

Taking an alginate impression

Suggested check-off sheet

Mark **S** for satisfactory completion or **U** for unsatisfactory completion of each criterion in the appropriate space

PERFORMANCE CRITERIA: Does the student	FACULTY	STUDENT
1. Assemble the armamentarium		
2. Prepare the patient		
3. Select the proper tray		
4. Apply beading wax		
5. Mix alginate properly		

Mandibular impression

	FACULTY	STUDENT
6. Fill the tray to the level of the beading wax		
7. Insert the tray properly by retracting one cheek with the fingers and the other with the side of the tray		
8. Have the patient raise his/her tongue		
9. Muscle mold		
10. Stabilize the tray		
11. Control gagging if necessary		
12. Remove the tray with a quick motion while protecting the opposing teeth		

Maxillary impression

	FACULTY	STUDENT
13. Fill the tray to the level of the beading wax		
14. Insert the tray properly by retracting one cheek with the fingers and the other with the side of the tray		
15. Muscle mold		
16. Stabilize the tray		
17. Control gagging if necessary		
18. Remove the tray with a quick motion while protecting the opposing teeth		
19. Take the interocclusal record		

EVALUATION:

	FACULTY	STUDENT
20. Impressions free of voids and tears		
21. All necessary structures included		

ADDITIONAL COMMENTS:

Pouring the impressions

Suggested check-off sheet

Mark **S** for satisfactory completion or **U** for unsatisfactory completion of each criterion in the appropriate space.

PERFORMANCE CRITERIA: Does the student	FACULTY	STUDENT
1. Assemble the armamentarium		
2. Mix the gypsum properly		

Mandibular impression

	FACULTY	STUDENT
3. Fill in the tongue area		
4. Flow a small increment into the teeth		
5. Gradually flow larger increments into the teeth and impression		
6. Fill the base former		
7. Invert the impression into the base former, and set it away from the vibrator		

Maxillary impression

	FACULTY	STUDENT
8. Flow a small increment into the teeth		
9. Gradually flow larger increments into the teeth and impression		
10. Fill the base former		
11. Invert the impression into the base former, and set it away from the vibrator		
12. Allow the casts to completely harden before separating the impressions from the casts		

EVALUATION:

	FACULTY	STUDENT
13. Impressions free of excessive voids, fractures, and/or air bubbles		
14. Impressions smooth and hard		

ADDITIONAL COMMENTS:

Trimming the casts

Suggested check-off sheet

Mark **S** for satisfactory completion or **U** for unsatisfactory completion of each criterion in the appropriate space.

PERFORMANCE CRITERIA: Does the student	FACULTY	STUDENT
1. Soak the casts in water		

Maxillary cast

	FACULTY	STUDENT
2. Trim the posterior border to be perpendicular to the midline		
3. Trim the top of the cast to be parallel to the occlusal plane		
4. Trim the sides to be parallel to a line from the cuspid to the last molar		
5. Trim the anterior portion from the cuspids to form a point over the central incisors		

Mandibular cast

	FACULTY	STUDENT
6. Trim the excess width		
7. Trim the posterior border to be even with the posterior border of the maxillary cast		
8. Trim the bottom of the cast to be parallel to the occlusal plane and the top of the maxillary cast		
9. Trim the sides to be parallel to a line from the cuspid to the last molar		
10. Trim the anterior portion to be rounded from cuspid to cuspid		
11. Trim the posterior angles of both casts to be even with the opposite cuspid		

EVALUATION:

	FACULTY	STUDENT
12. Proper outline form		
13. Anatomic structures undamaged		
14. Adequate art base—width and thickness		
15. Models remain occluded when positioned on posterior borders		

ADDITIONAL COMMENTS:

ACTIVITIES

1. View videotapes produced by the Quercus Corporation (*Taking an Impression,* 1976; *Trimming a Cast,* 1976).
2. Watch a more experienced clinician prepare study models—taking the impressions and pouring and trimming the models.
3. Prepare a set of alginate models for a partner; pour and trim the models (see check-off sheets).
4. After taking impressions for a partner and after being a patient for the procedure, discuss what it was like to be a patient during the procedure. In light of this experience, would either clinician like to modify his/her technique?
5. Secure a set of study models and chart as many findings as possible on the caries or periodontal chartings.
6. Read about health hazards and precautions of alginate material. See the ADA Council report (1981) listed in the references.

REVIEW QUESTIONS

1. What are the four uses of study models?
2. What three factors are important to remember when manipulating alginate and gypsum?
3. What is the criterion for determining if a tray is the proper size?
4. Describe how to place a maxillary tray filled with alginate into a patient's mouth.
5. What is muscle molding, and why is it performed?
6. What can the clinician do if a patient gags while the impression is being taken?
7. What is the danger in removing an alginate impression from the mouth with a slow rocking motion?
8. What is the purpose of an interocclusal record?
9. How should gypsum be flowed into the impression during the pouring procedure?
10. Draw and label the outline forms of the art bases for the maxillary and mandibular casts.

REFERENCES

ADA Council on Materials, Instruments, and Equipment. 1981. Dentist's desk reference, ed. 1. Chicago: American Dental Association.

Alginate impressions and diagnostic models. 1976. Haywood, Calif.: Quercus Corp., U.S. Department of Health, Education, and Welfare.

Appelbaum, M.B. 1981. Abused and misused—the alginate impression technique: a timely reminder. Quintessence Int. **12:**1051.

Brune, D., et al. 1978. Levels of airborne particles resulting from handling alginate impression materials. Scand. J. Dent. Res. **86:**206.

Buchan, S., and Peggie, R.W. 1966. Role of ingredients in alginate impression compounds. J. Dent. Res. **45:**1120.

Carlyle, L.W. 1983. Compatibility of irreversible hydrocolloid impression materials with dental stones. J. Prosthet. Dent. **49:**434.

Chasteen, J.E. 1978. Four-handed dentistry in clinical practice. St. Louis: The C.V. Mosby Co.

Craig, R.G., editor. 1980. Restorative dental materials, ed. 6. St. Louis: The C.V. Mosby Co.

Craig, R.G., O'Brien, W.J., and Powers, J.M. 1983. Dental materials: properties and manipulation, ed. 3. St. Louis: The C.V. Mosby Co.

de Freitas, J.F. 1980. Potential toxicants in alginate powders. Aust. Dent. J. **25:**224.

Eisner, S. 1976. Morphodynamics of the human dentition. Philadelphia: University of Pennsylvania.

Firtell, D.H., et al. 1972. Sterilization of impression materials for use in the surgical operation room. J. Prosthet. Dent. **27:**419.

Goldman, H.M., and Cohen, D.W. 1980. Periodontal therapy, ed. 6. St. Louis: The C.V. Mosby Co.

Graber, T.M. 1972. Orthodontics: principles and practice, ed. 3. Philadelphia: W.B. Saunders Co.

Greenlee, J.S. 1983. Review of currently recommended aseptic procedures. II. Dental instrument preparation. Dent. Hyg. **57**(12):12.

Hattab, F. 1981. Absorption of fluoride following inhalation and ingestion of alginate impression materials. Pharmacol. Ther. Dent. **6:**79.

Hattab, F., et al. 1978. The release of fluoride from alginate impression materials. Community Dent. Oral Epidemiol. **6:**273.

Hill, C.J., and Gellin, M.E. 1970. Impression taking for the young child who gags. J. Am. Dent. Assoc. **81:**161.

Hirshfeld, I. 1933. Importance of casts in periodontia practice. J. Am. Dent. Assoc. **20:**1223.

Hollenback, G.M. 1963. A study of the physical properties of elastic materials (the linear overall accuracy of reversible and irreversible hydrocolloids), IV. J. South Calif. Dent. Assoc. **31:**403.

Knapp, J.G., et al. 1981. Syringe application of alginate impression material. J. Mich. Dent. Assoc. **63:**220.

Jarvis, R.G., and Earnshaw, R. 1980. The effects of alginate impressions on the surface of cast gypsum. I. The physical and chemical structure of the cast. Aust. Dent. J. **25:**349.

Leung, R.L., and Schonfeld, S.E. 1983. Gypsum casts as a potential source of microbial cross-contamination. J. Prosthet. Dent. **49:**210.

Lorton, L. 1982. A method to facilitate impressions of orthodontically bonded teeth. J. Prosthet. Dent. **48:**356.

Miller, J.B., and Burch, J.G. 1973. Criteria and procedures for cast trimming. J. Prosthet. Dent. **30:**843.

Morris, J.C., et al. 1983. Effect on surface detail of casts when irreversible hydrocolloid was wetted before impression making. J. Prosthet. Dent. **49:**328.

Phillips, R.W. 1982. Skinner's science of dental materials, ed. 8. Philadelphia: W.B. Saunders Co.

Pouring study casts. 1977. Lexington: Dental Auxiliary Education, Department of Dental Hygiene, University of Kentucky.

Robson, E. 1973. Preparation of orthodontic study models. Dent. Tech. **26:**50.

Roswick, N.A., and Simon, W.J. 1974. Impression for study models. Dent. Assist. **43:**10. (a)

Roswick, N.A., and Simon, W.J. 1974. The pouring of models. Dent. Assist. **43:**9. (b)

Rowe, A.H., et al. 1978. The probability of contamination and a method of disinfection. Br. Dent. J. **145:**184.

Rudd, K.D. 1968. Making diagnostic casts is not a waste of time. J. Prosthet. Dent. **20:**98.

Sanad, M.E., et al. 1982. The repair of gypsum casts. J. Prosthet. Dent. **48:**492.

Selection and preparation of the impression tray for alginate impression. 1977. Lexington: Dental Auxiliary Education, Department of Dental Hygiene, University of Kentucky.

Skinner, E.W., and Hoblit, N.E. 1956. A study of the accuracy of hydrocolloid impressions. J. Prosthet. Dent. **6:**80.

Stankewitz, C.G., et al. 1980. Bacteremia associated with irreversible hydrocolloid dental impressions. J. Prosthet. Dent. **44:**251.

Storer, R., et al. 1981. An investigation of methods available for sterilizing impressions. Br. Dent. J. **151:**217.

Taking an alginate impression. 1977. Lexington: Dental Auxiliary Education, Department of Dental Hygiene, University of Kentucky.

Taking an impression. 1976. Haywood, Calif.: Quercus Corp.

Thompson, E.O. March 1963. Constructing and using diagnostic models. Dent. Clin. North Am., p. 67.

Thurow, R.C. 1977. Atlas of orthodontic principles. St. Louis: The C.V. Mosby Co.

Trimming a cast. 1976. Haywood, Calif.: Quercus Corp.

Trimming study casts. 1977. Lexington: Dental Auxiliary Education, Department of Dental Hygiene, University of Kentucky.

16 INTRAORAL PHOTOGRAPHY

OBJECTIVES: *The reader will be able to*

1. Discuss how intraoral photography can be used in dentistry.
2. List the objectives of a clinical camera system.
3. Describe a camera system that meets the objectives.
4. Identify the parts of a 35 mm camera used for clinical photography.
5. Define the following terms:
   a. Shutter speed
   b. Aperture setting
   c. Depth of field
   d. ASA film speed
6. State the purpose for using cheek retractors and mirrors as intraoral photographic accessories.
7. Load and unload a film cartridge for a 35 mm camera.
8. Describe the composition of the intraoral photographic series consisting of 12 views.
9. State the criteria for evaluating a slide.
10. Insert the cheek retractors with minimal patient discomfort.
11. Select the appropriate mirror for a particular photograph, considering not only the composition, but also the differences in patient oral antatomy.
12. Place the mirror for each view to aid retraction, light, and accessibility for the camera operator.
13. Handle photographic equipment properly.
14. Compose the picture through the viewfinder.
15. Compose a picture that is centered vertically and horizontally.
16. Compose a picture free of extraneous objects (fingers, retractors, mirror edges, excess saliva bubbles, mirror fog) to the best of the clinician's and patient's ability.
17. Focus the camera for each view.
18. Display concern for the patient through:
    a. Gentle insertion of mirrors and retractors
    b. Considerate direction and communications
    c. Efficiency in time required to take each view
19. Record the camera use as specified by clinic guidelines.

In recent years photography has become a part of dental practice. Clinicians in both general practice and specialties have found the pictoral representation of the patient's conditions to be an invaluable part of the patient's record (Dahlberg, 1968; Meister et al., 1978; Nuckles, 1975; Rosenfeld, 1976).

The photographic series captures the actual state of the patient as no other diagnostic aid can. Chartings of patient's restorations are useful for patient identification and reference, but these are time con-suming to complete and may be inaccurate because of human error. Chartings of this type are usually done on a diagram, making actual tooth morphology and alignment configuration difficult to illustrate. Study models capture the form of the teeth and adjacent soft tissues but are limited in that not all areas of the oral cavity can be subjected to the impression technique. Radiographs are excellent for assessing boney anatomy, caries, and restorations. A look at underlying conditions is provided, but representation of the soft tissue is lost.

Photography captures the color, shape, texture, and characteristics of the oral cavity. The camera objectively records its subject, revealing conditions that may be lost in notation when the patient is absent.

A complete series of intraoral photographs such as that in Plate 3 is useful for treatment planning. The series can be referred to at the clinician's convenience. With the series and the use of other diagnostic aids, the patient's presence may not be necessary for the clinician to assess treatment needs.

With the photographic series and treatment plan in hand, the clinician is ready for the case presentation. As the patient studies his/her oral conditions and considers treatment needs, the scope of his/her dental care is realized. With the help of intraoral photography, the patient is able to see his/her conditions from "the outside." This may encourage the patient to ask questions or discuss therapy from a less defensive position. If the clinician has photographic records of other completed treatment, the patient is able to study the before and after photographs of another person who underwent similar care.

Although identical results cannot be guaranteed, the photographs help the lay person visualize the proposed treatment. The visual communication of the clinician's work may enhance trust in the clinician's skills.

Photography is part of documenting a patient's care. This makes the patient record more accurate and complete. Images establish the patient's actual oral conditions prior to treatment. Made during treatment, the color slides record the progress of care (i.e., improvements in tissue or steps in restoration). At the completion of a phase of therapy, a final series establishes the treatment outcome. The entire series of images, which can be referred to at a future date, provides a record of treatment. Too often, when recall is necessary, the memory is inadequate, and written documentation is sketchy. Should a legal question concerning treatment arise, photographic records may provide invaluable information. Case documentation procedures are described in Chapter 36.

As an educational resource, photography has almost endless possibilities. Patients are motivated by seeing themselves in photographs before and after treatment. Tissue changes occur slowly, making day-to-day appreciation of the healing process difficult. Clinicians benefit in the same manner as the patient's improvement is monitored.

Kodachrome slides can be made to create an instructional series. From these slides quality color or black and white prints can be made. In this way educational materials can be developed in the clinic or office to present information particularly suited to one's clinical philosophy. Series depicting the use of brushing techniques, flossing principles, or the use of auxiliary aids are examples.

The slide collection rapidly becomes a resource for presenting information to groups of patients or peers for a variety of instructional or educational purposes. As the concept of peer review grows, photography may become even more important as a dimension for assessing quality care. Visual documentation of treatment may be required as third-party payment mechanisms increase.

Intraoral photography has become part of comprehensive oral health care. Photography is useful as an aid in:

Diagnosis
Treatment planning
Case presentation
Case documentation
Patient education and/or motivation
Instruction and/or peer review

SELECTING A CAMERA SYSTEM

There are many clinical camera systems on the market, and so few places to secure competent advice about what a quality system should consist of. For this reason, three types of clinical camera units are recommended in this chapter. With these units specific lenses, flash units, and a rotating 180-degree flash bracket are suggested. Excellent results can be assured with this known-quality equipment. Precise photographic images do not just happen; they are made with the proper equipment and photographic technique (Freehe, 1976, 1983).

Daniels and Sherill (1975) have summarized the objectives of a clinical camera system that provides excellent quality and the maximum in flexibility for photographing all aspects of the oral cavity by the following criteria. The camera system is able to:

1. Provide for a simple and repeatable clinical procedure requiring approximately 1 minute for taking a photograph at any image size.

2. Provide for minimum manipulation (i.e., does not require changing accessories or components) regardless of the subject area being photographed.
3. Provide for accurate focusing and composing of the subject.
4. Provide a continuous focusing range from very close (1 × 1) magnification to a "head-to-clavicle" size for maximum convenience and flexibility.
5. Provide for adequate working and lighting distance.
6. Provide for optimum photographic quality in the final result.

The components of such intraoral camera systems would include (Fig. 16-1):

35 mm camera body with single-lens–reflex (SLR) viewing system (manual or automatic)
100 mm macro-lens with extension adapter to achieve 1:1 magnification or
100 mm automatic short-mount bellows lens
Fully automatic bellows (not auto-bellows)
Electronic point-source, color-corrected flash unit mounted on rotating bracket
Proper color correction filters and ring on lens
Pistol grip attachment with single-cable shutter release

The function of a camera body is to hold the light-sensitive film. An SLR camera body is selected for its viewing system. The SLR viewing system allows the photographer to see through the view window exactly what the camera lens sees. This is accomplished by mirrors that form an image from light coming through the lens. Because of the accuracy of this viewing system, it is best suited to the demands of intraoral photography.

A 100 mm lens is selected for the camera system. A 50 mm lens is the standard lens that a 35 mm camera is purchased with. This lens is good for general, nonclinical photography, since it sees approximately what normal vision is. If used clinically for close-up photos, a 50 mm lens has to be used about 4 inches from the subject. This does not allow enough working space or room for proper lighting of the subject. At best, in a close frontal view, the anterior teeth would appear distorted and wider than normal. The 100 mm automatic lens does not distort the close-up subject and allows a working distance of approximately 8 inches from the camera lens to the subject. If images are made

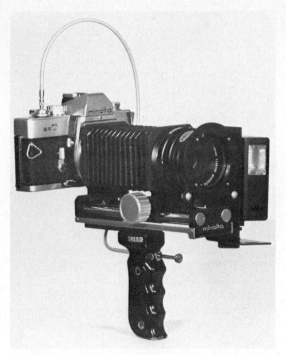

Fig. 16-1. Complete Minolta bellows clinical camera unit. (Courtesy C.L. Freehe, Sumner, Wash.)

during a clinical procedure, this distance provides a more appropriate working field for dental instruments and photographic accessories such as mirrors and retractors. A 135 mm short-mount lens may be used in some specific instances. All 35 mm camera lenses of 100 to 135 mm are perspective distortion free.

A 100 mm lens can be attached to the camera body or to an automatic bellows. A macro-lens attaches to the camera body and allows focusing from infinity to close-up. An adapter extension may be necessary to achieve full life size (1:1) magnification if desired. This adapter must be put on and removed as needed. The size of the macro-lens in relation to the camera body takes some practice to handle comfortably. This fact and the need to use an adapter occasionally may be important in deciding whether this type of camera system is best suited to the clinician's needs. Fitting a macro-lens unit with the appropriate flash attachment may also be difficult. In general, quality macro-lens systems are slower to use, weigh more, and cost more.

The 100 mm short-mount lens is attached to an automatic bellows system. The bellows is an adjustable accordion-type apparatus. The main characteristic of the bellows system is that it is continuously adjustable. The short-mount lens and bellows are capable of focusing from 4½ feet to 7 inches, achieving an orthodontic view ranging from a head-to-clavicle view to one consisting of four to five anterior teeth. No other parts need to be added or adjusted.

The bellows apparatus attaches to a pistol grip, which is helpful in providing stability when handling the camera. A cable release allows the shutter to be released by activating a trigger in the pistol grip. This enables the free hand to adjust the bellows, aid in focusing the view, assist the patient, or place an instrument in the view. The size of the bellows system may be considered by some to be a disadvantage. The 100 mm short-mount lens and automatic bellows camera system has been specifically designed for intraoral photography and is not suited for general photography. This camera can be recommended for use in other health, natural science, and research fields where quality close-up photography is desired.

Recommended camera parts

The purchase of a dental clinical camera can be frustrating even if one knows what to select. This type of camera unit is very specialized and should only be purchased from a company that can assemble and adjust the unit with the proper parts and accessories.

The bellows clinical camera (Minolta or Pentax) consists of:

Minolta body (any one, old or new style)
Automatic bellows (Washington Scientific Camera Co.)
Minolta F4 100 mm bellows lens
Rotating 180-degree flash bracket (Washington Scientific Camera Co.—C. Freehe design)
Maxwell 303H or Yashica Pro 50 DX flash unit with proper modification, accessories, and filter
Proper lens filters and ring
Pistol grip and 12- or 20-inch cable release

The Pentax bellows clinical camera unit is assembled from the same accessories made to fit a Pentax camera body.

A clinical camera using a macro-lens would con-

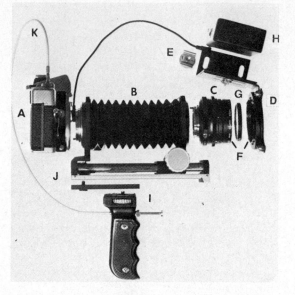

Fig. 16-2. Camera and parts needed for a fully automatic bellows clinical unit. *A,* Single-lens–reflex camera body; *B,* fully automatic bellows; *C,* 100 mm short-mount lens; *D,* Washington Scientific 180-degree rotating flash bracket; *E,* shoe and bolt for flash; *F,* S-7 lens adapter rings; *G,* S-7 color correction filter; *H,* vertical electronic flash unit; *I* to *K,* pistol grip with 20-inch cable release and balance bar. (From Freehe, C.L., 1983. Dent. Clin. North Am. **27:**3.)

sist of a 100 mm True macro-lens and all the same items except the bellows and bellows lens. Additional light unit accessories may also be necessary.

Clinical Research Associates have studied camera systems and have reported that the unit that most consistently produces quality intraoral photographs is the bellows clinical camera described in this text (Fig. 16-2). For more information and a reliable source of supply for units or accessories contact Washington Scientific Camera Co., P.O. 88681, Tukwila, Wash. 98188.

Image lighting

Lighting is the most critical component in the camera system. The proper type and style of lighting can truly *make* the image. The lighting for intraoral photography can be achieved by using:

Single side-mounted point-source flash
Single ring light flash
Ring light and point-source flashes together

The ring light attachment encircles the lens. In this way the light source moves with the focusing of the lens to provide adequate lighting for the photographic field. Some ring lights have a rheostatic power control and require adjusting the power up or down, depending on the view for proper exposure. In addition to the time it takes to make the proper adjustments, this can cause a change in slide color. The ring light produces an image that may lack definition, contrast texture, and good color. The center of the image has no shadow, whereas a hazy 360-degree shadow is cast around the subject. These images may appear flat when compared with point-source lighting, which provides a more natural, three-dimensional image by the contrast created by lighting the subject from one side. All quality art work or scientific images require some directed shadow to capture true form.

The point-source flash is mounted on a rotating bracket and adapter rings on the front of the lens. When attached in this manner, the flash unit moves with the bellows to provide correct lighting for the view and proper exposure. The light source can be rotated from the 3 o'clock position on one side of the lens to the 12 o'clock position at the top and to the 9 o'clock position on the other side of the lens to provide adequate illumination of the field and cast a shadow for definition. Obtaining the correct mount for the rotating light source and making the adjustments for position during shooting are necessary for successful photography (Freehe, 1983).

The proper side-mounted point-source light will produce excellent intraoral views. The bellows system uses a point-source light unit, and a few macro-lens systems use a ring light. With the proper modifications, a ring light and point-source flash could be used together on a camera system. The clinician's preference for lighting control and color and the adaptability of the camera/lens system will determine the best lighting solution.

Flash unit recommendations

The direction and power of the lighting actually create the image of the subject. Important points to consider about the electronic lighting unit for the clinical camera include position, color temperature, and flash exposure.

A side-mounted point-source flash is recommended as the first choice for lighting because this type of unit creates directed lighting to produce clear, well-defined images. When selecting this type of lighting over ring lighting, an analogy of the sun's lighting is appropriate. On an overcast, foggy day general sunlight has no direction; no positive shadows are cast for texture and definition of objects in view. Subtle tones of color in sunlight are lost, and objects that lack that dimension can be confusing to the viewer. Some clinical cameras do use ring lights, but these images as compared with similar views lighted with a point-source flash reveal important differences in capturing the subject's true form.

Positioning the point-source flash for a clinical camera was a problem until a side-mounted flash holder was designed by Freehe in 1959 and redesigned to a rotating flash holder a few years later. This rotating holder places the flash unit in a vertical position as close as possible to the lens and allows both a 180-degree rotation of the flash around the lens and forward-backward movement with the bellows lens as view composition is changed.

The position of the flash close to the lens is important, since a horizontal placement too far from the lens will produce too much shadow, creating a poor image.

The flash unit is selected for its small size. Most units, regardless of manufacturer, need some modification of the base, PC cord, and filter correction to fit the rotating bracket.

The flash unit should have a guide number of 45 to 50 for use with Kodachrome (ASA 64) film. The color output of the flash unit should be as close to 5500° Kelvin (K) as possible. Most flash units have a color output of 5600° to 6400° K, which produce images with blue or purple tissue color. If the color output is below 5500° K, tissue color will be red to yellow. Depending on the flash unit and the type of lighting in the clinical setting, color correction filters over the lens and flash are necessary to achieve ideal color. A light yellow filter is indicated if the films appear blue. A bluish filter will improve a yellow color.

Although a filter can be placed over a macro-lens, correcting the ring light flash is more difficult. If power output can be adjusted with a rheostat for the ring light, then the macro-lens filter must be adjusted. The mechanics of these adjustments are time consuming, and consistent results cannot be assured. The dental light can also affect the color tone of the slides. This light is directed on the cheek, and not on the area to be photographed.

Electronic flash units may be manual or automatic. An automatic flash is programmed for a specific exposure at each specific camera setting. These units cost more than manual flash units and are not practical for a clinical camera. To achieve the best consistent exposure for intraoral photographs at F-19 and F-22 at a distance of 8 to 10 inches, the flash unit should be set on manual with the shutter set at 1/60 second.

Flash units can be AC or battery operated. The AC power offers the convenience of always being ready to flash, but access to electrical outlets and maneuverability may be a consideration. Rechargeable batteries are recommended if battery operation is preferred. The flash should recycle within 5.7 seconds to aid in taking a series of pictures at one time. A flash duration of 1/800 to 1/1000 second is also recommended. Once the camera system is selected, a roll of practice film should be exposed in the clinical setting to determine the necessary corrections in lighting and color filtration.

CAMERA PARTS

Proper handling of a camera, as with every other piece of equipment, requires knowledge of its parts and their function. Depending on the camera model, the manufacturer's instruction booklet is most helpful in this regard. In general, it is important to be able to identify the following parts:

Shutter and ASA speed dial
Film advance lever
Shutter release button
Frame counter
Finder eyepiece
Aperture setting, f-stop
Lens and lens cover
Electronic flash unit attachment
Flash plugs connecting at "X" on camera and on flash attachment
180-degree rotating flash bracket
Flash "ready" light
Automatic bellows
Bellows adjustment knob
Pistol grip and trigger
Film rewind crank and back-cover release
Film cartridge chamber
Film take-up spool
Film pressure plate
Film rewind button on camera base
Battery cover and switch on camera

CAMERA ADJUSTMENTS

Adjustments for the camera include shutter speed (1/60 second), aperture setting (f-stop), and film speed (ASA number).

Shutter speed

The shutter speed (the period of time during which the shutter remains open) works in conjunction with the aperture (lens opening) to determine the amount of light striking the film. The higher the shutter speed, the more efficiently it will momentarily "stop" the action of the subject.

To set the shutter speed, simply rotate the shutter speed dial until the desired speed is aligned with the indicator on the camera body. For intraoral flash photography, the shutter speed is 60, or 1/60 of a second. This is the speed at which the electronic flash is automatically synchronized with the opening of the shutter. On some makes of cameras, the synchronized flash speed may be as high as 1/125 of a second. The shutter and flash must be synchronized, or less of the image will appear on the film.

Lens aperture setting

The lens aperture setting controls the amount of light reaching the film at any given shutter speed. The aperture setting, also known as the f-stop, indicates depth of field. The term *depth of field* refers to the area in which all objects are in focus.

The smaller the aperture opening, the greater the depth of field. The smallest aperture opening is indicated by the largest f-stop number (f-32). For example, f-22 sets a smaller aperture opening than f-16. As the aperture is closed from f-16 to f-22, the amount of light reaching the film decreases by 50%. In intraoral photography, a great depth of field (f-19 or f-22) is desired to achieve sharpness of all objects in the picture. With a camera system having a fully automatic lens and bellows (Washington Scientific Camera Co.), the automatic operation of the camera allows enough light for good viewing of the subject at f-4, but when the shutter is tripped, it causes the aperture to close to the proper predetermined f-stop just prior to the shutter opening and the flash going off. When one looks through the camera viewfinder with the lens wide open, the depth of field is very short (only one tooth); all other teeth appear out of focus. One should focus one third into the scene. For a full facial view on a normally curved arch, this means focusing on the midline of the cuspid. When the image is automatically recorded at f-19, the central incisors to the first molar will be sharp, and the second molar almost sharp. For a normal head-to-clavicle view taken at a distance of 5 feet, the aperture is set at f-8 and the focus is on the eyes. For most intraoral views consisting of approximately four to six teeth, the f-stop is 22. Intraoral views of dark-skinned or black people should be set one half-stop more open at f-19. Conversely, a pure white subject requires less light. When making a view of a set of plaster casts, one should select the setting that would close the aperture to f-27 (Freehe, 1983). The f-stop will also depend on the position and power of the flash and on the film speed.

Film selection

In dental photography, Kodachrome 64 color slide film is selected to reproduce the characteristic true color tones of the oral tissues. Color film available for slides is called *transparency film;* an example is Kodachrome film. Color print film, called *negative film,* such as Kodak Vericolor III Professional film, is available. The principal purpose of the photograph will determine the type of film to be used. Color negative film can be used to produce color prints, black and white prints, or fair color slides, but with each generation of processing a small amount of photographic quality is lost. If Kodachrome 64 film is used, this is a grainless color transparency. The film exposed in the camera is processed and mounted to make the slide, thereby preserving the greatest resolution of the original quality. When necessary, color or black and white prints can be produced from the original color slide by making an internegative. These copies are of the same quality as those from any negative film, since Kodachrome is a grainfree image. Kodachrome is the only permanent color film today. Its color can last 100 or more years. Ektachrome slides or negative film can last as little as 4 to 20 years.

The film is given an ASA number that refers to its light sensitivity. This is the amount of time the film needs to be exposed to light to create a quality image. This is also called film speed. A fast film with a high ASA number such as VR400 or VR1000 indicates that the film is extremely sensitive to light. Less light is necessary to produce an acceptable image. Although useful in some types of photography, these films are not practical for intraoral photography. A film speed that will produce slides with excellent color and detail is the main concern. As film speed increases, grain size increases and contrast decreases. An intermediate film speed such as Kodachrome 64 is ideal for slide production or color print copy because of its high sharpness and lack of grain. Kodachrome 25 could be used, but it has too much magenta for dental photography unless the proper light filters are used to correct for the excessive redness. This is not easy to do. When an electronic flash is used and is color corrected with filter for 5500° K, color daylight film should be used. Kodachrome (ASA) 64 with the proper electronic flash is the correct choice for medical and dental photography.

PHOTOGRAPHIC ACCESSORIES

Accessories for intraoral photography include cheek retractors and mirrors.

Cheek retractors

Cheek retractors are used to clear the area to be photographed of the lips and labial and buccal mucosa. This, in turn, improves visibility and allows the maximum amount of light to enter the oral cavity. Cheek retractors are available in clear plastic or metal (Figs. 16-3 and 16-4). Metal retractors are less attractive but can be autoclaved. This is of particular concern when photographing a patient who may transmit infectious pathogens to dental personnel or to the next patient. The main use of the metal retractor is to hold the mirror for a buccal view. Only one wire retractor is necessary, since a plastic retractor is used for retracting the lips on the other side (Fig. 16-5). The transparent plastic retractors are esthetically most acceptable. Natural tissue color shows through this retractor, limiting the potential for distraction.

Retractors are either single or double ended. The double-ended retractors provide a small curvature and a larger curvature. This feature allows adaptability to a variety of mouth sizes. The extra retractor end acts as a handle, which also enhances retraction. Single-ended plastic retractors (Fig. 16-6) have a longer, tapered handle for holding. The

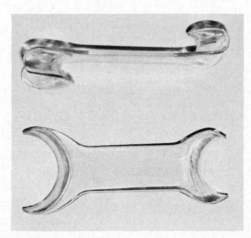

Fig. 16-3. Clear plastic cheek retractors, double ended.

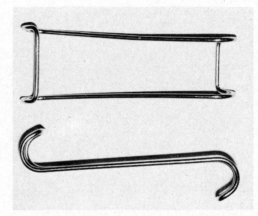

Fig. 16-4. Metal cheek retractors, double ended.

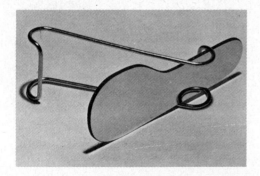

Fig. 16-5. Use of Columbia wire lip retractor with buccal mirror for posterior buccal view. Use one curved plastic lip retractor on opposite side. (From Freehe, C.L. 1983. Dent. Clin. North Am. **27**:3.)

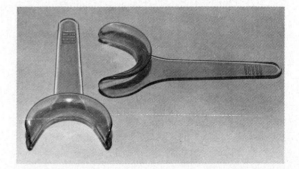

Fig. 16-6. Standard adult shape and size for long-handled blue plastic lip retractor. (From Freehe, C.L. 1983. Dent. Clin. North Am. **27**:3.)

curved end is larger for excellent lip retraction, and these can be cut down or modified to make smaller sizes.

Chemical sterilization procedures are necessary, since plastic retractors cannot be autoclaved. After sterilization, the retractors should be rinsed well to remove all traces of the chemical, which may be irritating to the patient. Directions should be followed for the timing of chemical sterilization because extended time in the solution may damage the plastic.

Technique for inserting retractors (Valentine, 1975)

1. Moisten the retractors in water.
2. Ask the patient to relax the lips and open the mouth slightly.
3. Place the rim of the retractor onto the edge of the lower lip (Fig. 16-17).
4. Rotate the handle of the retractor until it is parallel to the corner of the mouth (Fig. 16-8).
5. Repeat this for the other side of the mouth if necessary.
6. Instruct the patient to bite down on the posterior teeth. Pull out the retractors laterally and slightly forward (Fig. 16-8). Avoid pulling the retractor handles toward the ears. This will cause the buccal mucosa to be pressed onto the buccal surfaces of the teeth, as well as cause the patient discomfort when the retractor is pressed against the gingiva and alveolar process.

Intraoral mirrors

Intraoral mirrors are used to provide a reflected image for photographing. As one can imagine, it is impossible to obtain a direct view of many of the intraoral structures.

Glass mirrors that have been rhodium plated on both sides create an excellent reflective surface. Intraoral mirrors may be purchased in several sizes. The two mirrors shown in Fig. 16-9 allow the clinician flexibility with minimal equipment for general adult photography. For photography of the pedodontic patient, smaller-size mirrors are recommended, especially a child-size occlusal mirror.

Mirrors are washed with detergent and water and sterilized between patients. They should be rinsed thoroughly with plain water before being used in the patient's mouth. Care must be taken

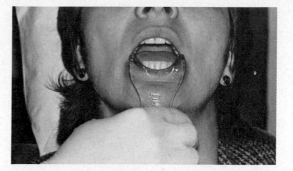

Fig. 16-7. Cheek retractor insertion. With patient's mouth open slightly and lips relaxed, place rim of retractor onto edge of lower lip. Gently rotate retractor to the side.

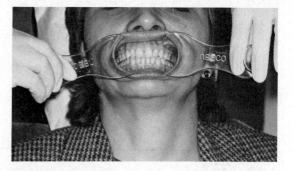

Fig. 16-8. Place second retractor onto lower lip and rotate to opposite side. Pull out laterally and slightly forward.

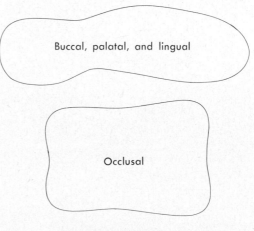

Buccal, palatal, and lingual

Occlusal

Fig. 16-9. Intraoral mirrors.

when using the mirrors because they can be easily scratched or broken. They should be wiped with a soft tissue or cloth and wrapped in cloth or felt for safekeeping.

Technique for inserting mirrors

1. Place the mirror in warm water prior to use to prevent fogging. Laying the mirrors on a small heating pad could also be used to keep them warm.
2. Insert the appropriate cheek retractor.
3. Select the mirror and the appropriate end for the desired view.
4. Place the mirror flat into the mouth, and as you retract with your fingers, rotate the mirror into position. Take care not to hit the teeth or press into the alveolar process, since this is annoying and uncomfortable for the patient.
5. Hold the mirror securely at the opposite end while maintaining retraction.
6. If fogging occurs, blow a gentle stream of compressed air onto the mirror.

Figs. 16-10 to 16-20 diagram that portion of the mirror used for the reflected image. Additional directions for mirror placement are given in the section on technique for individual views.

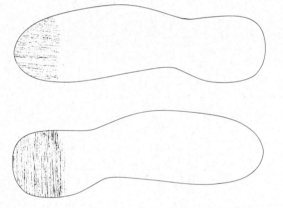

Fig. 16-10. Shaded area indicates portion of mirror that is used for the reflected image in anterior lingual views.

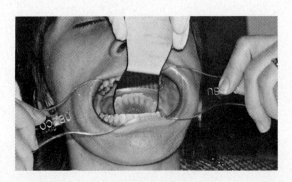

Fig. 16-11. Mirror and retractor placement for mandibular anterior lingual view (see Plate 3, *C*).

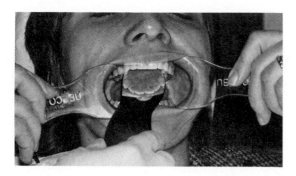

Fig. 16-12. Mirror and retractor placement for anterior palatal view (see Plate 3, *D*).

Fig. 16-13. Mirror and retractor placement for mandibular occlusal view. Rotate retractors down and defog mirror with compressed air (see Plate 3, *E*).

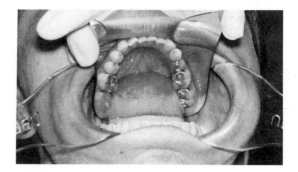

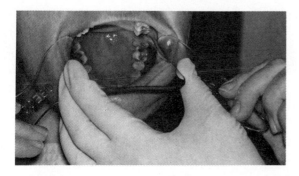

Fig. 16-14. Mirror and retractor placement for maxillary occlusal view. Rotate retractors up and depress mirror to 45-degree angle (see Plate 3, *F*).

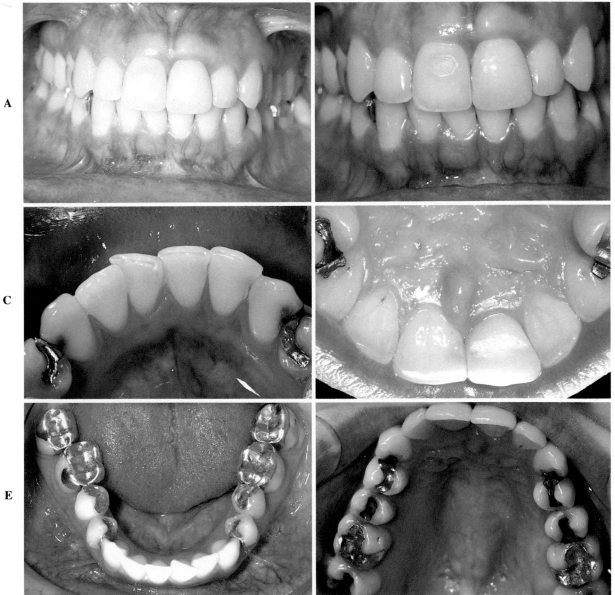

Plate 3. Complete intraoral series. **A,** Full direct view. **B,** Anterior direct view. **C,** Mandibular anterior lingual view. **D,** Anterior palatal view. **E,** Mandibular occlusal view. **F,** Maxillary occlusal view.

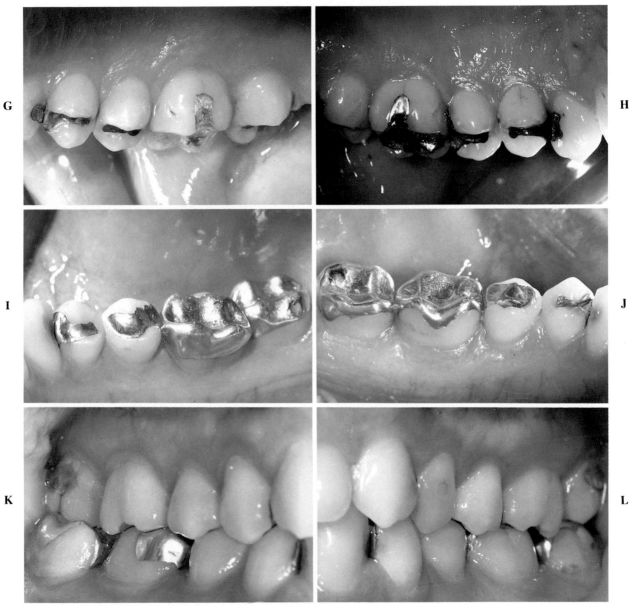

Plate 3, cont'd. **G,** Right posterior palatal view. **H,** Left posterior palatal view. **I,** Right posterior lingual view. **J,** Left posterior lingual view. **K,** Right buccal view. **L,** Left buccal view.

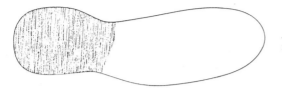

Fig. 16-15. Shaded area indicates portion of mirror used to reflect posterior palatal view.

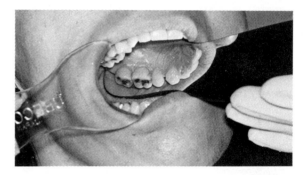

Fig. 16-16. Mirror and retractor placement for right posterior palatal view (see Plate 3, *G*). Person holding mirror may stand on either side of patient. Take care not to pinch lip between mirror and teeth. Retractor could be placed more anteriorly to aid retraction of lower lip.

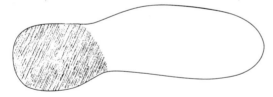

Fig. 16-17. Shaded area indicates portion of mirror used to reflect posterior lingual view.

Fig. 16-18. Mirror and retractor placement for right posterior lingual view (see Plate 3, *I*). Take care not to pinch lip between mirror and teeth. Retractor could be placed more anteriorly to aid retraction of lower lip. If possible, place mirror deeper into floor of mouth to provide excellent view of gingiva and aid tongue retraction.

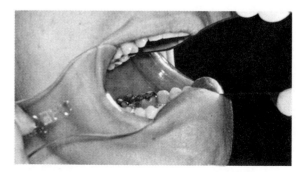

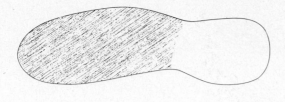

Fig. 16-19. Shaded area indicates portion of mirror used to reflect buccal view.

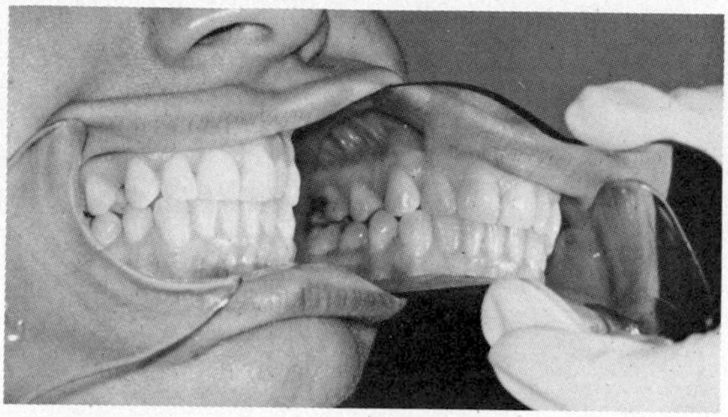

Fig. 16-20. Hand-held mirror and retractor placement for right buccal view (see Plate 3, *K*). Retraction can also be obtained by using wire retractor with mirror (see Fig. 16-5).

RECORD KEEPING AND STORAGE

A record book is placed in the case with each camera. The record book consists of pages that are numbered with the possible exposures available according to the film in use (i.e., 20 or 36 exposures). On the number line that corresponds to the camera frame number, the patient's name and the view that was exposed are recorded. Other information may include the date, the photographer's name, or the camera setting if adjustments were made.

Recording the date and name of the person who loaded and unloaded the camera is helpful in determining the status of the film in the camera. When a film cartridge is unloaded, the camera is reloaded out of courtesy to the next user. This ensures that the camera is ready to be used at a moment's notice.

When the film is processed, the slides are sorted according to the notation in the record book. For identification, each slide is labeled with the patient's name and the view. The clinician's name and the appointment at which the exposure was made are also helpful. The month the slide was processed is generally already imprinted on the slide mount.

Storage

Clear plastic sheets that hold 20 or 36 slides are available to fit three-ring binders. The labeled slides are arranged according to patient and either stored in a central location or incorporated in the patient's record (Barch, 1972). Slides should be projected or viewed on a color-corrected viewer. The radiographic view box will cause the slides to have poor color. Manual slide viewers that magnify the image are also available. Since color slides may fade with time, protection from unnecessary exposure or handling is advised. Since Kodachrome has permanent color, slides need only to be protected from dirt, dust, and finger oils. With quality processing and moderate attention to care and storage, the color quality of Kodachrome 64 film will remain stable for 100 years.

THE PHOTOGRAPHIC SERIES

A complete series of intraoral photographs is shown in Plate 3. It consists of 12 views of the teeth and adjacent soft tissues. The series does not include a full face or profile view, which may be incorporated depending on the clinician's preference. If the slides identify a person and are going to be used for display or educational purposes, a permission or release form can be developed for the patient to sign (Nuckles et al., 1975). A view of the teeth provides only necessary identification for dental personnel; it does not provide easy recognition of the patient by other observers.

GENERAL PHOTOGRAPHIC TECHNIQUE

Following are general principles for loading and unloading the film. Consult the manufacturer's directions for specific steps suited to the particular camera.

Loading the camera

1. Raise the back-cover release knob, and "pop" the back open.
2. Place the film cartridge in the cartridge chamber at the left. Replace the back-cover release knob to hold the cartridge, and feed the film leader onto the take-up spool.
3. Operate the film advance lever. The film will begin to wind around the spool. Watch that the film perforations are engaged on the *upper* and *lower* teeth of the sprocket gears.
4. Press the shutter release button when the advance lever locks. After approximately two shutter releases, the film should be well secured.
5. To make sure the film is flat against the pressure plate, as well as attached to the take-up spool, carefully rotate the film rewind crank in the top of the back-cover release knob to increase the tension slightly. *Always* move the crank in the direction of the arrow. At this point the back of the camera can be closed.
6. Continue to advance the film to the "1" position. As the film advances look to see if the rewind knob is moving, showing that the film is unwinding.
7. Record your name and the date the camera was loaded.

Removing the film

1. Press the rewind button on the bottom of the camera base.
2. Rotate the rewind crank in the top of the back-cover release knob in the direction of the arrow. This winds the film back into the cartridge.

3. As you wind toward the end of the film, you will feel resistance on the crank. Usually after a click that signals the release of the film from the spool, the tension is then released and the crank will move effortlessly. You can then assume that all the film is back in the cartridge.
4. Raise the back-cover release knob, and the back will open.
5. Place the film in its protective canister and send for developing.
6. Record your name and the date of unloading. It is camera courtesy to load the camera for the next person.

Making the photograph

The steps in making a photograph include checking the camera settings, placement of accessories, and composing the view.

1. Check the shutter speed—60 for intraoral photography.
2. Check that the f-stop is set at 22, 19, or 8, depending on the view.
3. Check that the electronic flash "ready" light is on.
4. Check that the film has been advanced.
5. Hold the camera with the pistol grip in the right or left hand. If a macro-lens is used with no pistol grip, place the safety strap from the camera body around your neck.
6. Insert the cheek retractors and mirrors if necessary.
7. When using mirrors and a rotating flash unit, make sure that the flash unit is placed on the same side as the mirror.
8. Dry the field with compressed air as needed.
9. Check the picture composition and the mirror reflection for any adjustments needed at this point.
10. Look through the viewfinder. The bellows is used to obtain the correct composition of the picture. Adjusting the bellows to the most extended position provides the most magnified, close-up view. Change the bellows position for each view as necessary. The bellows does not focus the image; it only provides image ratio or size changes for intraoral views.
11. Correct the mirror placement if necessary. For the best image, position the mirror so that only the reflected image is seen through

the viewfinder. Often the natural teeth are observed, which creates a confusing slide (Fig. 16-21). To correct this problem, move the entire mirror further away from the subject. Although it is not always possible to clear the natural teeth from the field, particularly on occlusal or buccal views, attempting to do so is generally beneficial. Often a movement of 1 or 2 mm is all that is necessary.

12. Focus the view. For maximum brightness during focusing, the automatic bellows lens is always at its largest opening (f-4). With the lens aperture set to f-19, etc., it is wide open during focusing but closes down to f-19 as the shutter is triggered. The view is focused by rocking the camera and photographer's body back and forth until the center image in the viewfinder is sharp. Focus on a point one third of the way into the scene of the subject. For example, use the mesial aspect of the first molar for focus on palatal or mandibular posterior lingual views.

13. Make a final check through the viewfinder for distracting fingers, mirror, or retractor edges, and natural teeth (Fig. 16-22). At this point, the photographer gives the assistant verbal directions for adjusting the accessories without taking his/her eyes away from the viewer. This eliminates additional time being used to compose the view and focus from the beginning again (Fig. 16-23).

14. While steadying the camera, gently squeeze the shutter release.

15. If correct exposure is uncertain, make the necessary adjustments and take the additional exposure. Film is inexpensive compared with the cost of setting up again or losing the record forever.

16. Record the exposure in the record book.

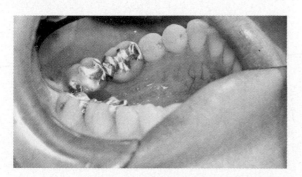

Fig. 16-21. Natural teeth and reflected image create a confusing picture. Adjust mirror by moving posterior end away from natural teeth. Capture only the reflected image.

Fig. 16-22. Fingers can often be distracting in final picture. Check edges of viewfinder just before shooting picture to make any necessary adjustments.

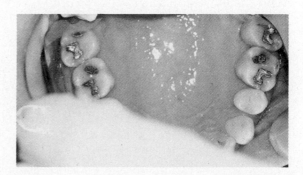

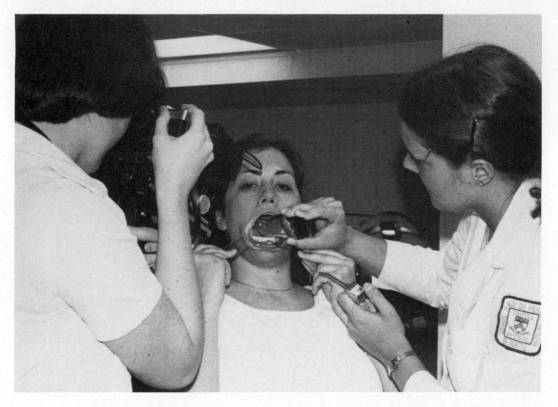

Fig. 16-23. Intraoral photography is a cooperative effort. Photographer gives directions to patient holding retractor and to person holding mirror while looking through camera.

TECHNIQUE FOR INDIVIDUAL VIEWS
Anterior facial views

Composition. Full direct view: The photograph includes all teeth in occlusion as far posteriorly as possible. The incisal and occlusal plane should run in a straight line horizontally across the middle of the slide. The midline is centered (Valentine, 1975) (see Plate 3, *A*).

Anterior direct view: The photograph includes the area from the distal aspect of the right cuspid to the distal aspect of the left cuspid, as well as an adequate zone of gingiva. The incisal plane should run in a straight line across the middle of the slide. The midline is centered (Valentine, 1975) (see Plate 3, *B*).

Patient position. The patient sits upright in the chair, with the head resting securely in the headrest.

The mandible is parallel to the floor when the teeth are in occlusion. The photographer approaches the subject from a position directly in front of the face. To prevent leaning over the dental chair, the photographer can ask the patient to turn his/her head toward the camera.

Retractors. Both retractors are pulled laterally when composing these pictures.

Mirror. None is required.

Flash. The point-source flash is in the 3 or 9 o'clock position for both the full direct view and the anterior direct view.

Helpful hints. Beware of the upper lip casting a shadow on the maxillary gingiva if the flash is used at the 12 o'clock position. If the cheek retractors are pulled too far posteriorly, the buccal mucosa will press into the buccal surfaces of the teeth.

Anterior lingual views

Mandibular anterior lingual view

Composition. The photograph contains a lingual view of the mandibular anterior teeth and gingiva from the distal aspect of the right cuspid to the distal aspect of the left cuspid. The incisal plane runs in a line horizontally across the slide, and the midline is centered (Valentine, 1975) (see Plate 3, *C*).

Patient position. The patient is tilted back slightly in the chair with the head resting securely in the headrest. The mouth is opened wide, with the tongue relaxed in the floor of the mouth.

Retractors. Both retractors are used in retracting the lower lip.

Mirror. Either end of the tapered mirror can be used in composing this picture, depending on the width of the patient's mandibular arch (see Fig. 16-10). It is placed one tooth distal to the teeth that are to be photographed and held as parallel as possible to the long axis of the anterior teeth (see Fig. 16-11).

Flash. The point-source flash is in its top position for this view, or if more light contrast is desired, the flash can be placed in the 3 or 9 o'clock position.

Helpful hints. To avoid an excess of saliva in the composition, ask the patient to swallow first.

Maxillary anterior palatal view

Composition. The photograph contains a palatal view of the maxillary anterior teeth and gingiva from the distal aspect of the right cuspid to the distal aspect of the left cuspid. The incisal plane runs in a line horizontally across the lower edge of the slide, and the midline is centered (Valentine, 1975) (see Plate 3, *D*).

Patient position. The patient should be tilted back slightly in the chair, with the head resting securely in the headrest. The mouth is opened wide, with the tongue resting against the mandibular anterior teeth.

Retractors. Both retractors are used straight out with a slight upward rotation to retract the upper lip.

Mirror. Either end of the mirror can be used in composing this picture, depending on the width of the patient's maxillary arch and the size of the palatal vault. It is placed one tooth distal to the teeth that are to be photographed and held as parallel as possible to the long axis of the teeth (see Fig. 16-12).

Flash. The point-source flash is in the 3 or 9 o'clock position for this view.

Helpful hints. To prevent inclusion of the patient's nostrils in the photograph, make sure that the lower edge of the mirror is depressed as far as possible against the mandibular teeth when the mouth is opened wide.

Occlusal/soft tissue views

Mandibular occlusal view

Composition. The photograph includes the mandibular arch around the perimeter of the mirror (occlusal surfaces) and the floor of the mouth or the tongue (Valentine, 1975) (see Plate 3, *E*).

Patient position. The patient is tilted back in the chair, with the mandible pointed up slightly. The occlusal plane is parallel to the floor when the mouth is opened wide. The tongue may be placed lightly on the soft palate or left to relax in the floor of the mouth.

Retractors. Both retractors are used for this view. Retract the lip downward as necessary.

Mirror. The occlusal mirror is used specifically for this view. Depending on the size of the patient's mouth, either the small or large end of the mirror is inserted posteriorly until the borders of the mirror rest on the retromolar pad. The mirror is then adjusted until it rests at a 45-degree angle to the plane of the occlusion. Blow a stream of compressed air to defog the mirror prior to taking the photograph (see Fig. 16-13).

Flash. The flash is in the 3 or 9 o'clock position for this view.

Helpful hints. To avoid seeing the fingers or retractors in your composition, hold the mirror at its very edge. Tilt the chair back slightly if necessary. In some cases the cheek retractors do not need to be used if the lips are not obscuring the view. Have the patient swallow to prevent pooling saliva.

Maxillary occlusal view

Composition. The photograph includes the maxillary arch around the perimeter of the mirror (occlusal surfaces) and the palate (Valentine, 1975) (see Plate 3, *F*).

Patient position. The patient is sitting in the chair with the head resting securely in the headrest. The mouth should be opened wide and the tongue relaxed against the mandibular teeth.

Retractors. Both retractors are used in this view.

Mirror. The occlusal mirror is used specifically for this view. Depending on the size of the patient's mouth, either the small or large end of the mirror is inserted posteriorly until the borders of the mirror rest on the retromolar pad. The mirror is then adjusted until it rests at a 45-degree angle to the plane of the occlusion (see Fig. 16-14).

Flash. The flash is in 3 or 9 o'clock position for this view.

Helpful hints. To avoid seeing the fingers or retractors in your composition, hold the mirror at its very edge. If the nostrils are still in view, depress the mirror more toward the mandibular teeth or have the patient open wider. Tilt the chair back slightly if necessary. In some cases the cheek retractors do not need to be used if the lips are not obscuring the view.

Posterior palatal views (right and left)

Composition. The photograph includes a palatal view of the maxillary posterior teeth and gingiva from the distal aspect of the cuspid to the maxillary tuberosity. The occlusal plane runs in a straight line horizontally across the slide (Valentine, 1975) (see Plate 3, *G* and *H*).

Patient position. The patient is tilted back slightly in the chair, with the head resting securely in the headrest and usually turned slightly to the side being photographed. The patient's head is turned slightly to the side to permit the best view of the mirror.

Retractors. Both retractors are used to retract the lips and provide access for the mirror on the specific side.

Mirror. The rounded end of the buccal mirror is preferred for this view (see Fig 16-15). It is placed along the midline of the palate until its distal portion is adjacent to the maxillary tuberosity. The anterior end may rest on the incisal surfaces of the lateral incisor of the opposite quadrant. For a direct palatal view, the mirror is maintained as parallel to the long axis of the teeth as possible (see Fig. 16-16).

Flash. The flash is rotated to the same side as the mirror for this view.

Helpful hints. To avoid simulating a gag reflex, do not rest the mirror on the soft palate. If the patient's natural teeth are in the composition, move the entire mirror toward the midline.

Posterior lingual view

Composition. The photograph includes the area from the distal aspect of the cuspid up to and including the retromolar pad. The view is a direct lingual view and shows as little of the occlusal surfaces as possible (Valentine, 1975) (see Plate 3, *I* and *J*).

Patient position. The patient is tilted back slightly in the chair with the head resting securely in the headrest. The mouth is opened wide with the tongue relaxed on the floor of the mouth.

Retractors. Both retractors are used to retract the lips and provide access for the mirror on the specific side.

Mirror. The more rounded end of the mirror is preferred for this view, with the arc toward the floor of the mouth (see Fig 16-17). The tongue is gently retracted away from the lingual surfaces of the teeth with the mirror as it is positioned just distal to the retromolar pad. The mirror will cross the arch diagonally, and the anterior portion of the mirror will rest as far posteriorly on the bicuspids of the opposite quadrant as possible. The mirror is held as vertically as possible to provide the best view. If the top edge of the mirror is tilted toward the teeth, too much of an occlusal view will be observed. The entire mirror is moved away from the teeth if the natural teeth are in the view (see Fig 16-18).

Flash. The flash is rotated to the same side as the mirror for this view.

Helpful hints. Work quickly with this view, since it is not only uncomfortable, but it is taken in an extremely wet field. Be careful not to retract the tongue too harshly, stimulating the gag reflex.

Posterior buccal views (right and left)

Composition. The photograph includes the area from the distal aspect of the cuspids to the distal aspect of the most posterior tooth in each arch, as well as a glimpse of the retromolar pad or the maxillary tuberosity. The occlusal plane runs in a straight line horizontally across the midline of the slide. The view is as direct a buccal view as possible, rather than a mesial view (Valentine, 1975) (see Plate 3, *K* and *L*).

Patient position. The patient is sitting upright in the chair, with the head resting securely in the headrest. With the teeth in occlusion, the mandible is parallel to the floor.

Retractors. One wire retractor is used to hold the mirror for the best view. A plastic retractor is used on the opposite side to retract the lip.

Flash. The flash is rotated to the same side as the mirror for this view.

Mirror. The long tapered end of the buccal mirror is preferred for composing this picture (see Fig. 16-19). The mirror is inserted into the frame of the wire retractor and placed between the buccal surfaces of the teeth and the buccal mucosa all the way to the distal aspect of the last tooth in the arch. It should be pulled laterally away from the alveolar process as much as possible (see Fig 16-5). An alternate technique does not use a wire retractor. The mirror is placed and positioned as described. A secure grip should be kept on the mirror to prevent the buccal musculature from pushing the mirror anteriorly or medially (see Fig 16-20).

Helpful hints. Retract the tissue firmly and as close to a 45-degree angle as possible from the natural teeth to provide the photographer with the best view.

Summary

These directions are intended as a guide for the beginner. Depending on the camera system and the clinical environment, experience will help each clinician determine the best technique. Slight adjustments in chair position and cheek retractor and mirror placement usually have to be made, depending on the patient's oral conditions.

EVALUATION OF SLIDES

The student is encouraged to evaluate the slides he/she has taken according to clinical criteria. Following are suggested criteria for slides:

Above average
1. Inclusion of all desired oral structures
2. Excellent photographic detail; excellent focus
3. Excellent lighting/color
4. No extraneous material
5. Structures well centered
6. Slide labeled properly

Average
1. Inclusion of desired oral structures
2. Adequate photographic detail

3. Lighting/color improvement needed
4. Extraneous material included, but not to distraction of slide's value.
5. Centering improvement needed
6. Slide labeled properly

Unacceptable
1. Omission of desired oral structures
2. Inadequate photographic detail
3. Inadequate lighting/color
4. Obvious extraneous material included
5. Subject completely off-center
6. Slide incorrectly labeled

Following the student evaluation, an instructor meets with the student to concur on the slide evaluation. Discussion focuses on suggestions to improve technique for forthcoming photography sessions. Positive comments and encouragement are helpful, since hours of practice are necessary to reach competency in this psychomotor skill.

CONCLUSION

Intraoral photography has become a part of modern dentistry. With this skill the clinician enhances the process of treatment planning and accurate documentation of the patient's care. Basic photographic skills have been presented for handling a clinical camera system and composing a series of intraoral views.

The criteria sheet on p. 290 is included for process evaluation of student progress during laboratory clinic instruction.

Almost all major photographic manufacturers make some of the components of a clinical camera. The cost of adapting some of this equipment greatly increases the cost of the unit. Unfortunately, most local camera shops do not have personnel who are clinical camera specialists, nor do they have the appropriate equipment to adapt.

The company listed is internationally known for its quality clinical camera and accessories. For the greatest flexibility and quality of detailed clinical photography, the cost of a complete clinical unit will be $550.00 and up. This will not include mirrors or other accessories.

After 10 years of field use by a number of evaluators, Clinical Research Associates (1983) have reported that the Washington Scientific Clinical Camera System is well planned, simple to use,

---

Intraoral photography

STUDENT: _____

DATE:

PERFORMANCE CRITERIA: Does the student

COMMENTS

1. Prepare all equipment for intraoral photography (camera, sterile mirrors, retractors, ASA 64 film, record book)
2. Make all adjustments on the camera to ensure a successful exposure. (1/60 shutter speed, electronic flash "ready", appropriate f-stop)
3. Position the electronic flash according to the area of the mouth to be photographed
4. Insert cheek retractors with a minimum of trauma to the patient
5. Correctly place the intraoral mirrors to obtain the desired composition
6. Use compressed air to dry the area to be photographed
7. Hold the camera securely
8. Focus the camera by adjusting the bellows and body position, or by adjusting the macrolens
9. Record all photos in the record book
10. Store the camera without cocking the trigger
11. Rack the bellows to the full "in" position for storage, or correctly position and store the macro-lens
12. Sterilize and store the cheek retractors and mirrors appropriately
13. Care for the photographic equipment in a responsible manner
14. Load and/or unload the camera properly
15. Evaluate the quality of slides and recommend variations in photographic technique to correct inadequate exposure

---

Modified from checklist supplied by University of Pennsylvania Department of Dental Hygiene.

relatively inexpensive, and has years of service experience to support acceptability of the concept and the device.

Dental equipment and accessories

Washington Scientific Camera Co.
P.O. Box 88681
Tukwila, Wash. 98188

Mirrors only

Evaporated Metal Films
701 Spencer Road
Ithaca, N.Y. 14850

Acknowledgment

Our sincere thanks to Mr. Clifford L. Freehe for his assistance in preparing this chapter. Mr. Freehe is available for questions and advice at the following telephone number: 206-863-7172.

ACTIVITIES

1. Identify the parts of a camera. Practice loading and unloading a "test" film cartridge.
2. View slides of the complete intraoral series, identifying the composition of each view. Unacceptable slides may be shown to illustrate common photographic errors.
3. Divide into lab groups of four students: photographer, patient, mirror holder, and an extra to hold retractors, position light, dry field, etc. Rotate being photographer and practice taking the intraoral views (1 hour per session is suggested). One faculty member per group of students is ideal. Eight to ten sessions are suggested for mastering basic skills.
4. When slides are returned from processing, meet as a group to critique the views and plan new technique strategies.
5. Practice photographic skills by taking complete series of intraoral photographs for clinical patients as a part of treatment and case documentation.

REVIEW QUESTIONS

1. State four ways in which intraoral photography can be useful in dentistry.
2. List the components of a clinical camera system.
3. Match the terms in column 1 with those in column 2 that are most closely related. Place the appropriate number in the space provided.

___ a. Single-lens reflex	1. Error in viewing
___ b. Aperture setting	2. 60
___ c. Focus	3. Controls photographic composition
___ d. Shutter speed	
___ e. Parallax	4. Produces shadow for definition
___ f. Depth of field	
___ g. Film	5. "Rocking" adjustment with body and camera
___ h. 100 mm	
___ i. Point-source light	6. Lens
___ j. Bellows position	7. ASA 64
	8. Plane of focus
	9. Mirror viewing system
	10. f-22

4. Give the steps for placement of intraoral cheek retractors.

5. Give the composition of the following views:
   a. Mandibular anterior lingual
   b. Buccal of right side
   c. Anterior direct
   d. Maxillary occlusal

REFERENCES

Barch, L. 1972. Storage and filing of dental color slides. J. Acad. Gen. Dent. **20**:24.

Clinical Research Associates. 1983. Camera for clinical photography. Newsletter, (Provo, Utah) **7**(5):1.

Dahlberg, W. 1968. Photography in periodontics. Dent. Clin. North Am., p. 763.

Daniels, T., and Sherill, C. 1975. Handbook of dental photography. San Francisco: University of California School of Dentistry.

Faucher, R.R. 1983. Dental photography in the graduate teaching program. Dent. Clin. North Am. **27**:109.

Freehe, C.L. 1968. Dental retractors and accessories. Dent. Clin. North Am. p. 731.

Freehe, C.L. 1976. Clinical dental photography: equipment and technique. In Clark, J., editor. vol. 1. New York: Harper & Row, Publishers, Inc.

Freehe, C.L. 1983. Photography in dentistry: equipment and technique. Dent. Clin. North Am. **27**:3.

Hamilton, A.I. 1983. Preparing text, tables, and illustrations for a journal editor. Dent. Clin. North Am. **27**:197.

Hetherington, W., and Freehe, C. 1968. Single lens reflex cameras and associated equipment for use in dental photography. Dent. Clin. North Am., p. 699.

Jordan, R., et al. 1983. A clinical lecturer's application of dental photography. Dent. Clin. North Am. **27**:121.

Meister, F., et al. 1978. The value of photography in a periodontal survey. Dent. Radiogr. Photogr. **51**:8.

Nelson, L.C. 1983. Photography: its uses in dental practice, lectures, and the home. Dent. Clin. North Am. **27**:171.

Nuckles, D., et al. 1975. Close-up photography in the dental office. J. Am. Dent. Assoc. **90**:152.

Rosenfeld, L. 1976. Periodontics: photos tell the tale. Dent. Stud. **54**:29.

Stern, N. 1973. Indexing and storing teaching slides. Dent. Radiogr. Photogr. **46**:86.

Tilly, D., and Hagen, A. 1983. Preparing graphics for visual presentation. Dent. Clin. North Am. **27**:75.

Tribe, H. 1983. Selecting and preparing illustrations for publication and presentation. Dent. Clin. North Am. **27**:95.

Valentine, R.M. 1975. Expanded duties: a self-determined pace laboratory program. Philadelphia: Department of Dental Hygiene, School of Dental Medicine, University of Pennsylvania.

PART THREE

PLANNING

Once assessment data are gathered, it is time to logically *plan* care for the patient. This includes developing an action plan to solve the problems that have emerged from the assessment phase and setting goals for the patient's health progress.

Involving the patient in planning is an important key to ensuring active participation and shared ownership of the plan. Therefore in Chapters 17 to 20 the patient is an integral part of the planning of care.

Some signs of implementation will begin to emerge in these planning chapters, since the line between planning and implementation is often difficult to define. The planning process in many ways triggers the patient's need to know and need to have care provided. The dental professional's responsibility is to ensure that planning is adequately defined and that the program moves into implementation at a point when the patient is most receptive.

17 PLANNING FOR THE CONTROL OF DENTAL DISEASE

OBJECTIVES: *The reader will be able to*

1. Discuss the role of the hygienist as dental health educator.
2. State how prevention of dental disease has moved from philosophic concept to reality.
3. State three types of research in which the investigation of dental plaque and related oral diseases is being continued.
4. State the best current preventive approach to plaque-related disease.
5. Provide a possible explanation for the popularity of preventive education programs in recent years.
6. Describe several preventive education formats.
7. Describe several important characteristics of the person responsible for carrying out preventive education.
8. Discuss the value of an individualized approach to patient education.
9. Prepare an individualized plan of preventive education with the component phases of assessment, planning, implementation, and evaluation.
10. State four basic guidelines for patient instruction.
11. Give examples of educational appeals that are successful for short-term and long-term patient motivation.
12. State the characteristics of a toothbrush that are important for effective oral cleaning.
13. Describe the usefulness of a disclosing agent in a patient education program.
14. Describe and demonstrate the following brushing techniques: roll stroke, modified Stillman's method, Bass method, and scrub brush method.
15. Discuss the need for interproximal cleaning.
16. Demonstrate interproximal cleaning techniques.
17. Identify patients who may need instruction with additional cleaning or massaging tools such as the following: floss holder, floss threader, yarn, gauze strip, periodontal aid, wood wedge, rubber tip, interproximal brush, modified or automatic brush, and oral irrigators.

In 1906 when Irene Newman became a dental auxiliary responsible primarily for instructing patients on the care of oral conditions in addition to her role in cleaning the teeth of patients, the tradition of the hygienist as dental educator was born.

Since that time, education of the general public and private patients has been a large part of the profession. Indeed, the role of educator has been emphasized more or less throughout the years in cycles of popularity (Woodall, 1983). Currently, public education is enjoying much attention. This is the age of being informed, of consumerism, and of getting the most valuable product for the time and money spent.

The dental health professional provides information on dental awareness, preventive home care methods, corrective therapy for oral habits, and nutritional counseling. As the team approach to planning treatment is emphasized, the clinician is called on to present a variety of modes of therapy. The dental health professional participates in the education of individual patients, families, institutional patients and staff, school students, community groups, and peers.

As the profession of dental hygiene expands in

clinical responsibilities, so it expands in educational opportunities. The expanded-function clinician will continue the tradition of the hygienist as oral health educator.

This chapter focuses on the clinician's role in educating patients in the prevention of dental disease.

It can be assumed that even in the early 1900s, the primary reason for educating the patient was to help the individual prevent further dental problems. With the advent of extensive oral science research, preventive education has become a much more tangible topic. Investigations in microbiology, histology, pathology, and related areas have provided valuable information regarding the nature of dental diseases (Ellen, 1976; Listgarten, Lai, and Socransky, 1975; Page and Schroeder, 1976). Such information has enabled the dental educator to share with the patient scientific evidence that supports the need for and benefits of home care measures. Preventive education is no longer a philosophic concept. Clinical evidence of a reduction in the number of caries and especially in signs of the inflammatory disease processes indicate that following preventive home care procedures is a sound practice (Axelsson and Lindhe, 1981; Cohen, 1975; Golub and Kleinberg, 1976; Loe, 1970; Loe, Theilade, and Borglum, 1965; Socransky, 1970).

When the patient is aware of the nature of dental diseases, has assistance in establishing appropriate home care techniques, and values this information by demonstrating motivation and practice of these skills, dental disease can be prevented.

THE PROBLEM

Dental plaque is accepted as a major factor in inflammatory gingival disease and in caries development (Cohen, 1975; Page and Schroeder, 1976).

Within recent years the prevalence of dental caries has been greatly reduced by water fluoridation programs. The regular use of fluoride in topical treatments, dentrifices, and mouthwashes and the development of pit and fissure sealant materials continue to have an important impact on decreasing dental caries.

Although much research has been completed, periodontal disease remains the leading cause of tooth loss. In a national health survey done in 1962, 75% of the adult population had some degree of periodontal disease. More recently, a survey following North Carolina's dental needs over the past 14 years indicates that even though total caries and the number of untreated caries in the population are declining, periodontal disease has increased. If this long-term study has broader implication for the nation as a whole, the 1981 report of the American Association of Public Health Dentists is correct in stating that the future emphasis of the dental profession must be on mobilizing an effective campaign against periodontal disease. Since few periodontal problems occur without previous gingival inflammation or gingivitis, the front line of prevention concerns dental plaque.

As described in Chapter 13, when subjects stop oral hygiene practices, microscopic signs of inflammation occur within 2 days, with clinical evidence of disease within 10 to 21 days. When oral hygiene practices are started again, plaque and gingivitis scores return to preexperiment levels within 2 days (Loe, Theilade, and Borglum, 1965). It seems that microbial plaque formation must be eliminated, reduced, or rendered harmless for inflammatory periodontal disease to be prevented.

Antimicrobial agents such as antibiotics and chemical irrigation products (chlorhexidine, enzyme rinses)—even common products such as fluorides, baking soda, and hydrogen peroxide—are being studied for use in control of bacterial plaque. Sanguinaria has emerged as a safe antiplaque agent that, in both rinse and toothpaste media, reduces plaque and gingivitis. The rinse can be carried into the sulcus with subgingival irrigation as part of the prophylaxis or included with the patient's routine. Research continues into other agents, but sanguinaria is considered an important agent for helping control periodontal disease (Bhaskar, 1984; Greenfield and Cuchel, 1984; Klewansky and Vernier, 1984; Lindhe, 1984; Nygaard-Oestby and Persson, 1984).

THE PREVENTIVE PROGRAM

The emphasis on education in home care methods, often called a plaque control program, is the foundation for all preventive education. The public's interest in preventing dental disease is influenced by the following factors:

1. Health care providers are focusing on the responsibility of preserving health instead of treating disease.

2. Scientific evidence of the benefits of plaque control methods are clear. Previously held beliefs, such as the loss of teeth being purely hereditary or that one tooth is lost for each pregnancy, are recognized as myths.
3. Health care, including dentistry, continues to increase in expense. The financial burden of treatment makes the economics of prevention the most sensible approach.
4. The population in general has become more health conscious, as evidenced by the current concern for diet modifications and exercise regimens. Individuals are taking the initiative in maintaining a healthier environment.
5. As life expectancy increases, so does the need to preserve one's natural health resources, including teeth.
6. Society places a high value on physical esthetics. An attractive smile with teeth in good repair and alignment is an asset. A clean, odor-free mouth is socially desirable.

Certainly, with the advent of efficient dental equipment, safe anesthesia, and better restorative materials, dental care is sought more frequently as a routine health service. The demand for preventive dental health education coincides with an era of self-awareness. More patients than ever before actively pursue information on what they can do for themselves to maintain their health. Dentistry, on the other hand, recognizes its obligation to make such preventive education available. A preventive program is often cited as one of the recommended qualities of a "good" dental office.

The preventive program can take many forms (Corn and Marks, 1978; Katz, McDonald, and Stookey, 1979; Woodall, 1983). Some practitioners try to complete a series of preventive visits prior to any dental treatment, if possible. The rationale here is that the patient is able to see the changes in oral health brought about by improved home care alone (Figs. 17-1 and 17-2). Additionally, the dental treatment will progress much more comfortably and effectively in an inflammation-free mouth. These preventive visits may be scheduled on consecutive days or perhaps once a week when only plaque control information or instruction in home care techniques is provided.

In other instances preventive education is incorporated along with the dental hygiene treatment. In these cases the prophylaxis is performed over

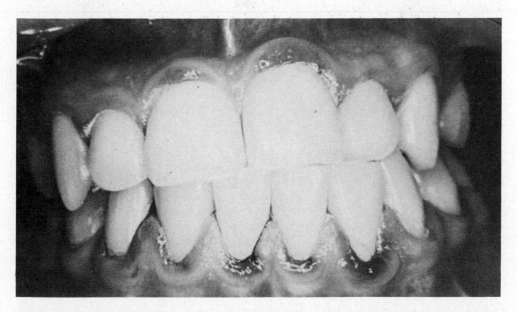

Fig. 17-1. Severe marginal inflammation, bleeding, and pocket formation extending beyond mucogingival junction in 17-year-old woman. (From Corn, H., and Marks, M. 1978. Continuing Dental Education, University of Pennsylvania School of Dental Medicine **1:** No.10.)

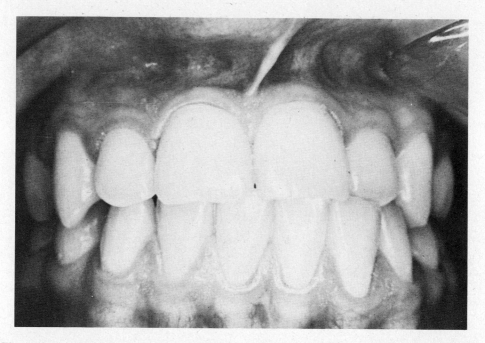

Fig. 17-2. Note dramatic repair that has occurred just by introduction of plaque removal techniques of flossing and brushing. It becomes obvious that in absence of calculus, instrumentation is not required. Plaque control procedures prior to scaling and root planing enable patient to observe significant changes that will occur with removal of toxic by-products of plaque. (From Corn, H., and Marks, M. 1978. Continuing Dental Education, University of Pennsylvania School of Dental Medicine **1:** No. 10.)

several visits as necessary to bring the patient's instruction, tissue evaluation, and hygiene therapy to completion.

In all cases patients requiring emergency care should have these problems attended to initially. Preventive education is of little value to anyone with an immediate dental problem.

There is some evidence that removal of heavy calculus and temporizing open lesions are essential before the benefits of home care are evident. In these cases, the bacterial population is so pathologically overpowering that expecting to eliminate inflammatory processes with home care alone is unrealistic.

Little evidence exists to show that one preventive education format is consistently better than another for improving and sustaining health care habits. Innumerable variables in dental care settings, personnel responsible for preventive education, and patient needs make scientific research of this aspect of dentistry difficult.

As the national focus on periodontal disease becomes clear, the dental profession will need to closely examine its priorities. The clinician with training in periodontal skills and the ability to direct preventive education efforts will have a strong position in delivering care.

Philosophy of prevention

Essential to any preventive program is a person with a sincere commitment to a preventive philosophy. Because the clinician selected a caring profession as a career, most likely the dedication to helping others is already present. Some choose to serve by becoming experts in reconstruction or in maintenance; others provide service by researching or by teaching the concepts of prevention. Realistically, the latter have the potential for the greatest impact. Treatment is essential, but by sheer prevalence, it is a losing battle to try to control dental disease by treatment alone.

Embracing a preventive philosophy and practicing one are two entirely different levels of commitment. Each practitioner must identify his/her own commitment.

On a personal level, this means maintaining one's own oral health status. Being a good example will model the benefits of prevention. In a broader sense, much of becoming an oral health educator is in seeing this as a primary career role. Often the clinician is defined by the skills dictated by the employment situation. If scaling and polishing teeth are the sole activities of the day, then seeing oneself as a health educator may be difficult. Ideally, the employment situation will allow the clinician to develop a personal approach to home care with each patient. During the day, time should be devoted to assessing oral conditions, providing educational information, and evaluating patients' efforts in addition to performing a variety of clinical services. These circumstances will permit practicing a preventive philosophy in an environment conducive to providing health education.

While remaining committed to a preventive philosophy, the person responsible for preventive education needs to be sensitive to the individuality of each patient. With this comes the realization that a program of prevention must be flexible and individualized to be effective.

Motivational strategies

While no particular preventive program is better or more successful than others, well-designed programs pay particular attention to identifying individual needs. Instructional formats and motivational appeals are selected for their appropriateness in each case, and long-term reinforcement strategies are included. Closely supervised teaching on a multiple-visit basis with periodic reinforcement can result in a significant, sustained improvement in oral hygiene, but there is a tendency for regression in performance as the period of time after the instruction lengthens (Melcer and Feldman, 1979). Boyer and Nikias (1983) surveyed 123 randomly selected adult patients who had participated in a plaque control program. Slightly more than one third of the patients were highly compliant in performing prescribed procedures. Another one third were moderately compliant, and one third were poorly compliant. Almost all patients had adopted the preventive dental procedures for varying lengths of time. Keeping the patient motivated

about oral health over the long term seems to be a key goal in any plaque control program.

Much has been written about Maslow's hierarchy of human needs in relation to motivation (Katz, McDonald, and Stookey 1979; Maslow, 1970; Pipe et al., 1972). A pyramid model is used to represent the levels of human need from the most basic level: the physiologic need for food, shelter, warmth, rest, and reproduction to the apex of the pyramid labeled self-realization. At this highest need level, a person aspires to be personally fulfilled by reaching his/her potential. The intermediate levels are security needs, social needs, and esteem needs.

Except under special circumstances, the physiologic and security need levels of the general population in our society are fairly well satisfied. Maslow proposes that higher-level needs do not emerge until lower-level needs are satisfied. One has little energy to spend on esteem needs if food or shelter needs are not satisfied. He also states that once a need has been satisfied, it no longer continues to be highly valued or to act as a motivating force.

If a person is suffering from a toothache or because of other conditions is in pain, this could be interpreted as a threat to the individual's security. The person has a need to be removed from physical peril. Certainly, at this point the need for help occurs and one becomes desperate to follow the steps necessary to remove the cause of the threat. Often, preventive education takes this opportunity to make its greatest appeal: "Ah-ha. These teeth are loose and causing you discomfort because of severe periodontal disease. This is caused by the accumulation of plaque, calculus, and the resultant bacterial toxins that have irritated and destroyed the ligaments in the supporting tissues which actually hold the tooth in the bone. If this continues, you will lose all your teeth." The patient gasps, "Can you help me?" "Yes, we can do something about this. First I'll show you a new or better way to care for your teeth to help remove the irritants. Then a thorough prophylaxis and possibly a bit of surgery will be done to remove the tissue that is beyond healing and reattachment." The patient's natural response is "Of course, anything." The follow-through with home care and the necessary treatment proceed smoothly.

After the "problem" has been resolved, the clinician may continue to motivate the patient by appealing to the security level. "You remember what happened before, don't you?'' For some reason, it is human nature to forget unpleasant or frightening experiences. The memory of the discomfort, time involved, money spent, and inconvenience may not be vivid. Second, the problem was essentially solved by treatment. The patient naturally assumes that treatment could resolve the problem again.

The point of this example is to show how effective the appeal to a security need can be as a motivator over a short period of time. It also points out the pitfalls of this appeal as a motivator over a longer term (Pipe et al., 1972). It is difficult to estimate how many patients who were motivated with short-term threats have become edentulous over the years. The hope that dental treatment (even if it is inconvenient and expensive) will save the patient's teeth in the nick of time eventually is proved false.

The two need-level appeals that do have potential as long-term motivators are those directed at social and esteem levels (Pipe et al., 1972). Throughout life a person generally wishes to remain socially acceptable and feel personally valued. A healthy mouth that projects an attractive smile and is free of disease makes anyone feel more comfortable in a social setting. Taking care of one's physical being often reflects the way a person values himself/herself. Because social and esteem needs tend to run the course of life, appeals to these levels are more appropriate long-term motivators to be incorporated in the preventive program.

In describing some sociopsychologic perspectives motivating change in oral hygiene behavior, Evans (1978) stresses the need to avoid the situation where the patient is dependent on the health professional for the focus of therapy. Motivating the patient to make new oral hygiene behaviors last means fostering long-term self-determination on the patient's part. A ''therapeutic alliance'' should exist between the patient and the health professional. Direct patient involvement should occur from the outset of treatment. The patient and clinician must work together to prevent dental disease. The professional role is as a reinforcer of the patient's desire to do something good for himself/herself.

After studying several plaque control programs, Weinstein (1982) identified seven common problems in the way preventive programs are structured and managed. The first three are:

1. Plaque control programs begin too early.
2. Plaque control begins without patient readiness.
3. The motivational appeal is often ''canned,'' not personalized.

Each of these problems is related to plaque control programs beginning before a relationship is established with the patient. The patient feels he/she is being plugged into a routine that everyone gets. An assessment of the patient's wants and needs has not taken place, making the patient feel that the program is not really designed for his/her dental condition.

Problems 4 through 6 are:

4. The dental staff's assumptions about the patient's nonperformance are often mistaken.
5. Patients receive feedback too infrequently.
6. Plaque control programs lack adequate follow-up.

These three issues deal with the way the dental staff follows the patient's progress. The dental health educator often fails to consider the effort it takes to establish and maintain a new habit. The clinician should recognize that lapses in the patient's skill or motivation do not mean the patient does not know how or does not care. It is necessary to provide regular feedback and to review skills without making the patient feel he/she has failed. Changes in oral health habits seldom last more than 6 months. Everyone has difficulty becoming proficient at and sustaining a new behavior. A positive attitude approaching the patient's problems with motivation is essential.

The seventh common problem of plaque control programs is that the time spent on them is not financially rewarding. When the practitioner is faced with the low probability of patient follow-through and a high likelihood of little financial reward for the dental staff's time, preventive activities are minimized or squeezed into treatment. Financial incentives need to be worked into a successful program. The health professional's time is valuable whether it is spent observing a home care technique or placing a fluoride tray. The issue is complicated by third-party payers who refuse to promote such preventive programs and by patients who are reluctant to pay for counseling time they feel is not a helpful personal service. By waiting for an indication from the patient that he desires to improve his oral health status, it may be assumed that the patient is ready to assume both the time and cost of a customized preventive program.

Of course, many aspects of patient education will never be paid for directly. Helpful advice the clinician provides during contact with the patient is a natural part of oral health care. All patients should be exposed to the opportunity to learn about good home care practices during the course of dental care regardless of entry into a specific plan of preventive visits.

A plaque control program that avoids some of the previously mentioned problems combines humanistic application of behavioral strategies in oral hygiene instruction. In this program the clinician is a skilled listener and provides information in line with the patient's concern for preventive education. When the patient expresses a desire to do something about the dental problem, the clinician is ready to assess the patient's skills and suggest changes. The patient becomes involved by collecting data at home about the new skill. The clinician and patient set some goals together and decide on techniques the patient can use to cue the new behavior. This could include such things as making a chart to place on the bathroom mirror, carrying dental floss in the lunch bag, or deciding to perform brushing and flossing at a particular time. Perhaps completing the oral hygiene routine *before* the usual morning shower will assure its place in the day more than if the routine is left to be done "if time permits." These kinds of steps will act as reminders to sustain the new skill long enough for the patient to see a positive change occurring. A written contract can be made with the patient to decide on the goals and time to be devoted to the program effort.

Habit formation is reviewed after about 2 weeks to make any modifications and provide positive feedback. The program ends with the patient and clinician planning how to avoid "backsliding" on the new behavior. The dental professional facilitates the patient's behavior change. The patient remains dependent on himself/herself to establish better home care that will influence his/her future dental needs.

In another conceptual model for patient motivation and education, Bakdash (1979) emphasizes the assessment of the patient's incoming behavior. Taking time to identify the patient's perceptions of his/her dental problems and recognizing the emotional aspects of the patient's behavior and the socioeconomic factors that contribute to the patient's attitudes will influence the type of information and style of the preventive education program best suited to the patient. Once this is done, a plan including appropriate motivational strategies can be followed. Providing frequent contact and positive reinforcement to encourage self-confidence in the patient is also stressed to gain a successful result.

Motivation is an important part of patient education on the part of both the learner and the instructor.

An unmotivated teacher rarely has motivated students. It is especially important for the preventive educator to stay enthusiastic about preventive goals. Over time, however, treatment of numerous dental problems associated with a variety of patient personalities can be extremely exhausting. In addition, it is often difficult to accept the fact that people do not always do what is good for them or will not learn what seems obvious. Such frustration does nothing to enhance the educator's motivation. The commitment to a preventive philosophy laced with patience and determination is the backbone to sustaining this energy. Staying enthusiastic means keeping the goals of disease prevention in mind. Helping patients achieve a better state of health and a greater degree of independence from dental disease continues to be the best reason to persist.

When patient education is individualized and the clinician and patient share an interest in the preventive plan, changing human behavior is merely difficult—not impossible.

INDIVIDUALIZED PREVENTIVE EDUCATION
Assessment

Initially, the patient's current health status and home care methods are assessed:
1. Examine the gingival tissue for signs of inflammation.
2. Examine the teeth for carious lesions.
3. Use current radiography for information regarding interproximal caries, periapical disease, and bone loss.

4. Perform a periodontal screening by gently walking the probe around the teeth. Recording specific pocket depths is not necessary at this time, since this is only a general survey. Note areas where the probe measures a pocket depth greater than 3 mm. Bleeding points may also be noted as the probe is used in this survey. The survey can be performed easily with or without the aid of an assistant and provides baseline data that will be helpful in planning the need for more extensive periodontal measurements.

5. Stain the teeth with disclosing solution for a plaque index and note the areas of particular plaque retention.

6. Allow the patient to perform his/her normal cleaning routine. Involve the patient in assessing the areas that may need improvement. Note the plaque index remaining after routine home care is performed.

7. Engage the patient in conversation regarding the frequency of brushing and other home care procedures. Seek additional information on the patient's general dental awareness and concern for oral conditions. This is valuable for determining the need for the guided self-assessment exercise (see Chapter 19) and for gaining an appreciation of the patient's wants, needs, and expectations (see Chapter 18). (See sample case on home care assessment, p. 303.)

Planning

At this point the preventive educator needs to reflect on the information gathered during the patient's assessment. The educator then plans a realistic approach for the preventive education the patient needs to improve home care routines, avoiding the temptation to demonstrate automatically sulcular brushing and flossing techniques to every patient. In general, patients need less help modifying cleaning methods than they do in understanding why cleaning the oral tissues is necessary. In essence, *helping the patient appreciate the value of prevention is the real goal.* Once this is accomplished, the patient is able to motivate himself/herself because prevention will seem the logical way to maintain his/her health.

In the planning phase it is important to identify some short-term and long-term goals. One of the most common mistakes is to expect too much of the patient too soon. Changing habits, particularly well-established ones, is extremely difficult, as any smoker who has tried to quit can testify. For the educational process to be successful, the learner must demonstrate a change in behavior. To do this, the learner moves through several stages as the commitment to a new behavior is established. These stages are awareness, interest, involvement, action, and, finally, habit (Katz, McDonald, and Stookey, 1979).

The preventive educator is a partner in this entire process. Too often, the educator feels that after the initial instruction the remainder of the work is the patient's responsibility. In actuality, the educator's role is only beginning. The individualized approach in a plaque control program characterized by frequent assessment, planning, implementation, and evaluation strategies helps keep the ongoing education process between the patient and the clinician vital, meaningful, and progressive. (See sample case on planning needs and goals, p. 304.)

Implementation

When the plan has been determined, it should be shared with the patient. Are the goals acceptable? What goals does the patient have? Is the patient committed to the plan? Usually when the patient has an investment in the preventive program, his/her cooperation is at a peak. Following are four accepted steps to keep in mind for the actual instruction (Katz, McDonald, and Stookey, 1979; Pipe et al, 1983):

1. *Small step size.* Provide the theoretical or factual information in increments that the patient can digest at points when the patient has expressed a *need* to know.

2. *Active participation.* Involve the patient in an activity that will enhance the learning and retention of the information.

3. *Immediate feedback.* Let the learner know the evaluation of his/her participation and progress. Of course, positive feedback is supportive and encouraging.

4. *Self-pacing.* Stay in tune with the learner's needs. If the learner cannot or will not handle more information, do not push. If interest is being shown, pursue the patient's signals.

Outline the dental health education plan and make accurate treatment notes at each appointment. (See sample case on implementation, p. 305.)

SAMPLE CASE

Dental health education—home care assessment

DATE: 10/10/84

PATIENT: Mr. John Johnson is a new patient who has not had regular dental care for the past 3 years. Age: 34.

CHIEF COMPLAINT: ''Painful back tooth''

CLINICAL FINDINGS:

1. *General:* Tooth No. 30 has a fractured amalgam. Teeth are lightly tobacco stained. Moderate calculus is obvious supragingivally in the mandibular lingual anterior area. Mandibular lingual gingiva in the posterior area appears red and edematous, especially in the interdental areas. Tongue is coated and stained.

2. *Periodontal survey:*

   a. Pocket depth: Highest readings (4 mm) ML and DL of Nos. 18 and 19, also Nos. 28 to 31.

Pocket depth	3					2						3				
Tooth number	1	2	3	4	5	6	7	8	9	10	11	12	13	14	15	16
Bleeding points			X												X	
Bleeding points		X	X		X	X	X		X					X	X	
Tooth number	32	31	30	29	28	27	26	25	24	23	22	21	20	19	18	17
Pocket depth			4					3						4		

   b. Bleeding index: 10 (signified by X)

   c. Plaque index: 48 areas of visible plaque

   d. Problem areas: Interproximal areas: mandibular lingual, posterior and anterior

HOME CARE: Combination roll stroke and scrub brush method. Completes maxillary teeth, then mandibular teeth; does not brush mandibular lingual or tongue. Demonstrates acceptable technique for flossing except in area of most posterior molars. Brushes twice a day to ''keep teeth clean and stop bad breath.'' Flosses occasionally ''because food gets caught sometimes.''

AWARENESS: Patient does not worry about gum disease. He believes his teeth will take care of themselves because he's generally a healthy person. Has had few problems in the past. He is unaware of dental plaque and does not know the purpose of a disclosing agent. He cannot remember ever being shown how to clean his teeth.

SAMPLE CASE
Dental health education—planning needs and goals

DATE: 10/12/84
PATIENT: Mr. John Johnson
TREATMENT: Temporize No. 30.

INSTRUCTION: Describe dental plaque.

ACTION: Demonstrate the use of a disclosing agent. Patient identifies plaque in his mouth.

INSTRUCTION: Discuss inflammation.

ACTION: Patient recognizes the signs of inflammation in his mouth.

INSTRUCTION: Discuss the etiology and chronic destructive nature of periodontal disease.
ACTION: Patient identifies problem areas in his current oral care and speculates on his future oral health.
REINFORCEMENT/INSTRUCTION: Stress
  1. *Brushing*
     a. Thoroughness
     b. Sequence
     c. Skill in lingual areas
  2. *Flossing*
     a. Regularity of interproximal cleaning
     b. Skill in posterior areas
TREATMENT: Remove calculus and stain.
INSTRUCTION: Evaluate efforts, provide encouragement, and discuss recall.
MOTIVATIONAL APPROACH: Capitalize on "the straight facts"—establishment of good habits to enhance appearance and sociability and to maintain health. Stress prevention of problems instead of slowly progressing disease that is costly in terms of the time and expense related to maintenance of repair.
GOALS OF PREVENTIVE EDUCATION:
  1. Patient will gain knowledge of the etiology of periodontal disease, particularly the nature of dental plaque and the process of tissue changes.
  2. Patient will be able to identify the signs of inflammation in his own mouth.
  3. Patient will establish home care techniques that will adequately reach the current problem areas—lingual of mandibular teeth, and interproximal areas.
  4. Patient will reduce his plaque index to fewer than 10 areas. Bleeding points will be reduced to 0 to 1.
  5. Patient will maintain the reduced plaque and bleeding indices over the period of recall.
  6. At the recall evaluation no inflammation will be present.
  7. At the recall evaluation current modifications in home care techniques will have become habitual.

Dental health education—implementation

PATIENT: Mr. John Johnson

| *Planned* | *Treatment comments* |

Appointment 1

Date: 10/17/84

1. Present preventive home care plan; agree on goals.
2. Temporize No. 30.
3. Complete guided self-assessment.
4. Identify signs of inflammation.
5. Explain etiology of inflammatory disease.
6. Take pretreatment photographs.
7. Have patient disclose and identify plaque.
8. Discuss patient's home care problems.
9. Work on brushing problem areas (lingual of mandible); suggest antiplaque agent.
10. Provide reinforcement.
11. Discuss what will occur at next appointment.

Patient agreed on preventive education goals. Treatment progressed as planned.

Patient was impressed with the information about the inflammatory process.

He was able to demonstrate lingual brushing without difficulty.

Appointment 2

Date: 10/24/84

1. Have patient check tissue; compare with slides from last visit.
2. Recheck periodontal survey.
3. Have patient perform home care routine.
4. Disclose and complete plaque index.
5. Work on interproximal problems with flossing.
6. Complete oral cancer examination.
7. Instruct on soft tissue cleansing.
8. Begin scaling.

Patient noticed change in tissue during the past week and pointed this out to me at the start of the appointment.

Plaque index: 30 areas

Bleeding index: 7

Tried loop method of flossing; patient will need to practice.

Appointment plan followed. Patient response is positive.

Appointment 3

Date: ~~10/31/84~~ 11/7/84

1. Check tissue; compare with previous visit.
2. Perform home care techniques.
3. Disclose and take plaque index.
4. Work on any skill problems; discuss establishing a habit of good methods; offer support; discuss roadblocks to habit formation.
5. Continue or finish prophylaxis.
6. Refer for restorative treatment.
7. Discuss evaluation in 1 month.

Patient cancelled original appointment because of illness.

Two weeks after appointment 2, the tissue contour and color is much improved.

Plaque index: 18 areas

Bleeding index: 4

The loop floss technique has worked well. Patient forgets to brush linguals sometimes so made a reminder sign for bathroom mirror.

Finished scale and root planing; delayed polishing.

1-month recall

Date: 12/7/84

1. Complete dental health education assessment (same as initial appointment).
2. Discuss success in relation to goals; identify areas that still need improvement.
3. Agree on a preventive recall plan.
4. Polish restorations.
5. Take photographs.

Assessment reveals pocket depth no greater than 3 mm.

Plaque index: 9 areas

Bleeding index: 2

Patient mentioned that he is pleased with himself and the treatment. He would like to be seen in 3 months for his first recall.

Checked scaling; polished teeth and restorations. Took photographs; patient can't wait to see these for comparison with initial visit.

Evaluation

Integrated in the individually prepared disease control plan is the process of evaluation. This is necessary to measure progress toward the patient's stated goals and can be used to assess the educational methods. Evaluation feedback is important for both the educator and the patient.

The clinical evidence of a decrease in inflammation, bleeding areas, and plaque retention is the best indicator of improved habits. This is especially true when a healthy state prevails in the absence of additional treatment (i.e., between recall visits). Evaluating the patient's skill level after practice is also important. Modifications in technique may be necessary as the educator and patient work together. Evaluation of changes in attitude and interest will be possible throughout interactions with the patient. (See sample case on evaluation summary below.)

HOME CARE TECHNIQUES

The goal in instruction is to aid the patient in practicing a nontraumatic method of cleaning the teeth and stimulating the gingiva. Both the patient and the clinician must be aware of the areas where plaque is causing irritation. These areas are assessed by using a disclosing agent.

Disclosing agents

Because dental plaque is not easily identified because of its colorless, or invisible, nature, an agent is necessary to make the plaque obvious to the patient. As described in Chapter 13, a disclosing agent stains plaque so that the patient is able to assess areas where plaque remains on the teeth.

Several materials are available that stain plaque. Armim (1963) discovered the first coloring that could be used routinely and safely as a dental disclosant. The food coloring erythrosine remains the most widely used agent and is dispensed in tablet or solution form. Erythrosine indiscriminately stains plaque, calculus, intraoral tissues, clothing, toothbrush bristles, towels, and skin (Yankell and Emling, 1978). This seems to be its only drawback, making instructions and warnings for its use advisable.

Color combinations such as FD & C red No. 3 and FD & C green No. 3 stain plaque differential-

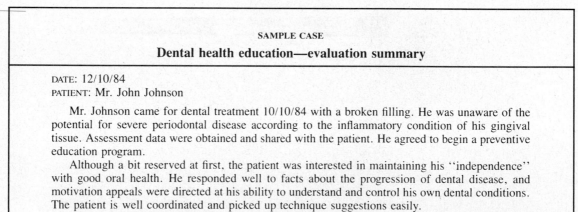

SAMPLE CASE

Dental health education—evaluation summary

DATE: 12/10/84
PATIENT: Mr. John Johnson

Mr. Johnson came for dental treatment 10/10/84 with a broken filling. He was unaware of the potential for severe periodontal disease according to the inflammatory condition of his gingival tissue. Assessment data were obtained and shared with the patient. He agreed to begin a preventive education program.

Although a bit reserved at first, the patient was interested in maintaining his "independence" with good oral health. He responded well to facts about the progression of dental disease, and motivation appeals were directed at his ability to understand and control his own dental conditions. The patient is well coordinated and picked up technique suggestions easily.

During the past 2 months, the patient has reduced his plaque index to the goal level. The bleeding index came close to the goal level, but malposed teeth continue to be a problem (Nos. 22 to 25). The patient recognizes signs of inflammation, readily identifies plaque, and can describe the process of dental disease. Mr. Johnson has practiced home care techniques and reports being much more regular about flossing. He never misses brushing the lingual surfaces any more. Overall, the goals of this initial phase of preventive dental health education were accomplished. The 3-month recall will be important for evaluating maintenance of health.

ly according to thickness of formation and maturation.

Another solution, sodium fluorescein, stains plaque but is only visible under ultraviolet light. This may be particularly useful in a dental practice in which patients may be returning to daily business where pink-stained oral tissues are unacceptable.

Any of the types of disclosing products are useful. The patient's preference is important.

It is important for the patient to use disclosing tablets or solution to assess plaque retention areas and to make self-evaluation of home care techniques possible. The routine use of disclosing agents has been shown to decrease periodontal disease as compared with the incidence of periodontal disease in groups who perform routine oral hygiene measures without the aid of a disclosing agent (Squillaro, Cohen, and Laster, 1975).

Disclosing agents may be most helpful in a preventive program initially. As the patient becomes more proficient in assessing his gingival status, the disclosing agent may be used less frequently to check the thoroughness of plaque removal (Tan, 1980; Melcer and Feldman, 1979).

The toothbrush

The primary tool in the removal of dental plaque is the toothbrush (Bass, 1948). Since areas that harbor plaque are mainly the tongue, the cervical one third of the tooth, and the gingival sulcus, a brush that is highly adaptable and that will not harm the soft tissue is most desirable. Synthetic or nylon bristles have the advantages of being manufactured in a consistent size. The diameter of the bristle determines its resiliency (Wilkins, 1982; Yankell and Emling, 1978). The smaller the diameter, the softer the texture. Soft bristles with polished ends are flexible and gentle on the oral tissues. To adapt the bristles with uniform pressure, the height of the bristles should be the same. Bristles can be clumped together to form a tuft, which may stand isolated, or several tufts can be placed close together (multitufted). The placement of the multitufted row may cover an area more completely than a brush with separated tufts. Either brush style is acceptable.

Brushes are manufactured in a wide variety of sizes and shapes. The most common configuration for adult brushes is three or four rows of bristles.

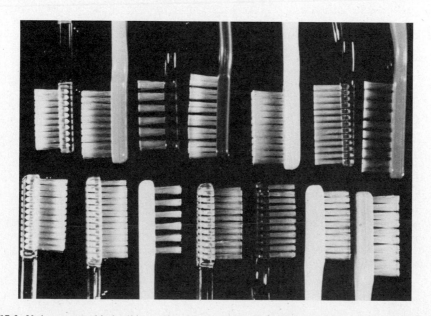

Fig. 17-3. Various acceptable brushing tools. (From Yankell, S., and Emling, R. 1978. Continuing Dental Education, University of Pennsylvania School of Dental Medicine **1:** No. 7.)

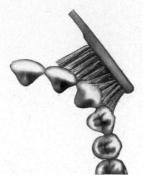

Fig. 17-4. Soft-textured brush adapts well to contours of dentition. (From Yankell, S., and Emling, R. 1978. Continuing Dental Education, University of Pennsylvania School of Dental Medicine **1**:18.)

In profile most brushes are flat. The individual manufacturer decides on the size of the toothbrush head. The profusion of sizes and shapes results from the lack of evidence as to which is the most effective brush. Perhaps there is no "most effective" brush (Fig. 17-3).

The most important feature of the brushing tool is that it adequately reaches all the areas to be cleaned. The brush should do this without causing tissue destruction as it disorganizes the dental plaque. This requirement is best satisfied by a soft-textured brush (Fig. 17-4).

In summary, the toothbrush of today has soft synthetic bristles with polished ends of uniform height in sharp contrast to the hard-textured, natural boar hair bristle brushes of the past.

Brushing methods

A few techniques for brushing the oral tissues are presented here. It is important to emphasize that although knowledge of specific techniques of brushing may be important for the health educator, the most important procedure for the patient to master is thoroughness in reaching all areas of his/her mouth. One method is not in and of itself better than another. One patient may need to use principles of several techniques to adequately clean his/her mouth. Guiding the patient toward methods that meet individual needs is more important than stressing the implementation of a particular technique.

Rolling stroke brushing. The rolling stroke method is designed as a general cleaning method to remove food and plaque primarily from the crowns of the teeth. This method places little emphasis on cleaning the sulcus.

Method: The patient is instructed to grasp the brush so that the bristles are pointed apically and placed on the gingiva (Fig. 17-5, *A*). With a sweeping motion, the bristles are gently rolled over the gingiva and teeth toward the incisal or occlusal surfaces (Fig. 17-5, *B*). The brush is replaced, and this roll stroke is continued in the same area five to ten times. Depending on the length of the brush head and the size of the teeth, two to four teeth may be cleaned with one brush placement. When the strokes for one section have been completed, the toothbrush is moved to the next area, with care taken to overlap at least one tooth. This rolling stroke should be performed in an overlapping sequence on the facial and lingual surfaces of both dental arches. *Sequence* refers to a systemic routine for brushing. With time this sequence becomes habit. For example, the patient starts on the buccal aspect of the most posterior tooth in the maxillary right quadrant and brushes to the most posterior tooth in the left quadrant. When the buccal aspect of the maxilla is completed, the patient starts on the lingual surface of the most posterior tooth in the right quadrant and brushes all the lingual surfaces to the most posterior tooth in the left quadrant. The mandible is completed in the same manner. With overlapping brush placement, the patient is much more likely to reach all areas than if a more random brushing technique is practiced.

Anterior lingual brushing. The narrow anterior lingual portion of the arch presents a problem because the brush head generally is too large to be

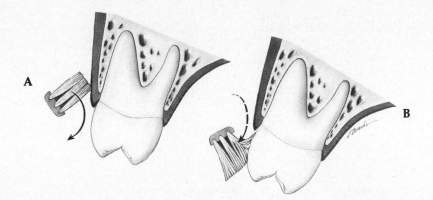

Fig. 17-5. Rolling stroke brushing method. **A,** Place bristles pointing apically on gingiva. **B,** Sweep bristles over teeth from gingiva toward incisal or occlusal surface.

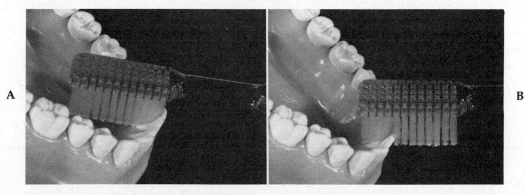

Fig. 17-6. Anterior lingual brushing method. **A,** Place brush vertically into narrow anterior portion of arch. **B,** Sweep brush from gingiva toward incisal edge.

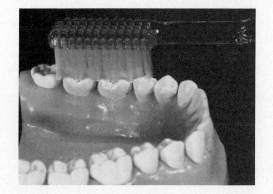

Fig. 17-7. Occlusal cleaning method. Flex, tap, or move bristles back and forth along occlusal surface to clean this portion of dentition.

placed horizontally. The patient is shown how to reposition the brush vertically and sweep from the gingival to the incisal edge (Fig. 17-6).

Occlusal cleaning. When both maxilla and mandible are completed on the facial and lingual surfaces, the occlusal surface should be scrubbed by moving the bristles back and forth. Flexing or tapping the bristles on the occlusal surface is an alternative method (Katz, McDonald, and Stookey, 1979) (Fig. 17-7).

Cleaning the tongue. The surface of the tongue is an ideal location for bacterial plaque and food debris to collect. The papillae of the tongue create a surface similar to a thick-piled carpet. The patient should be instructed to scrape or brush the tongue to clean it. By cleaning the tongue, the patient removes the deposits that may be causing odors or contributing to plaque formation in other areas of the mouth.

Method: While leaning over a sink, the patient extends the tongue. Using plenty of water, the tongue is cleaned by placing the brush as far posteriorly as possible and sweeping the brush anteriorly. After several strokes the patient inspects the tongue for coating.

Since gagging can be a problem, displacing the tongue as little as possible may be beneficial. Gagging is a natural reflex that generally creates a burst of salivary secretion, which may be helpful in flushing the oral pharynx areas. An alternate method is to clean the tongue in its normal resting position with the head erect.

Stillman's method (modified). Stillman's (modified) method is useful for stimulating and cleaning the cervical area. The roll stroke is then included for cleaning the clinical crowns.

Method: The toothbrush is grasped and the bristles, pointing apically at about a 45-degree angle, are placed on the attached gingiva. The bristles should be flexed with enough pressure to cause slight gingival blanching and are activated with a small rotary (circular) motion (Fig. 17-8). The rotation is repeated about eight to ten times. When this is completed, the brush is rolled from the gingiva toward the occlusal surfaces. With a soft-bristled brush, the bristles adapt to the interproximal areas as the roll is completed. The rotation/roll sequence if performed several times before the brush is placed in the next area, with care taken to overlap at least one tooth to ensure that the brushing sequence cleans all areas. The anterior lingual section is brushed by placing the toe of the brush on the gingiva, rotating, and sweeping toward the incisal edges. In this area only about two teeth at a time will be cleaned by each brush placement. The cleaning is completed by occlusal brushing and cleaning the tongue.

Bass method. The Bass method of brushing is generally accepted for effectively removing plaque from the sulcus area.

Method: The toothbrush is grasped and the bristles, pointing apically at a 45-degree angle to the long axis of the tooth, are placed at the gingival margin. Generally, only the first row will approximate the sulcus while the adjacent row will touch the gingival margin (Fig. 17-9, *A*).

By pressing lightly, the soft bristles will contour themselves into the sulcus and interproximal area. Without lifting the brush, about ten short back-and-forth vibration strokes are used to disorganize the plaque in the area. (Fig. 17-9, *B*). If the bristles make a scrubbing sound, the pressure of vibration is too great or the size of the back-and-forth stroke is too large. The pressure is relaxed, and the brush is moved to the next area, with care taken to overlap at least one tooth for each placement in the sequence. The main objective is sulcular cleaning. The buccal and lingual surfaces of the dental arches are completed in this manner. In the anterior lingual area the brush is inserted vertically, and the bristles of the toe of the brush are placed at the sulcular area and vibrated. The lingual surface is cleaned by the bristles being pulled over the tooth surface.

The occlusal surfaces and tongue are cleaned as described earlier.

The roll stroke method may be used in conjunction with this brushing method either as a procedure performed prior to the sulcular placement or afterward. This is called the *modified Bass method.*

Scrub brush method. This method is used for general cleaning. The brush is usually placed perpendicular to the long axis of the teeth. Vertical, circular, or horizontal strokes are employed. When a soft toothbrush is used, such a technique may adequately remove plaque on the clinical crowns. In general, vigorous brushing in such a random fashion is discouraged, since trauma to the teeth or gingiva may result. A brushing method such as this does not purposefully clean the interproximal or sulcular area, so critical areas may be missed.

However, this technique may work well with some patients. Children, patients with limited dexterity, or patients with specific tooth alignment problems may find this technique useful. After assessing the patient's needs, the hygienist should encourage a sequence of brushing and the use of other cleaning tools to complement this brushing method if necessary.

Summary of brushing methods. Brushing in an appropriate and thorough manner removes the food and plaque accumulation on the major portions of the clinical crowns of the teeth. The buccal, lingual, and occlusal areas are cleaned, in addition to a major portion of the sulcus and the gingiva. The tongue, palate, and buccal mucosa can be gently cleaned also. The tissue area that is yet un-

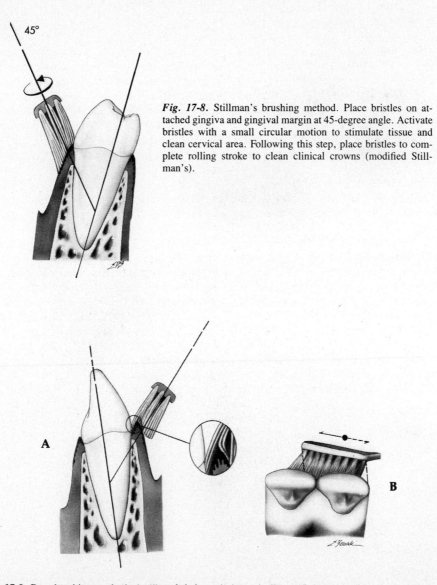

Fig. 17-8. Stillman's brushing method. Place bristles on attached gingiva and gingival margin at 45-degree angle. Activate bristles with a small circular motion to stimulate tissue and clean cervical area. Following this step, place bristles to complete rolling stroke to clean clinical crowns (modified Stillman's).

Fig. 17-9. Bass brushing method. **A,** Place bristles pointing apically at 45-degree angle to long axis of tooth. First row of bristles will approximate sulcus, and adjacent row will touch gingival margin. **B,** Activate brush with a short back-and-forth vibration to disorganize plaque in sulcus. Following this step, place bristles to complete rolling stroke to clean clinical crowns (modified Bass).

touched is the tooth surface protected by the interdental papillae in the interproximal area. This area collects plaque as easily as the other areas, but cleaning it with a brush is virtually impossible. The inflammatory and caries processes may occur here without interruption for long periods of time unless interproximal cleaning is performed.

Before addressing interproximal cleaning, the clinician determines the patient's skill level with brushing. The following questions are suggested for summarizing this aspect of the patient's preventive program.

1. Does the patient use a disclosing solution? Can the patient identify plaque in his/her own mouth?
2. Does the patient realize the relationship of plaque to dental disease?
3. Is the patient's brushing tool suited to his/her needs?
4. How effectively does the patient's cleaning method remove bacterial plaque and food from all surfaces?
5. Does the patient use a cleaning sequence?
6. Does the patient care for the oral soft tissues, gingiva, and tongue?

7. Does the patient recognize the limitations of brushing when caring for his/her oral health?

Interproximal cleaning

Dental floss and tape are the primary interproximal plaque removal tools. Basically, a material is needed that can easily fit through the tight contact areas of the teeth to clean the interproximal sulcus and the mesial or distal portion of the tooth untouched by the brush. Not all contact areas are the same. Consequently, several types of floss, from the thin, nonwaxed products to heavier, waxed tapes, have been marketed (Fig. 17-10). Even a variable-diameter floss that combines a stiff end for threading beneath contact areas, a section of regular unwaxed floss, and an area of yarn-type floss is available.

French and Friedman, (1975) found that both waxed and unwaxed products cleaned effectively. Stevens (1980) and Lobene and Soparkar (1982) have reported similar studies in which variable-diameter and mint-flavored floss removed plaque as well as other floss products. The floss type is selected according to the patient's specific conditions. Someone with normally firm contacts be-

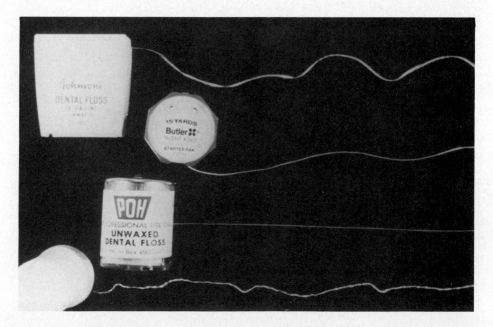

Fig. 17-10. Variation in acceptable interproximal plaque removal tools. (From Yankell, S., and Emling, R. 1978. Continuing Dental Education, University of Pennsylvania School of Dental Medicine **1:** No. 7.)

tween teeth may need an average-weight unwaxed floss. Someone else with crowded teeth, tight contacts, or rough interproximal restorations may be totally frustrated with interproximal cleaning unless a waxed floss, which resists fraying, is used. Manual dexterity may determine the appropriate type of floss. A very fine, threadlike floss may be impossible for a person who handles a heavier tape beautifully. The purpose of the tool is to remove the plaque in the easiest, safest, and most efficient way for the patient. Offering instruction for tools that the dental professional prefers may not be helping the patient if the patient is learning techniques that will not meet his/her needs.

Suggested flossing techniques. A piece of floss approximately 18 inches (45 cm) long is taken. Both ends are wound around the second or fourth finger of each hand (Corn and Marks, 1978, Wilkins 1982) (Fig. 17-11). The floss is secured with the index fingers and thumb of each hand with a length of ¾ to 1 inch (1.9 to 2.5 cm) between each hand. This length of floss will be manipulated into the contact area between the teeth. When floss is wrapped around the fourth finger, the excess floss is tucked out of the way, allowing maximum maneuverability for the index fingers and thumbs. In the maxilla, the floss is stretched over the thumbs, and these fingers are used to guide the floss (Fig. 17-12). On the mandible, the floss is stretched over the index fingers, and these are used to guide the floss (Fig. 17-13). One thumb or index finger is placed on the buccal side of the area being flossed, and the thumb or index finger from the other hand is placed on the lingual side (Figs. 17-14 and 17-15). Approximately 1 inch of floss is used to ''work'' through the contact area of the teeth. The span of floss is inserted into the contact area by sliding it against one of the interproximal surfaces (mesial or distal) of the tooth (Fig. 17-16). The floss is worked along the tooth with a back-and-forth motion at the contact area (Fig. 17-17). With the floss pulled firmly around the tooth surface, this seesaw motion flattens the floss as much as possible to ease it through the contact area. This part of flossing is often the most difficult, since control is needed not to slip through the contact too rapidly and cause trauma to the sulcular gingiva (Fig. 17-18). Once eased gently past the contact point, the floss is wrapped around the tooth and moved up and down against the tooth between the sulcus and the contact area of one tooth (Figs. 17-

19 and 17-20). Then the same cleaning is performed on the adjacent tooth in the interproximal space (Fig. 17-21). The floss is removed by being held against one of the teeth and using the seesaw motion again through the contact area. If the teeth are extremely tight or restoration margins are causing particular problems, one end of the floss is released. The remainder of the floss is pulled out of the interproximal area without struggling through the contact area and possibly breaking the floss. When moving to the next area, the used floss is wound around the finger to permit access to a clean, fresh span.

Another method for flossing is done with the floss tied in a loop (Katz, McDonald, and Stookey, 1979; Wilkins, 1982) (Fig. 17-22). It works the same way, but often the patient handles this better than the finger-wrapping technique. This can be especially good for parents flossing the teeth of a child or to allow persons with less nimble hands to maneuver the floss themselves.

Summary of flossing techniques. In general, flossing is best learned in a progressive way. Flossing the anterior teeth is practiced first so the patient can learn to manipulate the floss in an area that is easily viewed and accessible. When the clinician is assured of the patient's safe technique, the posterior areas are tackled.

This aspect of home care may be the newest to the patient. It should be understood that time, practice, and patience are critical to aiding the patient's realization that flossing is important and not impossible to make habitual.

The patient should be assisted with problem areas and allowed to experiment with different wrapping techniques. The emphasis for evaluation is on the success of plaque removal and the safety of the patient's method with whatever product he/she is most comfortable. The following questions are suggested for summarizing this aspect of the patient's preventive program:

1. Does the patient recognize the value of flossing in addition to brushing?
2. Has the patient identified a product that he/she can use effectively?
3. Has flossing been added to the patient's home care procedures on a regular basis? (If not, identify the reason. Chances are that the skill does not need to be retaught. Review planning work to identify and remove motivational roadblocks).

Text continued on p. 318.

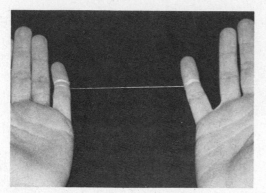

Fig. 17-11. Flossing technique. Wrap length of floss around fourth fingers of each hand.

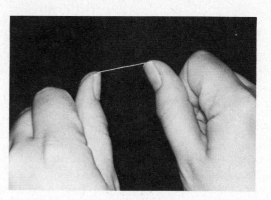

Fig. 17-12. Stretch floss over thumbs to clean maxillary teeth.

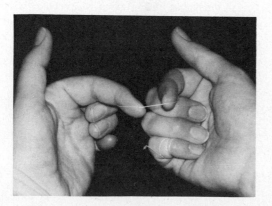

Fig. 17-13. Stretch floss over index fingers to clean mandibular teeth.

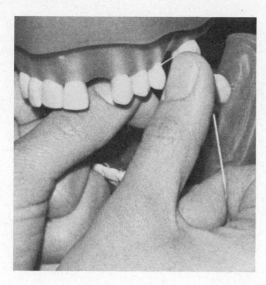

Fig. 17-14. Placement of thumbs and floss for maxillary technique. To clean interproximally, one thumb is placed on lingual side of tooth; other thumb is placed on facial side with approximately 1 inch (2.5 cm) of floss between the thumbs.

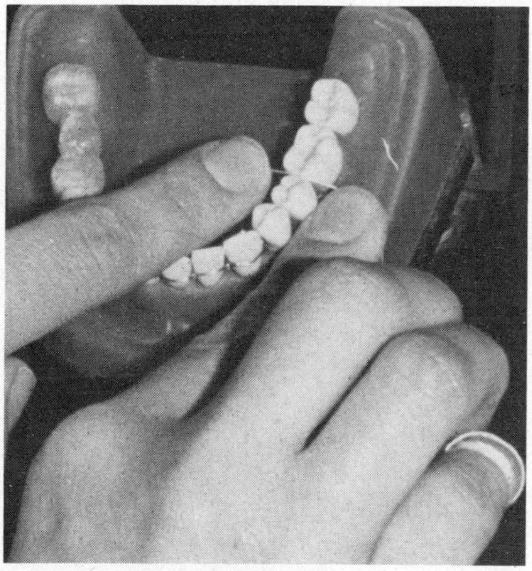

Fig. 17-15. Placement of index fingers for mandibular technique. To clean interproximally, one finger is placed on lingual side of tooth; other finger is placed on facial side with approximately 1 inch (2.5 cm) of floss between fingers.

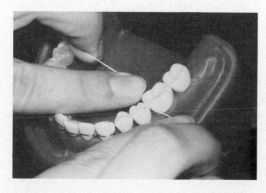

Fig. 17-16. Insert span of floss into contact area. Hold floss around one of the teeth to help ease past contact.

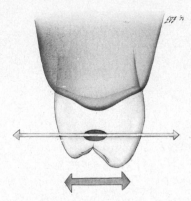

Fig. 17-17. Diagram illustrates back-and-forth, seesaw motion as floss is moved through contact area. (From Corn, H., and Marks, M. 1978. Continuing Dental Education, University of Pennsylvania School of Dental Medicine **1:**14.)

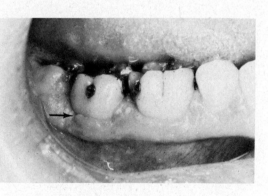

Fig. 17-18. With improper placement, a gingival cleft may result from dental floss being continually forced into sulcus. (From Corn, H., and Marks, M. 1978. Continuing Dental Education, University of Pennsylvania School of Dental Medicine **1:**16.)

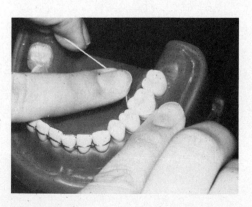

Fig. 17-19. Once past contact area, wrap floss around tooth and move floss up and down on proximal surface.

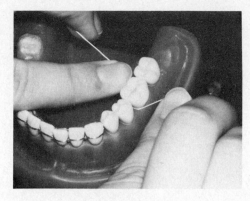

Fig. 17-20. Entire area from contact point to gingival sulcus is cleaned with floss well adapted to tooth.

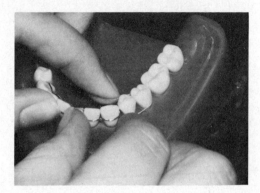

Fig. 17-21. When first proximal surface is completed, wrap floss around adjacent tooth, and use same cleaning stroke on this tooth.

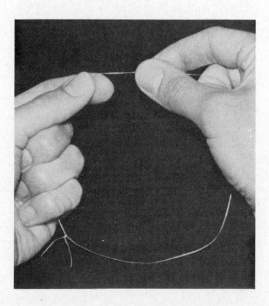

Fig. 17-22. Floss tied in a loop may be maneuvered more easily for some patients. Follow guidelines for finger placement and cleaning stroke as described in previous figures.

Additional cleansing tools

With thorough brushing and flossing, most patients will be on the way to preventing dental disease. However, some patients have conditions that require instruction in the use of special aids (Wilkins, 1982). Following are some of these conditions with the possible aids listed for each group:

1. Limited dexterity due to age, disability, or coordination
   a. Floss holder
   b. Electric toothbrush
   c. Modified brush
2. Areas of fixed bridges, splints for stabilization, or orthodontic wires that do not permit flossing as usual
   a. Floss threader
   b. Variable-diameter floss or yarn
   c. Oral irrigation
3. Wide interdental areas where the normal contour of the gingiva has been lost because of resolution of disease or surgery (These areas may be adequately cleaned by brushing and flossing methods, but sometimes the patient needs additional massage or cleaning assistance to maintain the area in a healthy state.)
   a. Yarn
   b. Periodontal aid
   c. Balsa wood wedge
   d. Interproximal brush
   e. Rubber tip stimulator
4. Sulcular areas with a pocket depth between 3 to 5 mm that cannot be adequately cleaned with the brush and floss but can be maintained with an additional aid or before surgical correction is instituted.
   a. Periodontal aid
   b. Toothpick holder
   c. Oral irrigator
5. Teeth that are isolated or are adjacent to edentulous areas.
   a. Yarn
   b. Gauze strip
6. Tooth contours that present difficulty because of access, furcations, or malposed or malformed teeth
   a. Periodontal aid
   b. Rubber tip
   c. Pipe cleaner

When advising the use of any of these aids, keep the overall home care armamentarium simple. Many of these aids can be used for the same problem. Select the one that the patient will have the least amount of trouble with and that the patient will enjoy using. Additional instruction or trial and error experience may be necessary to find the aid that works best for a particular patient. The more cumbersome home care methods become, the more difficult it is to motivate the patient to perform the skills. When unrealistic demands are made on a patient's performance, the patient will feel guilty and avoid further contact if possible. Following is a brief description of the aforementioned aids.

Floss threader. Several types are available that consist of a flexible material through which the floss can be threaded. These are used as a guide to insert the floss into the contact area so that cleaning may take place. Once the floss is threaded under the bridge or under the contact, the flossing technique described previously is used (Figs. 17-23 and 17-24).

Variable-diameter floss. This floss is used with the same technique as regular floss. The variation in the body of this floss allows it to be threaded under fixed bridges or below tight contact areas (Figs. 17-25 and 17-26). It may be used as yarn for wide embrasures or open contacts in addition to its regular flossing function (Figs. 17-27 and 17-28).

Floss holder. This device may be especially important for those patients who have limited dexterity or the use of only one hand. The holder is a frame that supports a length of floss. It holds the floss taut so that it can be manipulated between the teeth. Enough "play" exists so that by pressure against the tooth, the floss will adapt itself adequately around the interproximal area (Fig. 17-29).

Yarn. This is a thick, soft, and absorbent type of cleaner for wide interproximal areas or abutment teeth. Approximately 14 inches (35 cm) of synthetic yarn should be used. White is the best choice, since some dyes may run when moistened. If access between the teeth allows the yarn to be used as regular floss, previously mentioned techniques are followed. After the yarn is slid interproximally, a vertical stroke is used to remove plaque and polish the tooth surface. A floss threader may be used to assist in the yarn placement if necessary (Fig. 17-30).

Gauze strip. The cotton is removed from the gauze. The gauze is then folded and used as though shining a shoe; in the wide interdental or abutment area, the gauze is rubbed back and forth to clean and polish the interproximal surface (Figs. 17-31 and 17-32).

Pipe cleaner. These can be easily adapted to achieve access to furcation areas or malposed teeth. The pipe cleaner is used to rub the tooth free of plaque and food debris. Care must be taken not to damage the tooth or tissue with the wire of the pipe cleaner. The pipe cleaner is discarded after use (Fig. 17-33).

Periodontal aid. Generally, this consists of a toothpick and plastic holder. The toothpick is softened and applied to the gingival margin. With the tip directed at less than 45 degrees to the long axis of the tooth, it can be used to remove plaque in the sulcus. Another use is for stimulation and desensitization by the periodontal aid being used to massage fluoride or other desensitizing agents into the cervical third of the tooth (Figs. 17-34 and 17-35).

Rubber tip. This is a cone-shaped rubber tip that can be used to clean the tooth surface and massage tissues for stimulation and recontouring. Placing the tip on the interdental area with the tip end directed toward the occlusal surface, a rotation or back-and-forth motion with the side of the tip is used to massage the tissue. The tip can be used in a similar fashion in an exposed furcation area (Fig. 17-36).

Wood wedge. This is a wedge-shaped toothpick used for cleaning interdental areas and stimulation of tissues. The patient should soften the wedge and apply the base of the triangle to the interdental area with the tip directed slightly occlusally. The interproximal area is cleaned by using a vertical or horizontal stroke against the tooth surface. The proximal surface of one tooth should be cleaned and then that of the adjacent tooth. When the wedge begins to fray, it should be discarded (Fig. 17-37).

Interproximal brush. This is a small spiral brush or single tuft of bristles attached to a handle. The bristles are soft and adapt to the interproximal area of a wide embrasure. The brush is manipulated with a slight rotation or scrub motion and may be helpful for patients with appliances that present hard-to-clean areas (Fig. 17-38).

Modified toothbrush. An endless variety of brushes can be created with modified handles, bristle heights, or extensions. These are especially helpful for patients with a limited grasp, reach, or control in cleaning. Once an appropriate tool is designed, a brushing stroke is applied to meet the patient's needs (Fig. 17-39). (See Chapter 33 for more information on modifying toothbrushes for patients with special needs.)

Automatic toothbrush. This is an electrically or battery-powered brush and offers an alternative for patients unable or unwilling to use a manual toothbrush. Vibratory, reciprocating, and arcuate motion brushes are available with soft bristles (Fig. 17-40). Studies indicate that automatic brushes compare quite well with manual brushes; the degree of motivation and thoroughness in technique is most important. However, interproximal cleaning with floss or another aid is necessary as with manual brushing (Schifter et al., 1983).

Oral irrigator. This aid is excellent for stimulating tissues, cleansing by lavage, and removing food debris from the oral cavity (Arnim, 1976). Many devices are marketed either as faucet attachments or independent motorized units. The motor-driven irrigator is capable of creating a pulsating water jet, which is effective in creating a suction action that flushes oral debris and bacteria from the sulcus. In addition, the motor unit provides for regulation of the water pressure. The faucet-attached devices may not be as easily regulated.

Although oral irrigating devices do not remove the sticky plaque matrix, studies indicate that the harmful potential of plaque is reduced. These morphologic changes are seen in plaque that remains after the use of an oral irrigation device: (1) evacuation of bacterial cell content while the cell wall remains intact; (2) evacuation of content varying between total and slight, with the central portion of the cell content the last to disappear; (3) rupture of the cell-limiting membrane, usually accompanied by total loss of cell content (Brady, Gray, and Bhaskar, 1973).

The water jet is directed perpendicular to the long axis of the teeth (Fig. 17-41). In this way the margin of the gingiva is rinsed and massaged. In the interdental area, a suction-type force can be created that will remove food debris from the sulcus. The water spray *should not* be directed apically into the sulcus or used at a water pulsation level or pressure that could traumatize the tissue (Fig. 17-42), except when one is using some models' fine-diameter tips that enable sulcular insertion and introduction of antiplaque agents (Bhaskar, 1984).

Text continued on p. 326.

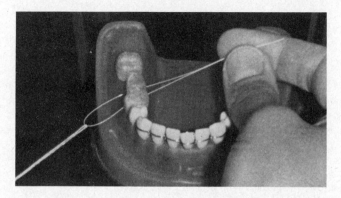

Fig. 17-23. Floss threader. Place floss through loop in threader (Butler), and feed floss under bridge or tight contact area.

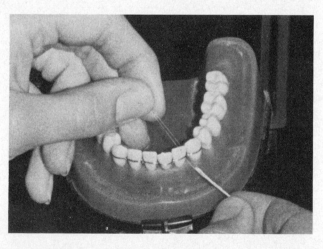

Fig. 17-24. Floss threader. Place floss through eye of clear plastic threader (Zons), and feed floss under appliance, tight contact, or bridge area.

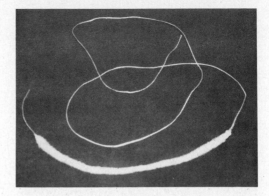

Fig. 17-25. Variable-diameter floss. This product combines a stiff end for threading, an area of yarn-type floss, and a large section of regular floss. This versatility may be well suited to some patients.

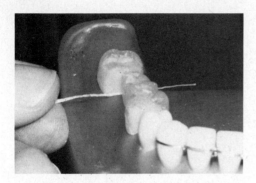

Fig. 17-26. Variable-diameter floss threader section being fed under bridge.

Fig. 17-27. Yarn section of variable-diameter floss for cleaning under bridge or in area where space permits.

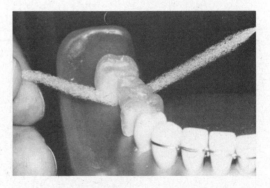

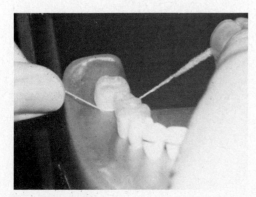

Fig. 17-28. Floss section of variable-diameter floss adapted for standard flossing technique.

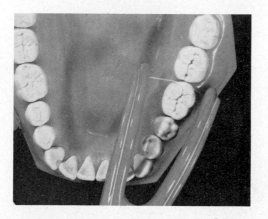

Fig. 17-29. Floss holder. Floss is stretched over frame and can be maneuvered for standard flossing with one hand.

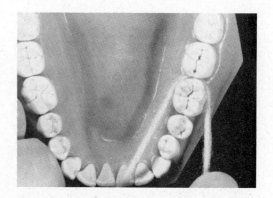

Fig. 17-30. White, synthetic yarn makes excellent cleaner for wide interproximal areas.

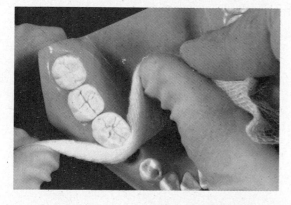

Fig. 17-31. Gauze strip can be folded and adapted to polish a wide interdental area.

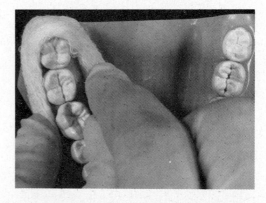

Fig. 17-32. Gauze strip becomes excellent polisher for hard-to-reach areas such as distal surface of last tooth in arch.

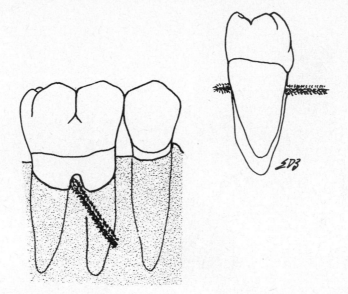

Fig. 17-33. Pipe cleaner can be bent and adapted to area of difficult access or to furcation area to remove plaque and food debris.

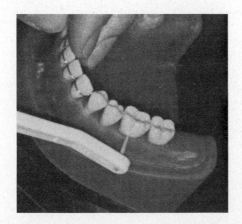

Fig. 17-34. Periodontal aid is toothpick in plastic holder. Toothpick is softened by wetting and applied to gingival margin. Tip can be moved gently in sulcus at less than 45-degree angle to remove plaque or can be adapted on cervical surface to massage fluoride for desensitization.

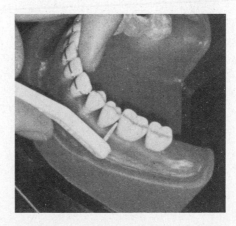

Fig. 17-35. Periodontal aid can be used to clean proximal surface of tooth. Tip is directed occlusally and moved along cervical area.

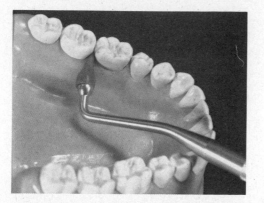

Fig. 17-36. Place rubber tip in interdental area pointed occlusally. Massage tissue by rotating tip against tissue.

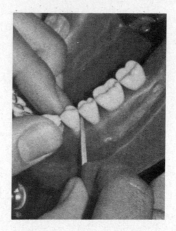

Fig. 17-37. Wood wedge is softened and placed with base of wedge on tissue. Point wedge occlusally and clean proximal surface by sliding wedge against tooth. At the same time, this stroke helps stimulate and recontour tissue.

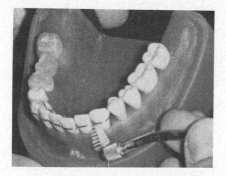

Fig. 17-38. Interproximal brush is spiral-shaped brush that can be placed in wide interdental areas to clean proximal surfaces and stimulate interdental tissue.

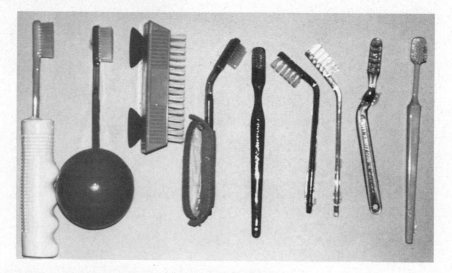

Fig. 17-39. Variety of modified brushes. Some patients have physical limitations that may require creation of a customized tool. Note variety in handles and bristle shapes.

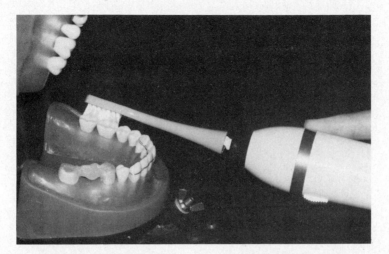

Fig. 17-40. Automatic brush is available in soft bristles and can be adapted to teeth for adequate cleaning.

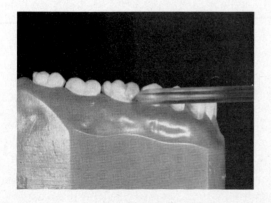

Fig. 17-41. Oral irrigator is helpful aid for stimulating tissues and flushing food from oral cavity. Oral irrigator tip must be held perpendicular to long axis of teeth to create most beneficial cleaning action.

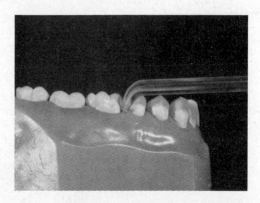

Fig. 17-42. *Do not* direct water spray apically into sulcus except with use of a specially designed fine-diameter tip intended for subgingival irrigation and introduction of antiplaque agents.

Patients should be educated concerning the therapeutic effects of irrigation, particularly in stimulating the gingiva and rinsing food debris. Instruction as to the limitations of plaque removal and the proper use of water direction and pressure is necessary. Patients who are susceptible to bacterial endocarditis (see Chapter 8) may require premedication to use this device, depending on the nature of the periodontal disease (Berger et al., 1974; Felix, Rosen, and App, 1971; Romans and App, 1971). Above all, patients must understand that oral irrigation is an aid and not a substitute for regular oral cleaning.

Beyond the basics

Approaching the patient with an individual plan for disease control is the basic principle of preventive education. Such a plan consists of a careful patient assessment initially and continued evaluation of the patient throughout treatment. Instruction in home care methods, which will benefit the particular patient as his/her needs and abilities change, is ongoing. The basic goals are (1) introducing the patient to the nature of oral disease and (2) fostering the patient's commitment to determining his/her future oral health.

A mirror, light, disclosing agent, and a variety of brushes, flosses, and aids in the hands of a willing instructor and participating patient are all that is needed for effective patient education. Beyond these basics, though, the clinician has available a variety of media to enhance the preventive program.

Preventive literature is abundant. A patient enjoys seeing a slide series or filmstrip that is relevant to his/her needs. Care and taste are part of selecting and presenting materials that are appropriate to the patient's age, intellectual level, and health goals.

In addition to focusing on more effective home care methods, the patient may benefit from activities that demonstrate caries susceptibility or plaque activity. The phase-contrast microscope is an instrument that allows the patient to view his/her own plaque. A slide is made from a small sample of plaque taken from the sulcus by a curette or explorer. The sample is diluted with a drop of saline or water to break up clumps of cells and spread the microorganisms in the pool. This simple procedure is effective in demonstrating "ownership" of viable organisms to the patient. When viewed under magnification, several types of bacteria can be identified. Loesche and Laughton (1982) have proposed the specific plaque hypothesis that suggests that the development and progression of periodontal disease is related to the presence of specific species of microorganisms in the dental plaque. Dental plaque associated with healthy periodontal conditions differs bacteriologically from dental plaque associated with periodontal diseases and dental caries (Listgarten and Hellden, 1978; Listgarten and Levin, 1981).

Keyes and Rams (1983b) have reported that subgingival dental plaque from diseased periodontal sites differs in five ways from that associated with healthy sites: (1) in the types of bacteria present, (2) in the number of microorganisms, (3) in the organization and interrelationships between cells, (4) in the coordinated dynamic behavior of bacterial populations, and (5) in inflammatory potential as indicated by crevicular leukocyte levels.

Patients with destructive periodontitis exhibit a highly organized colony of motile forms: especially spirochetes and gliding rods. Each microscopic field contains more than 125 crevicular leukocytes, and protozoa, amebas, and trichomonads can be seen in some individuals.

Patients with marginal gingivitis display a variety of unorganized motile rod-type organisms with fewer than 100 crevicular leukocytes per microscopic field. Periodontally healthy patients are characterized by the absence of motile forms and organized bacterial masses, few cocci, and low levels of crevicular leukocytes.

Using the microscope to monitor the patient's dental plaque may be helpful in identifying periodontal problems prior to the clinical signs of inflammation, bleeding, and increased sulcular depth. Such an indicator would provide valuable information that would influence the type of preventive program designed for the patient (Listgarten and Schifter, 1982).

A patient with high caries activity may be influenced by tests of his/her salivary flow, the buffering capacity of his/her saliva, or the rate of metabolic activity in the salivary bacteria (Katz, McDonald, and Stookey, 1979). Tests such as these continue to be investigated for their potential contribution to preventive dentistry and patient motivation.

The current status of dental disease prevention requires exploration of the scientific literature. The references listed at the end of this chapter include classic papers and current areas of investigation that will affect the approach to preventive care.

Providing health education to patients blends the science of the dental profession with the caring aspect of working with people. Influencing the way patients think, feel, and care for their dental health is one part of the career that should never become routine.

ACTIVITIES

1. Discuss the need for developing a preventive philosophy. Write down a few of the ideas you value, and share them with other students in small groups. Stress that with such values right or wrong is not an issue. Working in small groups, develop the components of a preventive philosophy, and present your group's philosophy to the entire class.
2. Investigate alternative methods of brushing. Demonstrate these methods and discuss the merits of all brushing techniques.
3. Make up several trays with samples of the additional tools for cleaning or providing oral physiotherapy. Practice with these aids on a typodont.
4. After sufficient practice with brushing techniques and the use of cleaning aids, divide in small groups. Each group is given an envelope filled with slips of paper asking for a demonstration of a particular facet of instruction. Select a slip of paper and demonstrate what is called for to the small group.
5. Present sample dental health education assessments. Discuss these and develop individualized education plans to meet the sample patient's needs. This can be done with the entire class or in small groups.
6. The following exercise may take several weeks to complete. It is designed to help each dental hygiene student bring his/her personal oral health to an optimal level. Complete a dental health assessment with a classmate. Plan for this patient's needs. Set aside one (or several) instruction sessions and a follow-up evaluation session. (Since these concepts and instruction methods are new to most students, instructor participation at each step is recommended.)
7. Provide individualized preventive education for a clinical patient. Keep a journal of events documenting the initial assessment, the educational plan, the instruction sequence, and the follow-up evaluation. Share this in a small group for feedback and suggestions.
8. Invite community hygienists, preventive therapists, or dentists to present a seminar on the preventive education format that is used in their practice settings. Share preventive education materials and discuss experiences.

REVIEW QUESTIONS

1. Discuss the hygienist's role as educator.
2. How has oral research had an impact on patient education?
3. What is the value of presenting an individualized approach to education?
4. During patient instruction, state the rationale for using:
   a. Small step size
   b. Active participation
   c. Immediate feedback
   d. Self-pacing
5. After three preventive visits the patient demonstrates good brushing techniques, but the plaque index is not improving and inflammation is still obvious. Which of the following responses is appropriate?
   a. Review brushing once again, emphasizing the need to place the brush in an overlapping sequence.
   b. Send the patient for medical consultation.
   c. Talk to the patient about what you have observed.
   d. Decide that you have tried, "it's his mouth," and finish the prophylaxis.
6. Which of the following are short-term motivators and which are long-term motivators? Also identify the need level appeal to which the statement is directed.
   a. You'll have more cavities the next time if you don't brush your teeth.
   b. You meet many people in your line of work; keeping your breath fresh with clean teeth and healthy gingiva must be important to you.
   c. The bleeding will continue unless you get serious about flossing.
   d. You really show you care about yourself by spending the time to clean your teeth after lunch at work.
7. Indicate whether you agree or disagree with the following statement and why: "Following a specific technique for brushing is the most important part of preventing dental disease."
8. Besides a soft brush and dental floss, what additional tools might you suggest for a patient who has wide embrasures after periodontal surgery, a fixed maxillary bridge, and a removable lower partial denture?
9. Why is it important to emphasize the following in patient instruction?
   a. Using a disclosing agent
   b. Brushing in a sequence
   c. Paying particular attention to the anterior lingual area
   d. Caring for the tongue and soft tissue

REFERENCES

ADA Council on Dental Therapeutics. 1982. Accepted dental therapeutics, ed. 39. Chicago: American Dental Association.
American Association of Public Health Dentists. 1983. Periodontal disease in America: a personal and national tragedy;

a position paper by the preventive periodontics sub-committee. J. Pub. Health Dent. **43**:106.

Arnim, S.S. 1963. The use of disclosing agents for measuring tooth cleanliness. J. Periodontal. **34**:227.

Arnim, S.S. 1976. Dental irrigators for oral hygiene, periodontal therapy and prevention of dental disease. J. Am. Soc. Prevent. Dent. **3**:10.

Axelsson, P., and Lindhe, J. 1981. Effect of controlled oral hygiene procedures on caries and periodontal disease in adults: results after six years. J. Clin. Periodontol. **8**:239.

Bakdash, M.B. 1979. Patient motivation and education: a conceptual model. Clin. Prevent. Dent. **1**(2):10.

Bass, C.C. 1948. The optimum characteristics of tooth brushes for personal oral hygiene. Dent. Items **70**:696.

Bergenholz, A., Bjorne, A., and Vikstrom, B. 1974. The plaque removing ability of some common interdental aids: an intra-individual study. J. Clin. Periodontol. **1**:160.

Berger, S.A., et al. 1974. Bacteremia after the use of an oral irrigation device: a controlled study in subjects with normal appearing gingivia: comparison with the use of a tooth brush. Ann Intern. Med. **80**:510.

Bhaskar, S. 1984. Clinical use of toothpaste and oral rinse containing sanguinarine. Comp. Contin. Educ. Dent. (Suppl.) **5**:S87.

Bowen, W., et al. 1975. Immunisation against dental caries. Br. Dent. J. **139**:45.

Boyer, E.M., and Nikias, M.K. 1983. Self-reported compliance with a preventive dental regimen. Clin. Prevent. Dent. **5**(1):3.

Brady, J.M., Gray, W., and Bhaskar, S. 1973. Electron microscopic study of the effect of water jet lavage device on dental plaque. J. Dent. Res. **52**:1310.

Cercek, J.F. 1983. Relative effects of plaque control and instrumentation on the clinical parameters of human periodontal disease. J. Clin. Periodontol. **10**:46.

Cerra, M.B., and Killroy, W.J. 1982. The effect of sodium bicarbonate and hydrogen peroxide on the microbial flora of periodontal pockets: a preliminary report. J. Periodontol. **53**:599.

Cohen, D.W. July-Aug. 1975. Preventive periodontics. J. Indiana Dent. Assoc. (Special Issue), p. 273.

Corn, H., and Marks, M. 1978. The integration of a preventive dentistry program into a dental practice. Continuing Dental Education, University of Pennsylvania School of Dental Medicine **1**: No. 10.

Ellen, R.P. 1976. Microbiological assays for dental caries and periodontal disease susceptibility. Oral Sci. Rev. **8**:3.

Evans, R.I. 1978. Motivating changes in oral hygiene behavior: some social psychological perspectives. J. Prevent. Dent. **5**(4):14.

Felix, J.E., Rosen, S., and App, G. 1971. Detection of bacteremia after the use of an oral irrigation device in subjects with periodontitis. J. Periodontal. **42**:785.

French, C.I., and Friedman, L.A. 1975. The plaque removal ability of waxed and unwaxed dental floss. Dent. Hyg. **49**:449.

Glavind, L., et al. 1983. Evaluation of various feedback mechanisms in relation to compliance by adult patients with oral home care instruction. J. Clin. Periodontol. **10**:57.

Golub, L., and Kleinberg, I. 1976. Gingival crevicular fluid: a new diagnostic aid in managing the periodontal patient. Oral Sci. Rev. **8**:49.

Greenfield, W., and Cuchel, S.J. 1984. The use of an oral rinse in dentifrice as a system for reducing dental plaque. Comp. Contin. Educ. Dent. (Suppl.) **5**:S82.

Greenwell, H., et al. 1983. Clinical and microbiologic effectiveness of Keyes' method of oral hygiene on human periodontitis treated with and without surgery. J. Am. Dent. Assoc. **106**:457.

Houle, B.A. 1982. The impact of long-term dental health on oral hygiene behavior. J. School Health **52**:256.

Katz, S., McDonald, J., and Stookey, G. 1979. Preventive dentistry in action. Upper Montclaire, N.J.: D.C.P. Publishing.

Keyes, P., and Rams, T. 1983. Clinical applications of microbiologically monitored and modulated periodontal therapy. N.Y. State Dent. J., p. 478. (a)

Keyes, P.H., and Rams, T. 1983. A rationale for the management of periodontal diseases: rapid identification of microbial therapeutic targets with phase contrast microscopy. J. Am. Dent. Assoc. **106**:803. (b)

Keyes, P.H., et al. 1982. Diagnosis of creviculoradicular infections: disease associated bacterial patterns in periodontal lesions. In Genco, R., and Mergenhagen, S., editors. Host-parasite interactions in periodontal diseases. Washington, D.C.: American Society of Microbiology. (a)

Keyes, P.H., et al. 1982. Microbial community structure as an indicator of therapeutic progress in treatment of destructive periodontitis. J. Dent. Res. (Special Issue) **61**:314. (b)

Klewansky, P., and Vernier, D. Sanguinarine and the control of plaque in dental practice. Comp. Contin. Educ. Dent. (Suppl.) **5**:S94.

Lindhe, J. 1984. Clinical assessment of antiplaque agents. Comp. Contin. Educ. Dent. (Suppl.) **5**:S78.

Listgarten, M.A., and Hellden, L. 1978. Relative distribution of bacteria at clinically healthy and periodontally diseased sites in humans. J. Clin. Periodontol. **5**:115.

Listgarten, M., Lai, C., and Socransky, S. 1975. Unusual ultra structure of plaque bacteria as an aid in their identification. J. Dent. Res. (Special Issue A) **54**:73.

Listgarten, M.A., and Levin, S. 1981. Positive correlation between the proportions of subgingival spirochetes and motile bacteria and the susceptibility of human subjects to periodontal deterioration. J. Clin. Periodontol. **8**:122.

Listgarten, M., and Schifter, C. 1982. Differential darkfield microscopy of sub-gingival bacteria as an aid in selecting recall intervals: results after 18 months. J. Clin. Periodontol. **9**:305.

Lobene, R., and Soparkar, P. 1982. Use of dental floss, effect on plaque and gingivitis. Clin. Prevent. Dent. **4**(1):5.

Loe, H. 1970. A review of the prevention and control of plaque. In McHugh, N.D., editor. Dental plaque. Edinburgh: E.S. Livingstone.

Loe, H., Theilade, E., and Borglum, J.S. 1965. Experimental gingivitis in man. J. Periodontol. **36**:177.

Loesche, W.J., and Laughton, B.E. 1982. Role of spirochetes in periodontal disease. In Genco, R., and Mergenhagen, S., editors. Host-parasite interactions in periodontal diseases. Washington: American Society of Microbiology.

Maslow, A.H. 1970. Motivation and personality. New York: Harper & Row, Publishers, Inc.

Melcer, S., and Feldman, S. 1979. Preventive dentistry teaching methods—improving oral hygiene: a summary of research. Clin. Prevent. Dent. **6**(1):7.

Nygaard-Oestby, P., and Persson, I. 1984. Evaluations of san-guinarine chloride in control of plaque in the dental practice. Comp. Contin. Educ. (Suppl.) **5:**S90.

Page, R.C., and Schroeder, H.E. 1976. Pathogenesis of in-flammatory periodontal disease: a summary of current work. International Academy of Pathology **33:**235.

Pipe, P., et al. 1972. Developing a plaque control program: a motivational approach to involving patients in dental care. University of California San Francisco, Berkeley, Calif.: Praxis Publishing Co.

Rams, T., and Keyes, P. 1983. A rationale for the management of periodontal diseases: effects of tetracycline on sub-gingival bacteria. J. Am. Dent. Assoc. **107:**37.

Romans, A.R., and App, G.R. 1971. Bacteremia, a result from oral irrigation in subjects with gingivitis. J. Periodontol. **42:**757.

Rosenberg, E.S., Evian, C.I., and Listgarten, M.A. 1981. The composition of the sub-gingival microbiota after periodontal therapy. J. Periodontol. **52:**435.

Rosling, B., et al. 1982. Topical chemical anti-microbial ther-apy in the management of the sub-gingival microflora and periodontal disease. J. Periodont. Res. **17:**541.

Schifter, et al. 1983. A comparison of plaque removal effec-tiveness of an electric versus a manual toothbrush. Clin. Prevent. Dent. **5**(5):15.

Slots, J. 1979. Subgingival microflora and periodontal disease. J. Clin. Periodontol. **6:**351.

Snow, L., Snow, R., and Schrott, J. 1983. Effect of nonsurgical periodontal treatment on different age groups and disease states with emphasis on chemical irrigation. N.Y. State Dent. J. **49:**475.

Socransky, S. 1970. Relationship of bacteria to the etiology of periodontal disease. J. Dent. Res. **49:**203.

Socransky, S. 1977. Microbiology of periodontal disease—present status and future considerations. J. Periodontol. **48:**497.

Squillaro, R.C., Cohen, D.W., and Laster, L. 1975. A com-parison of microbial plaque disclosants after personal oral hygiene instruction and prophylaxis. J. Prevent. Dent. **2:**3.

Stevens, A.W., Jr. 1980. Comparison effectiveness of variable diameter versus unwaxed floss. J. Periodontol. **51:**666.

Tan, A.E. 1980. The role of visual feedback by a disclosing agent. J. Clin. Periodontol. **7:**140.

Theilade, E., and Theilade, J. 1976. Role of plaque in the etiology of periodontal disease and caries. In Preventive den-tistry: nature, pathogenicity and clinical control of plaque. Oral Sci. Rev. **9:**23.

Weinstein, P. 1982. Humanistic application of behavioral strat-egies in oral hygiene instruction. Clin. Prevent. Dent. **4**(3):15.

Weinstein, P., and Getz, T. 1978. Changing human behavior: strategies for preventive dentistry. St. Louis: The C.V. Mosby Co.

Wilkins, E. 1982. Clinical practice of the dental hygienist, ed. 5. Philadelphia: Lea & Febiger.

Wolff, L., et al. 1982. Phase contrast microscopic evaluation of sub-gingival plaque in combination with either conven-tional or anti-microbial home treatment of patients with peri-odontal inflammation. J. Periodont. Res. **17:**537.

Woodall, I.R. 1983. Legal, ethical, and management aspects of the dental care system: issues for the dental team, ed. 2. St. Louis: The C.V. Mosby Co.

Wright, G.Z., Banting, D.W., and Feasby, W.H. 1977. The effect of interdental flossing on the incidence of proximal caries in children, J. Dent. Res. **56:**574.

Yankell, S., and Emling, R. 1978. Understanding dental prod-ucts: what you should know and what your patient should know. Continuing Dental Education, University of Pennsyl-vania School of Dental Medicine **1:** No. 7.

Zachowski, P. 1979. The effectiveness of dental floss in oral hygiene practice. Dent. Hyg. **53**(2):67.

18 FORMULATING A TREATMENT PLAN, CASE PRESENTATION, AND APPOINTMENT PLAN

OBJECTIVES: *The reader will be able to*

1. Given assessment data from a variety of cases, including medical history, vital signs, intraoral and extraoral examinations and chartings, radiographic surveys, diagnostic casts, and the patient's expectations:
   a. Design a treatment plan best suited to the specific needs of each patient.
   b. Design at least one alternative plan for each case.
   c. Design a case presentation format for each patient that meets (1) the legal requirements of *informed consent* and (2) the basic principles of interpersonal communication.
   d. Design a logical sequence of planned appointments to fulfill the treatment plan for each case.
2. Given a variety of treatment needs, identify priorities for treatment, including:
   a. Emergency needs
   b. Prevention of disease
   c. Restorative and surgical needs
   d. Maintenance needs

NATURE AND ROLE OF TREATMENT PLANNING

Treatment planning saves patients from an automated approach to dental and dental hygiene care. Completing an individualized treatment plan does not allow, for instance, for the assumption that all people need an oral prophylaxis or a fluoride treatment. It guides the health care provider in identifying specific *problems* and specific *health goals* and identifying treatment or other procedures to solve the problems and to meet the health goals. Careful planning allows these two foci to be accomplished in tandem.

In addition, treatment planning provides an opportunity for specifying those problems and goals so that they can be shared with the patient and explained in rational, understandable terms. It provides an opportunity to organize the sequence of care and to plan care so that the patient can identify with and participate in progress as it is made. Such organization maximizes time utilization and reduces frustration.

The written, agreed-on treatment plan is a legal contract that forms the basis of the legal relationship between the health care provider and the patient. It is an invaluable resource in a court of law as well as at the chairside. It provides a medium for discussing wants, needs, and expectations and for promoting a free exchange of perceptions (Clark and Morton, 1977).

PREPARING A TREATMENT PLAN

Once all of the assessment phases of care have been completed, the data from each of these procedures should be analyzed carefully and synthesized into a comprehensive picture of the needs of the individual patient (Clark and Morton, 1977; Fechtner, 1978; Fishman and Ortiz, 1977; Wood, 1978).

The medical history, review of systems, and vital signs should point out precautionary measures to ensure the general well-being of the patient. The need for a physician's clearance or referral to a physician should have been clearly identified prior to intraoral chartings. There should be special awareness of general signs of fatigue, unrest, anxiety, or other conditions based on this carefully collected data.

The significant findings of the examinations and chartings should be identified and compared with all the information gathered from various sources. Clinical evidence of health and disease should be compared with radiographic evidence. Evaluations of the conditions of the teeth should be compared with soft tissue findings in their respective areas of the dentition. Results of plaque indices should be laid alongside patterns of disease occurrence for the teeth and periodontium. A comprehensive picture of the objective clinical needs of the patient should emerge, or further questions about health status should be raised (Barsh, 1981; Morris, 1983).

A logical way to design a treatment plan is (1) to systematically review each assessment finding in terms of its significance; (2) to identify each significant finding as a problem or goal; and (3) to identify an appropriate course of action. Once these three steps are complete, then (4) a priority should be established for each procedure; from this, (5) a specific sequence in care should be assigned; and (6) estimated time needed should be identified for each step (Wood, 1978).

The treatment planning worksheet shown in Table 18-1 can be modified to meet the individual dental hygienist's approach to planning. Such a worksheet facilitates identifying critical needs, goals, phases of care, sequencing, and time needs. It minimizes the opportunity to overlook specific findings and displays groups of findings so that correlations among data are more apparent.

As objective needs emerge to form a series of preventive or treatment procedures appropriate for the patient, more subjective needs, particularly those expressed by the patient during the self-assessment of needs contribute to the overall picture of care that should be planned for the patient. The health care provider's attitudes toward these needs and expectations, as demonstrated in how they are accounted for in the treatment plan, can have a significant effect on how the patient perceives the health care provider and his/her ability to assist the patient in meeting long-term and short-term health goals (Goldberg, Plume, and Nacman, 1973).

The priority assignment is highly reflective of the philosophic approach of the dental hygienist to providing care. Most clinicians would agree that clinical problems that are causing pain or that are likely to cause pain in the near future are *emergency treatment* procedures that should receive top priority. Therefore deep caries, the presence of an apical radiolucency, or a suspicious oral lesion will delay preventive care.

Differences in philosophy are more apparent among health care providers when deciding whether *preventive* procedures or *restorative* and *surgical treatment* are the next highest priorities. Many clinicians believe that ensuring that the patient is in *control* of his/her dental health supersedes any treatment other than emergency procedures. Others believe that prevention should follow basic treatment procedures. Many combine this choice of priorities by integrating preventive procedures into each treatment appointment. *Maintenance* care, which ensures long-term periodic examinations and preventive procedures, logically follows the completion of therapeutic procedures.

The sequence of treatment does not necessarily follow the priority assignment, since some high-priority elements are more effective if they follow other preliminary procedures. For instance, curettage procedures to reduce chronic inflammatory periodontal disease may have a high priority but may be sequenced after thorough removal of hard deposits and after the patient has mastered brushing and flossing. Another example is the application of sealants, which may have a very high priority for a child with deep pits and grooves but which should follow other treatment needs such as those prompted by active caries.

Estimating the time needed to complete each procedure is an important step in treatment planning and should be noted while the assessment data are fresh in the clinician's mind. The large, subgingival deposits of calculus noted on the charting and visible on the radiographic survey can prompt more realistic estimates of time needed for debridement than can later recollections of the needs of the case.

Once the treatment plan is complete, the dental hygienist should review the patient's wants, needs, and expectations to ensure that his/her expressions of what the plan should include are met or at least addressed. A useful preliminary step is to imagine

Table 18-1. Treatment planning worksheet

Assessment tool	Significant findings	Problem or goal	Indicated course of action	Priority	Sequence in care	Time needed
Medical history						
Review of systems						
Vital signs						
Dental history						
Extraoral examination						
Intraoral examination						
Periodontal examination						
Calculus charting						
Dental charting						
Radiographic charting						
Guided self-assessment						
Plaque index						
Hemorrhage point index						
Nutritional self-assessment						
Patient's expressed wants, needs, and expectations						

oneself as the patient who will soon learn about this plan. A series of questions that may prove helpful in ensuring that wants, needs, and expectations as expressed at earlier appointments are met, and helpful in translating the treatment plan into a case presentation are:

Where in the plan are the patient's expressed needs addressed?

Is the *course of action* in meeting those needs and their *priority* likely to be satisfactory to the patient? Why or why not?

What additional phases of care are included in the plan that are related to needs of which the patient may be unaware?

How can those needs be described simply and accurately for the patient? How can self-assessment data be used to substantiate the findings?

Is the patient likely to be alarmed or upset by these additional findings? Is the patient likely to view these plans as a luxury or as unnecessary?

How can the proposed treatment and its likely outcomes be described so that the patient's confidence and trust are maintained? What questions is the patient likely to ask?

What specific goals for health should be emphasized? How can the patient become involved in helping realize those goals?

What alternative plans for care could be followed and with what consequences?

Is the patient likely to be concerned about appearance, pain, cost, and/or time? How does each of those concerns appear justified in terms of the proposed treatment plan?

What would be the likely outcome if the patient refused care or selected a modified plan?

The treatment plan, therefore, requires considerable knowledge of the implications of the assessment data as clinical and radiographic signs are interpreted. It is a critical point in individualizing and personalizing care and in applying knowledgeable professional judgment (Wood, 1978).

DESIGNING A CASE PRESENTATION

After having completed the planning worksheet and answered the aforementioned questions regarding the patient's likely perceptions, the dental hygienist should be prepared to define the treatment plan in an understandable case presentation. The primary purposes of the case presentation are to solidify the understanding of needs and plans and to formalize the contractual relationship between the patient and the dental hygienist for the treatment phase of care. *Informed consent* is the legal reason for the case presentation (Miller, 1979; Rosoff, 1981). *Mutual understanding* and *cooperation* are the more personal reasons for the case presentation.

The guidelines for establishing informed consent form a natural framework for explaining the case to the patient. First, the nature of the patient's condition should be described in understandable terms with ample opportunity for responding to the patient's concerns and requests for further explanation. It may be helpful to show the patient his/her study models and radiographs and to refer to other data gathered. The suggested plan of treatment should follow, with a discussion of the likely outcomes of the treatment. Risks involved should be described. The likely outcome of not proceeding with care should be described as well. Finally, alternative treatment approaches should be offered with a discussion of the advantages and disadvantages of such (Fishman and Ortiz, 1977; Miller, 1979; Rosoff, 1981).

If the patient is involved fully in the case presentation and agrees to proceed with care, informed consent is secured (Miller, 1979; Rosoff, 1981). The costs of care (usually expressed as a close estimate) and the time needed should be discussed also to minimize surprises and to further involve the patient in the decision-making process (Miller, 1979; Rosoff, 1981). The time estimates and sequence identified in the treatment plan should enable the hygienist to identify a logical order and number of appointments that are most compatible with the time constraints of the patient.

While the practice of including the requirements of informed consent in the case presentation is an important preventive approach in avoiding litigation and misunderstanding, two additional points are important in the legal ramifications of the contractual relationship. First, if any additional procedures are to be included in treatment, the patient's informed consent must be obtained for those new elements of care. If this is not done, the dental hygienist is liable for *technical assault* or *battery* (performing a procedure to which the patient did not consent) under tort law. Second, all procedures agreed to in the case presentation must be performed within a reasonable time with a reasonable standard of care. If a procedure is to be omitted or delayed, the patient first must be informed and agree. If this is not done, the dental hygienist can be subjected to a breach of contract suit (Fechtner, 1978; Miller, 1979; Rosoff, 1981).

More altruistic reasons for the case presentation are to decrease the patient's fear of the unknown, to build trust, and to form a helping relationship that maximizes positive outcomes. The case presentation should be thorough but simple, and it should be presented with a modicum of enthusiasm. Too much intensity can destroy the message (Keltner, 1973). The thorough, thoughtful case presentation should improve the patient's desire to cooperate by appearing for appointments, following preoperative and postoperative instructions, and paying for services. A sense of participation in care seems to promote this cooperation. The patient develops a sense of ownership of his/her needs and the methods to meet those needs (Cohen, 1975; Keltner, 1973). Likewise, the dental hygienist may derive great satisfaction from having learned about and cared for a person who needed his/her assistance.

The case presentation also helps the patient recognize the significance of the numerous assessment procedures in the beginning phases of care. The patient learns about good dentistry and good health care and experiences shared responsibility in care by having the opportunity to participate in the discussion.

Regardless of the quality of the assessments of the patient's needs, the logic of the treatment plan, and the interesting case presentation, the patient may decline treatment. A health care provider cannot force a patient to accept care (Fishman and Ortiz, 1977; Miller, 1979). While it may be shocking to hear the patient say, "I really don't think I want all this dental work," that kind of honesty is preferable to a nonverbal expression of the refusal to accept care—the broken appointment. It can be risky to ask, "Would you like to proceed with treatment?" It can be difficult to hear the response, "No." However, the direct positive response is usually a strong indicator of the patient's commitment to cooperate in care. It indicates that the pa-

tient accepts the described health needs as real and the proposed course of action as appropriate. A negotiated or compromised treatment plan, although it may not be ideal in the health care provider's view, is usually an even more positive sign of a solid partnership relationship with mutual respect between the patient and the health care provider (Clark and Morton, 1977; Keltner, 1973). With this kind of a relationship the "ideal" plan is more likely to be realized in the long run.

Hesitancy to accept the plan or a simple rejection deserve follow-up discussion (Fishman and Ortiz, 1977). Questioning the patient as to what his/her concerns are may bring out what the patient sees as roadblocks to care (financial problems, fear of discomfort or altered appearance, lack of time, etc.) or what appears to be a misunderstanding of the problem or the plan. The health care provider can serve as a facilitator in reducing or eliminating the roadblocks by further clarifying the specifics of the treatment plan. In any case, if the patient declines treatment, the reasons should be fairly clear, and the health care provider should be able to accept that decision as the patient's right. "Good persuasion endures and allows people to make intelligent choices; it does not take advantage of people's weaknesses" (Keltner, 1973).

With acceptance of the final plan, the development of an appointment plan solidifies the agreement and defines a set of expectations: when and for how long the patient and health care provider agree to receive and provide treatment, respectively. A commitment is made.

APPOINTMENT PLANNING

Translating the treatment plan into specific appointments requires several considerations. Using 15-minute increments (for example) as appointment units simplifies blocking out appointment time. Obviously, the estimated time needed for each procedure and the logic of grouping procedures that are interrelated are the primary determinants in designing appointments.

The patient's tolerance for long sessions in a dental chair (or for frequent trips to the dental office) is an important consideration. Children, for instance, usually should be scheduled for short appointments at a time of day when they are least fatigued. Some patients prefer a series of short appointments; other prefer fewer, longer appointments. For most treatment needs, sequencing of procedures can be made to accommodate patient preferences.

Tables 18-2 to 18-4 describe the translation of assessment data into treatment plans and then into appointment sequences. These examples reflect the time requirements of a hygienist who has achieved a satisfactory level of time-and-motion management. Beginning clinicians will define their time needs for treatment differently. Time needed to complete various procedures will decrease with greater skill and practice. Another important variable, regardless of the skill and experience of the clinician, is the amount of time that is spent waiting or participating in discussion with co-workers regarding the case. In health care delivery systems that require patient evaluation in several different clinics or departments, the time requirements in the beginning phases of care may be high. In less complex systems, time requirements for activities such as consultations, preparing release forms, and referral procedures may be less. Therefore, these examples are given primarily to illustrate how individual differences and needs can affect the planning of treatment and appointments and are not intended to reflect ideal time usage.

The case outlined in Table 18-2 describes an adult with what will probably be confirmed as chronic, inflammatory periodontal disease (Lynch, 1977). Medical complications are minimal. Assessment findings show a pattern of caries development and high plaque scores despite frequent dental visits. The indicated course of action focuses on monitoring the blood pressure, eliminating the periodontal problem, and instituting a strong preventive program for the patient. The key in motivation, and a factor to be kept in mind in planning, is the patient's concern for cost.

Table 18-3 outlines a case involving a leukemic patient who should be maintained on a solid, albeit low-pressure, preventive program to minimize irritants that could cause gingival problems (Lynch, 1977). Scheduling is based on the medical status of the patient, and traumatic procedures are minimized. The relative significance of good teeth for both this patient and the family should be kept in mind. The primary motivator is that teeth and their surrounding tissues should cause no additional problems. Therefore, an easily followed preventive routine is appropriate.

The third case (Table 18-4) is an outline for a patient with what will probably be confirmed as acute necrotizing ulcerative gingivitis (ANUG) (Lynch, 1977). The sequence of care is altered by the history of rheumatic fever. No probing or exploring could be performed until the patient had achieved satisfactory blood levels of antibiotics to counteract any microorganisms entering the bloodstream (bacteremia) through incidental hemorrhage. Once the premedication was assured, the periodontal examination was completed and debridement was begun (Lynch, 1977).

The fourth, and final case (Table 18-5) describes dental hygiene care planned for a postsurgical cancer patient, for whom the clinician needs to identify individualized needs, to coordinate efforts with other health care providers, and to reinforce oral hygiene procedures to reverse the progress of disease secondary to oral cancer therapy (Rose and Kaye, 1983). The changes in the oral tissues, the rise in the presence of caries and gingivitis, the reduction in oral fluids, and the patient's response to treatment all deserve careful attention and planning before any "routine" care is provided. (See Chapter 34 for further discussion.)

Dental hygiene treatment planning should always question the appropriateness of "routine" care. It seeks out and responds to the individual needs of patients, whether they are startlingly apparent or elusive. Such planning is an essential, professional responsibility of dental hygienists.

The ideal way to develop the ability to translate assessment data into a plan and then into an appointment sequence is to practice with a variety of hypothetical and real cases. Case presentations can then be role played with a student partner serving as a patient and with a student as an observer who reports regarding whether informed consent requirements were met and whether the "dental hygienist" listened to the expressed wants, needs, and expectations of the "patient" and responded to those concerns. Such practice facilitates clinical application of these basic skills in synthesis, planning, and communicating.

Text continued on p. 344.

Table 18-2. Case 1

Assessment tool	Significant findings	Problem or goal	Indicated course of action	Priority	Sequence in care	Time needed
Medical history	Within normal limits	—	—	—	—	—
Review of systems	Within normal limits					
Vital signs	130/86 right arm sitting (ras) Pulse: 75	Potential high bp	Record bp at each visit	A	First at each appointment	5 min per appointment
Dental history	Regular visits to dentists (every 6 months)	Maintain this habit	Reinforce behavior	—	6—at last appointment; recall system entry	5 min last appointment
Extraoral examination	Crepitus in TMJ	Determine its significance	Refer to dentist for assessment	D	At first treatment appointment	5 min first appointment
Intraoral examination	Within normal limits					
Periodontal examination	Red, edematous tissue—generalized Minimal attached gingivae 3 to 6 mm pockets	Normal gingivae	Plaque control Debridement Review for soft tissue curettage Refer for periodontal consult	C	4	2 hr (1-hr appointments)
Calculus charting	Generalized ledge and crustaceous calculus	Debride	Ultrasonic scaling	C	3	1 hr
Dental charting	Three suspicious areas of possible caries; one defective restoration (No. 30) Numerous restorations (24 total covering 60 surfaces)	Evaluate for need for restorative treatment	Refer to dentist for assessment	C	At first treatment appointment	5 min
Radiographic charting	None					
Guided self-assessment	Presence of numerous restorations despite regular dental visits Presence of red tissue	Reduce frequency of caries	Nutritional counseling Review brushing and flossing Consider phosphate fluoride treatment	B	2	15 to 20 min per appointment
Plaque index	Plaque on 60% of surfaces	Reduce plaque	Review brushing and flossing, antiplaque agents	A	1	5 min per appointment

Hemorrhage point index	30 areas of spontaneous hemorrhage	Reduce tissue inflammation	Debridement and improved plaque control	—	—	5 min per appointment
Nutritional self-assessment	High intake of refined sugars / Minimal intake of fruits and vegetables	Reduce sugar and add fruits and vegetables	Dietary counseling	B	3	10 to 15 min per appointment
Patient's expressed wants, needs, and expectations	Worried about cost	Minimize time needed and involve patient in self-care program to enhance healing	Teach control and dietary counseling early	A	1,3	5 min
			Use fluoride on suspicious carious lesions		5	

Appointment plan

Appointment 1 (postassessment)
1. Record bp — 5 min
2. Request dentist consult for
   Crepitus
   Carious areas (and decision to restore or treat with fluoride) — 10 min
3. Begin plaque control
   Brushing/antiplaque agents
   Flossing
   Dietary modifications — 30 min
4. Ultrasonically scale entire dentition — 60 min

SCHEDULE: 105 min (7 units)*

Appointment 2
1. Record bp — 5 min
2. Review plaque control
   Take indices
   Observe techniques of brushing, flossing
   Add oral physiotherapeutic aids (OPTA) as needed
   Review 3-day diet — 25 min
3. Root plane mandible — 45 min

SCHEDULE: 75 min (5 units)

Appointment 3
1. Record bp — 5 min
2. Review plaque control (see Appointment 2) — 20 min
3. Root plane maxilla — 45 min

SCHEDULE: 70 min (5 units)

Appointment 4
1. Record bp — 5 min
2. Record indices and discuss plaque control and diet as needed — 15 min
3. Evaluate for curettage
   Perform selected areas of curettage as needed
   Polish if curettage is contraindicated and apply fluoride
   Place on recall or refer for dental treatment — 30 min

SCHEDULE: 50 min (4 units)

Appointment 5 (if needed)
1. Remove periodontal pack — 5 min
2. Polish teeth — 15 min
3. Apply fluoride. — 5 min
4. Place on recall or refer for dental treatment — 2 min

SCHEDULE: 27 min (2 units)

*Each unit = 15 minutes.

Table 18-3. Case 2

Assessment tool	Significant findings	Problem or goal	Indicated course of action	Priority	Sequence in care	Time needed
Medical history	Leukemia	Avoid adding to medical problem	Treat during period of remission	A	—	—
			Seek physician consult and recommended procedures			
Review of systems	Blood dyscrasia due to leukemia 120/84 ras	Same as above	Same as above	—	—	—
Vital signs	Pulse: 80			—	—	—
Dental history	Pattern of numerous restorations at each visit (4 per year) Currently working with dietician	Reduce caries rate	Identify ways to improve diet—consult with physician and dietician	B	1	30 min
Extraoral examination	Palpable lymph nodes (cervical and submandibular) bilaterally	May be related to leukemia	Consult with physician	B	1	—
Intraoral examination	Within normal limits, but mucosa is generally a pale grey-pink	—	—	—	—	—
Periodontal examination	Gingivae are pale grey-pink with hemorrhage areas obvious in sulcus (*prior* to probing)	Characteristic of leukemia Attempt to improve gingival health and minimize irritation of tissues	Consult with dentist and physician regarding significance	B	2	30 min
			Emphasis on daily, gentle removal of irritants	C	2	30 min
			Oral prophylaxis	D	3	30 min
Calculus charting	None	Minimize recurrence of decay				
Dental charting	Numerous restorations (32 surfaces)	Restore area	Refer to dentist Dietary counseling	—	—	—

Assessment	Findings	Interpretation / Recommendation	Patient education	Priority	No.	Time
Radiographic charting	One new area of caries (D No. 30)	Same as above		—	—	—
Guided self-assessment	Confirms area of caries (D No. 30)	See soft tissue findings from intraoral and periodontal examinations	Plaque control	C	2	—
		Minimize emphasis on systemic causes; emphasize means of improvement				
Plaque index	Plaque on 30% of surfaces	Redo at each appointment. Decrease plaque	Plaque control. Antiplaque agents	C	2	5 min per appointment
Hemorrhage point index	Omitted due to generalized passive hemorrhage	Not necessary		—	—	—
Nutritional self-assessment	Frequent intake of sweets		Nutritional counseling	—	—	—
Patient's expressed wants, needs, and expectations	Dental care becoming an increasingly lower health priority	Keep at least minimal oral health habits easy and attractive as a routine	Keep simple	—	—	—

Appointment plan

Prior to appointment: Consult with physician, dentist, and dietician

Appointment 1 (postassessment)
1. Plaque control and dietary counseling — 30 min (or more as needed) — 30 min
2. Oral prophylaxis — 30 min

SCHEDULE: 60 min (4 units)

Appointment 2
1. Plaque index: review plaque control — 15 min
2. Review dietary counseling (3-day diet) — 15 min
3. Refer for restorative care

SCHEDULE: 30 min (2 units)

Table 18-4. Case 3

Assessment tool	Significant findings	Problem or goal	Indicated course of action	Priority	Sequence in care	Time needed
Medical history	Rheumatic fever at age 10	Possible subacute bacterial endocarditis from dental care	Prophylactic premedication	A	1	Delay in appointment
Review of systems	Cardiovascular: rheumatic heart; valve damage	Same as above	Same as above	—	—	—
Vital signs	124/82, ras Pulse: 90	—				—
Dental history	Complains of halitosis and bleeding and painful gums	ANUG	Debride and use antibiotic therapy Begin plaque control and nutritional education	B	2	1 hr
Extraoral examination	Within normal limits except for palpable submandibular lymph nodes	—	Consult with physician regarding nodes	—	—	—
Intraoral examination	Halitosis	Improve oral hygiene	Begin plaque control	C	3	30 min
Periodontal examination	Pain with probing; cratered interdental papillae; white membranelike appearance on gingivae; generally red and enlarged (probable ANUG)	Normal gingivae; reduce pain and debris	Use ultrasonic scaler for initial debridement; subsequent fine scaling and root planing	D	4	2 hr
			Refer for periodontal consult regarding gingival form	E	5	15 min
Calculus charting	Moderate amounts of supragingival and subgingival deposits	Debride	Ultrasonic and hand scaling	—	—	—
Dental charting	Caries free	Maintain	—	—	—	—

Radiographic charting	Minor loss of crestal bone height	Stop loss of bone	Refer for periodontal consult regarding gingival and bone form	—	—	—	—	—
Guided self-assessment	Red hemorrhagic gingivae; Halitosis; foul taste; Sound teeth	Improve soft tissue; maintain teeth	Plaque control; Antiplaque agents	—	—	—	—	—
Plaque index	Large amounts of visible plaque	Reduce plaque	Plaque control	—	—			
Hemorrhage point index	Generalized bleeding	Improve gingival condition	Plaque control	—	—			
Nutritional self-assessment	Total lack of green vegetables; minimal fruit and yellow vegetables; other groups adequate	Secure vitamins and minerals from missing foods	Dietary counseling; evaluate at each visit	F	6	30 min		
Patient's expressed wants, needs, and expectations	Eliminate bad breath; Stop gums from bleeding	—	Same as above	—	—			

Appointment plan

Appointment 1*
1. Periodontal evaluation — 15 min
2. Ultrasonically scale entire dentition — 60 min
3. Begin plaque control and dietary counseling; introduce antiplaque agent — 30 min

SCHEDULE: 105 min (7 units)

Appointment 2
1. Review plaque control and dietary modifications — 15 min
2. Scale and root plane mandible — 45 min

SCHEDULE: 60 min (4 units)

Appointment 3
1. Review plaque control and dietary modifications — 15 min
2. Scale and root plane maxilla — 45 min
3. Polish entire dentition — 15 min
4. Repeat periodontal evaluation and arrange periodontal consult — 15 min

SCHEDULE: 90 min (6 units)

*At the initial visit no procedures that could induce a bacteremia were performed. Antibiotic premedication was initiated after consultation with the physician. The patient returned for the periodontal examination, at which time relevant data were added and treatment as outlined commenced.

Table 18-5. Case 4

Assessment tool	Significant findings	Problem or goal	Indicated course of action	Priority	Sequence in care	Time needed
Medical history	Age: 48 yrs. Squamous cell carcinoma—hard palate and maxillary alveolus and sinus; chemotherapy and radiation	Watch for recurrence; help patient adjust; prevent secondary oral complications	Modify treatment; focus care to respond to this development and its ramifications	A	2	—
Review of systems	Receiving chemotherapy and radiation therapy; Low platelet count due to bone marrow suppression	Possible secondary complications; Possible clotting delay	Monitor oral conditions at each appointment; frequent oral recall; Consult with physician re platelet count	—	—	—
Vital signs	128/84 (ras); Pulse: 78	—	—	—	—	—
Dental history	Minimal caries or evidence of periodontal disease; Regular visits	Maintain at least historical level of oral health	Compare current with historical status	B	1	15 min
Extraoral examination	Skin on right side of face is red and dry; Slight loss of symmetry—right side	Proper care of skin during radiation therapy	Consult with dentist or physician regarding skin preparation recommendations; reinforce instructions for use	D	1	5 min
Intraoral examination	Obturator replaces right side of palate and portion of maxilla; Minimal saliva; tongue and mucosa abnormally dry and irritated	Maintain cleanliness of prosthesis and supporting structures; Improve oral lubrication and cleansing	Work with patient to establish a routine for oral self-care, with special aids as needed; Consult dentist or physician regarding saliva substitute or other measures to reduce dryness	B	1	15-20 min
Periodontal examination	Gingivae are red and tender; general inflammation and presence of irritants	Restore periodontal health and adjust oral care	Dental health education and initial periodontal treatment	D	3	30 min
Calculus charting	Moderate generalized supra- and subgingival deposits; recently formed	Restore periodontal health; Enable patient to resume or adjust oral health maintenance	Scale and polish; selective root planing and curettage (*requires* consult with physician, dentist given low platelet count)	E	5	60 min
Dental charting	Nos. 2, 3, and 4 replaced by obturator; Clinical evidence of 10 areas of new or recurrent caries; Numerous areas of decalcification, especially near cervical portion of crowns	Recalcify new areas of incipient caries; Ensure that caries requiring restoration are treated	Institute fluoride therapy program; Alert dentist to evidence of caries	C	4	15 min

Assessment	Findings	Goals	Actions	Code	No.	Time
Radiographic charting	None currently; complete set is 3 years old	—	Consult dentist and physician regarding need for exposure of diagnostic films	C	2	5 min
Guided self-assessment	Inadequate care of obturator and teeth; Decreased mouth moisture and oral hygiene frequency; Painful mucosa	Better self-care; Increased oral moisture	Involve patient in plans for better oral self-care and procedures for improving moisture	D	3	—
Plaque index	Plaque on 70% of surfaces	Improved gingival health	Plaque control	D	3	—
Hemorrhage point index	15 areas of spontaneous hemorrhage	Improved gingival health	Plaque control	D	3	—
Nutritional self-assessment	Diminished taste; chews sugared lemon drops; eats small amounts of food frequently; loss of appetite; eats soft foods; Working with dietician	Minimize sugar intake; continue good dietary habits	Substitute noncariogenic saliva stimulant	C	4	—
			Consult with dietician	D	3	15 min
			Reinforce good habits	C	4	—
Patient's expressed wants, needs and expectations	Afraid a new lesion will develop; dislikes having a prosthesis and does not like to look at it or postsurgical area	Reduced fear; acceptance of early detection procedures and self-care	Review oral cancer self-exam; Show acceptance of patient's state; Supportive watchfulness and acceptance	A	3	10 min

Appointment plan

Prior to appointment: Consult with dentist, physician, dietician, and psychologist; compare previous status with current and modify treatment as needed — 30 min or more as needed / 15 min — SCHEDULE: 45 min (3 units)

Appointment 1 (postassessment)
1. Review of self-care and plaque control; recommend lemon drop substitute — 30 min
2. Review oral cancer self-exam and care of appliance — 10 min
3. Begin fluoride therapy — 15 min
4. Scale (and polish) one quadrant — 15 min
   SCHEDULE: 90 min (6 units)

Appointment 2
1. Reassess oral self-care and reinforce plaque control and fluoride regimen — 10 min
2. Scale and polish remaining teeth — 40 min
3. Reinforce nutritional changes — 10 min
   SCHEDULE: 60 min (4 units)

Appointment 3
1. Reassess oral self-care, soft tissue health, plaque control, dietary habits, and use of fluorides — 15 min
2. Evaluate for further instrumentation — 15 min
Recall: 2 months (or less depending on recommendations of dentist or physician and on patient's desire to be seen more frequently)
   SCHEDULE: 30 min (2 units)

TREATMENT PLANNING AND DIAGNOSIS: LEGAL AND PROFESSIONAL RESPONSIBILITIES

In an era when the dental hygienist's role and responsibility are not uniformly defined by law, in clinical practice settings, or in educational programs, the use of the term *treatment planning* may raise concern among some persons that such a role is "beyond the scope" of the dental hygienist. Most licensing jurisdictions specifically reserve treatment planning and diagnosis for the dentist.

However, many dental hygienists arrange appointment sequencing and scheduling specifically for the dental hygiene care to be provided. For this to be done, assessment data must be gathered and translated into a meaningful summary and conclusions.

Generally, the dental hygienist prepares this initial synthesis and then discusses and confirms it with the dentist responsible for the overall dental needs of the patient. The dentist makes the final diagnosis before the patient is informed of the relative health and disease present. The keys to remaining within the law and to building and maintaining a cooperative team relationship with the dentist are (1) to perform thorough, reliable assessment, (2) to draw preliminary conclusions from the data, (3) to use the dentist as a resource and arbiter of decisions regarding the patient's status and proper treatment, and (4) to follow through with high-quality dental hygiene care, providing status reports for the dentist as the case progresses.

In this way the dental hygienist's understanding of basic, behavioral, and dental sciences can be fully used and grow with each case while the hygienist remains within the bounds of professional responsibility and maintains an interdependent relationship with the dentist. Maintaining this balance is critical, since the patient's well-being and the profession's credibility depend on it.

ACTIVITIES

1. Assemble assessment data from clinic patients who are receiving care from advanced dental hygiene students. Complete a treatment planning worksheet for three or more patients. Share your worksheets and appointment plans in groups of four or five, and develop composite plans in the group, which then can be shared with the entire class.
2. Role play case presentations derived from the plans generated in preceding activity. A "dental hygienist" should present the case to a "patient" while a third student serves as an observer, watching for the elements of informed consent and the presence of sensivity to the patient's wants, needs, and expectations. Rotate roles to give each student the opportunity to be an observer, patient, and dental hygienist.
3. Read Susan S. Miller's "Dental Hygiene Diagnosis" article in RDH **2**(4):46, 1982. As individuals, and then as a class, define dental hygiene diagnosis and develop a preliminary diagnostic nomenclature.

REVIEW QUESTIONS

1. What six elements must be included in a case presentation to meet the requirements for informed consent?
2. If a procedure is performed for a patient to which the patient did not give consent, the clinician may be charged with _____ .
3. What is a critical reason for integrating the patient's wants, needs, and expectations in the treatment plan?
4. The first priority in the sequence of care is treatment to meet any _____ needs of the patient.
5. How can a dental hygienist function responsibly and legally as part of the dental team when performing treatment planning for dental hygiene care?

REFERENCES

Barsh, L.I. 1981. Dental treatment planning for the adult patient. Philadelphia: W.B. Saunders Co.

Clark, J.D., and Morton, J.C. 1977. Behavioral assessment: an appraisal of beliefs and behaviors relating to treatment. Dent. Clin. North Am. **21:**515.

Cohen, D.W. 1975. Preventive periodontics. J. Indian Dent. Assoc. (Special Issue), p. 273.

Fechtner, J.L. 1978. Treatment planning. Dent. Clin. North Am. **22:**219.

Fishman, S.R., and Ortiz, E., Jr. 1977. Effective case presentation. Dent. Clin. North Am. **21:**539.

Goldberg, H.J., Plume, M., and Nacman, M. 1973. The importance of attitude in the delivery of health services. J. Public Health Dent. **33:**35.

Kagan, A.R., and Miles, J.W. 1981. Head and neck oncology: controversies in cancer treatment. Boston: G.K. Hall & Co. Publishers.

Keltner, J.W. 1973. Elements of interpersonal communication. Belmont, Calif.: Wadsworth Publishing Co., Inc.

Lynch, M.A. 1977. Burket's oral medicine. Philadelphia: J.B. Lippincott Co.

Miller, S.L. 1979. Legal aspects of dentistry. New York: G.P. Putnam's Sons.

Morris, R.B. 1983. Principles of dental treatment planning. Philadelphia: Lea & Febiger.

Rose, L., and Kaye, D. 1983. Internal medicine for dentistry. St. Louis: The C.V. Mosby Co.

Rosoff, A. 1981. Informed consent. Rockville, Md.: Aspen Systems Corp.

Wang, C.C. 1983. Radiation therapy for head and neck neoplasms. Boston: John Wright/PSG, Inc.

Wood, K.: 1978. Treatment planning: a pragmatic approach. St. Louis: The C.V. Mosby Co.

19 GUIDED SELF-ASSESSMENT OF ORAL CONDITIONS AND ORAL CANCER SELF-EXAMINATION

OBJECTIVES: *The reader will be able to*

1. Discuss the value of helping the patient become a self-assessor.
2. Assist the patient in:
   a. Identifying general anatomic structures of the oral cavity
   b. Recognizing existing conditions—restorations, stain, and obvious decay (caries)
   c. Identifying dental plaque
   d. Recognizing the signs of inflammation
3. Explain the importance of the oral cancer self-examination in the early detection of oral cancer.
4. Identify the predisposing factors that contribute to the risk of oral cancer and patients who are "at risk."
5. List the structures to be examined and the technique of examining each structure.
6. Develop approaches for explaining and teaching the oral cancer self-examination to a variety of patients.
7. Anticipate responses patients may have to be being introduced to the oral cancer self-examination and appropriate clinician responses.
8. Integrate the teaching of the oral cancer self-examination into patients' treatment plans as is appropriate.
9. Describe the signs and symptoms of oral cancer.

GUIDED SELF-ASSESSMENT OF ORAL CONDITIONS

The self-assessing patient is knowledgeable about basic oral conditions, understands his/her individual health needs, and accepts responsibility for his/her dental care. The objective of the self-assessment exercise is to directly involve the patient in an educational experience that will assist him/her in appreciating his/her oral status. When dental needs are understood, the patient is able to participate in decision making for dental care. This leads to accepting the shared responsibility of oral health care with the dental team.

Patient education through self-assessment assists the patient in becoming a knowledgeable dental care consumer. For many people, going to a dentist is much like taking a car to a mechanic. When the consumer has little knowledge of what needs fixing, he/she is often helpless in evaluating the me-chanic's decision for repairs. The cost of parts and labor is often shocking and frustrating, especially if the car develops a similar problem in a few months. A person might then try a new mechanic. So it goes, until the repairs solve the problem or a new car is purchased. A similar lack of knowledge about oral health may cause persons to pursue dentistry in this piecemeal fashion. Perhaps as patients become more aware of their oral conditions and more comfortable with modern preventive dental care, avoidance of comprehensive dentistry will be reduced.

Some professionals are reluctant to inform the public about medical/dental conditions. Primarily they fear that a little knowledge can be dangerous. Several years ago when breast self-examination was introduced, many thought that the public would be unwilling to perform the examination or would not do it properly. An additional concern was that scores of women would experience needless worry and consult the physician for every irregularity in tissue, which often occurs during the monthly hormonal cycle. More seriously, it was thought that a patient, fearing the worst, might actually delay professional evaluation. Some or all of these behaviors probably do occur, but the number of women's lives lengthened or saved by early identification and treatment is clearly significant. The oral cancer self-examination, discussed later in this chapter, is overcoming similar skepticism as it is being increasingly taught in educational institutions, clinics, and dental offices.

Before the topic of self-examination for oral cancer is addressed, it is our feeling that a basic awareness of oral conditions should be discussed with the patient. The idea of an examination for cancer may be too threatening to the patient to start with.

The guided self-assessment is designed to help the patient become familiar with the normal structures of the oral cavity and the current conditions of his/her mouth. The patient will become aware of general dental terms, the names of teeth, and major oral structures (Brand and Isselhard, 1977; Morgan, 1976).

The self-assessment of oral conditions is designed to be simple. Specific conditions are focused on by means of questions. The hygienist leads the exercise in the initial experience by asking the questions, but a handout for the patient to take home is helpful. The handout outlines the steps for the patient to perform, states questions, and provides general information about the structures to be viewed.

Learning is a cumulative experience. It will probably be necessary for most patients to complete the self-assessment exercise several times. At follow-up and recall visits, reviewing the exercise can occur quite naturally as the hygienist inspects the oral cavity, performs the intraoral and extraoral palpations, and provides treatment for the teeth and tissues. As the patient becomes comfortable with dental terminology and becomes aware of oral conditions, participation in the visit through questions and cooperation usually increases.

Not all patients will be enthusiastic about the self-assessment instruction. Some people would rather not know what their oral health is and do not wish to accept responsibility for dental care. In these instances the education process could be included in regular chairside instruction. The hygienist should be considerate of the patient's values and needs and should not expect the same response from all patients.

In this chapter a general format for self-assessment is presented. Each practitioner, whether in a private office or clinic, will develop a particular style suited to the needs of the practice. The entire process of educating a patient is one with immense latitude. The interest and ability demonstrated by the patient will affect the hygienist's judgment in this matter.

Preparation

A few moments should be taken to explain to the patient the design of the self-assessment exercise. The patient should understand that recognition of specific structures and conditions of the oral cavity that are normal for him/her is the goal (Fig. 19-1).

The tray setup includes a flashlight, a tongue depressor or mouth mirror, and a few gauze squares (Fig. 19-2).

Both the hygienist and the patient should wash their hands. The patient is then seated in front of a mirror. A large hand mirror can be used also.

Sequence. The patient is directed to observe the following structures. The listed questions are asked, or others are substituted that may be more appropriate for the patient. Often the patient will begin to make inquires that will guide the exercise. The following sequence is presented as the hygienist's dialogue.

1. First let's look at your face in general.
   a. Compare the relationship of one side of your face with the other. What do you observe about symmetry?
   b. Place your fingertips in front of your ears, and open and close your mouth. Feel the jaw move. Do you hear any clicking or popping?
   c. Look at your lips. Note the texture and color of the skin. Are there any signs of irritation (dryness, cracking at corners, blisters)?

This aspect of the self-assessment exercise allows the hygienist and patient to focus on the general function of the teeth in relation to the structure and appearance of the face. As the temporomandibular joint is pointed out, other topics such as the movements of the jaw and mastication can be addressed (Brand and Isselhard, 1977).

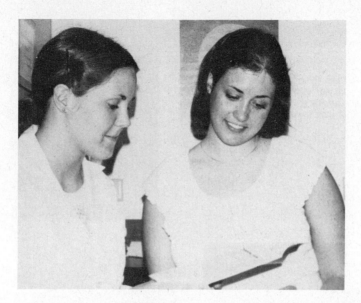

Fig. 19-1. Hygienist and patient reviewing self-assessment pamphlet.

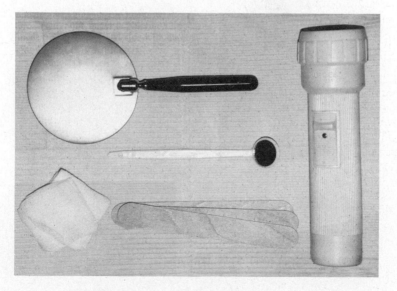

Fig. 19-2. Tray setup for guided self-assessment exercise.

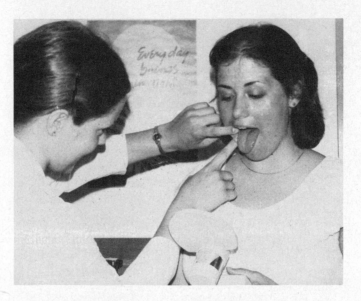

Fig. 19-3. Patient learns about her tongue, its surfaces, and types of papillae.

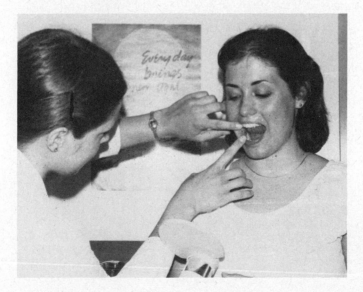

Fig. 19-4. First of several muscle attachments in oral cavity is pointed out—lingual frenum.

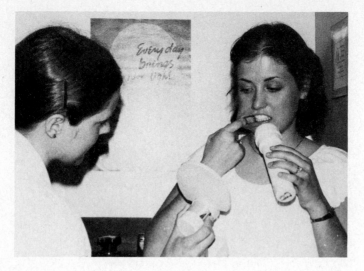

Fig. 19-5. With a light and mirror, patient inspects inside of cheek. Soft tissue characteristics are often noted in this area.

2. Now let's look into the oral cavity at your tongue. The tongue has three surfaces: the dorsum (top), ventrum (bottom), and lateral borders (sides).
   a. What color is your tongue?
   b. As you look over your tongue, do you see any changes in its texture or consistency (Fig. 19-3)?
   c. Lift your tongue up. Do you see where the tongue attaches to the floor of the mouth? This is called the lingual frenum (Fig. 19-4).
   d. Look for veins on the dorsum of the tongue and salivary glands under the tongue on the floor of the mouth.

At this point there is an opportunity to discuss the papilla of the tongue, taste buds, coatings, and perhaps the need to brush the tongue. The floor of the mouth has many other structures that the hygienist may wish to point out if the patient is curious (Brand and Isselhard, 1977; Katz, McDonald, and Stookey, 1979).

3. You can use the flashlight to look at the inside of your cheeks and lips. These structures are called the buccal mucosa and labial mucosa, respectively (Fig. 19-5).
   a. Describe the color and texture of the buccal mucosa.
   b. Do you see any signs of irritation (i.e., cheek biting)?
   c. Feel the buccal mucosa across from the molars of the upper teeth. Located here is Stensen's duct, or the opening of the parotid salivary gland.

d. Run your finger along the inside of your lips, or pull your lips out. Can you identify the labial frenum that attaches the lips to the dental arches?

This segment of the self-assessment exercise provides an opportunity for the hygienist to point out the linea alba, Fordyce granules, pigmentation, lichen planus, or other structures that may be characteristic for this patient.

4. Now look at your palate and the back of your throat.
   a. You have both a soft and a hard palate. Can you see and feel the difference between them?
   b. Some people have an extra bit of bone in the midline of the hard palate. This is called a palatal torus.
   c. Can you identify the uvula? This is the flap of tissue at the posterior of the soft palate.
   d. Point out your tonsils or the lack of them as you look toward the back of your throat. The tonsils lie between the anterior and posterior pillars.
   e. Does the back wall of your throat look red or feel irritated when you swallow?
5. Your teeth are the next structures to look at. The teeth sit in the alveolar bone of the dental arches. The upper arch is called the maxilla, and the lower arch is the mandible. There are four kinds of teeth: incisors, cuspids or canines, bicuspids or premolars, and molars (Fig. 19-6).
   a. Can you identify these kinds of teeth in your mouth?
   b. Are you missing any teeth?

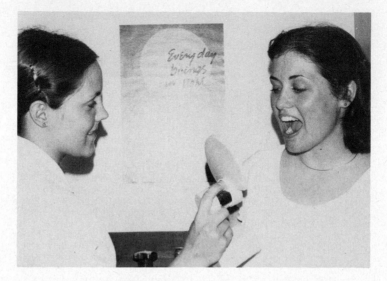

Fig. 19-6. Hygienist acquaints patient with names of teeth, noting characteristics of each, and discusses restorations, caries process, and dental plaque.

    c. Are any of your teeth discolored or stained?
    d. How many of your teeth have fillings (restorations)?
    e. Do you know what kinds of materials were used to fill, repair, or replace the teeth?
    f. Do you see or feel any obvious breakdown in structure of your teeth or the restorations?
    g. Dental plaque is the white or yellowish coating of bacteria and food particles that clings to the teeth especially at the gum line. Do you see any plaque on your teeth?
    h. Look at your teeth when they bite together. This shows your occlusion.
6. Finally, let's consider your gum tissue. The tissue that surrounds the teeth and covers the bone is called the gingiva. The gingiva fits around the neck of the tooth like a turtleneck collar. This collar area is called the sulcus. Plaque, which is a mass of bacteria, especially likes to collect here (Fig. 19-7).
    a. Describe the appearance of the gingiva around your teeth.
    b. Do you see any signs of inflammation (redness, swelling)?
    c. Does the gingiva feel tender?
    d. Does it ever bleed when you brush?
    e. Dry the gingiva off. Do you see firm tissue that looks like the skin of an orange peel? This is called stippled tissue.
    f. Does the gingiva change in appearance or consistency as it nears the labial mucosa? This is the mucogingival junction.

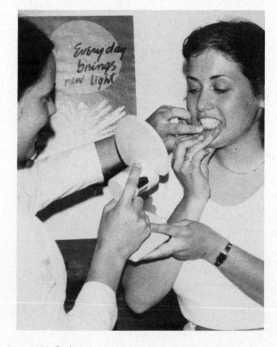

Fig. 19-7. Patient looks closely at teeth and tissue to identify plaque and other characteristics of soft tissue (e.g., gingival unit, inflammation).

As the teeth and gingiva are viewed, the hygienist has the opportunity to inform the patient about restorative procedures such as prosthetics, endodontics, and orthodontics. The question about stains introduces the subject of extrinsic and intrinsic staining factors. Assessing the gingiva, identifying plaque, and checking for inflammation create interest and the basis for further preventive education, including instructions for improving home care methods (Katz, McDonald, and Stookey, 1979).

An appropriate comment at the end of the self-assessment experience would be, "This completes the self-assessment exercise. May I answer any other questions you may have about the structures or conditions in your mouth?"

Conclusion

The guided self-assessment will probably require 30 minutes to 1 hour to complete, depending on the interest and participation of the patient. In the treatment sequence, it is helpful if this occurs prior to the case presentation. After performing the self-assessment exercise, the patient is familiar with his/her oral conditions and is probably ready to focus on treatment needs.

If an entire appointment cannot be devoted to the self-assessment exercise, the same information can be presented gradually to the patient at recall appointments. When this is the case, it is helpful to make notes of what is discussed at each appointment to avoid repetition and to guide the presentation of new information.

When a patient is aware of his/her own normal conditions, looking for changes in the oral cavity as part of the oral cancer self-examination is less difficult.

ORAL CANCER SELF-EXAMINATION

In the first portion of this chapter the guided self-assessment is described and recommended for all patients. Part of the rationale for the guided self-assessment is that educated, self-aware patients are more likely to be partners in care. Such patients will be more able to understand their oral conditions and needs and thus better appreciate necessary treatment.

Self-assessing patients are able to recognize the soft and hard tissue landmarks normal to their mouths. They are also able to recognize changes or out-of-the-ordinary, "abnormal" conditions. This ability is particularly important during another self-assessing exercise, the oral cancer self-examination. The oral cancer self-examination is a shorter, more specific examination that enables persons to inspect and palpate the soft tissues of the neck, face, and oral cavity to detect signs and symptoms of oral cancer. As mentioned earlier in the chapter, this examination is similar to the breast self-examination; both allow persons to examine parts of their bodies, in the privacy of their homes, at regular monthly intervals.

Incidence of oral cancer

It was estimated that in the United States in 1983 there would be 855,000 new cancer cases and 440,000 cancer deaths. Oral cancer, according to these estimates, would account for 27,000 of the new cases and for 9200 deaths in 1983 (American Cancer Society, 1982). Table 19-1 specifies the occurrence of oral cancer by site and sex. It was estimated that in 1983 oral cancer would account for 4% and 2% of all new cancer cases among men and women respectively, as well as 3% of cancer deaths among men and 1% of cancer deaths among

Table 19-1. Oral cancer estimates for 1983

Sites	Estimates, new cases			Estimates, deaths		
	Total	*Male*	*Female*	*Total*	*Male*	*Female*
Lip	4600	4100	500	175	150	25
Tongue	4900	3200	1700	2000	1400	600
Salivary glands, floor of mouth, other in mouth	9800	5800	4000	2775	1850	925
Pharynx	7800	5500	2300	4200	2900	1300
Total oral cancer	27,100	18,600	8500	9150	6300	2850

American Cancer Society, 1982. Facts and figures 1983. New York: American Cancer Society.

women. The overall 5-year survival rate for oral cancer is about 40%, but this varies according to site, from 22% for cancer of the pharynx to 84% for cancer of the lip (American Cancer Society, 1982). In other words, of the 27,000 persons estimated to be newly affected by oral cancer in 1983, 40%, or 10,800, will be alive in 1988 (barring deaths from other, unrelated causes). A person who survives for 5 years after the cancer was first diagnosed and treated is then, usually, considered to be cured.

Five-year survival rates for oral cancer are increased if the oral cancer is detected early (i.e., the lesion detected is less than 1.5 cm in size). Memorial Hospital for Cancer and Allied Diseases reported in an American Cancer Society publication (1975) a 5-year survival rate of 59% for oral cancers detected early as compared with a 17% rate for cancers that were greater than 3.0 cm in size when detected. Thus early detection, through regular self- and professional examinations, does save lives.

It is likely that the reader knows someone who has been affected by cancer—oral or another type. Cancer can be a devastating disease for the person as well as his/her family and friends. Many times, the treatments for cancer have very uncomfortable side effects. Certainly, anything that can minimize the extent of oral cancer and the necessary ensuing treatments is desirable. The oral cancer self-examination is one such procedure. By teaching patients this examination, the dental health professional will be helping patients minimize the effects of the cancer. In fact, the professional may even save lives.

Prevalence of oral cancer

Types. Approximately 96% of all oral malignancies are carcinomas (Silverman, 1981). A carcinoma is a malignancy arising from epithelial tissue. The other 4% of oral malignancies are sarcomas, lesions arising from other oral tissues (i.e., glands, muscles, nerves, blood, or lymph tissue) (Baker et al., 1973; Silverman, 1981). About 91% of all oral cancers are squamous cell carcinomas; thus control of squamous cell carcinomas is the primary objective in oral cancer efforts (Silverman, 1981). Determination of the type of malignancy is done through a biopsy. Not all oral lesions are malignant, and the only way to determine if a lesion is malignant is through a biopsy. Therefore, if a lesion is detected in a patient's mouth, it can only be considered suspicious until a biopsy has been completed.

Oral cancer can be localized, or it can spread (metastasize) through the blood, nerve, or lymph systems. Once oral cancer has metastasized, the treatment is much more involved, usually requiring extensive surgery and/or radiation, hormonal, or chemotherapy (American Cancer Society, 1982). The smaller the cancer is when detected, the more likely it is to be localized rather than metastasized. Once again, the importance of early detection is apparent.

Age. Oral cancer is a disease that tends to affect persons over the age of 45, with 60 being the average age of persons affected. In fact, about 95% of all oral cancers occur in persons over the age of 40 (Silverman, 1981). The "over-65" population is increasing; thus more and more people are at risk for oral cancer because of their age. The older population has the greatest need for learning the oral cancer self-examination. Consider though, that many older people (wrongly) do not seek routine dental care, because they may have dentures; they may not be able to afford care because of limited financial resources; they may be homebound because of illness or disability; or they may be confined to a nursing home. Certainly, teaching the oral cancer self-examination to older persons coming to a dental office or clinic should become standard procedure. Other approaches could be developed to reach persons who do not seek routine dental care. Marinelli (1983) reported that the well elderly living in a suburb of New York City identified an important role of the dental hygienist as teaching elderly patients to care for their mouths, including performing self-examinations. Perhaps it would be possible to teach the oral cancer self-examination in community centers frequented by the over-65 population.

Sex and race. Men are more likely to develop oral cancer than women by a ratio of 2.4 to 1 (American Cancer Society, 1982; Silverman, 1981). (The ratio used to be much greater, but because of the increased use of tobacco by women, it is believed that the ratio has decreased.) But, as Silverman (1981) noted, women outnumber men in the over-65 age group by 45%. Although men are twice as likely to be affected by oral cancer overall, a greater number of women are affected in the over-65 age group.

The incidence of cancer is higher among blacks than among whites. For example, the overall cancer incidence rate for blacks increased by 27%, whereas for whites it increased by 17% (American Cancer Society, 1982). Blacks have a higher oropharyngeal cancer rate than do other racial groups (Silverman, 1981). Another type of cancer, nasopharyngeal, is 20 to 30 times more prevalent in Chinese persons than in whites (Silverman, 1982). These examples show that the incidence of cancer rates and types varies among races. It is unclear if the difference can be accounted for on a genetic basis. It is more likely that the differences have to do with life-styles, exposure to carcinogens in the living and working environments, and cultural beliefs about health care (American Cancer Society, 1982; Silverman, 1981).

Site. The most common site for oral cancer is the tongue for both men and women (Silverman, 1981). Previously the lip was the most common cancer site for woman, but the increased use of protective lip agents during exposure to the sun has probably decreased the incidence of lip cancer (Silverman, 1981; Silverman and Galante, 1970).

Predisposing factors

Age has already been mentioned as a predisposing factor to oral cancer. The use of tobacco (smoking cigarettes, pipes, or cigars or chewing) seems to be the other major predisposing factor to cancer. Others include excessive use of alcohol, chronic irritation of the oral mucosa from a poorly fitting appliance or restoration, repeated trauma to the mouth, and overexposure to the weather (i.e., the sun or wind) (American Cancer Society, 1982).

Thus, considering the predisposing factors and the incidence of cancer, the oral cancer self-examination is indicated for persons over the age of 40, particularly those who use tobacco. Any other predisposing factor should be considered when the clinician is deciding whether the oral cancer self-examination should be taught. For example, if a 65-year-old black man who smoked a pack of cigarettes a day were being treated, teaching the oral cancer self-examination would be in order. If a 45-year-old white woman who smoked occasionally, drank alcohol excessively, and had a chronically irritated buccal mucosa from cheek biting were being treated, teaching the self-examination would also be a priority for her. Teaching the oral cancer self-examination could be included in the treatment

sequence but would not be a priority for a 20-year-old man who did not use alcohol or tobacco.

The above examples point out a possible dilemma for the clinician; namely, given the limited amount of time available during an appointment, should the guided self-assessment be taught before the oral cancer self-examination? This is a decision each clinician will have to make given a particular patient's circumstances. Ideally, the guided self-assessment should be performed, because it teaches the patient what is normal in his/her mouth. But, if a patient is a high risk for oral cancer, such as the first two patients described in the previous paragraph, the oral cancer self-examination should take precedence or be integrated with the guided self-assessment and receive special emphasis.

Signs and symptoms of oral cancer

Any swelling, red or white patches, or sores that do not heal within 2 weeks are considered suspicious. The American Cancer Society (1975) states:

Early signs of oral cancer occurring on the floor of the mouth, soft palate, and ventral or lateral tongue include red velvety (erythroplastic) or white (leukoplastic) patches. Any asymmetric, firm nodal enlargement or mass is a late sign and strongly suggests cancer, as does ulceration, fissures, or change in color or consistency.

As was stated previously, oral cancer must be diagnosed through a biopsy.

Oral cancer self-examination: teaching approach

The first time the patient performs the examination, the clinician can guide the patient through the steps of the examination and confirm the patient's findings. Ideally, the patient should sit in front of a large mirror, and the clinician should stand behind the patient or sit at the patient's side; from either of these positions, both the patient and the clinician can see into the patient's mouth. At the beginning of the examination, it may be helpful to remind the patient that he/she is examining the face, neck, and mouth to become familiar with the normal forms and structures so that any changes can be noticed during subsequent examinations. Also, the clinician will be helping the patient identify the normal structures within his/her mouth. The patient should follow the outline or pamphlet that he/she will be using at home and should perform as much of the examination on his/her own as possible. This is a difficult balance to strike because the clinician is playing the dual role of teaching the procedure and fostering some independence in the patient. Ultimately, at the end of the session, the patient will have learned the examination and be confident enough to perform the examination at home at regular intervals. In addition, the clinician has the challenging task of motivating the patient to want to perform the examination at regular intervals. The approaches for motivating a patient to perform the oral cancer self-examination are the same as the approaches for motivating a patient to perform home care procedures. In this situation, however, the potential benefits to the patient are even greater—his/her life.

The oral cancer self-examination is composed of several steps in which the face, neck, and mouth are examined (Atterbury, 1979; Burzynski, Moore, and DeJean, 1970; Carl et al., 1982; Engelman and Schackner, 1966; Glass, Alba, and Wheatley, 1975; Olszewski, 1976). A pamphlet such as *Early Detection of Oral Cancer May Save Your Life,* published by the American Cancer Society (Eastern Great Lakes, 1976), can be given to the patient. Many dental and dental auxiliary schools also have pamphlets outlining the steps of the oral cancer self-examination that can be used by the patient.

While the patient is learning to perform the examination, the clinician should point out the normal structures in each area and review with the patient the kinds of changes that should be noted.

At the completion of the examination, it should be emphasized to the patient that the earlier any changes are brought to the attention of the dentist the better. Any change or lesion that is present for 2 weeks should be checked by the dentist, waiting even until the next 6-month checkup may be too risky. It may be helpful to reassure the patient that the dentist would prefer to be asked to check a thousand changes in the patient's mouth that turn out to be normal rather than not being asked to check the one change that may lead to cancer.

The following outline for the lay person describes one way a dental hygienist can teach oral cancer self-examination (Atterbury, 1979; Burzynski, Moore, and DeJean, 1970; Eastern Great Lakes, 1976; Engleman and Schackner, 1966, Glass, Alba and Wheatley, 1975).

Oral cancer self-examination: outline for the lay person

This outline is to be used as a guide when you perform the oral cancer self-examination. The outline lists each of the areas to be examined and the kinds of changes that may be significant and should be brought to the dentist's attention. In general, you are looking for any of the following changes:

1. Any sores on the face, neck, or mouth that do not heal within 2 weeks
2. Any white, red, or dark patches in the mouth
3. Any swelling, lump, bump, or growth
4. Repeated bleeding for no apparent reason
5. Pain or loss of feeling in any area of the face, neck, or mouth

A mirror and good lighting are needed for the examination. Following are the steps of the oral cancer self-examination.

1. *Facial symmetry.* Look at yourself in the mirror. Both sides of your face and neck should be the same size, shape, and form. No person's face is absolutely symmetric, but the two sides are basically the same. Any swellings, lumps, bumps, or growths that appear on one side of your face should be noted; if they appear on both sides of your face, they are probably normal (Fig. 19-8).
2. *Face.* Look at the skin on your face and neck. You are looking for any changes in skin color, moles that have changed, lumps, or sores. If you wear glasses, take them off and examine the areas covered by them—the bridge of the nose. Finally palpate your face by gently pressing fingers from each hand against all areas of your face. By palpating both sides of your face at the same time, you will notice any differences between one side of your face and the other (Fig. 19-9).
3. *Side of neck.* With fingers of both hands, palpate both sides of your neck at the same time. As with your face, you are feeling for any lumps, bumps, or swellings that appear on one side of your neck but not on the other (Fig. 19-10).
4. *Center of neck.* Gently place your fingers against your "Adam's apple" and swallow; it should move when you swallow. Then grasp your Adam's apple and gently move it from side to side (Fig. 19-11). Once again check for any lumps or bumps, and note any hoarseness that does not clear up within 2 weeks.

Any dentures or partial dentures should be removed at this point.

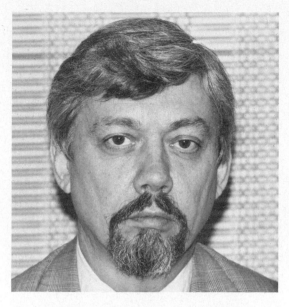

Fig. 19-8. Examining facial symmetry visually.

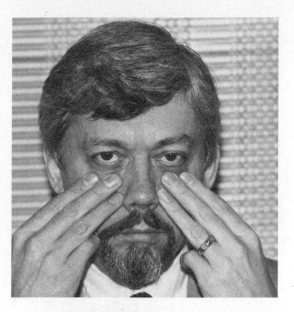

Fig. 19-9. Palpating face with both hands.

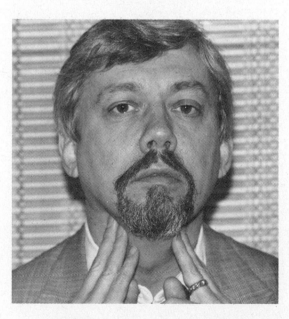

Fig. 19-10. Palpating neck with both hands.

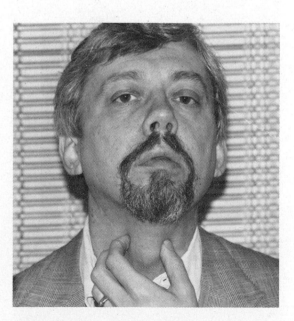

Fig. 19-11. Palpating center of neck (''Adam's apple'').

5. *Lips*. Pull your lower lip down and look for any sores or color changes. Gently squeeze your lip with your fingers to feel for any swellings, lumps, bumps, or tenderness. Repeat this procedure for your upper lip (Fig. 19-12).

6. *Cheek*. Pull back your cheek with your fingers so you can see the tissue inside your cheek. Look for any color changes—red, white, or dark areas. Place your thumb on the outside of your cheek and your index finger inside your cheek, and gently squeeze your cheek. Note any swellings, lumps, or bumps. Repeat this procedure for your other cheek (Fig. 19-13).

7. *Roof of mouth*. Tilt your head back and look at the roof of your mouth. Note any color changes—white, red, or dark areas—or any lumps. With your index finger gently press against the roof of your mouth to feel any lumps, bumps, or swellings (Fig. 19-14).

8. *Gums*. Look at your gums for any color changes—red, white or dark areas—lumps, bumps, or growths. Are there any sores that have not healed for longer than 14 days? Are there any areas that bleed without cause (Fig. 19-15)?

9. *Tongue and floor of mouth*. Place the tip of your tongue to the roof of your mouth. Look at the underside of your tongue and the floor of your mouth for any color changes, lumps, bumps, or growths. Palpate the floor of your mouth by gently pressing your finger against the floor area to feel any lumps, bumps, or growths. Extend your tongue and look at the top side of your tongue. Using a gauze square, grasp the tip of your tongue and gently pull your tongue to one side. Look at the side of your tongue and palpate your tongue. Note any color changes, lumps, bumps, or sores that have not healed. Repeat this procedure on the other side of your tongue (Figs. 19-16 to 19-19).

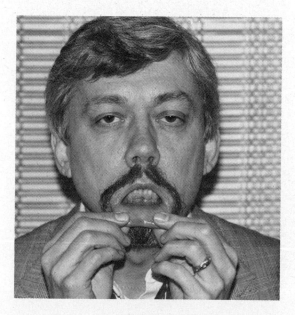

Fig. 19-12. Examining inner surface of lips.

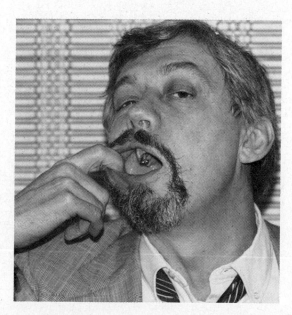

Fig. 19-13. Examining inner surface of cheek.

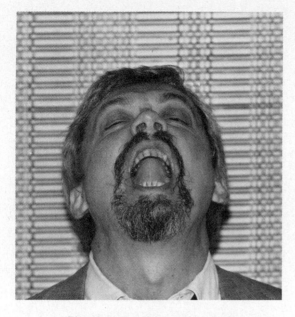

Fig. 19-14. Examining roof of mouth.

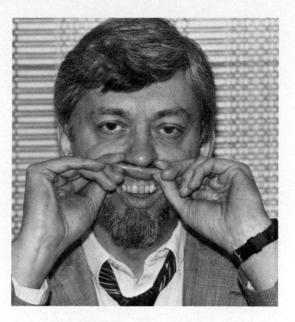

Fig. 19-15. Lifting lip to examine gums.

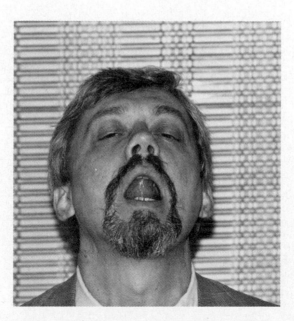

Fig. 19-16. Raising tongue to examine its undersurface and floor of mouth.

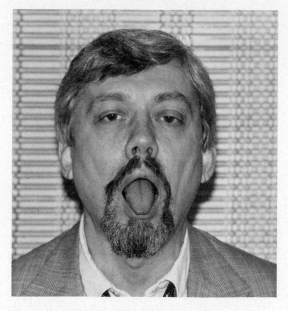

Fig. 19-17. Examining upper surface of tongue.

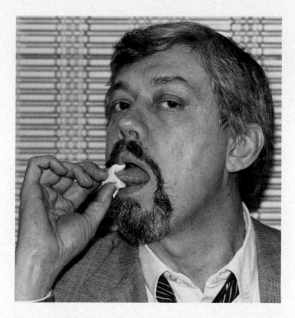

Fig. 19-18. Grasping tip of tongue with gauze and examining side of tongue.

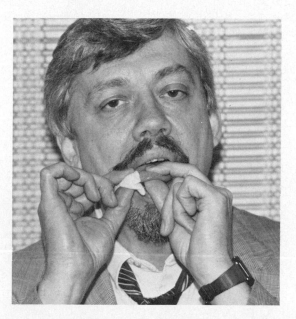

Fig. 19-19. Palpating tongue.

Summary

At the completion of the examination, the clinician can ask if there are any questions about the procedure. This is also a good time to ask patients if they have any concerns or hesitations about performing the examination. The clinician should be sensitive to patients' responses; some patients may express their concerns about actually finding oral cancer. Perhaps the patients' fears can be acknowledged and discussed as is appropriate. The patients should be encouraged to perform the examination routinely and to call the office as needed.

CONCLUSION

Teaching the guided self-assessment and oral cancer self-examination are important preventive adjuncts in dental hygiene treatment. The procedures and findings of the examination will need to be reviewed with patients at subsequent visits to ensure proper completion of the examinations. These examinations benefit both the patients and the dental health professional. The patients become knowledgeable about their oral conditions and able to detect oral cancer in its early stages. The professional is able to work with patients who are truly partners in care.

ACTIVITIES

1. Using the general format presented in the chapter, identify and discuss associated topics that the hygienist might address during the self-assessment exercise.
2. Individually or in small groups, create a guided self-assessment exercise with a patient handout for use in the clinic.
3. View a videotape of the self-assessment exercise or observe an actual encounter. Discuss the hygienist's and patient's participation in creating a valuable educational experience.
4. Perform the guided self-assessment for a lab partner or patient. (This exercise may be used as an introduction for beginning dental hygiene students. When the beginning student is paired with a senior student, this exercise is an opportunity for sharing information and experience, as well as helping the student become a self-assessor.)
5. Compare and contrast the instructions for the oral cancer self-examination presented in this chapter with the instructions for the oral cancer self-examination given in the American Cancer Society's pamphlet. Early Detection of Oral Cancer May Save Your Life (Eastern Great Lakes, 1976).

6. Role play teaching the oral cancer self-examination in each of the following situations:
   a. The patient's father has recently died of cancer, and she is obviously upset as soon as you mention the word "cancer."
   b. The patient is a 35-year-old man who smokes one pack of cigarettes each day. When you suggest performing the oral cancer self-examination, the patient says, "Cancer! I'm as healthy as a bull!"
7. Discuss the following situations:
   a. You have been asked by a local nursing home to teach the staff and some of the residents to perform the oral cancer self-examination. How would you organize this task?
   b. You are teaching a 65-year-old woman the oral cancer self-examination, and during the examination you notice a lesion on her tongue, which you strongly suspect may be cancerous. How would you handle this situation with the patient and the dentist?
8. Contact a representative from the American Cancer Society to speak to your group about cancer and to familiarize the group with the American Cancer Society's pamphlets and publications.
9. Review the oral cancer self-examination, and identify the normal structures in each area that could be shown to the patient. This would be a method of combining the oral cancer examination with the oral self-assessment.
10. Discuss the appropriateness of:
   a. Encouraging patients who use tobacco to abandon the practice.
   b. Health care professionals using tobacco despite the known association between tobacco use and cancer.

REVIEW QUESTIONS

1. State the purpose of the self-assessment exercise.
2. Why might a patient be reluctant to participate in the self-assessment exercise?
3. How will the patient's knowledge of the following items be useful in further dental treatment?
   a. Dental terminology
   b. Anatomic structures
   c. Presence of dental plaque
   d. Signs of inflammation
4. Why is the oral cancer self-examination an important part of the prevention regimen?
5. List the structures to be examined by the patient during the oral cancer self-examination.
6. What are the dental hygienist's goals for the patient who is learning to perform the oral cancer self-examination?

REFERENCES

American Cancer Society. 1975. The challenge of oral cancer. New York: American Cancer Society.

American Cancer Society. 1978. Facts of oral cancer. New York: American Cancer Society.

American Cancer Society. 1982. Facts and figures 1983. New York: American Cancer Society.

Atterbury, R.A. 1979. Self-examination of paraoral tissues for detection of early oral cancer. Dent. Surv. **55**:18.

Baker, H.W., et al. 1973. Oral cancer. New York: American Cancer Society.

Brand, R.W., and Isselhard, D.E. 1977. Anatomy of orofacial structures. St. Louis: The C.V. Mosby Co.

Browne, R.M., et al. 1977. Etiological factors in oral squamous cell carcinoma. Community Dent. Oral Epidemiol. **5**:301.

Burzynski, N.J., Moore, C., and DeJean, E. 1970. Basic steps in mouth-throat examination for cancer detection. J. Am. Dent. Assoc. **81**:932.

Carl, W., et al. 1982. Early detection of oral cancer: another aspect of preventive dentistry. Quintessence Int. **13**:1179.

Chesko, E.E. 1979. Detecting early oral cancer: the dentist's role is crucial. Oral Health **69**:42.

Dafoe, B.R. 1977. Dental self-assessment, module 2. Philadelphia: University of Pennsylvania, Department of Dental Hygiene.

Eastern Great Lakes Head and Neck Cancer Control Network and Department of Oral Medicine. 1976. Early detection of oral cancer may save your life. New York: American Cancer Society.

Engelman, M.A., and Schackner, J.S. 1966. Oral cancer examination procedure. Poughkeepsie, N.Y.: St. Francis Hospital.

International Dental Federation: Commission on Dental Research. 1971. Early detection of oral cancer, London: Federation Dentaire Internationale.

Glass, R.T., Abla, M., and Wheatley, J. 1975. Teaching self-examination of the head and neck: another aspect of preventive dentistry. J. Am. Dent. Assoc. **90**:1265.

Grabau, J.C., et al. 1978. A public education program in self-examination for orofacial cancer. J. Am. Dent. Assoc. **96**:480.

Hall, G.L., et al. 1980. Education in early detection of oral squamous cell carcinoma: a community outreach program. J. Am. Dent. Assoc. **100**:362.

Hill, M.W., et al. 1982. Influence of aging on oral cancer. Dent. Hyg. **56**(8):26.

Katz, S., McDonald, J., and Stookey, G. 1979. Preventive dentistry in action. Upper Montclair, N.J.: D.C.P. Publishing.

Laskin, D. 1978. The pitfalls of self-examination (editorial). J. Oral Surg. **36**:587.

Lumerman, H., et al. 1982. The oral soft tissue examination in the detection of oral cancer and other soft tissue lesions. N.Y. J. Dent. **52**:261.

Marinelli, R.D. 1983. Oral health care for the elderly: the role of dental hygienists. Dent. Hyg. **56**(10):14.

Morgan, P.A. 1976. Guided self-assessment of oral structures and conditions, module 2. Philadelphia: University of Pennsylvania, Department of Dental Hygiene.

Olszewski, V. April 1976. The role of the dental hygienist in oral cancer detection. Dent. Hyg. **50**:169.

Shugar, M.A., et al. 1982. Technique for routine screening for carcinoma of the base of the tongue. J. Am. Dent. Assoc. **104**:646.

Silverman, S., Jr, editor. 1981. Oral cancer. New York: American Cancer Society.

Silverman, S., Jr., and Galante, M. 1970. Oral cancer. San Francisco: University of California.

20   NUTRITIONAL SELF-ASSESSMENT AND MODIFICATIONS

OBJECTIVES: *The reader will be able to*

1. Describe the role of dietary assessment and planning in dental hygiene care.
2. Briefly describe the ways in which diet can affect the overall health of the body and specifically of the oral cavity.
3. Identify the basic role of each of the following nutrients in the health of the patient:
   a. Carbohydrates
   b. Proteins
   c. Lipids
   d. Vitamins
   e. Minerals
   f. Water
4. Describe the usefulness and limitations of the Recommended Dietary Allowances (RDAs) and the four food groups in assessing a person's diet and in recommending modifications.
5. Describe how carbohydrates and plaque promote caries.
6. Explain how diet has been shown to influence cancer formation.
7. Explain strategies for assessing a patient's diet using a 1-day diet review, or a 3-day or 7-day diary.
8. Conduct a dietary assessment for a patient, using the self-assessment strategy.
9. Given a variety of completed dietary assessments, assist each patient in determining which components of the diet could be changed, why they should be modified, and how the modification could be accomplished.
10. Identify several environmental factors that affect whether modifications are likely to occur following the self-assessment session.
11. Conduct a follow-up, reinforcement session as part of the dental care to evaluate the progress the patient is making and to assist the patient in identifying alternative approaches to diet modification.

The growing knowledge and awareness of the relationship between good dietary habits and good general health have brought nutritional assessment and dietary counseling into focus as essential components of dental hygiene care. Many of the effects of dietary habits are clearly reflected in the oral cavity, since poor nutrition has negative effects on the hard and soft oral tissues as well as on the person's general well-being. Dental hygienists see their patients more frequently and more regularly than do most other health care providers. Thus the hygienist has more opportunity to detect dietary problems and help the patient adopt changes (Poplin, 1981). The hygienist needs to know how to assess a patient's diet, what changes are indicated by the results, and when a patient's nutritional problems require the expertise of a dietitian.

Private dental practices that focus on prevention include nutritional assessment for new patients, with periodic review at recall intervals for established patients in the practice. Other sites, such as hospitals, nursing homes, day care centers, and other community-based settings include nutritional counseling as a significant part of the overall program to improve general and oral health.

Any dental professional who will be assessing patients' diets and helping patients identify changes needs a complete course in nutrition, a good grounding in communication and basic counseling skills, and supervised clinical experience with a range of patient cases. This can be accomplished as part of the educational preparation with clinic patients. This chapter provides only a survey of basic nutrition and an introduction to the philosophy of nutritional assessment and patient-centered dietary counseling.

For clinicians who understand the basics of proper nutrition in general and in oral health in particular and who include a dietary focus in their everyday clinical care, a dietary assessment for *every patient* is the best way to ensure that the focus is established and maintained.

The assessment can be a routine component of the overall assessment phase of dental hygiene care and can serve as the essential means for identifying patients for whom simple dietary counseling is necessary and those patients who may need referral to a dietitian or physician. It may also identify those patients whose diets are well within normal limits and who do not need modifications. The critical point, as with the gathering of all other assessment data, is that the "assumption" of need no longer determines how dietary or nutritional counseling is planned into care. Assessment information can help both the patient and the dental hygienist arrive at a well-informed decision about the need to proceed with further discussions of diet.

IMPORTANCE OF DIET IN GENERAL AND ORAL HEALTH

A well-worn, yet appropriate, cliche is "We are what we eat." Dietary patterns dictate how well the body grows and functions. Failure to consume appropriate amounts of carbohydrates, lipids, proteins, vitamins, minerals, and water can result in general fatigue, dysfunction, and disease (Katz, McDonald, and Stookey, 1979; Williams, 1982).

The first three nutrients—carbohydrates, proteins, and lipids—provide calories for the body. Most of the body's energy is derived from *carbohydrates*. They make up a major portion of most diets, since they are reasonably inexpensive, easily assimilated, and, frequently, quite palatable (Nizel, 1981; Williams, 1982).

Carbon, oxygen, and hydrogen are the three elements that make up carbohydrates. The simplest form of a carbohydrate is a monosaccharide (or simple sugar), such as glucose, fructose, or galactose. Disaccharides are double sugars made up of two of the simple sugars. Sucrose, lactose, and maltose are disaccharides. The most complex carbohydrates, polysaccharides, are made up of several units of one type of monosaccharide. Starch, dextrins, cellulose, pectins, and glycogen are examples of polysaccharides (Williams, 1982). Energy becomes available for use when complex carbohydrates, such as sucrose, lactose, and starch, are broken down to their simplest form (monosaccharides) and then are metabolized in the cells to form carbon dioxide and water with an accompanying release of energy taking place (Nizel, 1981; Williams, 1982). "Metabolism may be defined as the sum of the physical and chemical processes in a living organism by which energy is made available for the functioning of the organism and by which protoplasm, the basic substance of cells and tissues, is produced, maintained, or broken down" (Williams, 1982).

Carbohydrates serve other functions in the body also. They are an essential component of nerve tissue and can facilitate the oxidation of fats. They contribute to the structural elements of the body, such as collagen. Because complex carbohydrates, such as whole grains, contribute to food bulk, they assist normal digestion and elimination (Nizel, 1981; Williams, 1982).

If too much carbohydrate is ingested, the excess is converted to fat and deposited in the body's adipose tissues. Therefore a large intake of carbohydrates can lead to obesity. Since fermentable carbohydrates are essential for the development of dental caries, frequent ingestion, particularly of retentive carbohydrates (e.g., caramels, hard candies), promotes tooth decay and is unhealthful (Firestone, 1982; Nizel, 1981; Randolph and Dennison, 1981).

Proteins supply energy for the body, but their more critical role is that of being an essential component of body tissues, enzymes, and hormones. Approximately 50% of dry body weight is protein. It plays a major role in the body's chemical reactions in digestion, assimilation, and metabolism. A lack of protein in the diet can then, obviously, have major consequences if it is lost from the system and not replaced (Nizel, 1981; Williams, 1982).

Lipids, a term used for *fats* and fatlike substances, also have important functions in the body.

They are integral components of cells and cell membranes. They are necessary for normal growth and skin health, and they carry the fat-soluble vitamins A, D, E, and K. Additionally, they lend flavor to food, and they are digested slowly, thus reducing hunger sensations. They make up approximately 40% of the American diet, a figure that is too high in light of recent findings linking fats and cancer (to be discussed later in this chapter). They are an excellent source of energy and provide 9 calories per gram, whereas carbohydrates and proteins provide only 4 calories per gram. Stored fats help insulate and cushion the body (Williams, 1982).

Caloric intake from these three nutrients should balance with calories expended in daily activities. If intake exceeds energy used, the excess will be converted to and stored as fat deposits, and weight gain will occur. Conversely, if intake is lower than output, weight loss will occur. Based on the multiple functions that these three nutrients serve, it should be apparent that none of them should be strictly eliminated from the diet. Moderation in all three with the total calories consumed balanced with energy used is a healthier approach to weight control.

Vitamins, in constrast to carbohydrates, proteins, and fats, do not supply energy. They function as catalysts or as coenzymes to regulate metabolism and to assist in forming body tissues. As mentioned earlier, vitamins A, D, E, and K are fat-soluble vitamins. Any excess is stored and can cause an adverse effect if this excess reaches critical levels. The other vitamins are water soluble and thus are not readily stored in the body. Excess amounts are largely excreted (Williams, 1982).

The *vitamin B complex* consists of 11 different vitamins. All of them are water soluble and are found primarily in liver and yeast. All but three (inositol, choline, and para-aminobenzoic acid) are classified as necessary nutrients for human beings. The complete metabolism of carbohydrates depends on the presence of adequate amounts of each of the six energy releasing vitamins: niacin, thiamin, riboflavin, pantothenic acid, vitamin B_6, and biotin (Nizel, 1981; Williams, 1982).

Folic acid and vitamin B_{12} are essential in the formation of red blood cells. Vitamin B_6 (pyridoxine) is an energy-releasing vitamin, and it serves as an antianemic coenzyme (Nizel, 1981).

Because the B complex vitamins are so interrelated, there is probably never a discrete deficiency of any one of them; rather there is a deficiency of many. Therefore, in instances in which there are symptoms of Vitamin B deficiency, a supplement that includes the range of B vitamins is indicated (Williams, 1982).

Ascorbic acid, *vitamin C,* is also a water soluble vitamin and is found in citrus fruits, red and green peppers, parsley, and turnip greens and other leafy vegetables. Vitamin C plays an essential role in collagen synthesis, and therefore it is an important component in tissue formation, particularly in wound healing. A person with a vitamin C deficiency often bruises easily because of capillary fragility. Vitamin C is involved in phagocytosis and acts as a detoxifying agent. Its presence can increase the resistance of traumatized tissues to infection. In addition, it influences the formation of hemoglobin (Williams, 1982). Appropriate amounts of the vitamin (60 to 100 mg daily) are obviously essential for health, including oral health. The soft tissue of the oral cavity, particularly the gingiva, is less susceptible to irritation and bleeding if vitamin C in proper dosages is ingested.

Vitamin C is often mislabeled the "sunshine vitamin," probably because of its association with orange juice and that industry's advertising approaches. However, the "sunshine vitamin" is *vitamin D* because of its formation in the presence of ultraviolet light. It is absorbed through the digestive tract as it is ingested in food and drink. Less dietary vitamin D is required in the diet if there is extensive exposure to sunshine (Williams, 1982). It is commonly added to milk to ensure a dietary source. Since vitamin D is best absorbed in the presence of calcium and phosphorus, milk is an ideal medium.

The primary function of vitamin D relates to the absorption and homeostasis of calcium. It distributes calcium and phosphorus ions within the boney matrix. Therefore it is critical to the proper formation of teeth and their supporting bone.

Vitamin D can be extremely toxic if taken in excess. Large amounts can cause intense calcification of bone, formation of renal calculi, and calcification of blood vessels. This is one instance where megavitamin doses can be extremely harmful (Nizel, 1981; Randolph, and Dennison, 1981; Williams, 1982).

Vitamin A is another vitamin that can result in severe toxicity if it is ingested in large amounts. Yellow skin and oral mucosa (carotenemia), anorexia, hyperirritability, skin lesions, bone, decalcification, and increased intracranial pressures are signs of toxicity (Williams, 1982).

In its proper dosage it is essential for proper vision, control of the differentiation of epithelium in mucus-secreting structures, bone remodeling, normal activity of the reproductive system, and the activity of the body's enzymes. Therefore it is important to the oral cavity with its plethora of mucus-secreting structures and as bone is remodeled to adjust to occlusal patterns and orthodontic treatment. Milk is fortified with vitamin A, and this vitamin is found in many vegetables (Williams, 1982).

Vitamin K is produced by microorganisms in the intestinal tract. It also occurs in green vegetables, egg yolk, and liver. It is essential for the formation of prothrombin and other clotting factors. Blood will not clot without prothrombin, thus the importance of vitamin K in health and disease. Since it is produced in the intestinal tract, it is not given as a supplement except in instances where pregnancy or an imminent surgical procedure indicates the need.

The last of the four fat-soluble vitamins is *vitamin E*. Its primary functions relate to reproduction and membrane stability, probably because of its role as an antioxidant in reducing the destruction of lipids carrying other fat-soluble vitamins and necessary fatty acids (Nizel, 1981; Williams, 1982).

Several *inorganic elements* that are essential for health are found in quantifiable amounts in the human body. Calcium, phosphorus, magnesium, sodium, potassium, sulfur, iron and chlorine all contribute to the growth, development, and function of the body. Trace amounts of elements, including copper, manganese, zinc, iodine, cobalt, molybdenum, selenium, and fluoride affect the body's biologic systems. Besides these there are several other elements found in the body that are not considered essential for health or about which minimal data have been collected.

The most critical elements in terms of dietary intake are *calcium* and *phosphorus* for the development and health of bones and teeth, *iron* for hemoglobin formation, *iodine* for thyroid regulation, and *fluoride* for decay-resistant teeth. The others are critical as well, but usually are ingested in adequate amounts if the aforementioned specific elements are found in the diet (Nizel, 1981; Randolph and Dennison, 1982; Williams, 1982).

Water, which serves as the fluid medium for the body's chemical and physical reactions, is probably the most critical dietary component. Without water, all the other nutrients would be incapable of activity (Williams, 1982).

Consuming too much as well as too little of any of the nutrients can increase the body's propensity for disease. Obesity, scurvy, rickets, and dental caries are prime examples of conditions based largely on deleterious dietary habits.

With the mention of dental caries as a nutritional disease, it may become more apparent that nutrition may have a direct effect on oral health as well as on general physical well-being. The oral cavity has been described as a barometer of general health (Randolph and Dennison, 1977; Randolph, 1981). This is particularly true in relation to nutritional problems. The nature of the oral structures allows them to reflect the body's nutritional maladies. The oral mucosa may appear extremely pallid or quite red. The texture of the tissue may indicate edema or friability. Cracks or fissures in the corners of the mouth or a heavily coated tongue may be signs that the general health of the individual is less than ideal. The presence of a large number of carious lesions provides information about the patient's consumption of fermentable carbohydrates (Randolph and Dennison, 1981).

TOXICITY

In the preceding section the toxic effects that some vitamins can have if taken in large quantities are mentioned. This is true for the fat-soluble vitamins (A, D, E, and K), for vitamin C, and for pyridoxine (B_6), which was recently found to produce toxic effects, including severe sensory nervous system dysfunction and ataxia (Schaumberg et al., 1983). Minerals such as zinc, fluoride, and iron, essential in prescribed amounts, produce toxic effects in large doses (Hamilton and Whitney, 1982; Randolph and Dennison, 1981).

In recent years there has been a widespread trend, in particular, toward taking large doses of vitamin C to prevent or cure infectious diseases and cancer. No well-controlled studies have supported this practice, and several have failed to show significant differences between taking vitamin C and taking a placebo. In addition, large doses of vitamin C raise the uric acid level of urine (sometimes triggering gout in susceptible persons); they obscure the results of some medical tests; and they impair the ability of white blood cells to kill bacteria, actually worsening infections. They may cause kidney stones, affect fertility, and induce a deficiency rebound in newborns whose mothers routinely took large doses.

Toxic reactions to large doses of vitamins are becoming more of a problem since the awareness of good nutrition has grown among the general public. Some people have erroneously assumed that *more* of a good thing is *better*. Self-prescribed doses may far exceed needed amounts and may be seen as a substitute for eating proper foods. In addition, lay articles advocating the use of megavitamin doses are omnipresent, unwittingly recommending levels of vitamins or minerals that not only exceed what is needed for normal functioning, but that also produce negative effects. In some cases the toxic response is very similar to the deficiency symptoms, which may prompt the person to take even more of the nutrient. It is therefore very important during a nutritional assessment to inquire about what vitamin supplements are being taken, in what doses, and with what frequency (Hamilton and Whitney, 1981).

DENTAL CARIES AND DIET

Most research related to the nutritional impact on caries has centered on systemic fluorides' effect on teeth. Teeth with a high fluoride content are less susceptible to caries. Less research has centered on the impact of other dietary components (Hefferren, 1981). Still, there are many findings that influence the way patients should be guided.

There is a direct correlation between sugar intake and plaque. The more sugar consumed, especially the disaccharide *sucrose,* the thicker and more plentiful the plaque (Carlsson and Egelberg, 1965). When oral hygiene is poor, even low quantities of sugar consumption promote caries (Kleemola-Kujala and Räsänen, 1982).

Binns (1981) and Newbrun (1982b) have summarized the numerous epidemiologic and clinical studies that show that eating high-sugar diets predicts a high caries rate. People living in countries where sucrose is consumed in large quantities have higher caries rates than people living where intake is low. Sreebny (1982) confirms that a diet of manufactured or processed food that contains higher levels of sucrose promotes higher levels of caries activity.

Retentive, sticky sugars (such as caramels or taffy) that are not quickly diluted by saliva and flushed from the oral cavity promote caries to a greater extent than do liquid sugars (such as soda pop). Complex carbohydrates (such as whole grain cereals and breads) are less cariogenic than simple sugars, but even these carbohydrates promote caries if food particles are retained around the teeth. The complex carbohydrates are reduced by the amylase enzyme in saliva to more simple forms, and they then can be fermented by the bacteria in plaque.

Plaque can form on teeth even when carbohydrates are not ingested; but it is thin and is not as highly structured as the thick, dense plaque that is associated with a high-sucrose diet. Plaque that is not fed a carbohydrate diet does not promote caries, because acid is not produced: its presence is therefore more associated with periodontal disease resulting from the soft tissue inflammation caused by bacterial toxins, antigens, and enzymes.

Once plaque is present, any ingested carbohydrates can diffuse into it, wherein the bacteria, especially *Streptococcus mutans,* ferment the simple sugars, producing acid that demineralizes the teeth, initiating a carious lesion (Hefferren and Koehler, 1981).

Plaque is especially important in promoting smooth-surface caries, since it provides the matrix for holding the bacteria and fermenting sugars against a surface that does not otherwise easily retain food. Pit and fissure caries formation relies less on plaque, since the anatomy of the tooth enhances sugar retention and access to acid-forming bacteria.

The longer sucrose is in contact with plaque, the lower the interdental plaque pH (i.e., the greater the acidity of the plaque). Therefore all-day suckers or lollipops, chewing gum, or slowly dissolving hard candies and mints pose a major risk in caries formation. So does the slowly sipped drink of cola or other sugared beverage. The passive, continual availability of sucrose keeps the acidity of the plaque high, enhancing ongoing tooth dissolution (Firestone, 1982; Newbrun, 1982a).

This point is especially evident in cases where babies are put to bed with a bottle of formula, milk, juice, or other substance that contains or is easily converted to simple sugars. The liquid, which stays in the infant's mouth with periodic replenishment as the child sucks during sleep, is chemically reduced and fermented, causing rampant tooth destruction, referred to as baby bottle caries or nursing caries (Randolph and Dennison, 1981).

Thus a major emphasis in dietary counseling is the reduction of the frequency and duration of ingestion of fermentable carbohydrates and the elimination of sticky sweets. Patients who have a high rate of smooth-surface caries (usually on the gingival third of mandibular teeth) are prime candidates for reviewing snacking habits. A patient with this clinical evidence may keep a box of cookies in the desk drawer at work, eat sugared mints or lozenges, chew gum, or frequently consume sugared drinks such as sweetened coffee or tea, soda pop, lemonade, etc.

Sreebny (1982) has concluded, based on epidemiologic data, that the "safe" upper limit of daily sugar consumption may be 50 g. For many individuals even this may be too much. Ingesting more than this raises the risk of caries considerably. This amount takes on more significance when the amounts of sugar in typical portions of commonly ingested foods are known: ketchup, 5g; fruit yogurt, 18 g; canned fruit, 46 g; milk chocolate bar, 26 g; hot chocolate, 12 g; cola, 32g (Wykeham-Martin, 1981).

Foods with a sugar content of 15% to 20% or higher are poor snack food choices because they are highly cariogenic. Even items that are 10% to 20% sugar should be restricted from between-meal use (Newbrun, 1982a). Any item that lists sugar or sucrose early in the list of ingredients on the label should be avoided.

A large number of sugar substitutes have been introduced over the past 20 years, in particular, in order to satisfy the public's demand for sweeteners that do not add calories and that do not promote tooth decay. Cyclamates, saccharin, and aspartame have all come under scrutiny for their links with cancer in laboratory animals. Cyclamates were banned in 1969. Saccharin-containing products are labeled as hazardous. Aspartame has been given approval for some foods, but the Food and Drug Administration ordered a temporary stay on its

marketing in 1975 (Hefferren, Ayer, and Koehler, 1981).

In recommending a reduction in sugar intake, the proposed alternatives should be evaluated for their safety in general health as well as for their role in dental health. Every clinician should be current on what is available, what is "safe," and what foods or snacks it is found in. Replacing sucrose with the sweetness of fruit or of sweet vegetables may be asking too much of some patients, but it is an alternative that avoids the folly of replacing cariogenic foods with carcinogenic additives.

DIET AND CANCER: NEW FOCUS IN NUTRITIONAL ASSESSMENT

Dental professionals help promote good general health when they help patients replace highly caloric, caries-promoting food with nutritionally well-balanced choices. This can be accomplished by targeting snack foods and the high sugar breakfast choices many people make (doughnuts, sweet rolls, processed cereals), and for the most part dental professionals limit their nutritional guidance to this sphere. They may emphasize the need for vegetables and fruits and protein sources but the diet in general has been less of a focus for most.

New evidence of the importance of diet in relation to cancer in general raises, however, the consideration of how far a dentist or hygienist should extend advice in counseling patients. The Committee on Diet, Nutrition, and Cancer of the National Academy of Sciences reviewed hundreds of published research findings to identify those pointing *conclusively* to the influence of dietary habits on cancer formation.* They reviewed epidemiologic studies of population groups with varying dietary patterns. They linked the findings of those studies with laboratory and case study results. Having identified several series of studies repeatedly pointing to the influence of diet, they released interim guidelines that should be followed in reviewing one's own diet as well as diets of patients:

---

*The complete report can be found in National Academy of Sciences. 1982. Diet, nutrition, and cancer. Washington, D.C.: Committee on Diet, Nutrition, and Cancer Assembly of Life Sciences, National Research Council. The Palmer and Bakshi citation in the text is a summary report of the 500-page original document.

Reduce the percentage of both saturated and unsaturated fat to approximately 30% of total calories. This represents a 25% reduction from the typical U.S. diet percentage. An even lower percentage is indicated by the data; the committee saw this reduction as more "moderate and practical."

Minimize consumption of salt-preserved, smoked, or salt-pickled food.

Persons who drink alcohol should do so in moderation.

The committee also recommended that carcinogenic and mutagenic contaminants in food be prevented through regulation and continued study of food additives and processing (Palmer and Bakshi, 1983).

Many of the findings relating fat consumption to cancer have come from studies designed to investigate fats and cardiovascular disease. In addition to linking high fat intake, especially of saturated fats, to heart and blood vessel problems, they have found that diets rich in either saturated or unsaturated fats are highly correlated with cancer of the breast, colon, and prostate gland. Cancers of the testis, uterus, ovary, and pancreas have also been associated with high dietary fat levels (Palmer and Bakshi, 1983).

In these studies persons who had a high fat intake but who also consumed large quantities of vegetables had a lower risk of colon cancer. Several other studies have shown that "consumption of vegetables in general, raw vegetables (e.g., lettuce and celery), or cruciferous vegetables in particular (e.g., cabbage, cauliflower, brussels sprouts, and broccoli)" is inversely related to cancer of the alimentary tract (e.g., esophagus, stomach, or colon). It is difficult to determine the mode of their anticarcinogenic activity. Some attribute it to their high fiber content, whereas others cite their vitamin A content or suspect some yet unknown biochemical function (Palmer and Bakshi, 1983).

Fresh fruit consumption or estimated vitamin C intake has also been shown to be inversely related to cancer incidence, especially of the stomach, esophagus, and larynx, and to uterine cervical dysplasia.

Bacon, ham, and other foods preserved with salt, smoke, or salt pickling are now known to be highly carcinogenic. But vitamin C tends to reduce their harmful effects (Palmer and Bakshi, 1983).

Numerous studies have shown a correlation between alcohol and cancer of the esophagus, tongue, pharynx, hypopharynx, larynx, lung, lip, glottis, and the supraglottic region. Studies also have shown "an interactive role between tobacco and alcohol in tumorigenesis of the oral cavity, larynx, lung, and esophagus" (Palmer and Bakshi, 1983).

Given that dental professionals have the most regular and frequent contact with healthy people, and given the convincing evidence of dietary contributions to cancer, hygienists can assume a role of major importance in reviewing individual's diets and moving them toward more healthful choices that are likely to reduce the risk of cancer.

CLINICAL ASSESSMENT: INTRAORAL AND EXTRAORAL EXAMINATION

During the complete intraoral and extraoral examination phases, the appearance of the gingivae, the teeth, lips, and oral mucosa, plus the texture of the hair and the skin may provide some clue that the patient has nutritional problems that should be carefully assessed (Christakis, 1973). Therefore it should be obvious that the dental hygienist is in an ideal position to identify potential nutritional and other general health problems by virtue of his/her role in the complete examination of patient's head and neck.

When a nutrient is not present in the diet, blood and tissue levels are maintained by reserves in specific tissues. No clinical signs are evident until the reserve stores are depleted and biochemical changes occur. Thus a person with obvious clinical symptoms can be assumed to have a relatively long-term deficiency rather than a poor diet for a day or two (Chipponi et al, 1982). Similarly, rampant caries reflects nutritional patterns that have existed for more than a few days.

However, the examination procedures are only one step in the nutritional assessment component of care. Just as the patient learns to conduct a self-assessment of oral structures and observe healthy structures as well as those that have changed in appearance or texture over time, the patient should learn how to self-assess dietary habits as well. Leading a patient through the self-assessment procedure is a learning procedure in itself. Additionally, it provides key data for making a decision regarding the need for dietary modifications and/or referral.

NUTRITIONAL SELF-ASSESSMENT

One way to include nutritional self-assessment routinely in dental hygiene care is to develop a simple questionnaire that can be used to determine what a "usual" day's diet is like (Nizel, 1981, Randolph, 1977). This can be done by asking a patient what he/she ate the day before, including the time of day each element was ingested and the approximate amounts eaten. The questionnaire can be given to the patient to complete; after the questionnaire has been completed, a discussion can follow, or the hygienist can ask the questions in an interview format.

Generally, a patient can be expected to recall with reasonable accuracy the previous day's intake. As with any questionnaire that seeks to gather information but not place any particular values on what is a right or wrong behavior, the questions should be phrased in such a way that the patient does not begin to be embarrased, angry, or puzzled by his/her failure to comply with a pattern of activities that fit into the questionnaire (Randolph, 1977). For instance, asking "What did you have for breakfast?" implies that breakfast should have been eaten. An alternative question is, "What was the first thing you ate or drank yesterday?" Then the following question can be, "What time of the day did you eat (drink) that?" and "How much of it did you consume?" A series of such questions can elicit the approximate kinds of foods and beverages consumed, the times of day they were ingested, and the approximate amounts taken. Keeping cups, spoons, drinking glasses, and plastic containers handy can help the patient identify more precisely the amounts ingested (Christakis, 1973). It is important to ask the patient about between-meal snacks, glasses of water that were ingested, and any kind of pills or other medications that were consumed. People often feel that snacks do not count in a dietary assessment and may ignore water or vitamin pills as sources of nutrients.

The question regarding pills and other medications may help expose a noncompliance with prescribed dosages of drugs. For instance, if the patient reports during the medical history that a drug to control high blood pressure has been prescribed, the hygienist might assume that the patient takes the medication. However, if during the dietary assessment the patients fails to report having taken the medication during an entire day, this may be a sign that the patient takes the medication sporadically or not at all, regardless of the fact that it has been prescribed. This is also one way to determine if the patient has adopted any other habits related to prescribed drugs or over-the-counter medications. In any case, just as the other phase of patient assessment can yield valuable clues regarding nutritional problems, the dietary assessment can provide valuable information regarding the medical status of the patient.

Once all the suggested questions have been answered and the dietary form completed, the hygienist should ask, "Is this a typical day's eating pattern? Would you normally eat and drink this amount of food at these times of day?" Further questioning should be, "What about on days when you are at work?" (or, "What about on days when you are at home?") A person's eating habits may differ greatly from the weekday to the weekend or from days spent at work to days spent off work (Randolph, 1977; Randolph and Dennison, 1981). If the day described is atypical, the assessment should be repeated at a subsequent visit for a more valid assessment (Christakis, 1973).

According to Randolph (1977), "We tend to choose food and beverage on the basis of where we are, who we are with, the time of day, the next scheduled activity, the way we feel, the money we have and are willing to spend, and what is available." A homemaker may have a substantially different pattern of eating when the family is home as opposed to when he/she is home alone. A question regarding this may ferret out information about the hoard of chocolate bars in the bed stand or the secret supply of beer hidden in the old refrigerator in the attic. With the right questions, the hygienist can learn a great deal about the patient's dietary habits.

Once a full day's inclusions have been identified and verified as representing a pattern in the patient's daily living, the hygienist should ask the patient to circle in *red* all those *solid foods* that he/she knows *contain sugar*. Most patients can identify a large number of foods that contain sugar (Katz, McDonald, and Stookey, 1979; Randolph, 1977; Randolph and Dennison, 1981). An *orange* pencil should then be used to circle *liquids that contain sugar. Dairy foods* should be identified by the patient and circled in *yellow. Meat* can be identified and circled in *blue,* and *vegetables and fruits* circled in *green*. *Bread and cereals* should be circled in *brown*. Observing the patient circling the items according to each of the food groups and identifying sugar-containing products should provide the hygienist with a great deal of knowledge about how aware the patient is of nutrition.

Once the circling is complete, the hygienist should ask the patient if there is anything he/she would like to change about his/her diet. In most instances, this too will be a strong indicator of what the patient knows but does not necessarily practice. Hearing the patient say all the right things about what to increase and what to decrease can be quite an awakening. In most instances, preplanned lectures on proper diet and nutrition are abandoned in counseling people about their diets. There no doubt will be considerable evidence regarding the patient's attitude about changes. For instance, if the patient can identify what should be changed but says, "There's no way I'm going to change it, however," the hygienist may need to be reasonably cautious about offering multiple suggestions for change. Not all patients want this kind of help; many may resent it.

Once the patient has had an opportunity to assess what should (or could) be changed in the diet, the hygienist can begin to provide a few insights into the patient's diet of which the patient may not be aware. For instance, most patients are not aware of the vast number of foods that contain refined

sugars. Therefore several additional items on the day's menu may need to be circled in red or orange to reflect their actual contents. Keeping common food items in the dental operatory or counseling room can be helpful in showing the patient that ketchup, many canned vegetables, and crackers, for instance, contain sugar. By pointing out how foods are labeled, the patient can learn about concentrations of sugar and salt in the product. In all instances the approach should be "You might be interested to know that. . . ." rather than "Well, there are several you missed in circling the sugar foods."

In many instances the four foods groups will be marked accurately, although they, too, should be reviewed to ensure reasonable accuracy. Table 20-1 provides an overview of these food groupings.

Two steps that are helpful in determining the effect of the day's diet on the patient's well-being include identifying the amount of time sugar has been active in the oral cavity and identifying how closely the patient's diet adheres to the Recommended Dietary Allowances (RDAs) (Table 20-2) and/or each of the four food groups. The former determination involves counting the number of times sugar was consumed and multiplying by 20. Each time sugar is ingested, it provides 20 minutes of acid production to promote tooth decay and the proliferation of plaque. Therefore calculating the number of minutes (or hours) that acid has been

Table 20-1. The four food groups

Food group	Recommended servings
Meat Poultry Fish Dried beans and peas Nuts Eggs	One serving of 3 to 4 ounces of cooked meat or fish or 3 to 4 ounces of beans, lentils, or other vegetables high in protein twice daily. It is best to choose lean meat and to limit the intake of egg yolk to three times per week.
Vegetables Fruits	One serving of ½ cup at least four times weekly, including green leafy vegetables, dark yellow vegetables, and fruits or fruit juices. Citrus fruits should be included daily.
Bread Cereals	Whole grain or enriched breads recommended: one serving (slice) four times daily, Muffins, pasta, biscuits, cereal, and rice are included in this group.
Milk products	One serving (usually an 8-ounce glass of milk) three times daily for children to age 12, four or more times daily for teenagers, and twice daily for adults. Cheese, cottage cheese, ice cream, and buttermilk are included in this group.

The four food groups are useful for assessing dietary intake with recommended dietary standards. They are not, however, a recommended mechanism for preparing a detailed dietary analysis with specific amounts of nutrients identified in measurable quantities. Food value charts that identify the specific nutrients present in a wide variety of foods provide a more detailed resource for such an analysis.

Table 20-2. Food and Nutrition Board, National Academy of Sciences–National Research Council Recommended Daily Dietary Allowances,[a] revised 1980: designed for the maintenance of good nutrition of practically all healthy people in the U.S.A.

	Age (yr)	Weight (kg)	Weight (lb)	Height (cm)	Height (in)	Protein (g)	Fat-soluble vitamins Vitamin A (μg RE)[b]	Fat-soluble vitamins Vitamin D (μg)[c]	Fat-soluble vitamins Vitamin E (mg α-TE)[d]	Water-soluble vitamins Vitamin C (mg)	Water-soluble vitamins Thiamin (mg)
Infants	0.0-0.5	6	13	60	24	kg × 2.2	420	10	3	35	0.3
	0.5-1.0	9	20	71	28	kg × 2.0	400	10	4	35	0.5
Children	1-3	13	29	90	35	23	400	10	5	45	0.7
	4-6	20	44	112	44	30	500	10	6	45	0.9
	7-10	28	62	132	52	34	700	10	7	45	1.2
Males	11-14	45	99	157	62	45	1000	10	8	50	1.4
	15-18	66	145	176	69	56	1000	10	10	60	1.4
	19-22	70	154	177	70	56	1000	7.5	10	60	1.5
	23-50	70	154	178	70	56	1000	5	10	60	1.4
	51+	70	154	178	70	56	1000	5	10	60	1.2
Females	11-14	46	101	157	62	46	800	10	8	50	1.1
	15-18	55	120	163	64	46	800	10	8	60	1.1
	19-22	55	120	163	64	44	800	7.5	8	60	1.1
	23-50	55	120	163	64	44	800	5	8	60	1.0
	51+	55	120	163	64	44	800	5	8	60	1.0
Pregnant						+30	+200	+5	+2	+20	+0.4
Lactating						+20	+400	+5	+3	+40	+0.5

From Recommended Dietary Allowances, revised 1980. Washington, D.C.: Food and Nutrition Board, National Academy of
[a]The allowances are intended to provide for individual variations among most normal persons as they live in the United States which human requirements have been less well defined.
[b]Retinol equivalents. 1 retinol equivalent = 1 μg retinol or 6 μg β carotene.
[c]As cholecalciferol. 10 μg cholecalciferol = 400 IU of Vitamin D.
[d]α-tocopherol equivalents. 1 mg d-α tocopherol = 1 α-TE.
[e]1 NE (niacin equivalent) is equal to 1 mg of niacin or 60 mg of dietary tryptophan.
[f]The folacin allowances refer to dietary sources as determined by *Lactobacillus casei* assay after treatment with enzymes (conjugases)
[g]The RDA for vitamin B_{12} in infants is based on average concentration of the vitamin in human milk. The allowances after weaning intestinal absorption.
[h]The increased requirement during pregnancy cannot be met by the iron content of habitual American diets nor by the existing iron substantially different from those of nonpregnant women, but continued supplementation of the mother for 2-3 months after parturition

active in the mouth can provide an interesting summary of the impact of the diet on the teeth. Likewise, each of the other items circled in various colors should be tabulated to determine if frequency and amount relate to that suggested by federal standards. The Food and Nutrition Board of the National Research Council of the National Academy of Sciences has the responsibility for recommending a specific optimum quantity, based on sex and age, for each nutrient. Recommendations are issued every 5 years. The quantities suggested provide a *margin of safety* and are designed for an *average* person; therefore they do not address individual differences or the nutritional needs of medically compromised people. As a basic reference, the RDAs provide overall useful guidelines in quantitating a diet. If specific amounts of nutrients ingested can be identified, they can be compared with RDA standards to determine if the intake approximates the optimum level (Hamilton and Whitney, 1981; Randolph and Dennison, 1981).

Many nutrition texts include comprehensive listings of food values that make it possible to perform a detailed analysis of a diet. For purposes of dietary

Water-soluble vitamins					Minerals					
Riboflavin (mg)	Niacin (mg NE)[e]	Vitamin B_6 (mg)	Folacin[f] (μg)	Vitamin B_{12} (μg)	Calcium (mg)	Phosphorus (mg)	Magnesium (mg)	Iron (mg)	Zinc (mg)	Iodine (μg)
0.4	6	0.3	30	0.5[g]	360	240	50	10	3	40
0.6	8	0.6	45	1.5	540	360	70	15	5	50
0.8	9	0.9	100	2.0	800	800	150	15	10	70
1.0	11	1.3	200	2.5	800	800	200	10	10	90
1.4	16	1.6	300	3.0	800	800	250	10	10	120
1.6	18	1.8	400	3.0	1200	1200	350	18	15	150
1.7	18	2.0	400	3.0	1200	1200	400	18	15	150
1.7	19	2.2	400	3.0	800	800	350	10	15	150
1.6	18	2.2	400	3.0	800	800	350	10	15	150
1.4	16	2.2	400	3.0	800	800	350	10	15	150
1.3	15	1.8	400	3.0	1200	1200	300	18	15	150
1.3	14	2.0	400	3.0	1200	1200	300	18	15	150
1.3	14	2.0	400	3.0	800	800	300	18	15	150
1.2	13	2.0	400	3.0	800	800	300	18	15	150
1.2	13	2.0	400	3.0	800	800	300	10	15	150
+0.3	+2	+0.6	+400	+1.0	+400	+400	+150	h	+5	+25
+0.5	+5	+0.5	+100	+1.0	+400	+400	+150	h	+10	+50

Sciences–National Research Council.
under usual environmental stresses. Diets should be based on a variety of common foods in order to provide other nutrients for

to make polyglutamyl forms of the vitamin available to the test organism.
are based on energy intake (as recommended by the American Academy of Pediatrics) and consideration of other factors, such as
stores of many women; therefore the use of 30-60 mg of supplemental iron is recommended. Iron needs during lactation are not
is advisable in order to replenish stores depleted by pregnancy.

assessment and most dietary counseling in dental hygiene care, qualitative assessments using the four food groups may be more useful than detailed quantitative analyses. In any case, the patient should be able to determine if his/her food selection is reasonably appropriate.

In addition to these two basic assessments, estimates of caloric intake may be made. The texture of the foods should be identified, since a diet of soft, nonfibrous foods can adhere to the teeth and cause problems with digestion and elimination. The distribution of eating during the day should be identified as well.

It is sometimes preferable to draw a line between assessment of need and implementation of dietary counseling. This is especially true if the patient appears to be apprehensive or reluctant to participate. If the assessment shows a need for such counseling, it can be included in a treatment plan and discussed at the case presentation.

In a number of instances, the patient may be able to identify at the time of assessment the kinds of modifications that are important for improved health. The patient may say, "I guess I never realized that I ate so few vegetables." Or the patient may say, "I knew I was a nibbler, but I would never have said that I could be found eating at 10 different times during a given day!" If the patient comes to one of these conclusions about his/her diet, then it may be appropriate to ask, "Would you like some suggestions for modification?" In all likelihood, the patient who has just had a revelation about his/her daily eating patterns will be open to at least a few suggestions for change.

The next question would be, "Where do you think you need guidance?" This question gives the patient the opportunity to say, for example, "Well, I know I can handle adding a few vegetables to my diet, but I really don't know what I'm going to do about all the sugared beverages I drink." This cues the hygienist to ignore the missing vegetables for the moment and turn the patient's attention to substitution foods that will make the decrease and possibly the eventual elimination of sugared beverages from the diet more tolerable. Once this patient-identified priority is addressed, the hygienist may return to the issue of the vegetables and ask, "What kinds of vegetables do you like? How do you usually prepare them?" Even though the patient may believe he/she can resolve a certain dietary problem, the verbal expression of plans for improvement and discussion of potential difficulties and varieties of ways in which to resolve the problem can help clarify the patient's goals and increase the likelihood of change. Another way of bringing the planned change closer to reality is to ask, "What can you do tomorrow to implement the changes you think you need?" The patient may decide that he/she needs to purchase the different foods today to make change possible for tomorrow. In almost all behavior changes, the goals need to be reduced to definable short-range steps that the patient can identify and accomplish, one by one. In any case the patient should be given ample opportunity to think and reply.

Merely giving instructions and information without including incremental behavior change strategies may improve the patient's *knowledge and awareness* of dietary needs but will have no more than a negligible effect on acutal performance (Morasky and Lilly, 1980).

If, after several moments of silence, the patient seems to be at a loss as to how his/her diet should change, the hygienist can provide missing information. The stock of canned and bottled goods can be brought into view for an assessment of what those foods contain. The hygienist can discuss the retention of food and the frequency of intake of sugar in terms of the total amount of time acid is produced in the mouth. Or he/she may point out the vitamins and minerals that are included in the dietary plan, making obvious those that are missing. A brief discussion of how those missing elements affect health and well-being may have an added impact on the patient's perception of his/her diet. The hygienist may find it appropriate to discuss the effects of an imbalance of caloric intake and utilization. It may be that the patient will decide to expend more calories through exercise as well as decrease the intake if obesity seems to be a problem.

In some instances the patient may inquire about what kinds of foods he/she should eat to fulfill a nurtitional recommendation. A wise response is to list a number of foods that are appropriate and ask the patient to specify which foods he/she enjoys and are available. It is important to remember that many food choices may not be available to patients because of financial and/or cultural barriers (Hamilton and Whitney, 1981; Nizel, 1981; Randolph and Dennison, 1981). Patients may have allergies to certain foods. And, most important, there are some foods a person simply does not like and will not eat.

As mentioned before, it is important for the patient to express what he/she could do the next day to alter the diet in the ways the patient had previously suggested. It is also wise to suggest incremental changes (Katz, McDonald, and Stookey, 1979). One small change over a few weeks followed by other small changes may actually result in long-term major changes. A crash program to change the entire structure of a person's diet is often shortlived, as can be verified by the numbers of people who have each gained and lost and gained back again hundreds of pounds over the years on fad approaches to weight loss. Ideally, the specific changes can be identified in writing for the patient and placed in the patient's record. Each change should be identified in a time frame. As each change is implemented, the patient can identify the date and time of day the change was implemented, thus tracking whether or not real change has occurred.

Finally, the hygienist should integrate follow-up

assessments of progress into each dental hygiene visit. People do not always do everything they say they will do; a supportive, helpful hygienist will remember to identify the areas in which even minor success has been achieved and reinforce that change. If recommended changes did not occur, the hygienist might ask, ''What seemed to be the biggest roadblock to making the change?'' Setting out to remove or diminish each roadblock as it appears can be an effective way to facilitate change over an extended period of time.

REFERRALS

Even though the dental hygienist has courses in nutrition and feels confident about proper dietary intake, there will be times when it is essential to refer the patient to a dietitian or a physician for more complete nutritional aanalysis and counseling (Nizel, 1981; Randolph and Dennison, 1981). In most instances if the patient's health history indicates diabetes, alcoholism, an obvious chronic nutritional debility, or any other complicated combination of disease and nutritional problems, the hygienist should recommend that the patient see a person more qualified to make recommendations and work with the patient. A protocol for these kinds of referrals should be established for the practice site so that co-workers are able to ensure rapid, safe referral for the patient. Subsequent to such referrals, the hygienist should inquire whether the patient was able to obtain assistance from the dietitian or the physician. Just as medication to control high blood pressure can remain in the bottle, appointments with other health care providers to whom the patient is referred may not always occur. A helpful step is to contact the person to whom the patient was referred to ensure that the patient complied with the recommendation and to determine if the hygienist's findings were accurate. This is one way to establish whether assessment skills in patient observation and history preparation are adequate. A dialogue with co-professionals can be beneficial to the dental hygienist as well as to the patient under discussion.

SUMMARY

With a solid knowledge of basic nutrition and its relationship to health and disease, a dental hygienist can play a valuable role in helping improve the dietary patterns of patients. The use of simple patient self-assessment procedures and the approach of guiding the patient in identifying necessary modifications can result in improvements in health and in patient cooperation in all phases of care. Perhaps the most essential point is for the hygienist to assume the facilitator role rather than the directive role. Decisions that the patient makes are most likely to lead to actual behavior change. The hygienist's role is to ensure that the decisions are guided properly and that roadblocks to their fulfillment can be identifed and reduced.

ACTIVITIES

1. Prepare 1-day, 3-day, and 7-day dietary assessments with a student partner. Use nutritional texts and articles to prepare a comprehensive evaluation of the records to reveal:
   a. Caloric intake and expenditure
   b. Consumption of bulk foods
   c. Consumption of liquids
   d. Degree of compliance with the four food groups and the RDAs
   e. Frequency and form of carbohydrates ingested
2. Videotape the dietary assessment encounter with a student partner to reveal the process of communication, verbal and nonverbal cues, and the approach used by the student dental hygienist.
3. Read Binns' (1981) article listed in the references at the end of this chapter.
4. Critique the General Mills ad placed on pp. 142-143 of the January 1981 issue of the *Journal of the American Dental Association*. How are research results manipulated to convince readers that they should counsel patients to eat processed cereals, regardless of their sugar content?
5. Form groups of five. Visit a grocery store and review labels on products in each of the following categories for the presence of sugar:
   a. Breakfast cereals
   b. Bread
   c. Juice
   d. Canned fruits, vegetables
   e. Tomato sauce and prepared spagetti sauces.
   Compare findings, identifying brand names of products high in sugar as well as those that are low in sugar or contain none.

REVIEW QUESTIONS

1. Identify the three nutrients that provide calories for the body.
2. Which of the three nutrients given in response to 1 can cause weight gain if consumed in excess?
3. Match the following nutrients with their important functions in the health of the human body.

___ a. Protein	1. Contributes to thyroid regulation
___ b. Fat	2. Serves as fluid medium for the body's chemical and physical reactions
___ c. Carbohydrate	
___ d. Vitamin B complex	3. Essential for development of healthy bones and teeth
___ e. Vitamin D	4. Helps teeth become resistant to decay
___ f. Vitamin A	
___ g. Vitamin K	5. Essential component of nerve tissue
___ h. Vitamin E	6. Essential component in body tissues, enzymes, and hormones
___ i. Iodine	
___ j. Fluoride	
___ k. Calcium and phosphorus	7. Helps cushion and insulate the body
___ l. Iron	8. Important in collagen biosynthesis and wound healing
___ m. Water	

9. Critical for the complete metabolism of carbohydrates and for energy release
10. Formed in the presence of ultraviolet light; important for the absorption and homeostasis of calcium
11. Essential in prothrombin formation
12. Essential in hemoglobin formation
13. Primary functions relate to reproduction and membrane stability
14. Essential for vision and control of differentiation of epithelium in mucus-secreting structures and in bone remodeling.

4. Why is it a useful strategy to ask the patient to identify the presence or absence of specific foods in his/her diet?
5. What role do the RDAs and the four food groups play in dietary assessment?
6. How does plaque aid caries formation?
7. What foods have been proved to be highly associated with cancer?
8. What foods tend to reduce the incidence of cancer?

REFERENCES

Binns, N.M. 1981. Caries and carbohydrates—a problem for dentists and nutritionists. Dent. Health **20**(4):5.

Carlsson, J., and Egelberg, J. 1965. Effect of diet on plaque formation and development of gingivitis in dogs. II. Effect of high carbohydrate versus high protein-fat diets. Odontol. Rev. **16**:42.

Chipponi, J.X., et al. 1982. Deficiencies of essential and conditionally essential nutrients. Am. J. Clin. Nutr. (Suppl. 5) **35**:1112.

Christakis, G. 1973. Nutritional assessment in health programs. Am. J. Public Health (Suppl.) **63**.

Firestone, A.R. 1982. Effect of increasing contact time on sucrose solution of powdered sucrose on plaque pH in vivo. J. Dent. Res. **61**:1243.

Hamilton, E.M.N., and Whitney, E.N. 1982. Nutrition concepts and controversies. St. Paul, Minn.: West Publishing Co.

Hefferren, J.J. 1981. A look ahead: diet and nutrition research. J. Am. Dent. Assoc. **102**:624.

Hefferren, J.J., Ayer, W.A., and Koehler, H.M., editors. 1981. Foods, nutrition, and dental health, vols. 1-3. Park Forest South, Ill.: Pathotox Publishers, Inc.

Katz, S., McDonald, J.L., and Stookey, G.K. 1979. Preventive dentistry in action, ed. 3. Upper Montclair, N.J.: D.C.P. Publishing.

Kleemola-Kujala, E., and Räs'auanen, L. 1982. Relationship of oral hygiene and sugar consumption to risk of caries in children. Community Dent. Oral Epidemiol. **10**:224.

Morasky, R.L., and Lilly, K.P. 1980: Nutrition management for dental health: a behavioral approach. Clin. Prevent. Dent. **2**(4):7.

Newbrun, E. 1982. Sugar and dental caries. Clin. Prevent. Dent. **4**(3):11. (a)

Newbrun, E. 1982. Sugar and dental caries: a review of human studies. Science **217**:418. (b)

Nizel, A.E. 1981. Nutrition in preventive dentistry: science and practice. Philadelphia: W.B. Saunders Co.

Palmer, S., and Bakshi, K.: 1983. Diet, nutrition, and cancer: interim dietary guidelines. JNCI **70**:1151.

Poplin, L.E. 1981. Cautions in nutritional counseling. Dent. Hyg. **55**(2):40.

Randolph, P.M. 1977. Dietary counseling. In Boundy, S.S., and Reynolds, N.J., editors. Current concepts in dental hygiene, vol. 1. St. Louis: The C.V. Mosby Co.

Randolph, P.M., and Dennison, C.I. 1981. Diet, nutrition, and dentistry. St. Louis: The C.V. Mosby Co.

Schaumberg, H., et al. 1983. Sensory neuropathy from pyridoxine abuse. N. Engl. J. Med. **309**:445.

Sreebny, L.M. 1982. Sugar availability, sugar consumption and dental caries. Community Dent. Oral Epidemiol. **10**:1.

Williams, S.R. 1982. Essentials of nutrition and diet therapy. ed. 3. St. Louis: The C.V. Mosby Co.

Wykeham-Martin, J. 1981. Hidden sugar. *Dent. Health* **20**(3):14.

PART FOUR

IMPLEMENTATION

Implementing care in dental hygiene practice is defined in the following 15 chapters in terms of periodontal care (Chapters 21 to 26), caring for appliances (Chapter 27), using chemical agents for the prevention of dental caries and for the control of tooth hypersensitivity (Chapters 29 to 31), evaluating occlusion (Chapter 28), controlling pain (Chapters 32 and 33), modifying dental hygiene care for patients with special needs (Chapter 34), and performing restorative procedures (Chapter 35).

Most of the highly technical skills of dental hygiene practice are further developed and expanded in these chapters, with a firm grounding given in the scientific basis for these procedures. During this phase of development the student may begin to recognize that the cycle of assessing, planning, implementing, and evaluating is not limited to one large cycle, but occurs in a series of minicycles throughout implementation and each of the other phases. Even while a clinical procedure is being implemented, the thinking clinician is assessing the state of the tissue and its response, planning the next move, carrying out each sequence of the procedure, and evaluating the performance of each procedure.

21 REMOVING HEAVY DEPOSITS: HAND SCALING

OBJECTIVES: *The reader will be able to*

1. Use a pen grasp, fulcrum, wrist rock, and a variety of stroking patterns to remove calculus from teeth with:
   a. Sickle scalers
   b. Universal curettes
   c. Hoes
   d. Chisels
   e. Files
2. Given a variety of calculus deposits, use exploratory and working strokes to identify deposit location and size and to engage the deposit for removal.
3. Differentiate exploratory and working strokes.
4. Differentiate vertical, horizontal, oblique, and circumferential stroking patterns.
5. Identify instances in which the selection of a sickle, universal curette, hoe, chisel, or file for calculus removal is appropriate.
6. Describe the uses and limitations of each of the calculus removal instruments.
7. Describe an order of instrumentation for effective utilization of the calculus removal instruments, based on effective clinician and patient positioning and effective time and motion economy.
8. Demonstrate four alternative fulcrum placements.
9. Identify methods for evaluating complete deposit removal.
10. Explain briefly why removing calculus and ensuring good oral hygiene are not sufficient to stop periodontal disease.

Removing calculus deposits from the teeth is still a large part of what a clinical dental hygienist does in his/her daily routine. This is an important role in the initial therapy that patients receive, and it is an integral part of maintenance care or prevention. The very term, *prophylaxis,* which is the profession's term for scaling and polishing teeth, means *prevention.* This procedure is viewed as part of a total regimen of professional and self-care that can prevent most instances of dental caries and periodontal disease. Yet, there has been considerable controversy regarding exactly how much the oral prophylaxis is able to prevent. Does oral prophylaxis in itself prevent disease? In most instances, dental hygienists and other health professionals would agree that it does not in itself prevent disease. At least, the periodic recall prophylaxis administered every 6 months is unlikely to do so.

Certainly, the single event of a complete oral prophylaxis in initial periodontal therapy does not in itself prevent periodontal disease. However, most practicing dental hygienists can show that in combination with thorough, habitual plaque removal and proper diet, the oral prophylaxis is one contribution to maintaining oral health.

Research findings support this belief. Periodontal patients who receive initial therapy including these procedures show significant decreases in oral disease over a 1-month period (Morrison et al., 1980). Similar results have been reported for maintenance periods of 13 months (Badersten et al., 1981) and 6 years (Axelsson and Lindhe, 1981). Periodontal patients maintained with regular prophylaxes *without* surgical intervention over an 8-year period have shown no significant difference in oral status from patients with comparable conditions for whom surgery was performed (Knowles et al., 1980). Thus scaling, root planing, and soft tissue curettage have been shown to be efficacious modes of treatment when combined with a high degree of oral hygiene.

Taken in its proper perspective as part of a complete program of prevention, the oral prophylaxis is an important service for the patient. It removes irritants from the teeth, smooths surface irregularities that enhance plaque formation and growth, and provides the patient with a clean feeling that he/she is more likely to want to preserve. Also, the teeth may look better as a result of the oral prophylaxis.

If the oral prophylaxis is given too much significance by the patient or the hygienist, it may become a flimsy crutch. A preoccupation with the short-term cosmetic effects, an acceptance of the recurrent deposits on the teeth, and the patient's reliance on the dental hygienist as the source of clean teeth are all signs of abuse of the procedure and are a certain pattern for supervised neglect. Teeth that are cleaned every 6 months but that have no regular daily care in the form of plaque removal and that are subject to cariogenic foods will not be safe from caries, slow periodontal destruction, and eventual loss.

The dental hygienist's goal is to be so effective as a health educator and as a motivator that the oral prophylaxis becomes basically nonessential for the patient. Over the course of a few months or years, the patient should become increasingly interested in self-care and in long-term health. As deposits are not allowed to reaccumulate between professional appointments, less and less scaling and polishing will be needed. Maintenance becomes a process of evaluating tissue health (both hard and soft tissues, intraorally and extraorally) and of providing the patient with information and suggestions for maintaining optimal oral health (Parr et al., 1976). The dental hygienist becomes a resource rather than a "tooth cleaner."

In initial care and for those patients who have not yet achieved control of oral health, the dental hygienist needs to have skills in deposit detection and removal. In Chapter 5 the basic principles of detection are presented.

In this chapter the basic principles of deposit removal are presented, and in later chapters the principles of root planing and curettage, as well as other procedures supportive of complete periodontal care, are discussed. The oral prophylaxis procedure and more advanced periodontal instrumentation need to be learned so that they can be performed safely, efficiently, and thoroughly. At this point the dental hygienist begins to develop as a therapist as well as a data gatherer and health educator.

COMMON PRINCIPLES OF INSTRUMENTATION FOR EXPLORING AND REMOVING CALCAREOUS DEPOSITS

The basic principles of instrumentation presented in Chapter 5 will be extremely useful in learning the principles of deposit removal. For nearly all the calculus removal instruments the modified pen grasp, fulcrum placement, wrist rock, and stroking patterns discussed in Chapter 5 are the same as those used in detecting deposits and in probing subgingivally.

Recall that the instrument is held between the thumb and the first *two* fingers (a *modified pen grasp*), with the first two sections of the index finger flat against the instrument for maximum control. The third finger, or ring finger, is used as a *fulcrum,* giving the movements of the instrument control and stability. Usually the fulcrum (also called a finger rest) is on the occlusal or incisal surfaces of the teeth, near the operative site. The *wrist rock* is the unified lateral or vertical hand and arm motion that causes the instrument to move in a prescribed *stroking pattern* on the tooth for detecting calculus or for removing it and other irregularities from the tooth. The stroking pattern can be vertical, oblique or diagonal, or circumferential. *Exploratory strokes* require minimal pressure against the tooth, since nerves in the fingers need to detect the slight variations in the texture and morphology of the teeth that cannot be seen when working subgingivally, but that can be felt with a fine explorer or probe. The *adaptation* of the instrument tip against the tooth as it moves around the circumference of the tooth is critical in detecting root variations and in preventing accidental piercing of the soft tissue with the point. All of these principles are important in exploring and probing. They also are important in removing deposits. In addition, two new principles of instrumentation require mastery for safe removal of de-

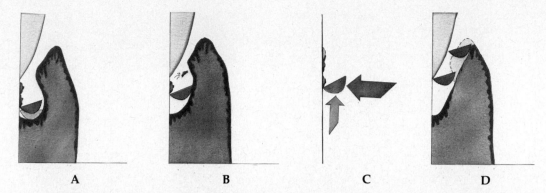

| A | B | C | D |

Fig. 21-1. A, Scaler inserted to base of sulcus and beneath a calculus deposit. **B,** Calculus being removed by properly angulated blade (more than 45 degrees and less than 90 degrees to tooth). Calculus is removed by increased horizontal pressure against tooth as working stroke is activated, **C,** and motion out of sulcus is completed, **D.** Coincidental curettage of sulcus wall occurs in some instances as cutting instrument moves out of sulcus. (Adapted from Seibert, J.S. 1978. Continuing Dental Education, University of Pennsylvania School of Dental Medicine **1:** No. 8.)

Fig. 21-2. Instrument may merely chatter over or smooth down a calculus deposit if insufficient horizontal pressure is used or if blade is dull. (Adapted from Seibert, J.S. 1978. Continuing Dental Education, University of Pennsylvania School of Dental Medicine **1:** No. 8.)

posits: working stroke and angulation. The principle of a working stroke is described here. Angulation is discussed following a description of the parts of a scaler and an introduction of the necessary terminology.

Working stroke

One critical difference between probing and removing deposits relates to the type of stroke used. Although the same gentle stroke is used with a scaler in moving into the sulcus, once a deposit is located with the scaler, the motion out of the sulcus becomes a *working stroke*. A working stroke involves increased pressure laterally against the tooth at the edge of the deposit as the instrument is brought out of the sulcus with the wrist rock motion. The increased pressure against the tooth forces the deposit to fracture away from the tooth (Fig. 21-1). The goal is to fracture away the entire deposit if possible. It is *not* to chip away or wear down the deposit. If adequate pressure is not maintained against the tooth, the instrument will slide over the deposit, smoothing it down but not removing it from the tooth (Fig. 21-2). Also, the horizontal pressure against the tooth prevents the instrument from being pulled from the sulcus with a jerk. All alternating exploratory and working strokes should remain under solid control and generally be maintained subgingivally until the surface feels smooth with the scaler. As with the probe and explorers, the instrument should not exit completely from the sulcus with each stroke. Rather, the instrument should remain subgingivally until the area being scaled feels smooth. Then the instrument can be used to scoop out any loose calculus or other debris, and the area can be flushed thoroughly with an air-water spray. When an entire sextant or quadrant is scaled and feels smooth to the scaler, the clinician should then reevaluate the areas with a fine explorer or periodontal probe for more definitive detection of deep deposits or residual pieces of deposits.

A critical element in ensuring a light-handed approach to instrumentation is to use working strokes only when calculus or roughness is detected on the tooth. Otherwise it is best to use exploratory strokes with cutting instruments.

The horizontal pressure against the tooth is effective only if the instrument doing the calculus removal has a sharp blade (Parr et al., 1976; Seibert, 1978). The sharp blade on the cutting instruments used in deposit removal distinguishes them from the probe and explorers used thus far in instrumentation. Similar to the explorers, the cutting instruments must be designed so that they have access to all areas of the mouth and so that they will not damage healthy tooth structure and soft tissue during proper use. There is a wide variety of instruments that meet these criteria and from which an experienced dental hygienist may select his/her instruments of choice.

A solid working knowledge of the types available and their general use in deposit removal makes it possible for each individual to try a wide range of instruments suitable for the variety of cases that challenge the clinician (Parr et al., 1976; Seibert, 1978). Deposit location, size, tenaciousness, and accessibility place limitations on the variety of instruments that may be selected for use.

Sickle scaler

The basic design of the working end of a sickle scaler is shown in Fig. 21-3. The working end is formed by two blades terminating in a point. Each of the two blades is formed by the bevel or facial surface and a lateral surface. The two lateral surfaces join at the bottom of the instrument to form an unused third edge. It should be obvious that two hazards in using the instrument are the potential trauma caused by the point (just as with the point on the explorer) (Fig. 21-4) and by the edge on the bottom of the instrument. Careful adaptation of the sickle scaler can ensure that the point does not wander into soft tissue. Generally, the third edge can be made less of a problem by dulling the underside with a sharpening stone. A few strokes directly over the bottom of the scaler reduce potential difficulty.

The relatively short shank and relatively long straight working end limit the sickle scaler's usefulness) Seibert, 1978). Generally, it is limited to removing supragingival calculus or subgingival

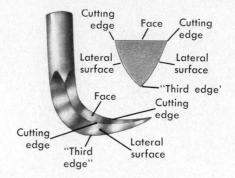

Fig. 21-3. Sickle scaler has two cutting edges. Lateral surfaces join at back of instrument to form a third "edge" that should be dulled to reduce possible tissue trauma. Face (or bevel) of instrument is surface between the two blades converging to form a point. (Adapted from Seibert, J.S. 1978. Continuing Dental Education, University of Pennsylvania School of Dental Medicine **1:** No. 8.)

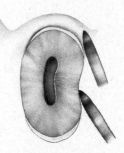

Fig. 21-4. Side of point of sickle must be carefully adapted to tooth to ensure that it does not pierce soft tissue, particularly as it is guided around line angles of tooth. (Adapted from Seibert, J.S. 1978. Continuing Dental Education, University of Pennsylvania School of Dental Medicine **1:** No. 8.)

calculus that is only 1 to 2 mm beneath the margin of the gingiva. It is not effective for deep deposits and may cause tissue trauma if an attempt is made to use it in deep pockets.

The solid design of the instrument makes it strong enough to remove reasonably heavy deposits as long as it is sharp and is used with adequate pressure against the tooth during the working stroke.

Selecting the proper end is a reasonably easy

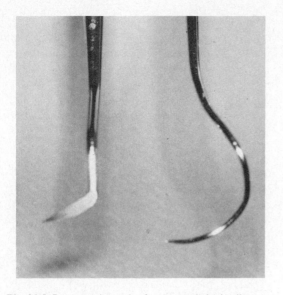

Fig. 21-5. By comparing ends of contra-angled (pigtail or cowhorn) explorer and sickle scaler, it is possible to find matching ends that curve in same direction. Sickle scaler can then be selected for use in areas of dentition by following same principles as for selecting appropriate end of contra-angled explorer.

task once proper end selection with the cowhorn or pigtail explorer has been mastered (Chapter 5). The best way to determine the proper end is to place the double-ended sickle next to the cowhorn or pigtail and determine which ends match. One end of the cowhorn will curve in the same direction as one end of the sickle scaler (Fig. 21-5). The other ends will match likewise. Careful comparisons will reveal that the terminal shank of the instrument adjoining the working end matches the terminal shank of the explorer. Therefore the process used to establish which end of the explorer to use is also the appropriate process for selecting the proper end of the sickle scaler. The end of the explorer used on the mandibular right buccal, for instance, provides a model for the end of the sickle scaler that is appropriate for that area of the mouth. Without referring to the explorer's matching end, it is possible to place either end of the sickle against the mesial surface of a tooth in the mandibular right sextant and determine which end is aimed across the mesial surface and also has a terminal shank in parallel relation to the long axis of the tooth. Its pair should be usable on the lingual surface of the mandibular right sextant, with the shank parallel

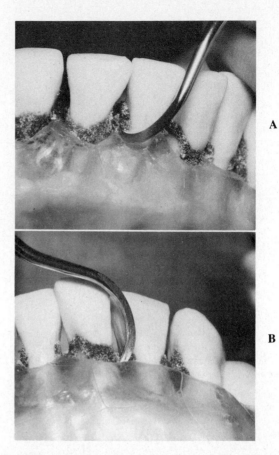

Fig. 21-6. A, Anterior sickle with less angular working end in this case is shown adapted to mandibular anterior tooth on proximal surface. Shank is angled in toward midline of tooth to ensure that angle of blade to tooth is less than 90 degrees. Side of tip is carefully adapted to tooth to avoid piercing soft tissue with point of sickle. **B,** Anterior or straight-shanked sickle can be used with circumferential or horizontal stroke on direct facial and lingual surfaces to remove deposits that are otherwise inaccessible. Extreme care is necessary in adapting blade and in ensuring use of short strokes to prevent tissue trauma.

to the long axis of the tooth. Thus the basic principles of instrument selection for explorers should be useful in selecting paired contra-angled sickle scalers.

Anterior sickles have a straight shank. *The simpler the shank, the more anterior the intended area of use for the instrument* (Fig. 21-6). Anterior sickles can be adapted on anterior proximal surfaces or on the direct facial and lingual surfaces of teeth using a horizontal or circumferential stroke.

Angulation

While basic principles of end selection, grasp, fulcrum, wrist rock, and stroke are basically the same as for explorers (except for the increased horizontal pressure with the working stroke), *angulation* is a critical difference that is important to learn when using cutting instruments. The blade must be angled to the tooth so that it can engage the deposits optimally and so that the edge that is not placed against the particular tooth surface is not engaging soft tissue (Parr et al., 1976; Seibert, 1978). To ensure that these two needs are met, the blade should be angled so that it is less than 90 degrees and more than 45 degrees to the tooth. If the angle of the blade is less than 45 degrees to the tooth, the blade is "too closed," and the facial aspect of the working end is almost completely in contact with the tooth. Instrumentation is therefore ineffective. If the angle of the blade is at 90 degrees or more to the tooth, the angle of the blade is "too open," therefore posing a hazard of tissue damage as well as decreased effectiveness in deposit removal.

Universal curette

A universal curette is shown in Fig. 21-7. It, too, is a paired instrument. Universal curettes come in a variety of sizes and shank lengths for use in heavy calculus removal and in fine scaling (Parr et al., 1976; Seibert, 1978). The shape of the working end of curettes allows them to be used safely in subgingival areas. The universal curette has a rounded toe instead of a point and does not have a third edge on the back. It is generally more spoon shaped and thus is less hazardous to surrounding soft tissue. Yet it is a relatively strong instrument that can be extremely useful in removing heavy, deep deposits. The curved blade (which extends around the toe to form two useful cutting edges) allows it to be more readily adapted to curved root surfaces.

When inserting the universal curette for subgingival scaling, the blade should be closed against the tooth to 0 degrees and inserted to the base of the sulcus past the deposit with this same closed angle. At the base of the sulcus the angle is opened to between 45 and 90 degrees and prepared for the working stroke to remove the deposit (Seibert, 1978) (Figs. 21-8 and 21-9).

The stroking pattern can be a series of vertical

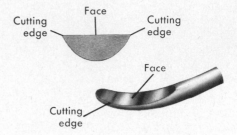

Fig. 21-7. Universal curette has rounded back and rounded toe, which enhance its use in subgingival areas, since this back and toe are less likely to cause inadvertent trauma than are sharp-edged back and pointed toe of sickle scaler. (Adapted from Seibert, J.S. 1978. Continuing Dental Education, University of Pennsylvania School of Dental Medicine **1:** No. 8)

or oblique strokes that overlap (Fig. 21-10) to cover the root or crown surface (Parr et al., 1976; Seibert, 1978). This stroke is used for initial scaling around the tooth and is highly successful in removing most deposits. A second kind of stroke is the circumferential or horizontal stroke (Fig. 21-11). The stroking pattern engages the deposits on the sides and allows another approach to calculus that will not come off with a vertical stroke. It also is a useful stroke for removing small pieces at the line angles of teeth and for gaining access to the very base of the pocket and to furrows and grooves on root surfaces that may be incompletely scaled by vertical strokes (Fig. 21-12).

The same process used in selecting the paired explorer and the paired, contra-angled sickle is used in *selecting the proper end* for the universal curette. Placing the universal curette next to the contra-angled sickle and the explorer allows the clinician to match ends based on direction of curvature and location of the terminal shank. When the universal curette is placed intraorally, the terminal shank should be parallel to the long axis of the tooth as the toe of the instrument is aimed across the proximal surface of the tooth to be scaled (Fig. 21-13). The same principles of grasp, fulcrum, wrist rock, and stroke are used with this type of instrument.

In general, the shank design and working end design of the universal curette allow the instrument to be used with a slightly less restricted pattern of adaptation in the dentition than that allowed by the sickle. Just as with the cowhorn explorer and the

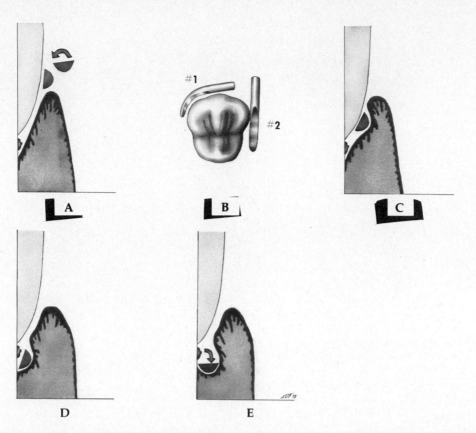

Fig. 21-8. Curette is inserted into sulcus at 0 degrees angulation. **A,** so that it resembles curette No. 1 in **B.** Curette is moved into sulcus and past calculus with exploratory stroke, **C** and **D.** At base of sulcus, blade is opened to between 45 and 90 degrees before beginning working stroke, **E.** If 90-degree angle (as shown here) is used, soft tissue will be removed also. Closing it to 75 to 80 degrees minimizes this hazard. (Adapted from Seibert, J.S. 1978. Continuing Dental Education, University of Pennsylvania School of Dental Medicine **1:** No. 8.)

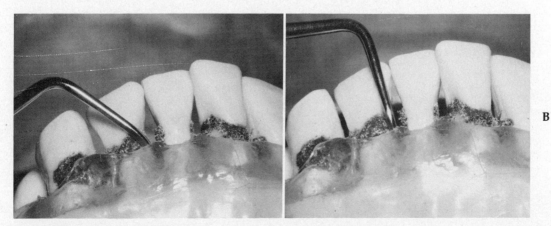

Fig. 21-9. **A,** Curette inserted at 0 degrees and, **B,** then opened to approximately 75 degrees in sulcus.

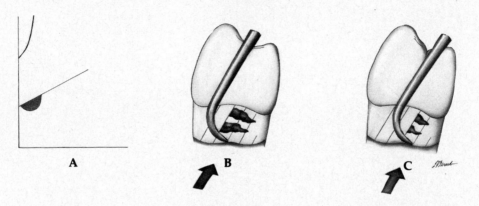

Fig. 21-10. Once blade is engaged at proper angle to tooth, as suggested in **A,** vertical or oblique overlapping working strokes can be used to remove calculus deposits in **B** and **C.**. (Adapted from Seibert, J.S. 1978. Continuing Dental Education, University of Pennsylvania School of Dental Medicine **1:** No. 8.)

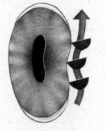

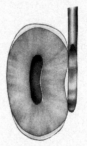

Fig. 21-11. Horizontal or circumferential stroke uses blade with toe aimed more apically so that blade engages lateral side of deposit rather than the most apical aspect of deposit. Horizontal stroking is useful when vertical strokes are not successful and for removing deposits from line angles and from the very base of a pocket. Horizontal stroking also helps obtain adaptation in root furrows and grooves. (Adapted from Seibert, J.S. 1978. Continuing Dental Education, University of Pennsylvania School of Dental Medicine **1:** No. 8.)

Fig. 21-12. Often a vertical stroke will not be adequate in scaling convoluted roots, especially in furrows and deep grooves. Adaptation is critical, since calculus often forms in these protected areas. Rather than trying to adapt full length of blade to proximal surface as shown, adapt first 2 mm of blade and follow contours of root as shown in Fig. 21-4. (Adapted from Seibert, J.S. 1978. Continuing Dental Education, University of Pennsylvania School of Dental Medicine **1:** No. 8.)

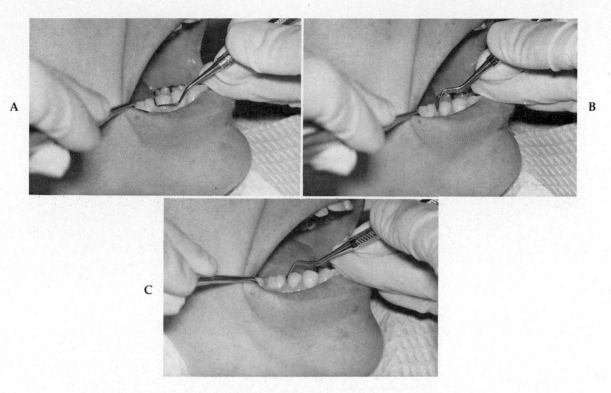

Fig. 21-13. A, Universal curette is adapted with toe directed proximally but with terminal shank perpendicular to long axis of tooth. **B,** Universal curette is adapted with terminal shank parallel to long axis of tooth. **C,** Angulation is closed to less than 90 but more than 45 degrees before beginning working stroke.

paired contra-angled sickle, the instrument can be used in any given sextant from the facial or lingual surfaces, *with one edge adapting against the mesial aspect and the opposite edge on that same end adapting on the distal aspect.* In other words, the same end of the instrument is used for all proximal surfaces in a given sextant from the buccal aspect. And, of course, the opposite end is used in that same sextant from the lingual aspect on all proximal surfaces. The two edges on a given end of the instrument make it possible to scale the mesial surface and then the distal surface and so on by merely changing the edge being used and the orientation of the shank in relation to the long axis of the tooth.

With the universal curette it is possible to use the *opposite end* of the instrument to scale most distal surfaces as well. That is, the end that normally would not be used on a given sextant from a particular aspect can be used on the distal surfaces safely and with the proper angulation. For example, one end can be used on the mandibular right area from the buccal aspect; the other end can be used in that quadrant from the lingual aspect. With the universal curette the end used from the lingual aspect can also be used on distal surfaces from the buccal aspect. The terminal shank, however, will not be parallel to the long axis of the tooth in this case. Return to Fig. 21-13, *A,* which shows the position for using the *opposite end.* By raising the shank to a 45-degree angle to the long axis of the tooth, the instrument can be adapted on the distal surface safely. Generally, this particular use of the instrument is an adjunct to regular patterns of instrumentation largely because it necessitates an additional change of ends of the instrument, which is not necessary if the opposite edge of the same end is used as usual. It is helpful to know that this adaptation can be safely accomplished, since there are times when a slightly different approach to an area will allow the right adaptation to remove a particularly challenging deposit.

Selecting a curette: design variations

There are many varieties of universal curettes and therefore considerable opportunity for selecting a specific curette for a particular patient's need. Variations in shank angle, shank strength, and shank length allow for an appropriate curette to be selected to use in remote or more anterior areas of the dentition, for heavy tenacious deposits, and for very deep or relatively shallow pockets. Tissue tightness to the tooth often dictates the size of the shank or blade that may be selected. Extremely tight tissue will not allow a heavy, large instrument adequate access to remove subgingival deposits.

The length of the blade is another variable in selecting a universal curette. Longer blades are needed to gain access across the relatively broad proximal surfaces of posterior teeth but may be quite inappropriate for use on the narrow mandibular anterior teeth.

While the universal curette is often the instrument of choice for removal of moderate or heavy amounts of calculus and when the width and depth of the pocket can accept the heavier shank, there are other curettes that are more appropriate for adaptation in deep, tight pockets and for removal of fine deposits and root planing. Gracey curettes are examples of instruments with longer, thinner shanks and with more delicate blades. They are characterized by a preangled blade design. The blade and bevel are set at the correct angle to the terminal shank so that the shank can be kept parallel to the long axis of the tooth throughout instrumentation. The universal curettes (and the sickle scalers) require that the blade be angled to between 45 and 90 degrees after it is inserted; the shank is then angled toward the long axis of the tooth during instrumentation. The Gracey curettes are introduced in Chapter 23.

General guidelines for selection of universal curettes include (1) reserving heavy, large curettes for heavy deposits and finer, smaller curettes for finer deposits or for access to tight subgingival areas; (2) using long-shanked instruments for deep

pockets; and (3) selecting the blade length according to the amount of tooth surface to be scaled.

Sequence

Whether the universal curette or the sickle scaler is being used for removing moderate to heavy amounts of calculus, the same general sequence is followed as described in detail in Chapter 5.

The mandibular posterior sextant closer to the clinician (mandibular right for right-handed clinicians; mandibular left for left-handed clinicians) is scaled first, moving from the most posterior tooth through the first premolar. The distal, facial, and mesial surfaces are scaled using overlapping exploratory and working strokes as calculus is detected and engaged for removal. The stroking pattern should carry the instrument past the proximal midlines of each tooth to ensure that typically elusive deposits are not left.

The clinician then scales the mandibular sextant on the opposite side of the mouth, approaching it from the lingual surfaces. The lingual surfaces on the side of the mouth nearer the clinician are next, and then the buccal aspect of the opposite side of the mouth is scaled. At this point all the posterior teeth are scaled. If the instrument has reached sufficiently far across the proximal surface, and if the instrument has reached under the deposits to engage and remove them with overlapping strokes, few deposits should remain. With either a posterior sickle or a universal curette, this can be accomplished with only one position change (moving to the rear position for the buccal surfaces on the side away from the clinician) and with only one instrument change (changing ends when moving from the lingual surfaces of the distant sextant to the lingual surfaces of the near sextant).

The anterior teeth can then be scaled either from the rear or front position.

Many clinicians stop and explore the mandibular teeth for remaining deposits before moving to the maxilla. If considerable deposits remain on these teeth, time will be needed to return to these locations and remove the calculus and recheck.

Once no deposits can be detected on the mandibular teeth, the clinician moves to the buccal aspect of the maxillary sextant closer to the clinician and then to the lingual aspect of the distant posterior maxillary sextant. The clinician changes ends and positions (to a rear position) and scales the lingual surfaces of the nearer maxillary sextant, followed by the buccal aspect of the distant sextant. The anterior teeth are then scaled from the rear position. The maxilla is explored for residual deposits and rescaled as needed.

Particularly difficult deposits may require the use of adjunct instruments such as a hoe or file. Deposits located in areas defying access may need to be approached with an unconventional adaptation or fulcrum placement.

Hoe

The hoe is an instrument that is usually limited to removal of large ledges of calculus (Seibert, 1978). Calculus that rings the tooth, particularly on the facial, lingual, and distal surfaces of teeth that have no posterior tooth adjacent to them, can be removed relatively easily with a hoe.

Fig. 21-14 shows the design of a hoe. It has one blade. The angle of the shank determines the area of use. Generally, the instruments are paired so that one end can be used on the facial surface and its pair can be used on the lingual surface of a given tooth. The companion instrument has one end that can be adapted on the distal surface of a tooth, while its pair can be adapted on the mesial surface of the tooth. The mesial and distal pairs are useful when the adjacent tooth is missing. Thus they are especially helpful in removing ledge calculus from the distal surface of the last tooth in the quadrant and on the direct lingual surface of lower

anterior teeth, especially when a large bridge of calculus is present.

The same modified pen grasp, fulcrum, and wrist rock are used with hoes as are used for the previously described instruments. However, in implementing the stroking pattern, the instrument is limited to a vertical pattern of strokes (Fig. 21-15). The instrument is placed into the sulcus and moved apically past the deposit of calculus. It is not possible or advisable to force the instrument near the

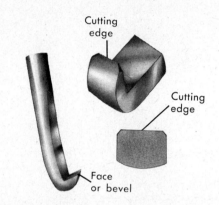

Fig. 21-14. Hoe has one blade and firm shank. When placed beneath a ledge of calculus, a vertical stroke will usually be successful in removing deposit. As shown, corners of blade should be clipped off with sharpening stone. (Adapted from Seibert, J.S. 1978. Continuing Dental Education, University of Pennsylvania School of Dental Medicine **1:** No. 8.)

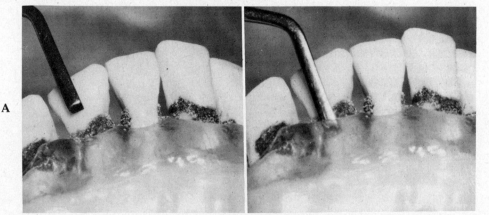

Fig. 21-15. **A,** Hoe with shank parallel to long axis of tooth. **B,** Instrument is moved below edge of calculus with exploratory stroke. Vertical working stroke pattern will engage and remove deposit.

attachment because of its bulk. Once the instrument has moved past the ledge of calculus, it should be held firmly against the tooth with the horizontal pressure of a working stroke and moved coronally out of the sulcus. The blade should engage the deposit and remove it in large pieces. The instrument can be used to detect any residual pieces of calculus, but it is not known for fine detection potential. It is a heavy working instrument that generally precedes additional scaling with fine curettes.

Most clinicians maintain a sterile set of hoes for those times when a heavy case requires their use. They are not regular inclusions in a standard tray setup for scaling, however, because of their limited use.

Chisel

The chisel is another instrument that is usually maintained as an adjunct instrument. The Zerfing chisel is illustrated in Fig. 21-16. It is used solely to remove large ledges of calculus from the lingual surfaces of the anterior teeth. It is used with a horizontal push stroke with the blade held against the proximal surfaces of the anterior teeth and entering from the labial aspect (Fig. 21-17). The blade is adapted against the distal surface, then against the mesial surface, and so on with a gentle push stroke between the teeth until the large bridge of calculus is adequately loosened and can be removed from the lingual aspect of the teeth. It is never to be pushed down into the gingival sulcus, and it is not designed for a pull stroke out of the sulcus. Its sole function is in the anterior areas, where most instruments would crumble the deposit, and more time would be required to remove a bridge formation of heavy calculus.

File

When an area of subgingival calculus defies removal with universal curettes, sickles, hoes, and other instruments generally used for universal scaling, a file can be used effectively to crush the deposit and roughen it so that other instruments can remove the fine remnants of calculus (Fig. 21-18). The size of files varies, but generally speaking the small fine files that can be readily adapted subgingivally provide the greatest flexibility and accessibility. In design, files are like several small hoe blades placed in a row on a flat head. They are

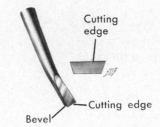

Fig. 21-16. Chisel has single blade and straight shank. Cutting edge is at end of instrument so that when it is pushed against a deposit, leading cutting edge will engage calculus. It is sharpened with flat stone on bevel.

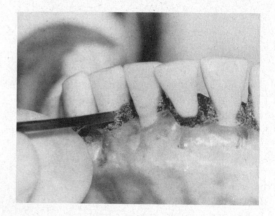

Fig. 21-17. Chisel is used solely to remove lingual calculus on anterior teeth by placing blade against proximal surfaces from labial aspect and pushing toward lingual aspect.

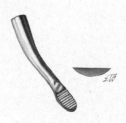

Fig. 21-18. Files are composed of a series of parallel blades on a flat working head. Heavy files have a few large blades, whereas fine files have many small blades.

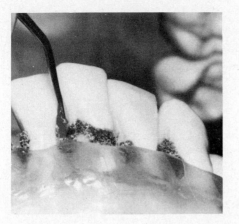

Fig. 21-19. File is adapted to tooth to crush calculus and smooth area. Follow-up strokes with a curette are important for removing small fragments and smoothing tooth structure.

usually paired to allow access on direct facial and lingual surfaces with one pair of instruments and on mesial and distal surfaces with the other pair of instruments. Thus, in basic design and in areas of access, files are quite similar to hoes. However, the instruments designed for mesial and distal surfaces can be used even in areas where there is an adjacent tooth. Fig. 21-19 illustrates a file approaching the mesial surface of a tooth. The instrument is carefully inserted between the papilla and the tooth, is used to find the tenacious deposit, and is engaged against the deposit with the head of small blades pressed against the deposit and ground into the deposit, crushing it. Horizontal and vertical strokes can follow this crushing motion. A universal curette or a finer curette can be used to finish the area.

Files are usually placed in the category of adjunct instruments and therefore may not be used routinely in general practice or in a recall program.

Other instruments

There are many other kinds of shank designs, working end sizes, and shank strengths available. However, the basic designs apply to most instruments and can be helpful in selecting instrument ends and in selecting which type of instrument to use for each type of case. Regardless of the type of instrument presented, a careful analysis of the position of the blade(s), shank size and angulation,

and size of the head of the instrument will determine the usefulness and limitations of the instrument. While the student of dental hygiene functions with a limited set of instruments, it is helpful to have a wide variety of instruments available for advanced instrumentation in the later phases of clinical development.

EVALUATING FOR COMPLETE DEPOSIT REMOVAL

While the working instruments provide some amount of tactile sense in determining the presence of deposits in the mouth, all scaling procedures should be carefully evaluated with instruments that provide maximum tactile sensitivity. The explorer or probe should be used at the completion of scaling in each quadrant or arch to determine whether deposits are completely removed. These finer instruments may uncover deposits located just apical to the contact area, a location difficult to reach with heavy instruments, or the explorer may detect a small portion of a deposit at the corner of the tooth or just above the attachment, both of which easily can be missed with a heavier instrument.

During the scaling procedure itself, it is wise to use exploratory strokes with the working instruments to detect relative smoothness of the tooth surface before moving on to another area. However, it is essential that all areas be thoroughly evaluated with explorers or a probe before an area is declared complete.

As mentioned in Chapter 12 it is sometimes possible to detect calculus in subgingival areas by directing a stream of compressed air into the sulcus. The tissue, particularly if not tight to the tooth, can be deflected from the tooth, allowing the clinician to look into the sulcus. Also, after a period of healing, the tissue can be evaluated to identify any particular areas of continued inflammation. Often, isolated areas of poor healing identify the location of residual calculus deposits. Sometimes those deposits will be visible as a dark shadow at the margin of the gingiva. A stream of air can confirm that finding, along with thorough follow-up exploring.

Supragingival calculus is best detected with air and with a well-directed beam of light. The calculus will appear as a chalky white layer across the tooth surface. It will feel crusty and soft to the explorer rather than smooth and hard, as enamel is. Disclosing solution will usually stain this crustaceous calculus. Even the fine grains that cannot be seen clearly with air and light will be visible with a disclosant. It is important to differentiate calculus deposits from plaque, since even repeated polishing will not remove them from the teeth. A sharpened curette or sickle is necessary to remove the fine, residual grains of calculus. If they remain on the teeth, they provide an opportunity for new plaque to adhere, and they can be felt by the patient's tongue.

Whether the deposits are visible or not, it is essential to remove all deposits from the teeth and use thorough evaluation procedures to ensure their complete removal. The time-honored goal in the profession is 100% removal of all deposits—subgingival as well as supragingival. At some point in a clinician's career, particularly when he/she is at the point of believing that clinical skills are quite well developed, it may be useful to observe a periodontal surgery being performed for one of the patients the clinician has had the opportunity to scale. A great deal can be learned about adequacy and thoroughness as a clinician by seeing a flap laid in the area of scaling and seeing if areas of calculus remain despite even the most careful efforts. Research shows that it is extremely difficult to remove all calculus, especially when it is embedded in irregularities and when it is in deep pockets (Nishimine and O'Leary, 1979; Rabbani et al., 1981). Complete scaling and evaluation is a skill that develops with time; the goal of 100% removal for all patients may be a value to be strived for rather than a valid measure of day-to-day success.

ALTERNATIVE FULCRUM PLACEMENT

As described in Chapter 5 and earlier in this chapter, the usual location for a fulcrum or finger rest is on the occlusal surfaces of teeth. The tooth surface should be dry so that the clinician's finger is less likely to slip, particularly during a working stroke, when control is absolutely essential. If the finger rest is lost, the instrument may accidentally traumatize the patient's palate, lip, gingiva, or the clinician's hand. The first choice for a finger rest or fulcrum is on a dry, stable tooth. Slippery mucosa or no finger rest is an unsafe choice.

There are instances when an alternative fulcrum is needed (1) in order to reach inaccessible areas, (2) when even slight pressure against the lip or stretching of the lips is not easily tolerated, (3) when there are not enough teeth in the sextant to provide a fulcrum, or (4) when removing a particularly tenacious calculus deposit demands the greater leverage available from having a more distant fulcrum.

Fig. 21-20 shows an alternative rest for the lingual aspect of the maxillary left quadrant for a right-handed clinician. The left index finger is laid across the mandibular arch in the area of the premolars, and the fulcrum finger of the right hand rests stably on it. This is a useful approach for patients with small mouths or in instances when there are few teeth in that sextant to provide a fulcrum.

Fig. 21-21 shows the fulcrum finger placed on the left index finger, which is resting securely in the labial vestibule, retracting the lip. This alternative is useful when using circumferential strokes on the facial surfaces or when there are inadequate numbers of teeth to provide a ready fulcrum site. It is the fulcrum of choice when using a horizontal, facial-to-lingual push stroke with a chisel.

In Chapter 5 there is considerable discussion regarding access to the buccal aspect of the maxillary teeth in the sextant closest to the clinician. Two rests are described: one posterior to the operative site and one anterior to the site. The two approaches require different wrist rocks (see Fig. 5-21—right-handed clinician—or 5-33—left-handed clinician). The finger rest posterior to the operative site is described as using the orbicularis oris muscle at the corner of the mouth to provide much of the

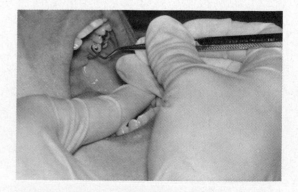

Fig. 21-20. Alternative fulcrum placement for maxillary left lingual sextant uses left index finger resting on mandibular arch.

stability, particularly for extreme posterior instrumentation sites. When the last tooth in the quadrant is being explored or scaled, all fulcrum support is localized on the elastic resistance of the corner of the mouth.

There are two other alternatives for access to this area. Fig. 21-22 shows a rest where the backs of the third and fourth fingers are pressed firmly against the cheek, serving as an extraoral fulcrum. Or, the left index finger can be used to retract the cheek, with the right fulcrum finger resting on it (Fig. 21-23).

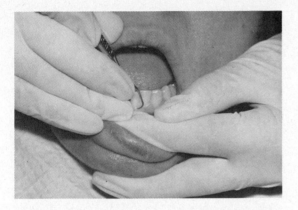

Fig. 21-21. Fulcrum finger rests on index finger placed in mandibular anterior vestibule.

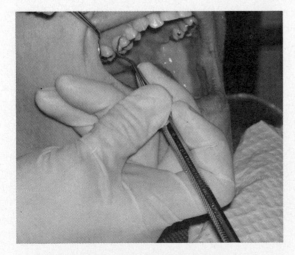

Fig. 21-22. Backs of third and fourth fingers are pressed extraorally against cheek for fulcrum for access to maxillary right buccal area.

BEYOND CALCULUS REMOVAL

This chapter has focused on removing calculus deposits with hand instruments. As noted in Chapter 12, it is important to remove calculus in order to create an environment less conducive to the accumulation of plaque. However, initial and maintenance therapy for patients with periodontal involvement requires more than just calculus removal. It requires that all plaque and the endotoxin by-products of plaque be removed from the root surfaces so that the surrounding soft tissues can repair and generate reattachment. It requires that surrounding soft tissue be prepared for healing, which may necessitate soft tissue curettage.

It is now clear that simply removing calculus and polishing teeth, even when combined with good patient oral hygiene, are not adequate to halt the disease. The subgingival plaque front can progress apically, and the cementum-bound endotoxin will continue to irritate the soft tissues, causing continued subclinical destruction despite the deceivingly healthy appearance of the gingivae (Daly et al., 1982; Aleo et al., 1974; Waerhaug, 1978a, 1978b).

In the next few chapters other instrumentation procedures are introduced for removing calculus, for debriding the root surfaces, and for performing curettage. Given our growing understanding of the progress and prevention of periodontal disease, these functions are essential components of the scope of practice of a dental hygienist.

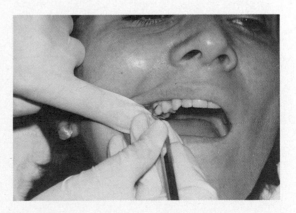

Fig. 21-23. Left index finger retracts cheek; right fulcrum finger rests on it for access to maxillary right buccal area.

ACTIVITIES

1. Compare the contra-angled sickle and the universal curette with the cowhorn or pigtail explorer. Identify which ends match in terms of the direction of the shanks. Given either end of the contra-angled sickle or universal curette, identify all areas in the dentition where that end may be used so that the point aims across the intended proximal surface, the terminal shank is parallel to the long axis of the tooth, and the handle exits the mouth from the front.
2. Use the suggested sequence of position to adapt the contra-angled sickle, straight sickle, and universal curette in each sextant of the dentition. Be certain to:
   a. Use a modified pen grasp.
   b. Establish a firm fulcrum.
   c. Use all fingers as a unit to generate a wrist rock, pivoting on the fulcrum finger.
   d. Adapt the side of the tip to the tooth to avoid piercing the tissue with the point or toe of the instrument.
   e. Angulate the face of the instrument at greater than 45 degrees and less than 90 degrees to the tooth.
   f. Execute exploratory strokes around the tooth with the scaler or curette, using horizontal pressure against the tooth when engaging a deposit (working stroke).
   g. For the universal curette: use the *opposite end* on distal surfaces and analyze its usefulness.
3. Adapt the hoe, chisel, and file on a typodont and on calculus-laden teeth set in plaster. Explore apically with the hoe and file to detect calculus and engage horizontal pressure apically to remove it. Use a push stroke from labial to lingual surfaces to loosen a bridge of calculus by engaging the blade of the chisel on the proximal surfaces.
4. Scale a quadrant for a more advanced student's patient. Have the advanced student watch the procedure and offer suggestions. Observe as the student uses air, light, explorer, probe, and/or disclosant to evaluate for residual calculus.
5. Role play ways of responding to hypothetical patients, employers, and peers who describe the dental hygienist as a person who cleans teeth.
6. Develop a role definition of dental hygiene that adequately describes the class's perception of how the oral prophylaxis fits into the scope of practice.
7. Compare the effects of a dull blade and a sharp blade for calculus removal from plaster-mounted calculus-laden teeth.
8. Compare the shank sizes and shapes and the sizes of the working ends for a variety of:
   a. Universal curettes
   b. Hoes
   c. Files
9. Given descriptions of clinical conditions such as amounts and location of calculus, sulcus or pocket depth, and gingival tissue conditions, practice selecting appropriate scalers for removing the deposits.

REVIEW QUESTIONS

1. What are two major differences between scaling with a cutting instrument and exploring?
2. True or false. Correct the false statements.
   a. A chisel is useful for removing large bridges of calculus from the lingual surface of the mandibular anterior teeth.
   b. The chisel is used with a pull stroke.
   c. The hoe is useful for removing ledge calculus that is readily accessible to a heavy instrument.
   d. The file is used to crush calculus.
   e. The universal curette is used primarily for deep calculus removal.
   f. The sickle scaler is the most versatile instrument, since it is effective for deep scaling as well as supragingival scaling.
   g. As long as calculus is removed from the teeth, the soft tissues will be able to heal with time.
3. What are the three methods for evaluating complete calculus removal?

REFERENCES

Aleo, J.J., et al. 1974. The presence and biological activity of cementum-bound endotoxin. J. Periodontol. **45:**672.

Axelsson, P., and Lindhe, J. 1981. The significance of maintenance care in the treatment of periodontal disease. J. Clin. Periodontol. **8:**281.

Badersten, A., et al. 1981. Effect of nonsurgical periodontal therapy. J. Clin. Periodontol. **8:**57.

Daly, C., et al. 1982. Histological assessment of periodontally involved cementum. J. Clin. Periodontol. **9:**266.

Knowles, J., et al. 1980. Comparison of results following three modalities of periodontal therapy related to tooth type and initial pocket dept. J. Clin. Periodontol. **7:**32.

Morrison, E., et al. 1980. Short-term effects of initial, nonsurgical periodontal treatment (hygienic phase). J. Clin. Periodontol. **7:**199.

Nishimini, D., and O'Leary, T.J. 1979. Hand instrumentation versus ultrasonics in the removal of endotoxins from root surfaces. J. Periodontol. **50:**345.

Parr, R.W., et al. 1976. Subgingival scaling and root planing. San Francisco: University of California School of Dentistry.

Rabbani, G.M., et al. 1981. The effectiveness of subgingival scaling and root planing in calculus removal. J. Periodontol. **52:**119.

Seibert, J.S. 1978. Incorporating root planing and gingival curettage into a clinical practice. Continuing Dental Education, University of Pennsylvania School of Dental Medicine **1:** No. 8.

Waerhaug, J. 1978. Healing of the dento-epithelial junction following subgingival plaque control. I. As observed in human biopsy material. J. Periodontol. **49:**1. (a)

Waerhaug, J. 1978. Healing of the dento-epithelial junction following subgingival plaque control. II. As observed on extracted teeth. J. Periodontol. **49:**119. (b)

22 REMOVING HEAVY DEPOSITS: ULTRASONIC INSTRUMENTS

OBJECTIVES: *The reader will be able to*

1. Given information about oral conditions and general health status, identify those patients for whom ultrasonic scaling is or is not an appropriate choice.
2. Describe the advantages and disadvantages of ultrasonic scaling.
3. Briefly describe how the ultrasonic scaler removes deposits.
4. Identify precautions that must be taken to minimize cross-contamination during ultrasonic scaling.
5. Given a patient for whom ultrasonic scaling is indicated, describe the procedure for the patient's information to ensure patient confidence, informed consent, and sufficient information to enable the patient to decide whether or not to proceed.
6. Identify four important measures for helping the patient cope with water flow.
7. Given an ultrasonic unit, prepare it for operation by connecting:
    a. Electrical outlet
    b. Foot control
    c. Water supply
    d. Handpiece
8. Describe the procedure for preparing an instrument tip for use in a manual tune unit.
9. Identify the design and usefulness of each of the following tips:
    a. Chisel
    b. Beaver-tail
    c. Universal curette style
    d. Periodontal probe style
10. Describe the best sequence and stroking pattern to produce a smooth tooth surface with an ultrasonic scaler.
11. Describe the length and speed of the stroke used with an ultrasonic instrument.
12. Contrast ultrasonic instrumentation principles with those employed with hand instruments.
13. List three functions of the water lavage in ultrasonic scaling.
14. Describe the procedure for adjusting temperature of the water lavage.
15. Given a series of patients for whom ultrasonic scaling is indicated:
    a. Prepare the patient for maximum comfort and with sufficient information for informed consent.
    b. Prepare the equipment and take precautions to minimize microbial cross-contamination.
    c. Select an appropriate area for completion.
    d. Use appropriate tips in a sequence that removes stain and calculus both supragingivally and subgingivally.
    e. Explore all areas for removal of deposits.
    f. Root plane all areas to completion, obtaining a hard, smooth surface.
    g. Ensure that plaque control measures are being learned and employed by the patient to ensure the best possible tissue resolution.
16. Briefly describe research findings related to effectiveness, tissue response, tooth structure smoothness, and safety precautions when ultrasonic instruments are used.

A complete intraoral assessment of a patient may reveal large amounts of calculus. Some patients have calculus that bridges the teeth, especially in the mandibular anterior and maxillary posterior areas. Large, tenacious deposits may prevent the patient from adequately flossing interdental areas, and if they are visible, their presence may be of major concern to the patient, especially since they are an esthetic problem.

From a treatment planning point of view, many clinicians feel it is advantageous to remove as much of the calculus as possible early in treatment so that the patient is able to begin a new routine of self-care and to feel better about his/her mouth immediately. Additionally, thorough early removal of the heavy deposits makes it possible to more accurately assess pocket depth and establish a prognosis.

To remove heavy deposits with minimal trauma to soft tissues in a relatively short amount of time, an ultrasonic scaling device can be used. Although hand instruments designed for heavy deposits such as chisels, hoes, and heavy universal curettes can be used, the ultrasonic scaler requires less time and results in less clinician and patient fatigue and discomfort (Green and Sanderson, 1965). Depending on the type of deposit and the expertise of the clinician, scaling with ultrasonic instruments may require only 20% to 60% of the time required to complete the procedure with hand instruments alone.

Less chair time for the patient is usually valuable to both the patient and the clinician. The patient who has accumulated large amounts of calculus has usually had a long sabbatical from dental care and is pleased to have preliminary appointments that are brief and maximally productive.

Likewise, the clinician who is confronted with several years' accumulation of calculus can anticipate a proportionate amount of hand fatigue when using hand scalers. In contrast, the ultrasonic scaler results in almost no hand fatigue, since it requires only a light grasp and virtually no pressure against the tooth. Two arches of supragingival and subgingival scaling can be accomplished by the experienced clinician in a 45-minute to 1-hour appointment. Less experienced operators may select one arch to complete during an appointment, with re-evaluation of the scaled arch and scaling of the remaining arch reserved for a later appointment.

One major advantage of ultrasonic scaling is its positive influence on tissue responses. The water lavage that accompanies the calculus removal is apparently largely responsible, along with a co-agulation of the necrotic soft tissue wall adjacent to the tooth surface (Ewen, 1961). The lavage flushes most small calculus fragments and dislodges necrotic tissue from the sulcus so that the site has few if any local irritants remaining to retard healing. It is frequently described as the instrument of choice for patients with acute necrotizing ulcerative gingivitis (ANUG), a painful, inflammatory disease. Symptoms disappear more rapidly when ultrasonic scaling is used, and patients report less discomfort immediately following treatment (Fitch et al., 1963). One study has reported that after 8 weeks there was no statistically signficant difference between tissue healing after hand scaling and tissue healing after ultrasonic scaling (Torfason et al., 1979).

Ultrasonic scaling is, however, not without controversy. For the 30 years that it has been used in dentistry, research regarding its impact on the teeth and surrounding tissues has resulted in mixed reports (Green and Sanderson, 1965). Most of the studies that question its long-term merit focus on the changes the instrument makes on root structure, particularly in contrast to the results obtained from using hand instruments in root planing procedures. A more complete discussion of these controversies is given at the end of this chapter.

ORIGINS AND MECHANISM

Ultrasonic instrumentation was first used in dentistry in the 1950s. An ultrasonic drill was used to prepare teeth for restorations, but it relied on an abrasive slurry to cut the tooth and therefore reduced visibility considerably. High-speed turbine drills were developed about that time as well. Since the turbine drill was found to be quite effective, the ultrasonic drill was phased out (Ewen and Glickstein, 1968; Green and Sanderson, 1965).

An ultrasonic instrument reappearaed in 1955 for periodontal instrumentation and was first described by Zinner (1955). It has undergone many changes in design and usefulness since that time. The bulky, complex units are now compact and easy to adjust. The variety of tips has increased, and many tips carry the needed water supply through an internal tube rather than by means of an external tube, which can easily bend out of alignment with the tip. Several manufacturers have developed units, each with unique features. Air-driven units that generate less heat are available for direct connection to air turbine hoses, competing with the ultrasonic devices largely because of their ease of operation and simple storage (Woodruff, Levin, and Brady, 1975).

Ultrasonic instruments use high-frequency sound waves to fracture deposits from teeth and to cavitate the accompanying water supply to mechanically flush the area. The instrument tip vibrates approximately 25,000 cycles per second, with the water spray creating a halo of tiny bubbles surrounding the tip in a fine mist (Green and Sanderson, 1965).

Because the ultrasonically "vibrating" tip and cavitating water cleanse the tooth, there is no need for sharp instruments. In fact, for purposes of scaling and curettage, the tips must be dull. There is no need to engage a sharp blade against the deposit or tissue; the vibrations from merely placing the activated tip on the operative area cause the deposits to fracture away and necrotic tssue to coagulate. Placing the tip against the deposit and moving it over the surface result in a calculus-free area and a smoother tooth surface. No pressure against the tooth is necessary. Usually the instrument will simply stop if pressed against the tooth, although damage to the tooth can sometimes occur.

INDICATIONS, CONTRAINDICATIONS, AND PRECAUTIONS

When the ultrasonic scaler was first introduced, overly zealous users employed it for all prophylaxis procedures, since it was much easier than hand scaling. However, indiscriminate use is a mistake. It is best reserved for patients with large amounts of calculus. Since hand planing should, according to most investigators, follow ultrasonic instrumentation, the patient with almost no calculus will need more chair time than necessary if the ultrasonic scaler is used. And, of course, there are instances in which the medical history or certain oral conditions preclude its use.

Generally, the ultrasonic scaler should be used for those patients who have large, tenacious deposits and stains on their teeth. It can be used to remove deposits from teeth that will be extracted, minimizing the possibility that calculus will lodge in the extraction site. But its greatest usefulness is in preparing teeth for definitive periodontal therapy. Teeth with heavy deposits can be cleansed so that only the final stages of root planing are necessary. As mentioned previously, patients with ANUG frequently commence treatment with ultrasonic debridement (Ewen and Glickstein, 1968; Fitch et al., 1963).

Ultrasonic scaling is extremely useful for clearing local irritants in pericoronitis and gingival and periodontal abscesses. It can be used to clear deposits in cases of chronic marginal gingivitis, periodontitis, idiopathic fibrous hyperplasia, drug-induced hyperplasia, and hormonal gingivitis such as that associated with pregnancy, puberty, or menopause (Ewen and Glickstein, 1968).

Composite resins, especially Class IV and V restorations, should be avoided when scaling ultrasonically, since the action of the instrument tends to cause margin leakage leading to marginal staining and loss of retention (Pollack and Kronenberg, 1981).

Ultrasonic scaling is contraindicated for any patient with a pacemaker, since the sound frequencies of the scaler may disrupt the electronic mechanism with electromagnetic interference. Although most newer models of pacemakers have shielding to prevent such interference, it is unwise to subject the patient to such a risk. It is also not to be used for patients with local osteomyelitis, chronic cyclical gingival infections, gingivosis of menopause, nutritional deficiencies of a chronic debilitating nature, severe uncontrolled diabetes, and local neoplasms of metastatic nature. It should not be used on young, growing tissues or for patients undergoing immunosuppressive or prolonged antibiotic and/or corticosteroid therapy (Ewen and Glickstein, 1968; Gross, Divine, and Cutright, 1976).

The ultrasonic scaler generates heat, which is cooled by water. However, if insufficient water is used to reduce heat or if the instrument is held against one area of a tooth for more than a few seconds, the temperature in the pulp chamber can rise to hazardous levels. The thermal conductivity of restorations and the thickness of tooth structure separating the instrument from the pulp affect the likelihood of a rise in pulp temperature. Usually the patient will feel discomfort and alert the clinician, preventing continued trauma. But if the operative site is anesthetized, damage could be considerable (Abrams et al., 1979). Water flow must be maintained, and the instrument must be kept moving at all times in order to reduce the possibility of pulp trauma.

Since the water spray that accompanies the procedure creates an aerosol of water and microorganisms that contacts the clinician and settles on adjacent equipment surfaces, it is *essential* that the clinician wear protective lenses and a face mask. The entire area sould be disinfected thoroughly after each use. It is also recommended that the air in the operatory be continually flushed with a laminar airflow system, which circulates and filters the air of microorganisms (Williams, 1970). When the ultrasonic device is being used, there is a thirtyfold increase of airborne microorganisms, most of which are known to be normal flora of the mouth (Holbrook et al., 1978). Of the airborne contaminants that could cause infection of the clinician or subsequent patients, 97% can be removed with laminar airflow (Williams, 1970). Obviously, it would be unwise to use the ultrasonic device for patients known to have hepatitis or tuberculosis, when the aerosol of pathogens would be extremely dangerous, but precautions should be taken to ensure that even the less virulent organisms are contained.

Another potential hazard of the ultrasonic device is the microbial contamination that can be carried to the surgical site by the water lavage itself (Gross, Devine, and Cutright, 1976). Public water supplies with high counts of microorganisms inoculate the surgical area. Also, the narrow tubing in the unit provides an ideal site for bacterial growth. Water valve connections in the unit may be a site of growth of microbes and of the accumulation of mucin and debris. The results of one study suggest that sterile water should be used (Ballinger, Brasher, and Maupin, 1976). A more recent study has shown that there are no statistical differences in postoperative infections between patients treated with ultrasonic scaling using sterile water and those treated with ultrasonic scaling using regular tap water (Reinhardt et al., 1982). With or without separate water supplies, it is important to assess for backwash of bacteria into the unit and subsequent contamination of the water.

Since ultrasonic scaling has been shown in one study to cause temporary tinnitus (ringing in the ears) and hearing shifts, it is probably wise to avoid extremely prolonged, repeated use for any patient (Möller, Grevstad, and Kristoffersen, 1976).

Once the patient's conditions have been established and it is apparent that the ultrasonic scaler is the instrument of choice, there are several specific procedures that should be followed if the patient is to be comfortable, if the procedure is to be efficient, safe, and effective, and if the equipment is to be properly maintained.

PREPARATION OF THE PATIENT

Perhaps the most important phase of preparation is readying the patient for the procedure. Most patients look warily at humming machines that are rolled into view. Therefore the first step is to briefly explain to the patient the condition that warrants a scaling procedure, why scaling should be done, the consequences of not having complete scaling, the likely aftereffects of the procedure, and the time and cost involved. Included with this explanation should be an introduction to the machine itself.

Following is a typical case presentation in preparing the patient for ultrasonic scaling:

Presentation: I'd like you to take a look in the mirror while I show you something. (Patient grasps mirror; clinician retracts lips to expose gingivae and heavy calculus, using a mouth mirror.) These dark, crusty deposits are hard, chalklike pieces of calculus that are firmly attached to the teeth. They usually go hand in hand with disease of the gum tissue (or gingiva) and bone. Their presence makes it difficult for you to use floss and to adequately cleanse your teeth. (Pause to answer any questions and to follow up on the patient's nonverbal responses.)

One of the first things that needs to be done is to remove these deposits. Once they are gone, your tissue should begin to feel better, and it should be easier to keep up your home care routine. Besides, your teeth will look better.

Sometimes right after the deposits are removed, your teeth will be sensitive to cold. You've had all that crusty insulation for a few years, and once it is gone, the teeth will need to generate their own internal insulation. Other than the sensitivity and a couple of days of tender gingiva, the properly performed procedure has no known harmful effects.

There are two ways in which we can complete the procedure. One is with hand instruments, which you may have had used on your teeth some time ago. Have you ever had your teeth cleaned with metal instruments? (Pause for response and discussion.) The other way is to use the ultrasonic scaler. This latter method should take a good deal less time, since sound waves from this tip remove the deposits (rather than hand pressure) and since it is constantly flushing the area to clear away the loosened debris. Usually it feels a good deal better both during and after the procedure, since there isn't extensive pressure and the instrument is gentler on the soft tissues. Healing time may be less also, since the soft tissue is disturbed less and because the water lavage creates a clean site for the tissues to respond.

One problem you may encounter is tooth sensitivity during the procedure. Some patients do experience this sensation—although many feel it with hand instruments as well. (Pause for questions and discussion.)

If we use hand instruments, it may take up to three or four 1-hour appointments to remove all deposits and smooth the roots. If we use the ultrasonic instruments, the first appointment should result in removal of almost all deposits. Two more appointments will involve fine smoothing of the roots of the teeth to ensure that all irritants are removed and to produce a hard root surface. The cost per visit, as mentioned earlier, is $ _____.

Do you have any questions about your condition or the procedure? (Most patients will ask how the ultrasonic device works. It is usually helpful to let the patient see the tip work with the water spraying around it and to let them feel a tip that is kept handy for demonstration purposes. However, you do not want the patient to contaminate sterile equipment with his/her fingers. Also, you can try the sterile tip on a readily visible area while the patient observes in the mirror as the deposits are removed. Usually, contrasted with one or two areas of hand scaling, the patient will opt for ultrasonic scaling.)

It is a maxim that fully informed, consenting patients are more cooperative and generally more relaxed. Participation in their own care seems to make the difference. Many patients feel uncomfortable when they feel they are the *objects* of care, *to whom* instead of *for* or *with whom* care is being provided.

Other preparations for patient comfort include placing a plastic drape and an absorbent napkin, giving the patient a wipe to catch any stray trickles of water, and placing the patient in a full supine position. The "halfway" position usually stimulates considerable gagging. *In all cases,* be certain to have *adequate suction.* The passive suction of the saliva ejector is inadequate. High-volume suction manipulated by an assistant or linked to a saliva ejector is essential.

Also, it is important to explain to the patient that the water can be adjusted if it is too warm or too cold. Sensitivity associated with the procedure often can be reduced by means of a simple adjustment of water temperature or by lowering the power setting used with the tip that is selected.

PREPARATION OF THE EQUIPMENT

The equipment for most units includes a control box, foot control, water connector, and handpiece. Insert tips for the handpieces are separate.

The control unit should be moved close to the chair for easy access for adjustments. It should be plugged into the electrical outlet. If the foot control is separate, it usually plugs into the back of the unit (Fig. 22-1). Matching the shape of the plug prongs with the shape of the holes in the unit determines the correct outlet. The plug must be securely attached. Next the water hose is attached to the unit. Usually it is either a "quick disconnect" clip-on junction (Fig. 22-2) or a junction with

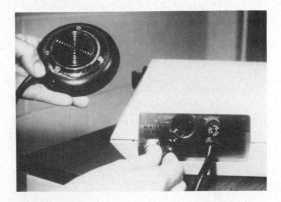

Fig. 22-1. If foot control is separate from unit, it usually plugs into back of unit.

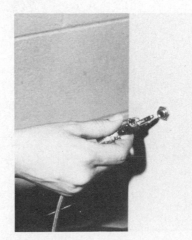

Fig. 22-2. Water source for ultrasonic unit is hose that connects to dental unit with either a quick disconnect "clip-on" (as shown) or with a screw-on nozzle.

threads for screwing the hose endpiece into the unit. Again, it is important that this connection be secure.

Many ultrasonic units have the handpiece attached. If the handpiece is separate, matching the prongs with the outlet (usually found on the front of the control box) is again important.

Once the electrical connection, foot control, water source, and handpiece are attached, the unit is turned on. It is essential to follow the manufacturer's directions for any of the variety of units available.

For a commonly used unit with manual tuning, the procedure is as follows (Clark, 1969):

1. Turn the unit on by setting the power to *high*.
2. Hold the handpiece upright (*without* tip in place).
3. Activate the foot pedal until water emerges from the handpiece opening. (This clears air from the line to reduce heat buildup.)
4. Tip the handpiece to the side, and adjust the water flow control until the water trails from the edge in a steady flow of nearly contiguous drips (Fig. 22-3). Two minutes of water flow will help clear stagnant water from the unit and should reduce the likelihood of direct inoculation of proliferating microorganisms. This procedure is essential if the unit has been standing unused for several hours or more.
5. Remove foot from the pedal. Disinfect the handpiece, and wash hands thoroughly to remove contaminants.
6. Insert the sterilized tip selected for the initial phases of scaling (Fig. 22-4). Lock it firmly in place (Fig. 22-5). Select the power setting suggested for the tip.
7. Hold the tip over a sink. Turn the tune control to 10. Depress the foot pedal (Fig. 22-6).
8. Activate the tune knob from 10 back to the point at which the highest pitched squeal is heard and the water sprays into a halo around the tip (Fig. 22-7). If this point is passed, return the knob to 10 and proceed down the scale again, while listening carefully and watching the spray.

Once the aforementioned steps have been accomplished, the unit is ready to function. For self-tuning units, omit steps 7 and 8. The unit will tune itself after it operates for a few seconds.

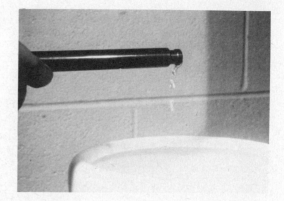

Fig. 22-3. Before placing tip insert, activated handpiece should be held upright until water emerges from opening. It should then be turned to the side and water flow adjusted until water trails from edge in steady flow of nearly contiguous drips.

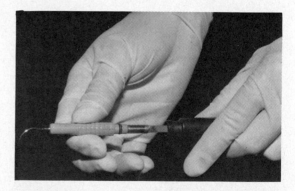

Fig. 22-4. After water has run freely from handpiece for at least 2 minutes, first tip to be used may be inserted into handpiece. Many different methods of insertion are used by different manufacturers. In this case, insert slides into handpiece.

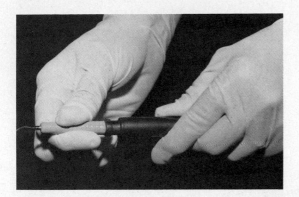

Fig. 22-5. Insert is locked firmly in place prior to tuning.

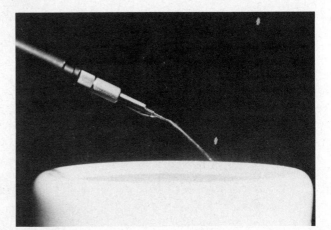

Fig. 22-6. Prior to proper tuning, water runs or sprays off end in a stream.

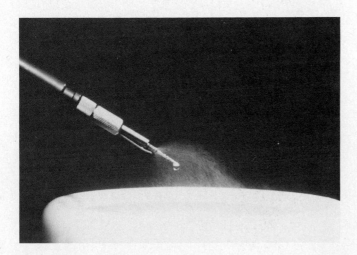

Fig. 22-7. When tip is in tune, water should spray around tip in a ''halo.'' High-pitched squeal is heard at this point. One or two shakes of handpiece will eliminate drop from tip.

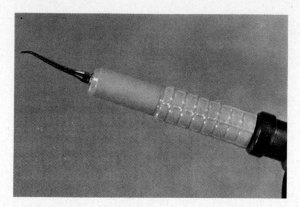

Fig. 22-8. Tip shaped like Zerfing chisel can be used to loosen and remove lingual bridges of calculus. Water flows through instrument and strikes working end at correct angle to create cavitation.

Fig. 22-9. Chisel-shaped tip is used with "blade" against proximal surfaces from labial aspect with horizontal push stroke. As it is applied to each surface, bridge of calculus on lingual surfaces is gradually loosened and can be lifted out in one or two pieces.

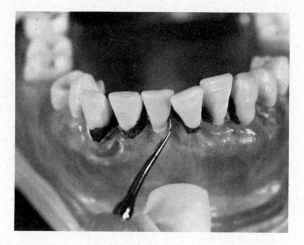

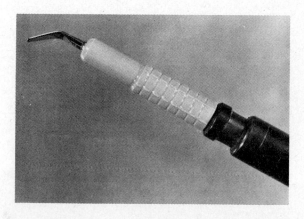

Fig. 22-10. Flat-tipped beaver-tail tip is used to remove large, tenacious deposits throughout mouth.

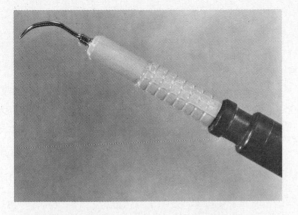

Fig. 22-11. Universal curette tip is probably most commonly used in practice. This tip has greater access to 3 to 4 mm pockets and adapts more readily to curved tooth surfaces.

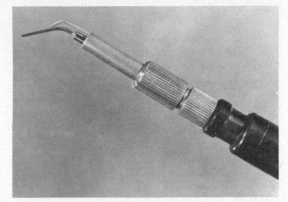

Fig. 22-12. Tip shaped like periodontal probe removes fine deposits. It has best access to deep pockets and furcation areas. This tip has external tube water source targeting working end. All tips shown are available with either internal or external tubing.

INSTRUMENT SELECTION

The selection of an appropriate tip is an important component of ultrasonic scaling. It is just as essential as the selection of appropriate hand instruments for scaling and root planing.

The tip should be heavy enough to adequately remove the deposits but not heavier than necessary. The tip should readily adapt to tooth surfaces.

Just as in hand scaling, the heaviest instruments are used to remove the heaviest deposits. For a patient who has bridges of calculus linking the teeth together, the tip shaped like a Zerfing chisel can be employed to loosen the bridge in one or two pieces (Fig. 22-8). The chisel is applied horizontally with a push stroke, flat against the proximal surfaces, and moved from labial to lingual aspects (Fig. 22-9). Once the heavy bridges are removed, the flat-tipped instrument, often referred to as a *beaver-tail* tip, can be used on all surfaces to remove large deposits (Fig. 22-10). This tip should be used until the heaviest and most tenacious chunks are dislodged. Because of its size and shape, it is not the tip of choice for deep or small deposits.

After using the beaver-tail tip, clinicians often use the universal tip, which is most commonly used in practice. Its shape is similar to that of a Gracey 7/8 curette, except, of course, for the fact that it has no cutting edge. This tip can be inserted into 3 or 4 mm pockets, adapts more readily to curves, and still can remove relatively heavy deposits (Fig. 22-11).

Once the quadrant, arch, or other designated segment of the mouth has been thoroughly scaled with the beaver-tail and universal tips, it is appropriate to move on to the tip with a shape similar to that of the periodontal probe (Fig. 22-12).

This tip removes fine deposits and helps smooth clinically detectable root roughness. It is used to remove small residual irritants and is extremely useful in furcations, root furrows, and other anatomic depressions. It is, however, basically ineffective in the removal of heavy deposits.

Other tips are useful adjuncts and may meet the individual preferences of experienced clinicians. There are, for instance, contra-angled versions of the universal tip that are useful on proximal surfaces of posterior teeth. Each manufacturer has a selection of tips. It is important to assess the variety of available tips before purchasing such a unit, since poorly designed tips will not result in a thorough scaling.

TREATMENT PLANNING AND ORDER OF INSTRUMENTATION

A patient for whom ultrasonic instrumentation is indicated can usually have the entire mouth scaled by an experienced clinician in 1 hour, unless the deposits are particularly firmly attached. A beginning clinician should select one quadrant to complete or, at most, one arch.

As each tip is used, the entire designated area to be completed in the appointment should be scaled before tips are changed. A common error is to scale all areas and then change to a finer tip before the area has been evaluated for deposits remaining and before all heavy deposits have been removed. The unactivated tip can be used to detect the presence of deposits in each area as it is scaled. However, detection with an explorer or periodontal probe will provide a more accurate and thorough evaluation.

Therefore, once the chisel and beaver-tail tips have been used both supragingivally and subgingivally, the areas should be explored and air should be used to deflect the tissue to examine the areas. If deposits remain, it is wise to leave the heavy tip in place and remove them. Then the tip can be changed.

Another error is to use one tip to remove "gross deposits" throughout the mouth with no single area brought to completion at the appointment. This can lead to difficulty in future scaling appointments if the tissues close down over deep deposits. Also, there may be an added danger of periodontal abscesses forming. The best rule is to complete the predetermined areas. At subsequent appointments the areas can be rechecked to ensure completion.

Ewen and Glickstein (1968) have described a stroking pattern that ensures the smoothest surface. It involves a series of vertical, horizontal, and cross-hatching strokes on each area. If the instrumentation moves from the heaviest to the lightest tips, following the suggested stroking pattern, the first set of strokes on an area (excluding the infrequently used chisel) are made with the beaver-tail tip, the second set of strokes is done at a right angle to the first set with the universal tip, and the final cross-hatching strokes are done with the probe tip.

Regardless of the tip selected, the terminal end of the blade (or point) should never be applied at a perpendicular angle to the tooth. The cycle and direction of motion would hammer the tooth, causing pain and structural damage to the tooth. The terminal end should be maintained at an angle between 10 and 30 degrees to the tooth to ensure that the direction of motion is working tangentially to the tooth rather than hammering at it (Clark, 1969; Stapff, 1975).

If this sequence is followed, it is possible to follow a logical order of instrumentation that minimizes tip changes and maximizes the cleansing of the tooth structure. Such an order is the following:
1. Use the *chisel* tip to break out bridges of calculus.
2. Use the *beaver-tail* tip with horizontal strokes on proximal surfaces and with vertical strokes on direct facial and lingual surfaces (Fig. 22-13). The sequence is:

Horizontal on distobuccal No. 32
Vertical on buccal No. 32
Horizontal on mesiobuccal No. 32
Horizontal on distobuccal No. 31
Vertical on buccal No. 31
Horizontal on mesiobuccal No. 31

3. Use the *Universal curette–style* tip with vertical strokes on proximal surfaces and with horizontal strokes on facial and lingual surfaces (Fig. 22-14). The sequence is:

Vertical on distobuccal No. 32
Horizontal on buccal No. 32
Vertical on mesiobuccal No. 32
Vertical on distobuccal No. 31
Horizontal on buccal No. 31
Vertical on mesiobuccal No. 31

4. Use the *periodontal probe* tip with diagonal cross-hatching strokes in the following sequence (Fig. 22-15):

Diagonal toward lingual on distobuccal No. 32*
Diagonal toward mesial on buccal No. 32
Diagonal toward distal on buccal No. 32
Diagonal toward lingual on mesiobuccal No. 32*

Rapid short strokes should be used. The tip should be constantly moving, since some units generate heat that can damage soft tissue and heat the pulp if it contacts the tooth for longer than 1 or 2 seconds. The wrist rock used for most hand scaling is replaced by finger motion to generate the strokes. The speed of the stroke is approximately two sets of back-and-forth strokes across a surface per second. Short strokes enable the tip to fracture away deposits at their most vulnerable point—their edges. As the edges break away, the stroke moves further across the surface to engage more of the deposit.

*Diagonal strokes on proximal surfaces angled toward the buccal aspect are completed from the lingual side of the tooth.

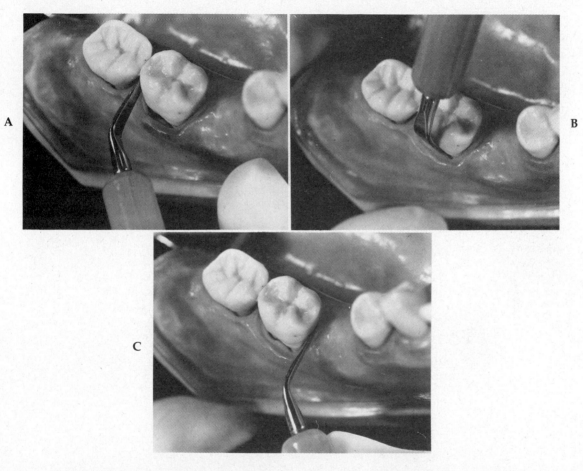

Fig. 22-13. In beginning a pattern of strokes, beaver-tail tip is used on distal surface of tooth No. 31 from buccal aspect with horizontal stroke, **A;** on facial surface with vertical stroke, **B;** and on mesial surface from buccal aspect with horizontal stroke, **C.**

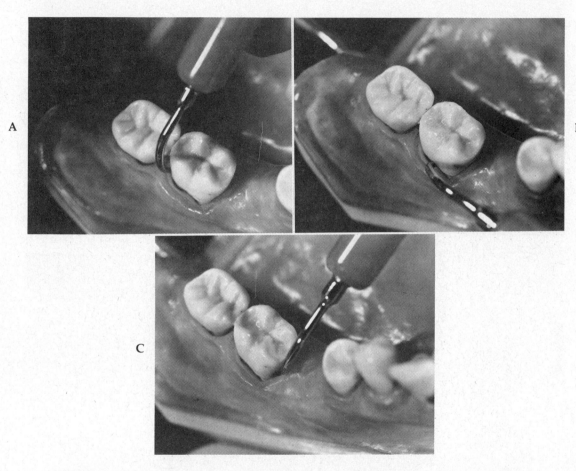

Fig. 22-14. Second pattern of strokes is vertical on distal surface with universal curette–style tip, **A;** horizontal on facial surface, **B;** and vertical on mesial surface, **C.**

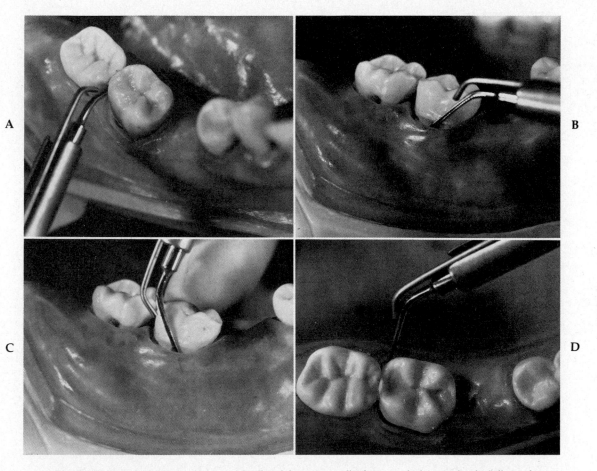

Fig. 22-15. Periodontal probe tip is used in diagonal pattern on distal aspect, **A;** in cross-hatched diagonal pattern on facial aspect, **B** and **C;** and in diagonal pattern from lingual surfaces on distal aspect, **D.** Mesial and lingual surfaces are scaled similarly.

WATER LAVAGE/TEMPERATURE REGULATION

Since most units generate heat and since water is essential to adequately flush away debris, a water spray must accompany ultrasonic scaling. With many types of units it can be harmful to use a tip on the tooth without a flow of water. Water serves as a coolant, lubricant, and cleansing agent. When it is cold, it reduces hemorrhage. When it is warm, it aids in dissolving debris and in floating out fatty substances.

As the water meets the vibrating tip, it cavitates into a spray of bubbles that collapse inward. This is what causes the halolike appearance of the water at the tip.

If the patient complains about cold water, the recommended procedure is to *reduce* the flow of water past the tip to allow more time for the working tip to warm the water. Conversely, if the water is too warm, the water flow should be increased (Ewen and Glickstein, 1968). If the teeth are hypersensitive even though there is a moderate water temperature, the power setting on the unit should be reduced so that sensitivity is also reduced, but so that the tip is still effective. Most manufacturers recommend power settings for various tips, but often these tips can and should be operated at the lowest effective power setting. It is not wise to operate the tips at power settings higher than that recommended by the manufacturer because they may be damaged.

FINISHING PROCEDURES

When the designated area is completed, each surface should be evaluated for remaining deposits. Definitive exploration should follow any ultrasonic scaling to ensure that remaining fine particles or especially deep deposits are detected and removed. A universal curette is usually the instrument of choice for such needs.

The results of one study suggest that intentional curettage of the wall of the pockets should be done immediately after ultrasonic (and hand) scaling to remove loose calculus that is embedded in the wall of the sulcus. The study showed that some of the wall is removed unintentionally; therefore it was suggested that the curettage procedure be performed. The study concluded that water lavage and exploring procedures alone do not ensure removal of loosened calculus, and remaining calculus combined with a partially curetted sulcus wall may hamper healing (Schaeffer, Stende, and King, 1964).

If curettage is indicated after ultrasonic scaling, it may be easily accomplished with the ultrasonic tip, since the instrument has been demonstrated to be highly effective for this purpose (Sanderson, 1966).

When all areas have been completed, the patient should receive postoperative instructions to brush all areas with a soft brush several times a day and to rinse with warm saline if necessary. Flossing may be recommended depending on the case.

The equipment should be stored, with water flushed and then drained from the hoses and the tips sterilized for future use.

The surrounding area should be swabbed thoroughly with a disinfectant after the visit.

At a subsequent appointment the areas that were scaled should be thoroughly reevaluated, and the roots should be planed to ensure that no roughness remains. The objective is to create the smoothest, hardest surface possible to prevent continued disease.

CONTROVERSY: THE IMPLICATIONS OF RESEARCH FINDINGS

Early investigations demonstrated that ultrasonic scaling devices did not harm soft tissues of the periodontium (McCall, and Szmyd, 1960; Zinner, 1955). Many subsequent studies have shown that considerable benefit in terms of improved healing of gingivae is derived from the use of ultrasonic instrumentation. It has been established that the instrument should not be used *on* bone (Ewen, 1961). However, in a study on cats, there was no greater postsurgical bone loss when the ultrasonic scaler was used to scale the teeth (*adjacent* to bone) than when hand instruments were used (Glick and Freeman, 1980).

Controversy is focused on the impact of ultrasonic scaling on tooth structure, particularly that of the root. Early investigations relied on histologic sections of teeth and on the profilometer, a mechanical device used to measure tooth roughness. Later the scanning electron microscope allowed researchers to photograph tooth surfaces at extremely high power so that minute structures and defects could be seen for purposes of contrasting ultrasonically prepared teeth with teeth prepared by a variety of other techniques.

Researchers generally agree that ultrasonic devices remove calculus, subgingival plaque, and endotoxin as well as do hand instruments (Lie and Meyer, 1977; McCall and Szmyd, 1960; Moskow and Bressman, 1964; Nishimine and O'Leary, 1979; Stende and Schaffer, 1961; Thornton and Garnick, 1982; Wilkinson and Maybury, 1973). Disagreement centers on how smoothly roots can be prepared with ultrasonic instrumentation and whether it is effective in root planing.

Many studies using one or more of the three basic techniques of investigation have shown that curettes result in a smoother planed surface (Kerry, 1967; Van Volkinburg, Green, and Armitage, 1976; Wilkinson and Maybury, 1973). A few report actual root "damage" that can be improved only with subsequent thorough root planing. Others report undamaged surfaces but do not advocate ultrasonic root planing. A few report that surfaces as smooth as curetted ones are attainable with ultrasonic instrumentation (Moskow and Bressman, 1964; Pameijer, Stallard, and Hiep, 1972). Most of the recent articles concur that variance in the methods of assessing root structure as well as variance in pressure, power, tip selection, and strokes may account for the mixed results (Clark, Grupe, and Mahler, 1968; Wilkinson and Maybury, 1973; Woodruff, Levin, and Brady, 1975).

A thorough review of the literature can lead to any number of conclusions. The most logical seem to be that the benefits of the instrument warrant its use in *selected cases* as described earlier; that the instrument can be safely and effectively used subgingivally on root surfaces; that the instrument can approximate root planing, depending on the skill of the clinician; and since clinicians are limited in most instances to clinical evaluation of success, that each such procedure should be followed with hand root planing with a curette. The skilled clinician should have to perform less hand instrumentation following ultrasonic scaling than the less experienced clinician.

The research clearly demonstrates that using the lowest effective power for a given tip and a limited number of light strokes (Ewen et al., 1976) will result in less tissue trauma (Clark, 1969; Clark, Grupe, and Mahler, 1968). Research comparing commercial brands of equipment shows little significant differences in their effectiveness (Pearlman, 1982; Van Volkinburg, Green, and Armitage, 1976; Woodruff, Levin, and Brady, 1975). Tip de-

sign does limit access to various tooth surfaces. Two studies have shown that the vibrating air-driven turbine blade causes less surface damage to teeth than ultrasonic instrumentation (Allen and Rhoads, 1963; Lie and Meyer, 1977).

Regardless of the type of instrument, experience and careful attention to precautions and protocols will increase positive results.

OTHER USES

In addition to removing deposits, ultrasonic tips can be used for soft tissue curettage (Sanderson, 1966), periodontal surgery, irrigating periodontal abscesses, recontouring restorations, removing orthodontic cement (Shaver, Siefel, and Nicholls, 1975), administering drugs, cleansing root canals (Martin et al., 1980), and stripping contact areas of crowded teeth (Clark, 1969).

Ultrasonic instrumentation has also been used for condensing amalgam, but the cavitation of expressed mercury is a health hazard; thus the use of ultrasonic instrumentation in amalgam restorations has been virtually eliminated (Chandler, Rupp, and Paffenbarger, 1971).

The most frequent use of ultrasonic instrumentation is in periodontal procedures. It can be a valuable adjunct to therapy when the patient and clinician understand its usefulness as well as its limitations (Forrest, 1967; Green and Sanderson, 1965).

ACTIVITIES

1. Debride extracted teeth with an ultrasonic scaler using the sequence of tips and the stroking pattern suggested. If possible, submit the teeth for scanning electron microscopy (SEM) evaluation.
2. Role play the process of informing the patient about his/her periodontal conditions and the relative merits of selecting ultrasonic scaling to remove hard and soft deposits.
3. Conduct a clinical evaluation of the usefulness and efficacy of ultrasonic scaling for one or more patients by preparing one half of the mouth with ultrasonic scaling and the other half with hand scaling alone. Document immediate preoperative and postoperative results with intraoral photographs. Rephotograph the areas after 3, 7, 10, and 15 days of healing time.
4. Investigate the variety of ultrasonic and air turbine scaling devices, comparing:
   a. Ease of operation
   b. Variety of tips available
   c. Cost and maintenance needs

REVIEW QUESTIONS

1. Ultrasonic scaling should be limited to patients (select the best answer):
   a. With large deposits of calculus and stain
   b. Who have basically healthy oral tissues
   c. Who show signs of tooth sensitivity
   d. Who have limited time for treatment
   e. Who have extremely resilient teeth
2. A patient who has generalized subgingival ledge calculus, chronic marginal gingivitis, severe diabetes, and oral tori is *not* an appropriate case for ultrasonic scaling. Which of the above factors contraindicates ultrasonic scaling?
3. A 10-year-old patient has drug-induced hyperplasia with large amounts of hard and soft deposits. Is this patient appropriately treated if ultrasonic scaling is performed? Why or why not?
4. What are four safety precautions that should be followed to minimize the danger of cross-contamination from the microbial aerosol created by the ultrasonic scaler?
5. How does the ultrasonic scaler remove deposits?
6. Place the following steps for the preparation of a manual tune unit in their correct sequence:
   a. Turn the tune control to 10.
   b. Insert the tip; select the correct power setting.
   c. Activate the foot pedal until water emerges from the upright handpiece.
   d. Flush water from the handpiece for 2 minutes while adjusting the water flow so that the water trails from the edge of the handpiece in a steady flow of nearly contiguous drips.
   e. Turn the unit on by setting the power to high.
   f. Activate the tune control from 10 back to the point of highest pitch squeal.
   g. Remove foot from the pedal. Disinfect the handpiece and wash hands thoroughly to remove contaminants.
7. If the water is too cold, the water flow should be _____ ; if it is too hot, the water flow should be _____ .
8. List the four most commonly used tips in the sequence of their use (first to last).
9. Mark those statements *true* that accurately summarize research findings related to ultrasonic scaling:
   a. Ultrasonic scaling is very effective in removing hard and soft deposits.
   b. Some studies have shown that roots planed ultrasonically are as smooth as hand-curetted roots, but most have concluded that hand planing must follow ultrasonic scaling.
   c. Some minor temporary tinnitus and hearing shifts have been detected in patients who were treated with an ultrasonic scaler.

d. Using the lowest effective power and a limited number of light strokes minimizes root trauma.
e. Ultrasonic debridement yields excellent results in treating patients with ANUG.

REFERENCES

Abrams, H., et al. 1979. Temperature changes in the pulp chamber produced by ultrasonic instrumentation. Gen. Dent. **27**(5):62.

Allen, E.F., and Rhoads, R.H. 1963. Effects of high speed periodontal instruments on tooth surface. J. Periodontol. **34**:352.

Ballinger, M.E., Brasher, W.J., and Maupin, C.C. 1976. Water contamination and the ultrasonic scaler. Va. Dent. J. **53**:10.

Chandler, H.H., Rupp, N.W., and Paffenbarger, G.C. 1971. Poor mercury hygiene from ultrasonic amalgam condensation. J. Am. Dent. Assoc. **82**:553.

Clark, S.M. 1969. The ultrasonic dental unit: a guide for the clinical application of ultrasonics in dentistry and in dental hygiene. J. Periodontol. **40**:621.

Clark, S.M., Grupe, H.E., and Mahler, D.B. 1968. The effect of ultrasonic instrumentation on root surfaces. J. Periodontol. **39**:135.

Ewen, S.J. 1961. The ultrasonic wound—some microscopic observation. J. Periodontol. **32**:315.

Ewen, S.J., and Glickstein, C. 1968. Ultrasonic therapy in periodontics. Springfield, Ill.: Charles C Thomas, Publisher.

Ewen, S.J., et al. 1976. A comparative study of ultrasonic generators and hand instruments. J. Periodontol. **47**:82.

Fitch, H.B., et al. 1963. Acute necrotizing ulcerative gingivitis. J. Periodontol. **34**:422.

Forrest, J.O. 1967. Ultrasonic scaling: a five-year assessment. Br. Dent. J. **122**:9.

Glick, D.H., and Freeman, E. 1980. Postsurgical bone loss following root planing by ultrasonic and hand instruments. J. Periodontol. **51**:510.

Green, G.H., and Sanderson, A.D. 1965. Ultrasonics and periodontal therapy—a review of clinical and biologic effects. J. Periodontol. **36**:232.

Gross, A., Divine, M., and Cutright, D.E. 1976. Microbial contamination of dental units and ultrasonic scalers. J. Periodontol. **47**:670.

Holbrook, W.P., et al. 1978. Bacteriological investigation of aerosol from ultrasonic scalers. Br. Dent. J. **144**:245.

Kerry, G.J. 1967. Roughness of root surfaces after use of ultrasonic instruments and hand curettes. J. Periodontol. **38**:340.

Lie, T., and Meyer, K. 1977. Calculus removal and loss of tooth substance in response to different periodontal instruments. J. Clin. Periodontol. **4**:250.

Martin, H., et al. 1980. Ultrasonic versus hand filing of dentin: a quantitative study. Oral Surg. **49**:79.

McCall, C.M., and Szmyd, L. 1960. Clinical evaluation of ultrasonic scaling. J. Am. Dent. Assoc. **61**:559.

Möller, P., Grevstad, A.O., and Kristoffersen, T. 1976. Ultrasonic scaling of teeth causing tinnitus and temporary hearing shifts. J. Clin Periodontol. **3**:123.

Moskow, B.S., and Bressman, E. 1964. Cemental response to ultrasonic and hand instrumentation. J. Am. Dent. Assoc. **68**:699.

Nishimine, D., and O'Leary, T.J. 1979. Hand instrumentation versus ultrasonics in the removal of endotoxins from root surfaces. J. Periodontol. **50**:345.

Pameijer, C.H., Stallard, R.E., and Hiep, N. 1972. Surface characteristics of teeth following periodontal instrumentation: a scanning electron microscope study. J. Periodontol. **43**:628.

Pearlman, B.A. 1982. Ultrasonic root planing. Aust. Dent. J. **27**:109.

Pollack, B.F., and Kronenberg, E.B. 1981. A pilot study on the effects of ultrasonic instrumentation on composite resins. N.Y. J. Dent. **51**:151.

Reinhardt, R.A., et al. 1982. Effect of nonsterile versus sterile water irrigation with ultrasonic scaling in postoperative bacteremias. J. Periodontol. **53**:96.

Sanderson, A.D. 1966. Gingival curettage by hand and ultrasonic instruments: a histologic comparison. J. Periodontol. **37**:279.

Schaeffer, E.M., Stende, G., and King, D. 1964. Healing of periodontal pocket tissues following ultrasonic scaling and hand planing. J. Periodontol. **35**:140.

Shaver, R.L., Siefel, I.A., and Nicholls, J.I. 1975. Effect of ultrasonic $ZnPO_4$ cement removal on band adhesion and cement solubility under orthodontic bands. J. Dent. Res. **54**:206.

Stamps, J.T., and Muth, E.R. 1978. Reducing accidents and injuries in the dental environment. Dent. Clin. North Am. **22**:389.

Stapff, K.H. 1975. Debridement with ultrasonics, I. Quintessence Int. **6**:57.

Stende, G.W., and Schaffer, E.M. 1961. A comparison of ultrasonic and hand scaling. J. Periodontol. **32**:312.

Thorton, S., et al. 1982. Comparison of ultrasonic to hand instruments in the removal of subgingival plaque. J. Periodontol. **53**:35.

Torfason, T., et al. 1979. Clinical improvement of gingival conditions following ultrasonic versus hand instrumentation of periodontal pockets. J. Clin. Periodontol. **6**:165.

Van Volkinburg, J.W., Green, E., and Armitage, G.C. 1976. The nature of root surfaces after curette, Cavitron and Alphasonic instrumentation. J. Periodont. Res. **11**:374.

Wilkinson, R.F., and Maybury, J.E. 1973. Scanning electron microscopy of the root surface following instrumentation. J. Periodontol. **44**:559.

Williams, G.H. III. 1970. Laminar air purge of microorganisms in dental aerosols: prophylactic procedures with the ultrasonic scaler. J. Dent. Res. **49**:1498.

Woodruff, H.C., Levin, M.P., and Brady, J.M. 1975. The effects of two ultrasonic instruments on root surfaces. J. Periodontol. **46**:119.

Zinner, D.D. 1955. Recent ultrasonic dental studies, including periodontia, without the use of an abrasive. J. Dent. Res. **34**:748.

23 REMOVING FINE DEPOSITS AND ROOT PLANING

OBJECTIVES: *The reader will be able to*

1. Define root planing.
2. Identify the objectives for performing root planing.
3. Contrast root planing techniques with scaling of heavy deposits in terms of instrument selection and number, length, direction, and pressure of working strokes.
4. Describe design differences between Gracey curettes and universal curettes.
5. Discuss the importance of irrigation as part of root planing.
6. Describe adaptation of Gracey curettes to the teeth.
7. Discuss the criteria used to evaluate the root planing procedure and their application.
8. List the factors that may complicate implementation of root planing and suggest ways of eliminating or responding to them.
9. Discuss five contraindications for performing definitive root planing for a patient.

The use of hand instruments for fine scaling and root planing is an effective method of treatment for patients with gingival and periodontal inflammation. The two procedures, scaling and root planing, complement each other in treating the hard tissue side of the sulcus or pocket by removing the foreign and diseased substances that are attached to the tooth and that cause inflammation and destruction of the adjacent soft tissues and supporting bone. *Fine scaling* involves the use of hand instruments and ultrasonic devices (see chapters 21 and 22) to detect and remove deposits of plaque and calculus from the surface of the enamel or cementum. During scaling, the emphasis is to remove soft and hard deposits and to smooth plaque-retentive surfaces (e.g., overhanging amalgam restorations) but no intentional attempt is made to remove the surface cementum completely. *Root planing* extends the treatment of the root surface that has been exposed to the oral environment of the periodontal pocket as a result of the loss of previously attached gingival fibers. This exposed cementum, which has been altered by the disease process, is carefully and completely planed, or shaved away, from the root surface during root planing to ensure the removal of all embedded calculus, plaque, and its toxic by-products (endotoxins), as well as any surface cementum that may still harbor inflammatory substances.

It is important to have a clear understanding of the inflammatory process of periodontal disease when one is considering its treatment. Many studies have underscored the importance of plaque as the primary etiologic agent in periodontal disease. Chief among these studies is the one by Loe et al. (1965) in which it was demonstrated that normal healthy tissues became inflamed after 21 days when plaque removal procedures were not employed. The inflammation was reversed when plaque control was reinstituted in these same subjects. Later studies confirmed the role of plaque as the etiologic agent in gingival inflammation and periodontal disease (Theilade et al., 1966; Waerhaug, 1977, 1978a).

Supragingival plaque control measures such as brushing, flossing, and the use of auxiliary plaque control aids have been emphasized as effective means of preventing inflammatory disease. In the patient who has not experienced any prior irreversible inflammatory disease, these measures can be effective in preventing its onset. The situation is different, however, for the patient who has already suffered the loss of gingival attachment and bone as a result of inflammation. Once plaque has formed submarginally, it is no longer accessible to removal by routine home care procedures such as those mentioned above. It is unlikely that the bristles of a toothbrush will clean more than 1 mm below the gingival margin (Waerhaug, 1981). Waerhaug (1976) reported an effective cleaning depth of no more than 2.5 mm for the small interdental brush. Once plaque has migrated along the tooth surface to a submarginal depth of 2 to 3 mm, it becomes inaccessible to these methods of removal. Several studies have described the effect of subgingival plaque on the dentogingival junction and indicated that it is the presence of this subgingival plaque that leads to the inflammatory tissue reactions that result in loss of gingival attachment and periodontal destruction. Supragingival plaque that had not been removed completely gave rise to an advancing plaque front that moved apically into the sulcus area. This plaque front was estimated to move at a speed of about 1 to 2 μm a day toward the dentogingival junction. Once it reached the level of the gingival attachment, it began to destroy the attachment apparatus, which then migrated apically along the root of the tooth. The loss of attachment kept speed with the advancing plaque front. Waerhaug emphasized the need for complete subgingival plaque removal through scaling and root planing in order to reestablish a healthy dentoepithelial junction and prevent further destruction. In addition to being formed from available supramarginal plaque, submarginal plaque can also reform from remnants that are left behind following ineffective subgingival scaling and root planing. It was noted that the speed of reformation of subgingival plaque from these sources will occur just as rapidly as from supragingival sources. These studies stressed the necessity of performing complete submarginal plaque control in addition to daily, effective supramarginal plaque control (Waerhaug, 1978a, 1978b).

Aleo et al. (1974) demonstrated the presence of plaque endotoxin or endotoxin-like substance on the cemental surfaces of periodontally involved teeth. This substance was toxic for gingival fibroblasts and prevented their growth and proliferation (Aleo et al., 1975). These studies generated interest in the role of plaque endotoxins as the major etiologic factor in periodontal disease. Jones and O'Leary (1978) demonstrated that thorough root planing of the cemental surfaces of periodontally

involved teeth was effective in removing the cementum-bound endotoxin and restoring the root surface to endotoxin levels that were comparable to those of healthy teeth with no periodontal disease. Thus it would seem that root planing is an effective means of treating the root surfaces of periodontally involved teeth through its ability to produce a clean, endotoxin-free environment that is conducive to the repair and regeneration of the adjacent soft tissues.

The role of calculus as an etiologic agent in periodontal disease has been studied over the years. One theory stated that the calculus acted as a mechanical irritant to the soft tissues, producing an inflammatory response. Later studies demonstrated, however, that the mere presence of calculus alone was not a primary factor in the incidence of gingival inflammation. Rather, it was the plaque that covered the calculus deposits that induced the inflammation. Baumhammers et al. (1973) performed a scanning electron microscopic study of calculus and described how the rough and porous nature of calculus makes it suitable for plaque accumulation and permeable to penetration by endotoxins. It is these plaque-retentive characteristics of calculus, then, that make it incompatible with the achievement of a healthy gingival sulcus. In order to restore periodontally affected tissues to health, all such plaque retentive surfaces, including calculus and improperly contoured restorations, must be removed from the environment. They not only harbor plaque and its endotoxins, but also make it difficult, if not impossible, for the patient to practice effective supragingival plaque control measures.

Calculus removal by scaling alone is not always possible because of the ways in which calculus can attach to the root surface (Chapter 12). Canis et al. (1979) reviewed the nature of this attachment and identified three ways in which it could occur. One method involved attachment of calculus into cemental irregularities in such a way that a mechanical locking of the deposits and the cementum occurred. Another method of attachment was by direct contact of the intercellular matrix and the root surface. Either of these two methods of attachment would require removal of the cementum in order to guarantee complete calculus removal. This finding is significant because it indicates that even if the clinician scales the root surface until it feels smooth, remnants of undetectable calculus can still remain embedded in the surface itself. Root planing of the cementum surface is necessary to remove the remnants of calculus that remain after fine scaling has been accomplished. There have been many reports of the ineffectiveness of scaling in removing all calculus from the root surface (Jones et al., 1972; Kerry, 1967; Rabbani, et al., 1981; Volkinbrug, et al., 1976; Wilkinson and Maybury, 1973). Many reasons for this have been proposed, including the impossibility of detecting calculus that lies embedded in depressions and resorption lacunae in the cemental surface, or that has been smoothed or burnished during scaling. Even the finest tactile sense and sensitive exploration cannot discriminate between calculus and cementum under these circumstances. The only guarantee that these root surfaces are clean of toxic substances is removal of the cementum itself.

It should be clear by now that no matter how well the patient performs self-care and even if scaling and polishing are accomplished, the affected root surface will remain an irritant to the soft tissue wall of the pocket unless the diseased cementum, which contains viable endotoxins, is removed and all plaque-retentive qualities of that surface have been eliminated (Jones and O'Leary, 1978). In summary, the problems that exist here are (1) an inflammatory process that is causing destruction of tissues; (2) a root surface environment that favors the inflammation; and (3) an inability by the patient to affect these conditions by regular home care methods. What is needed is a means of removing the irritants from the root surface so that the tissues can heal and a method for preventing this situation from recurring.

Fine scaling followed by root planing can be successful in treating periodontally involved root surfaces, but it must be accompanied by the ability and willingness on the part of the patient to perform daily, effective plaque control. Both procedures must occur in order to produce long-term improvements in the oral health of the periodontal tissues. Root planing can create an environment that favors healing in the soft tissues, but lack of effective supramarginal plaque control will undermine these efforts in only a short period of time by allowing the plaque and associated endotoxins to reform again in the pocket area. The objectives of root planing include:

1. To eliminate plaque and associated endotoxins or endotoxin-like substances from the root surface
2. To remove all calculus and other plaque-retentive surfaces from the root
3. To produce a smooth, hard root surface that may be less likely to attract and retain plaque and calculus deposits, and one that enhances the patient's ability to remove accessible plaque
4. To promote gingival healing and the resultant shrinkage and reduction in pocket depth
5. To provide an environment that favors the new attachment of epithelial and gingival tissues to the surface of the tooth

COMPARISON OF FINE SCALING AND ROOT PLANING

To accomplish the goals of scaling, the clinician must detect and recognize the presence of plaque, calculus, and plaque-retentive surfaces both supramarginally and submarginally. Then, with the aid of hand instruments or the ultrasonic scaler, these deposits and/or surfaces can be removed so that the tooth and root feel smooth to an explorer and the deposits can no longer be detected visually. To accomplish the goals of root planing, the entire root surface must be thoroughly cleaned of affected cementum by shaving away the root surface until it feels "polished" (e.g., exceptionally smooth, hard, and homogeneous). Scaling should always precede root planing. The more obvious deposits must be removed before the clinician can evaluate the nature of the root surface itself. The clinician may choose to use the same or different instruments for scaling and root planing, depending on the type and amount of deposits that are present initially. Scaling procedures can be accomplished with the use of ultrasonic devices, curettes, sickle scalers, hoes, files, or a combination of any of these instruments. Root planing is best accomplished with instruments designed for optimal adaptation to deep submarginal areas and for delivery of sensitive tactile transmissions to the clinician.

The instrumentation skills that are employed for fine scaling must become highly developed and refined to facilitate effective root planing. The clinician must have mastered the principles of adaptation, insertion, and angulation and must be able to direct working strokes effectively to avoid injuring the inflamed soft tissues. While this is certainly important for all submarginal instrumentation, it is especially crucial during root planing because of the large number of strokes that are employed to treat every portion of the root surface during this procedure. The ability of the clinician to control the amount of pressure applied to each working stroke must also be developed so that the root surface is not gouged or overplaned, resulting in unnecessary loss of cementum. The clinician must be able to apply the instrument to the cementum with a constant pressure and effective angulation. In addition, the clinician is required to evaluate the progress of the procedure continuously and to determine if adjustments in pressure or angulation are needed either to accelerate or to minimize the removal of cementum depending on the quality of the surface.

The most important skill required for root planing is the clinician's ability to receive a wide variety of delicate tactile sensations, to discriminate among them, and to interpret them accurately. The clinician must detect roughness, graininess, or subtle abnormalities of the root surface that indicate the presence of fine or burnished calculus deposits, diseased cementum, or ridges and gouges created by earlier instrumentation. Because of the nature of these surface irregularities, they will be less obvious to the tactile sense than were the larger deposits and plaque-retentive surfaces that were encountered during the preceding scaling procedures. At other times the clinician may be unable to detect any surface roughness at all, but must still perform some root planing of the surface cementum in order to remove plaque and its associated endotoxins from the root surface. It has not been established exactly what type of attachment exists between endotoxins or endotoxin-like substances and the cementum surface, so it is difficult to determine how deeply these substances have penetrated into the affected cementum. Clinicians should avoid unnecessary removal of the cementum during root planing and must monitor the gingival response to determine if the root surface has been made biologically acceptable to the adjacent soft tissues.

Since most root planing occurs submarginally, unless there has been gingival recession, the cli-

nician must have a reliable mental picture of root morphology to assist the tactile sensations in guiding the adaptation of the instruments. It should be added, however, that no matter how well the clinician knows "normal" root morphology, there is no guarantee that all teeth will fit the "normal" mold. This awareness of root morphology, coupled with a keenly developed tactile sense, will allow the clinician to detect and to navigate the contour of root surfaces, including depressions, grooves, line angles, and furcation entrances. The curette blade and explorer must follow the irregular contour of root surfaces exactly, delivering both exploratory and working strokes that cover every square millimeter of the root surface. In addition, this task must be accomplished without traumatizing the inflamed soft tissues with which the instruments are in close contact.

One critical area for instrumentation during root planing is the apical extent of the pocket at the dentogingival junction. Waerhaug (1978a) studied the effect of subgingival plaque removal on this dentogingival junction and reported that the proximity of the plaque front to this junction could be as close as 0.5 mm. This means that the instrument must be located at the very base of the pocket and in some cases must compress the apical soft tissues in order to remove effectively plaque and calculus that have formed there. Since it is the presence of this plaque that results in destruction of the gingival fiber apparatus, it is crucial that it be removed during instrumentation. Effective plaque and calculus removal at the base of all pockets is a challenge that exists for all clinicians, since it is precisely this part of the pocket in which calculus deposits are often missed. Waerhaug (1978b) issued the ultimate challenge to clinicians when he stated that "removal of 99% of subgingival plaque is likely to be just as bad as no plaque control at all in the long run." It should be clear that definitive root planing is an exacting and time-consuming procedure that demands a great deal of skill, diligence, and patience on the part of the clinician.

ROOT PLANING
Armamentarium

The instruments and supplies used for root planing are much the same as those that might be used for scaling heavier deposits. Instruments that may be used are curettes, hoes, and files. Any of these instruments can successfully remove light deposits and cementum in accessible areas. Several studies comparing the three have shown that different types of instruments produce the smoothest root surface and inflict the least amount of damage to the cementum and the surrounding soft tissues (Kerry, 1967; Wilkinson and Maybury, 1973). In light of these studies, curettes are recommended for use in root planing. Hoes and files may be used as supplemental instruments for heavy and fine scaling in preparation for root planing by the curette. Clinicians who are skilled in the use of hoes and files can adapt them submarginally with good results. The size of the working ends of these instruments has decreased over the years, improving their accessibility to submarginal areas. Although they may speed the scaling and smoothing process, the use of these supplemental instruments should always be followed by the use of a curette to achieve the smoothest surface possible. Not only does the curette design facilitate optimal adaptation to the root surface, but the rounded toe and back also protect the soft tissues from trauma during the procedure.

In choosing the best type of curette for the root planing procedure, there are several factors to be considered. The clinician needs an instrument that will adapt to a wide variety of pocket depths and shapes. The curette design must be versatile enough to be used in any part of the mouth and to reach apically into deep pockets. It must have a blade design that facilitates its use in small, confined areas such as furcations (Bower, 1979). The curette must also be designed with maximum ability to transmit minute vibrations from light calculus deposits and rough cementum and yet be rigid enough to remove these deposits effectively. A narrow blade is necessary because in many cases the deepest pockets are also very tight and allow only limited access to instruments. The Gracey curette designs meet all of the criteria mentioned and are preferred for root planing by many clinicians. Examples of the various area-specific Gracey curette designs are shown in Fig. 23-1.

There are several differences between the design of a Gracey curette blade and that of a universal curette blade. One major difference is that the two cutting edges are not parallel to each other. Instead, the Gracey curette has offset cutting edges so that one edge appears to be lower than the other. In the universal curette design, both cutting edges could be correctly adapted for use on a tooth (as discussed in Chapter 21), but only the lower cutting edge of the Gracey curette should be adapted to the tooth for working strokes. The Gracey curette also has a characteristic beveled surface adjacent to one of its cutting edges, which universal curettes do not have. The different blade design of the Gracey curette gives it what is called a *self-angulating* capability. This means that when the Gracey curette is correctly adapted to the tooth so that the terminal shank or last bend in the shank nearest the blade is parallel to the long axis of the tooth, the blade is already aligned at the optimal working angulation and further adjustments are unnecessary.

Gracey curettes also differ from universal curettes in that there are a variety of shank designs available for the Gracey curettes. Each shank design permits optimal access of that instrument to a specific area of the mouth or to specific tooth surfaces. This means that more than one of these instruments is needed in order to fine scale and root plane the entire mouth thoroughly. In contrast, each universal curette is designed so that it can be used "universally" throughout the mouth. The following list designates the design numbers of the Gracey curettes shown in Fig. 23-1 and the areas for which optimal adaptation can be obtained:

Gracey 1/2 and 3/4: anterior teeth

Gracey 5/6: anterior and premolar teeth

Gracey 7/8 and 9/10: posterior teeth, buccal and lingual surfaces

Gracey 11/12: posterior teeth, mesial surfaces

Gracey 13/14: posterior teeth, distal surfaces

Those Gracey curettes that were designed for use in anterior segments of the mouth have a rather straight and simple shank design, whereas those designed for harder-to-reach areas in the posterior segments of the mouth have shanks with more complex and convoluted designs. Although each of these curettes is useful in its own way, the efficient clinician will limit the choice of instruments for the root planing tray setup to only those designs that are absolutely required to get the job done. Too much time can be wasted hunting for essential instruments among a tray cluttered with extras. A good "starter set" of Gracey curettes that will provide accessibility to any area of the mouth includes the 1/2, 7/8, 11/12, and 13/14.

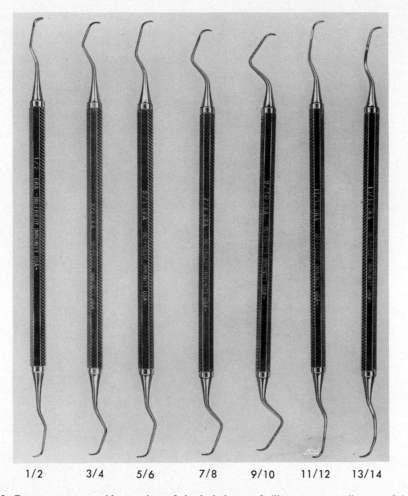

1/2   3/4   5/6   7/8   9/10   11/12   13/14

Fig. 23-1. Gracey curettes provide a variety of shank designs to facilitate access to all areas of dentition. Working-end design is well suited to root planing and removal of fine deposits.

Other instruments or supplies that are necessary for the root planing procedure include a mouth mirror, explorer, probe, and anesthesia setup. The clinician should carefully choose the explorer to be used for evaluating root planing. A fine, long-shanked explorer should be used because this procedure requires optimal tactile sensitivity for detection of fine deposits and root irregularities. The design of the explorer should allow the clinician access to even the deepest pockets. Curved explorers (e.g., the pigtail or cowhorn) cannot reach the apical extent of all pockets. The length of the explorer's working end, its ability to be maneuvered in deep pockets, and its ability to transmit subtle vibrations (i.e., diameter of the working end) must all be considered. Some explorers that fit these criteria, such as the fine No. 17 or No. 20 design shown in Chapter 5 (see Fig. 5-1), may not easily adapt to the distal surfaces of posterior teeth because of their straight design. For these surfaces, the clinician may elect to use a periodontal probe or another instrument for exploration.

The experienced clinician can also use a sharp curette blade to accomplish much of the detection. There are many advantages to developing tactile sensitivity with the curette blade for definitive exploration. According to basic instrumentation principles, this ability is necessary as a prelude to each working stroke performed with the instrument. The student should take time to practice and develop skill in using the curette for exploration because it will increase operating efficiency. This skill will not only facilitate deposit removal because the clinician will have a more accurate idea of where the deposit is located and what type of deposit it is, but it will also require less time and motion expenditure than continually switching from curette to explorer and back. Beginning students should continue to depend on an explorer to evaluate the tooth surface until they have developed their tactile sensitivity to the curette. In addition, the final check or evaluation of the procedure always should be performed with an explorer, even though earlier evaluations with the curette blade indicated completion. This allows the clinician to perform a definitive evaluation of all areas of the root surface for optimal results.

Use of topical or local anesthesia, or nitrous oxide and oxygen conscious sedation during root planing is dependent on individual patient needs. Many patients find any kind of instrumentation performed in inflamed areas somewhat uncomfortable, and because of the exacting requirements of this procedure it may be necessary and advisable to administer some type of pain control. Use of pain control should not be a cover-up for poor instrumentation technique but only introduced in consideration of patient comfort when even safe and effective techniques produce symptoms of pain.

Technique

Root planing employs many of the same principles of basic instrumentation already described for scaling and builds on them. Some comparisons of fine scaling and root planing techniques are discussed earlier on pp. 412 to 413. In addition, some of the specific modifications of the scaling technique as presented in Chapter 21 are discussed below as they pertain to root planing. These modifications include the number of strokes, the direction of the strokes, tactile sensitivity, pressure, the length of the strokes, and time required.

Strokes for root planing usually require less pressure against the wall of the tooth than those for scaling. Because cementum is significantly softer than enamel, there is more chance of gouging the root surface if too much pressure is used. Root planing is essentially a shaving process that re-

moves diseased cementum, attached calculus, and endotoxins layer by layer. The desired root surface is one that feels smooth and free of root irregularities that would attract and retain plaque and calculus. Lateral pressure of the blade against the root surface should be moderate at first until the surface debris of nonvital cementum and calculus is removed. These strokes should be followed by lighter strokes, which remove less cementum while continuing to smooth the root surface. The clinician should be careful not to apply heavy pressure at the onset of the stroke; instead, the same amount of pressure should be applied through the entire stroke. This will prevent ditching of the cementum at those areas where the strokes begin. Strokes used while root planing may also be longer than the ones required for scaling. In scaling the objective is to fracture calculus away from the tooth, and the working stroke can end as soon as the deposit is dislodged. In root planing the initial strokes should be relatively short, overlapping, and controlled until the area is smooth. As more and more of the tooth surface has been planed and the root is approaching smoothness, the planing strokes can be lengthened to blend the completed areas into each other. Short strokes are used initially because they are somewhat easier to control and adapt. Adaptation and control of instruments is especially important during root planing because of the wide variations in root morphology that may be encountered and the close proximity of soft tissues to the cutting edges of instruments.

The application of different types of stroking patterns over a given area is likely to produce a smoother surface than the use of only one stroke direction. For instance, if initial root planing is done with vertical strokes, an even smoother surface will be produced by also applying a series of overlapping oblique and horizontal strokes over the same area (Fig. 23-2). Instrument adaptation for vertical and horizontal strokes is shown in Figs. 23-3 and 23-4. This pattern of strokes is identical to the pattern recommended for ultrasonic scaling (see Chapter 22).

One major difference between scaling and root planing is the time required for each. Hand scaling a tooth usually requires only a few well-executed strokes in given areas, whereas root planing requires complete coverage of the entire root surface of the pocket with short, overlapping, continuous,

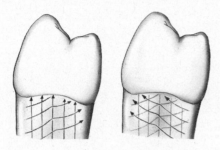

Fig. 23-2. Representation of overall smoothing effect that is produced during root planing through use of a wide variety of overlapping strokes. Result of this cross-hatching pattern of strokes is a surface that is completely planed and polished.

Fig. 23-3. Gracey 7/8 curette is properly adapted for implementation of vertical stroke on mesiobuccal line angle of tooth No. 30. Note that terminal shank is parallel to long axis of tooth for this stroking pattern. This adaptation ensures proper working angulation of lower cutting edge against tooth surface.

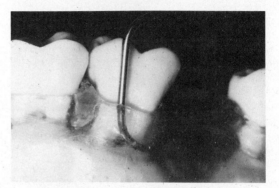

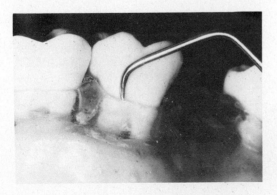

Fig. 23-4. Gracey 7/8 curette is being inserted in preparation for horizontal stroke. Note that toe will be along base of pocket and that terminal shank is not parallel to long axis of tooth.

and repeated strokes. Therefore, it takes much longer to root plane a tooth than to scale a tooth. While a whole mouth may be scaled in 1 hour, it may take the same amount of time to root plane only a few teeth carefully and completely. Obviously, root planing is a much more exacting and definitive procedure requiring a great deal of precision. It cannot be mastered after a few experiences, and many clinicians will admit this is the most difficult treatment procedure to perfect. Students will increase their appreciation of this fact as they perform some of the activities recommended at the end of this chapter. A variety of approaches to root planing are shown in Figs. 23-5 to 23-11.

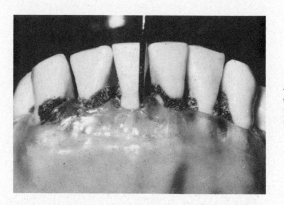

Fig. 23-5. Gracey 1/2 curette is being adapted to mesial surface of lower right incisor. Again note that terminal shank is adapted parallel to long axis of tooth. Deviation from this orientation will result in working angulation being too open or too closed.

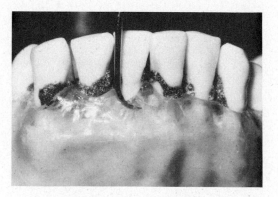

Fig. 23-6. Adaptation of curette blade along narrow labial surface of mandibular incisors is difficult and must be done with a great deal of tactile sensitivity to ensure that toe does not gouge into soft tissues.

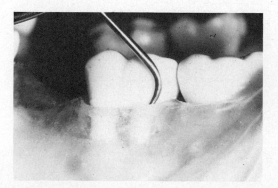

Fig. 23-7. First in a series of photographs demonstrating a variety of approaches to scaling and root planing buccal surface of mandibular left molar tooth in which furcation opening poses additional work. One approach is to use Gracey 7/8 curette on all surfaces except distal surface of mesial root, where it will not adapt. Starting at distal line angle and using vertical and oblique strokes, Gracey 7/8 curette can be used easily in this illustrated buccal area.

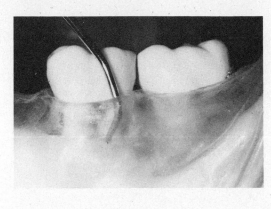

Fig. 23-8. Gracey 11/12 curette is adapted to mesial surface of distal root and into furcation area. This instrument can also be adapted on buccal surfaces of tooth and root with success. As with Gracey 7/8 curette, this instrument will not adapt to distal surfaces of either root.

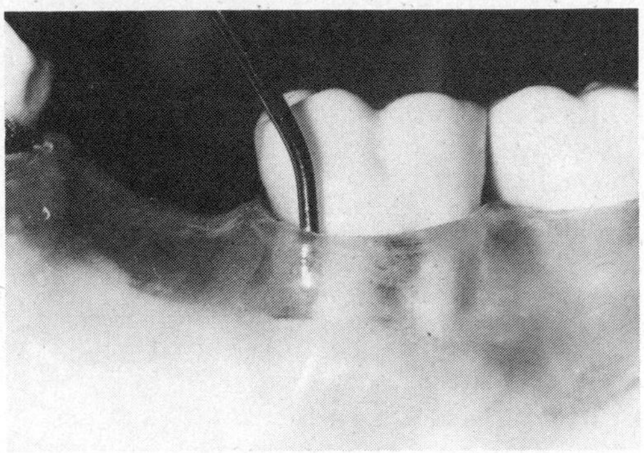

Fig. 23-9. Gracey 11/12 curette is used to continue root planing on mesial surface of tooth and mesial root. It is optimally designed to serve this surface. Note that terminal shank is always parallel to long axis of tooth when this instrument is correctly adapted.

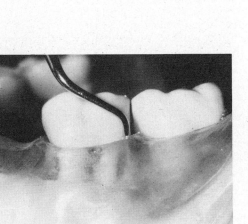

Fig. 23-10. Correct adaptation of Gracey 13/14 curette. Again, terminal shank, which is somewhat buried submarginally, is oriented as parallel to long axis of tooth as possible to facilitate adaptation and angulation.

Fig. 23-11. Gracey 13/14 curette allows adaptation of blade into furcation area so that distal surface of mesial root can be treated. This is instrument of choice for this area on tooth.

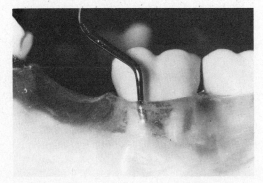

Evaluation

How does the clinician determine when to *stop* root planing? The best evaluation of the success of root planing lies in the response of the soft tissue side of the pocket. If, after a healing period, the clinical signs of inflammation subside and reduction of the pocket depths has occurred, then some of the objectives have been met. Waerhaug (1978, 1978b) warned that if a patient's *supragingival* plaque control is effective, gingival conditions may appear normal even though subgingival plaque is still present. Therefore the external appearance of the soft tissues can be misleading regarding the disease process, which is still occurring subgingivally. A more reliable test for the presence of inflammation is gingival sulcus bleeding. If there is no bleeding on probing in the areas that were root planed when the patient returns for reevaluation and if home care has been optimally maintained, then it can be assumed that the newly prepared root surface is now *biologically acceptable* to the adjacent soft tissues. Soft tissue evaluation cannot be reached until after several days of healing.

The clinician must be able to provide an ongoing evaluation of the root planing procedure to identify whether treatment objectives are being reached. How, then, can it be determined that the tooth is *clinically acceptable* and that root planing should cease? In making this determination the clinician can rely on several visual, audio, and tactile clues.

Visual. There are many more visual clues when part of the root surface to be planed is exposed to the oral cavity as a result of gingival recession than when it is submarginal. The clinician can see the color and texture of the exposed root surface and determine whether or not pieces of calculus or diseased cementum are still visible. The use of an air syringe to dry the tooth will aid in this evaluation. If drying reveals white flecks of calculus, diseased cementum, or extrinsic stains, more root planing is indicated. A root surface with a smooth, shiny appearance and homogeneous color is indicative of effective root planing. The clinician should also evaluate the root surface for signs of ditching or overplaning from previous instrumentation. This was a common result of root planing in the 1950s when it was thought that the only way to prepare the root surface adequately was to cut well into the healthy dentin, leaving the teeth with roots that were narrow and had an hourglass appearance (Riffle, 1956). (In cases where substantial root planing from previous treatment has removed a great deal of hard tissue, the clinician must evaluate whether additional removal of cementum and dentin will be beneficial or detrimental to the patient in the long term.) That practice has become outdated, but a controversy still remains as to how much of the cementum and dentin must be removed to ensure that the root surface is biologically acceptable to the soft tissue wall of the pocket. More research is necessary to determine exactly how the toxic substances that are thought to provoke the inflammatory response (endotoxins) attach to the root surface and how deeply they penetrate into cementum and dentin before this controversy can be resolved. Another way of visually assessing the root surface is to disclose the exposed portions and identify those areas that still attract the disclosant because of plaque or root irregularities. The clinician must remember, however, that the toxic by-products of plaque are not clinically visible and are frequently located submarginally. Therefore the only reliable method for evaluating the removal of these substances is by observing the gingival response to treatment.

Audio. A rough root surface produces a rough, scratchy, coarse sound when it is being root planed. As the root gets smoother, the sound of the curette blade against the root begins to diminish or take on a higher, squeaky pitch. By listening to the sound produced by the curette, the clinician will receive some clues as to whether or not a smooth, hard surface is being achieved. This sound can be amplified for the beginning student by placing the handle end of a single-ended curette in the rubber tube of a stethoscope from which the bulb has been removed. With the stethoscope the student should hear the change of pitch as the root goes from rough and irregular to smooth (Seibert, 1978). After hearing the amplified sound changes, it may be easier for the student to detect these same audio changes without the aid of the stethoscope.

Tactile. The most frequently used and most important of all clues for evaluating the clinical acceptability of root planing is the tactile sense of the clinician. Most root planing occurs submarginally where visual and audio clues are not available. Therefore the clinician must rely on an acute sensitivity to vibrations transmitted through the instruments to the fingers to recognize surface changes that are occurring as a result of the root planing procedure. The tactile sense must also guide the clinician carefully around the root morphology during all working and exploring strokes to ensure optimal adaptation and angulation of the instrument against the root surface. It takes a great deal of time and experience to distinguish between the rough, bumpy, irregular, somewhat sticky feel of the diseased root surface embedded with calculus and plaque and a thoroughly prepared root surface.

The beginning clinician must develop an acute tactile sense by learning to concentrate on tactile sensations and to interpret accurately the vibrations that are transmitted through the instruments to the fingers. Reception of tactile vibrations is easiest when a light grasp is maintained on the instrument for all exploration of the root surface. Another aid in developing and maximizing the tactile sense is the use of fine instruments; these include explorers with small-diameter working ends as described in Chapter 5 and curettes with fine blades and thin, light shanks, such as the Gracey finishing curettes. Many clinicians also find that instruments with hollow handles transmit more vibrations that those with solid handles. The fingers can detect more subtle vibrations with a sharp curette than with a dull one. Sharpening skills are of utmost importance in root planing for optimum efficiency of the procedure. Much time can be wasted by root planing with dull curettes; the procedure can be performed much faster and easier if the instruments are kept optimally sharp.

Exploring exercises on extracted teeth will help the beginning student develop and improve detection skills for root planing as well as calculus detection. One such exercise, described at the end of Chapter 12, p. 202, is to explore an extracted tooth with the eyes closed, concentrating on the different textures and curves of the root surface. Comparisons also can be made using different instruments and a variety of root surface irregularities. After the surface is explored and a mental image of what it looks like is formed, the eyes can be used to evaluate the accuracy of the tactile impression. Students should continue to test their tactile sense while working with clinic patients by comparing the feel of different root morphologies, deposits, and restorations and analyzing what it is that makes them feel different from each other. With continual practice a fine, discriminatory tactile sense will eventually develop.

Clinicians frequently evaluate the effectiveness of root planing on the basis of tactile information, since this is often the only source of information available during the procedure. The "finished" root surface has been described as velvety smooth, glasslike, or hard to an explorer, because these clinical characteristics seem to accompany the removal of calculus and diseased cementum. The concepts of smoothness and hardness, however, should be examined more closely as to their validity and reliability for predicting that a root surface is biologically acceptable and that an optimal healing response will occur. Both of these qualities can be measured only subjectively, since they are evaluated according to the tactile skills, clinical experience, and interpretation of each clinician. It is difficult, therefore, to explain to the beginning clinician exactly what is meant by a smooth or a hard root surface. The following discussion should help the reader review the significance and limitations of each of these clinical parameters.

The effect of periodontal disease on the surface cementum that is exposed because of apical migration of the dentogingival junction is variable. Cementum that is adjacent to the inflamed soft tissues of the pocket undergoes demineralization, reducing the microhardness of the cementum. Cementum that has been exposed to the oral cavity, however, by means of gingival recession may become remineralized to the extent that its microhardness approaches normal levels (Ruben and Shapiro, 1978). The exposed cementum has the apparent ability to absorb minerals such as calcium, phosphorus, and fluoride from the pocket environment and saliva. Unfortunately, this tendency to absorb also extends to the toxic substances within the pocket environment, which inflame the adjacent soft tissues. This information would lead the clinician to believe that the resistance of pocket cementum to planing might be less than that of normal cementum. Rautiola and Craig (1961), however, measured the microhardness of cementum and dentin in extracted teeth that had never been scaled. Their results indicated that there is no significant difference between the hardness of cementum that has been exposed to periodontal inflammation versus cementum that is unexposed. The study also indicated that there are no significant differences in the hardness of inner versus outer layers of cementum and that outer layers of dentin that interface with cementum have hardness values similar to that of the cementum. Several critical questions remain to be answered in light of these conflicting reports. If there is a difference in the hardness of periodontally affected cementum as compared with healthy cementum, is it a large enough difference to be clinically detectable to the extent that the clinician can determine exactly when intact, healthy cementum or dentin has been reached and root planing should cease? Is root hardness a reliable measure of the extent to which toxic substances have penetrated the root surface? Until answers to these questions are available, the clinician should use tactile information regarding root hardness only as supplemental feedback regarding the progress of the root planing process.

What is the risk of overplaning the cementum surface and removing excessive amounts of acellular cementum in the quest for a hard surface? Stahl (1977) studied the mechanisms of repair of the soft tissues to the treated root surface and concluded that by removing the acellular cementum, which is unlikely to regenerate, the clinician is more likely to achieve a repair involving the close adherence of the new junctional epithelium to the root surface rather than actual new attachment of connective tissue fibers—the preferred method of repair. The results of this study imply that excessive removal of cementum can reduce the chances of gaining this type of new attachment during the healing process. A dilemma is created for clinicians, since all diseased cementum must be removed to make the root surface biologically acceptable, yet the actual removal also reduces the chances of gaining new attachment.

If there is no clinically detectable difference between cementum and dentin, as reported by Rautiola and Craig, then it is impossible to determine when all cementum has been removed and dentin is being encountered. The decision as to how much to plane away from the tooth is a difficult one. Although it is necessary to remove all the endotoxin-bearing hard tissues, most clinicians try not to proceed any further into dentin than necessary to avoid distortion of the root surface or unnecessary hypersensitivity of the root surface caused by overplaning. It is apparent, however, that because of the need to prepare the root surface thoroughly, it is likely that the patient may experience some sensitivity from the root planing procedure. When this occurs, the patient should be referred to special home care techniques designed to diminish the sensitivity. Chapter 31 deals with the treatment of hypersensitivity in greater detail. The cementum is especially thin near the cementoenamel junction, and extensive root planing in this area is likely to result in sensitivity.

The degree of root smoothness should be used only as a clinical indicator of the presence of calculus and cannot be depended on as a valid measure of the effectiveness of the root planing procedure. Clinicians should be wary of relying too heavily on this criterion alone as a predictor of the success of root planing. Although the relative smoothness of the root can provide tactile feedback to the clinician regarding the progress of the root planing process and the presence of remaining calculus deposits, it cannot provide any assurance that the root surface is free of the toxic by-products of plaque or that the root is biologically acceptable to the soft tissues. Several studies have demonstrated that root surfaces that feel smooth to an explorer still harbor calculus deposits that can be detected visually (Jones and O'Leary, 1978; Jones et al., 1972; Moskow and Bressman, 1964; Nishimine and O'Leary, 1979; Rabbani et al., 1981; Walker, 1976). The remaining deposits may be either burnished or simply too small to be detected tactilely.

It is frequently assumed that one of the reasons for producing a smooth root surface is that it will be less plaque retentive, more easily maintained by the patient, and therefore less susceptible to gingival inflammation. Rosenberg and Ash (1974) tested this assumption by comparing the plaque accumulation and gingival inflammation scores for roots that had been root planed with hand instruments versus roots that had been ultrasonically scaled. They found that although there was a statistically significant difference in the roughness values of the two groups of teeth, there was not a significant difference in the amount of plaque accumulation or gingival inflammation scores for the two treatment groups. This study has caused researchers to question the validity of promoting root smoothness as a means of preventing future plaque accumulation and gingival inflammation.

Interest in the significance of root roughness to

periodontal repair has generated investigations of the role of root roughness in promoting the reattachment of connective tissue fibers. Results indicate that in some cases areas of root roughness appear to facilitate this reattachment (Khatiblou and Ghodssi, 1983). More research is necessary to clarify this relationship.

Major research efforts have recently studied the effect of acids on periodontally affected root surfaces. This treatment, known as *acid demineralization,* involves the application of an acid to root surfaces that have been previously scaled and root planed. Although several different acids have been studied, citric acid seems to be preferred (Lasho et al., 1983; Nightingale and Sheridan, 1982; Register and Burdick, 1976). The effect on the root surface is one of demineralization or dissolving of surface minerals from the exposed dentin, resulting in a roughened or etched surface. Scanning electron microscope studies have shown that these roughened surfaces are caused by dissolution or decalcification of dentin around the dentinal tubules, resulting in extensions of the dentinal tubules and exposure of dentinal collagen fibers on the root surface. These changes in the root surface seem to promote the reattachment of new connective tissues to the treated areas. It is uncertain exactly how and why this reattachment occurs. These studies lend credence to the assumption that excessive root planing simply for the sake of achieving a smooth root surface may have been overemphasized as a means of promoting healing and repair of the soft tissues. Additional research on this subject is needed, and clinicians should follow current information about the potential impact of root demineralization as a method of treating the root surface. Unlike root planing, this clinical treatment of the root surface may be able to offer a means of accomplishing pocket reduction by actual reattachment of new connective tissue fibers. Acid demineralization is not likely to eliminate the need for root planing, however, since studies have indicated that acid demineralization requires root planing as a preparatory step (Garrett et al., 1978; Lasho et al., 1983). There is also a question regarding the ability of several acids, including citric acid, to remove bacterial endotoxin from periodontally involved root surfaces that have not been previously root planed (Sarbinoff et al., 1983). Unless these problems are solved, root planing will continue to be part of initial therapy prior to acid demineralization treatment of root surfaces.

It is important that clinicians understand the limitations regarding to use of root smoothness as an indicator of the completion of root planing. Although it is the best clinical indicator available for determining the presence of calculus, it can be unreliable. If a surface that feels smooth can still harbor calculus, then it certainly can harbor plaque and its by-products. Clinical smoothness of a root surface cannot be relied on as a means of preventing plaque accumulation or gingival inflammation, nor can it or any other clinical clue be relied on as a final test of the effectiveness of the root planing procedure. In fact, some research indicates that a rough root surface that is biologically clean may be preferred as a means of gaining clinical attachment. Although clinical indicators or clues provide helpful feedback regarding the progress of root planing, the only valid and reliable measure of the success of root planing is the response of the soft tissues to the treatment when supported by effective mechanical and chemical supragingival plaque control by the patient.

Complicating factors

There are a number of factors that complicate the root planing process: limited access to the root surface, bleeding, sensitivity, and root texture. There are many situations in which access to the affected area is difficult if not impossible.

Exposed furcation entrances and the complex anatomy of root surfaces not only play a significant role in the pathogenesis of periodontal disease, but also pose a difficult clinical challenge in the treatment of that disease (Bower, 1979b; Gher and Vernino, 1980). Furcation involvements may be large enough to permit the accumulation of plaque and its endotoxins but too small and too confined in area for access with a curette. Bower (1979a) compared the width of several commonly used curettes and determined that 58% of the furcation entrances that he studied had entrance widths that were smaller than the width of most curette blades. He concluded that it was unlikely that curettes would be able to clean the entrance area to furcations in a clinical situation. Access to furcations in maxillary molars and premolars is especially limited. Unlike the buccal and lingual furcations of mandibular teeth, these maxillary teeth have furcations opening

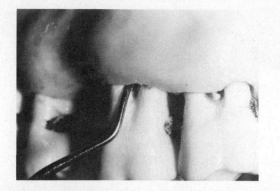

Fig. 23-12. With transparent gingiva removed, it can be seen that access to furcation areas is limited and that there is little room for maneuverability even with narrow blade of Gracey curette. Add to this the fact that normally this area is not visible during instrumentation, and it is easy to see why these areas complicate root planing procedures.

on mesial and distal surfaces adjacent to other teeth. In addition, there may be trifurcation involvements rather than bifurcation involvements. Certainly, the clinician must be well aware of the root morphologies of these teeth to treat these difficult areas (Fig. 23-12).

Another access problem is that of maneuvering even a small curette blade to the bottom of a deep, tight pocket. To ensure the removal of subgingival plaque and calculus, the curette must be inserted all the way to the dentoepithelial junction at the base of the pocket. Since most pockets become narrower at their apical extent, the pressure of the sulcular tissues against the instrument blade as it is inserted may fool the clinician into thinking prematurely that the base has been reached. Not only must the curette reach the base of the pocket, but slight compression of these tissues may also be necessary to locate the cutting edge near the pocket base and below the plaque and calculus that has formed there (Waerhaug, 1978b). This does not mean, however, that instrumentation should go on at the base of the pocket without consideration for the soft tissues. Excessive damage to the gingival fibers underlying the junctional epithelium and damage to the deeper periodontal ligament could result in the formation of an even deeper pocket after healing. The clinician must walk the fine line between damaging underlying soft tissues and al-

lowing calculus and plaque deposits to remain subgingivally. The goal is the removal of the plaque and calculus with as little soft tissue damage as possible. An almost certain result of the root planing procedure will be some *coincidental curettage*. This is the unintentional removal of soft tissue from the pocket wall adjacent to the treated root surface. It is impossible for the opposite cutting edge of the curette to avoid contact with the pocket wall. In many cases coincidental curettage is considered to be more beneficial than detrimental to the patient because it assists in the removal of inflamed soft tissues and aids the wound healing process. The clinician should be aware that any manipulation of inflamed soft tissues may be painful for the patient.

Another access problem is posed by the close proximity of roots, as in the lower anterior areas, making instrumentation in these confined areas difficult. Additional access problems may be experienced in distal pockets of posterior teeth where there is not much room for manipulation of an instrument to gain leverage for working strokes.

Bleeding is another complicating factor during root planing. Bleeding can be expected anytime instrumentation is done in an inflamed area. Bleeding serves a useful purpose during scaling and root planing by clearing loosened calculus, plaque, and other debris from the pocket, thereby promoting healing. The disadvantage of bleeding is that it hampers visibility and fulcrum stability. For optimal working conditions the area should be kept as free of blood as possible. This can be accomplished easily with water irrigation and suctioning devices. Slight bleeding can be controlled by blotting and light pressure to the wound site with a sterile gauze sponge. More profuse bleeding can be controlled through the use of irrigation and suctioning during the procedure. A stream of water from the water syringe may be directed at the area, followed by suction evacuation of the fluids. A forced spray of water and air combined should not be used to rinse the area, since it increases the production of blood-contaminated aerosols, which are then propelled at the operating team and can serve as sources of cross-contamination (see discussion of aerosols in Chapter 3). For patients who need anesthesia, the vasoconstrictor in the anesthetic solution will provide some hemostasis or control of bleeding to the area where it is injected. Control of bleeding will make the patient more comfortable and increase tolerance of the procedure. Patients may not realize that bleeding is a normal response to instrumentation in inflamed areas, and they should be assured in advance that it is expected and beneficial to the healing process. This explanation may help avoid a misunderstanding about the cause of bleeding.

Patient sensitivity often accompanies the root planing procedure. This sensitivity may arise from the inflamed soft tissues or from the root surface. Because patient cooperation and comfort are concerns, this sensitivity should be reduced as much as possible. Optimal instrumentation skills will minimize the pain and trauma for the patient but often are not sufficient to eliminate all sensitivity. Nitrous oxide and oxygen conscious sedation and/or a local anesthetic should be available to reduce the patient's discomfort during root planing if requested. The tolerance of pain varies greatly among patients, and while some may tolerate the procedure well without anesthesia, others may need it. The use of any type of anesthesia must not be a cover-up for poor instrumentation technique; all treatment should be performed with concern and respect for the soft tissues whether or not anesthesia is used. Damage caused by inappropriate instrumentation will not only hinder wound healing and repair of the gingiva, but also will destroy patient trust and confidence in the clinician.

As a result of root planing, the patient may also experience increased root sensitivity to stimuli such as hot or cold temperatures, resulting from the removal of cementum or dentin on the root surface. The patient should be informed that this might be a complication of treatment and why it may occur. In many cases this is only a temporary discomfort for the patient, and with proper desensitization procedures and home care it should diminish. (See Chapter 31 for more detailed instructions regarding the treatment of hypersensitivity.) Extreme hypersensitivity that does not respond to normal treatment may be a contraindication to further extensive root planing. This complication must be weighed against the extent of disease and the prognosis of the affected teeth in determining the best treatment for the patient.

Contraindications

The contraindications for root planing include the following: (1) lack of motivation to perform home care procedures; (2) teeth with severe periodontal disease and mobility; (3) severe pocket depth requiring some form of surgery or osseous recontouring; (4) patient with extreme hypersensitivity; and/or (5) acute periodontal infections.

Root planing is a time-consuming and exacting effort to provide an environment in the periodontal pocket that will promote healing. If the patient will not maintain home care, the results of root planing will be short-lived, and the conditions of the pocket will soon return to a diseased condition. No matter how clean and plaque-free the pocket may be at any one time, it will reverse itself in the presence of plaque and its endotoxins. A patient who does not make any effort to maintain supramarginal plaque control will soon have the plaque front again migrating apically into the pocket, and the disease process will recur. Patients must be informed that the success of the treatment is dependent on their ability and willingness to perform effective daily plaque removal. Without their complete cooperation, the benefits of any surgical treatment, including root planing, will be short-lived.

Patients exhibiting severe periodontal destruction such as deep infrabony pockets, mucogingival involvement, and mobility, require more definitive periodontal treatment than root planing alone can provide. Fine scaling and root planing should be part of initial therapy for these patients since removal of the etiologic factors will provide some reduction in pocket depth and reduction of inflammation in the soft tissues. In less severe cases root planing may produce significant healing prior to surgery so that the indications for surgery no longer exist. In more severe cases the initial therapy, which includes root planing, can improve the tissue condition so that there is less bleeding and less damage to tissues during surgical manipulation. Occasionally cases of severe periodontal destruction may be treated by conservative measures such as root planing and curettage because other surgical procedures are contraindicated because of medical complications, economic limitations, or stress factors. Even though root planing alone cannot resolve the periodontal problems in these patients, it may be the treatment of choice if both the practitioner and the patient decide that the risks of surgery outweigh the benefits.

When root planing is part of initial therapy prior to other surgical interventions, it is often accomplished under *open-flap* conditions. This means that a flap is raised so that the soft tissues can be retracted away from the root surfaces. In this way the clinician can benefit from visualization of the root morphology and the presence of calculus deposits, increasing the effectiveness and efficiency of the root planing procedure.

Dentinal hypersensitivity may exist in some patients, especially those who have undergone previous root planing treatment. Although the root planing itself can be accomplished with the patient under local anesthesia in these cases, the clinician should consider the possibility of increasing the patient's discomfort after the procedure by exposing additional dentin to the oral environment. The pain and discomfort of extreme hypersensitivity is likely to override any benefits that the patient perceives as the result of root planing and also may interfere with effective home care procedures. Root planing should be postponed until this situation can be brought under control.

Patients with acute periodontal inflammation, such as acute necrotizing ulcerative gingivitis (ANUG), should be treated for the acute condition before there is extensive manipulation of the tissue as in root planing. When acute infections occur, the tissue is friable and prone to traumatic injury until the condition subsides. There is also an increased chance of a bacteremia developing because of the number of bacteria and other infective microorganisms present at the site. Extensive instrumentation will increase the patient's discomfort and pain. These procedures should be postponed until the acute condition of the tissues is relieved.

Soft tissue response to root planing

The primary goal of root planing is to provide a biologically clean root surface on the hard tissue side of a periodontal pocket that will encourage healing and repair of the inflamed soft tissues. With removal of irritants both within the pocket and on the tooth surface, the body can work to reverse the inflammatory process and repair the damaged gingival tissues. The coincidental curettage that occurs as an indirect result of root planing assists in the healing process. In most cases some amount of coincidental curettage cannot be avoided and results in the partial removal of the ulcerated sulcular epithelium, the junctional epithelium, and superficial layers of the underlying inflamed connective tissues. The inadvertent removal of these diseased

tissues facilitates wound healing. Coincidental curettage should not be confused, however, with intentional curettage, which is described in Chapter 24.

Another result of the root planing process that is not beneficial to tissue healing is the entrapment of calculus, bacteria, and debris in the pocket and adjacent soft tissues following their removal from the root surface. These foreign particles are irritating to the soft tissues and will hinder healing if allowed to remain. Although bleeding and the curette may bring out much of the debris, the pocket should still be thoroughly irrigated with a stream of water to cleanse the area further (Moskow, 1962). Since water with high bacterial counts could result in a bacteremia when applied to wounded areas, the water supply to the dental unit should be tested for microbial contamination. In addition, water lines from the dental unit should be flushed for several minutes at the beginning of each day. The risk of cross-contamination between patients will be reduced if the trisyringe (air-water syringe) is flushed for 1 to 2 minutes between patient appointments (see Chapter 3). To minimize the risk of infection, all surgical wounds should be irrigated with a sterile normal saline solution rather than tap water. Oxygenating rinses may also help cleanse and debride these areas. Following irrigation, healing is further enhanced by the application of gentle compression and readaptation of the tissues to the teeth. This will assist in stopping the bleeding and in forming a thin blood clot against the tissues. Healing is enhanced by the formation of a thin, rather than a thick, blood clot. Performing these procedures immediately after root planing will help accelerate tissue healing and achieve an optimal tissue response.

Root planing has been shown to produce periodontal improvement in the treatment of slight, moderate, and severe periodontitis. Although the ideal result of periodontal treatment would be the creation of new attachment of connective tissue fibers along the root surface, this does not normally occur as a result of root planing. Following root planing, pocket depth reduction occurs as a result of gingival recession (shrinkage) and a secondary gain in the clinical attachment level. The gain in clinical attachment should not be misinterpreted as the creation of a new attachment of connective tissue fibers to the root surface at a more coronal level, since this is a rare and unpredictable occurrence. This gain in the clinical attachment level is caused by the creation of a new, longer junctional epithelium and the healing of the connective tissue fibers. The repaired gingival fibers consist of healthy, intact tissues that have the ability to provide resistance against the probe tip so that it cannot penetrate as far apically as it could when the tissues were inflamed.

In the presence of inflammation the connective tissue fibers that are located apical to the junctional epithelium are destroyed and replaced by inflammatory cells. Several studies have shown that this destruction allows the tip of a periodontal probe to pass through the junctional epithelium and come to rest only when it encounters intact gingival fibers, at an approximate depth of 0.25 to 0.4 mm beyond the apical extent of the junctional epithelium (Listgarten, 1980; Listgarten et al., 1976; Powell and Garnick, 1978; Silvertson and Burgett, 1976; Spray et al., 1978). When these tissues are permitted to heal, they offer increased resistance to the probe, so that the tip of the probe comes to rest at a point coronal to the junctional epithelium. The clinical probing depth will therefore reflect an apparent gain in attachment levels, although the histologic pocket depth remains the same.

In addition to the secondary gain in clinical attachment, healing also results in shrinkage of the gingiva caused by the reduction of tissue edema. When these two factors are evaluated following treatment, the clinical result is a decrease in the depth of the clinical pocket. The amount of pocket depth reduction seems to be related to the initial severity of the periodontal destruction. Deeper pockets show more depth reduction following root planing than do shallow pockets (Cercek et al., 1983; Hellden et al., 1979; Listgarten et al., 1978; Tagge et al., 1975).

Histologically, the healed pocket is characterized by the presence of a long junctional epithelium (Caton and Zander, 1979). The ability of a long junctional epithelium to provide effective protection against subsequent inflammatory attacks has been questioned in the literature (Barrington, 1981). This question was studied by Magnusson et al. (1983), who concluded that the presence of a long junctional epithelium offers the same resistance to plaque infection as an epithelial junction of normal length.

Root planing in shallow pockets (1 to 3 mm) can result in an actual loss of connective tissue attachment, followed by a corresponding loss of bone (Badersten et al., 1981; Knowles et al., 1980; Lindhe et al., 1982a, 1982b; Pihlstrom et al., 1981). One reason proposed for this loss of attachment is that it is a result of mechanical wounding and detachment of attached gingival fibers caused by repeated instrumentation (Lindhe, 1982b).

CONCLUSION

Supragingival plaque control performed regularly by the patient is vital to the success of the root planing treatment. In the absence of effective plaque control, root planing can provide only short-term benefits to the patient. Long-term maintenance of the improved gingival condition depends on the patient's willingness to cooperate by performing daily removal of bacterial plaque (Stahl et al., 1971; Tagge et al., 1975). Although plaque control alone contributes to some reduction of pocket depth as a result of gingival shrinkage, maximal pocket reduction is produced by a combination of both plaque control and root planing procedures (Cercek et al., 1983). If a combination of root planing and plaque control is not successful in reducing pocket depths to levels that allow the patient to maintain them without recurrence of disease, then other types of surgical treatment for pocket elimination may be indicated.

Root planing is definitely one of the most exacting tasks that a hygienist must perform. It is extremely valuable in the treatment of patients with periodontal disease and resultant bone loss. It does have limitations, however, and is not the treatment of choice for all periodontally involved cases. The hygienist and dentist must carefully assess each patient's needs to determine whether or not root planing will assist in the restoration of periodontal health and in the provision of long-term benefits.

ACTIVITIES

1. Practice root planing on extracted molar teeth. Use disclosant and a light microscope to help evaluate changes in the root surface as a result of the planing.
2. Remove the end from a stethoscope and insert the handle end of a single-ended curette. Root plane the teeth of clinic patients while listening for audio changes through the stethoscope.
3. Discuss which teeth would be the hardest to treat

because of their root morphology. Discuss approaches to treating various grooves and furcations.

4. If the facilities and personnel are available, root plane a tooth to completion for a patient who will be undergoing periodontal surgery. Observe the surgery to see the effectiveness of the root planing when the tissues are flapped away from the tooth.

REVIEW QUESTIONS

1. Compare scaling and root planing in terms of:
   a. Instrument selection
   b. Number of strokes
   c. Direction of strokes
   d. Pressure of strokes
2. Compare Gracey curettes and universal curettes in terms of:
   a. Blade size
   b. Cutting edges
   c. Shank design
3. Name four criteria that aid the clinician in determining the completion of root planing.
4. Write a brief response to the following statements, indicating whether or not you agree and your rationale:
   a. You should always root plane a surface until it is hard and glassy smooth.
   b. A skilled clinician never removes healthy cementum during root planing.

REFERENCES

Aleo, J.A., et al. 1974. The presence and biologic activity of cementum-bound endotoxin. J. Periodontol. **45:**672.

Aleo, J.A., et al. 1975. In vitro attachment of human fibroblasts to root surfaces. J Periodontol. **46:**639.

Badersten, A., et al. 1981. Effect of nonsurgical periodontal therapy. I. Moderately advanced periodontitis. J. Clin. Periodontol. **8:**45.

Barrington, E.P. 1981. An overview of periodontal surgical procedures. J. Periodontol. **52:**518.

Baumhammers, A., et al. 1973. Scanning electron microscopy of supragingival calculus. J. Periodontol. **44:**92.

Bower, R.C. 1979. Furcation morphology relative to periodontal treatment: furcation entrance architecture. J. Periodontol. **50:**23. (a)

Bower, R.C. 1979. Furcation morphology relative to periodontal treatment: furcation root surface anatomy. J. Periodontol. **50:**366. (b)

Canis, M.F., et al. 1979. Calculus attachment. J. Periodontol. **50:**406.

Caton, J., and Zander, H. 1979. The attachment between tooth and gingival tissues after periodic root planing and soft tissue curettage. J. Periodontol. **50:**462.

Caton, J., et al. 1982. Maintenance of healed periodontal pockets after a single episode of root planing. J. Periodontol. **53:**420.

Cercek, J.F., et al. 1983. Relative effects of plaque control and instrumentation on the clinical parameters of human periodontal disease. J. Clin. Periodontol. **10:**46.

Cogen, R.B., et al. 1983. Effect of various root surface treatments on the viability and attachment of human gingival fibroblasts. J. Periodontol. **54:**277.

Garrett, J.S. 1983. Effects of nonsurgical periodontal therapy on periodontitis in humans: a review. J. Clin. Periodontol. **10:**515.

Garrett, J.S., et al. 1978. Effects of citric acid on diseased root surfaces. J. Periodont. Res. **13:**155.

Gher, M.E., and Vernino, A.R. 1980. Root morphology—clinical significance in pathogenesis and treatment of periodontal disease. J. Am. Dent. Assoc. **101:**627.

Glick, D.H., and Freeman, E. 1980. Postsurgical bone loss following root planing by ultrasonic and hand instruments. J. Periodontol. **51:**510.

Hellden, L.B., et al. 1979. The effect of tetracycline and/or scaling on human periodontal disease. J. Clin. Periodontol. **6:**222.

Jones, S., et al. 1972. Tooth surfaces treated in situ with periodontal instruments. Br. Dent. J. **132:**57.

Jones, W.A., and O'Leary, T.J. 1978. The effectiveness of in vivo root planing in removing bacterial endotoxin from the roots of periodontally involved teeth. J. Periodontol. **49:**337.

Kerry, G.J. 1967. Roughness of root surfaces after use of ultrasonic instruments and hand curettes. J. Periodontol. **38:**340.

Khatiblou, F.A., and Ghodssi, A. 1983. Root surface smoothness or roughness in periodontal treatment: a clinical study. J. Periodontol. **54:**365.

Knowles, J., et al. 1980. Comparison of results following three modalities of periodontal therapy related to tooth type and initial pocket depth. J. Clin. Periodontol. **7:**32.

Lasho, D.J., et al. 1983. A scanning electron microscope study of the effects of various agents on instrumented periodontally involved root surfaces. J. Periodontol. **54:**210.

Lindhe, J., et al. 1982. Healing following surgical/non-surgical treatment of periodontal disease. J. Clin. Periodontol. **9:**115.(a)

Lindhe, J., et al. 1982. Scaling and root planing in shallow pockets. J. Clin. Periodontol. **9:**415. (b)

Listgarten, M.A. 1980. Periodontal probing: what does it mean? J. Clin. Periodontol. **7:**165.

Listgarten, M.A., and Ellegaard, B. 1973. Electron microscopic evidence of a cellular attachment between junctional epithelium and dental calculus. J. Periodontol. **44:**143.

Listgarten, M.A., et al. 1976. Periodontal probing and the relationship of the probe tip to periodontal tissues. J. Periodontol. **47:**511.

Listgarten, M.A., et al. 1978. Effect of tetracycline and/or scaling on human periodontal disease. J. Clin. Periodontol. **5:**246.

Loe, H., et al. 1965. Experimental gingivitis in man. J. Periodontol. **49:**337.

Lopez, N.J., and Belvederessi, M. 1977. Subgingival scaling with root planing and curettage: effects upon gingival inflammation: a comparative study. J. Periodontol. **48:**354.

Magnusson, I., et al. 1983. A long junctional epithelium—a locus minoris resistentiae in plaque infection? J. Clin. Periodontol. **10:**333.

Morrison, E.C., et al. 1980. Short-term effects of initial, nonsurgical periodontal treatment (hygienic phase). J. Clin. Periodontol. **7:**199.

Moskow, B.S. 1962. The response of the gingival sulcus to instrumentation: a histological investigation. I. The scaling procedure. J. Periodontol. **33**:282.

Moskow, B.S., and Bressman, E. 1964. Cemental response to ultrasonic and hand instrumentation. J. Am. Dent. Assoc. **68**:698.

Nakib, N.M., et al. 1982. Endotoxin penetration into root cementum of periodontally healthy and diseased human teeth. J. Periodontol. **53**:368.

Nightingale, S.H., and Sheridan, P.J. 1982. Root surface demineralization in periodontal therapy: subject review. J. Periodontol. **53**:611.

Nishimine, D., and O'Leary, T.J. 1979. Hand instrumentation versus ultrasonics in the removal of endotoxins from root surfaces. J. Periodontol. **50**:345.

Pihlstrom, B.L., et al. 1981. A randomized four-year study of periodontal therapy. J. Periodontol. **52**:227.

Pihlstrom, B.L., et al. 1983. Comparison of surgical and nonsurgical treatment of periodontal disease: a review of current studies and additional results after 6½ years. J. Clin. Periodontol. **10**:524.

Powell, B., and Garnick, J.J. 1978. The use of extracted teeth to evaluate clinical measurements of periodontal disease. J. Periodontol. **49**:621.

Proye, M.P., and Polson, A.M. 1982. Effect of root surface alterations on periodontal healing. I. Surface denudation. J. Clin. Periodontol. **9**:428.

Proye, M., et al. 1982. Initial healing of periodontal pockets after a single episode of root planing monitored by controlled probing forces, J. Periodontol. **53**:296.

Rabbani, G.M., et al. 1981. The effectiveness of subgingival scaling and root planing in calculus removal. J. Periodontol. **52**:119.

Rautiola, C.A., and Craig, R.G. 1961. The microhardness of cementum and underlying dentin of normal teeth and teeth exposed to periodontal disease. J. Periodontol. **32**:113.

Register, A., and Burdick, F. 1976. Accelerated reattachment with cementogenesis to dentin demineralized in situ. II. Defect repair. J. Periodontol. **47**:497.

Riffle, A.B. 1956. Radical subgingival curettage. J. Periodontol. **27**:102.

Rosenberg, R.M., and Ash, M.M. 1974. The effect of root roughness on plaque accumulation and gingival inflammation. J. Periodontol. **45**:146.

Ruben, M.P., and Shapiro, A. 1978. An analysis of root surface changes in periodontal disease—a review. J. Periodontol. **49**:89.

Sarbinoff, J.A., et al. 1983. The comparative effectiveness of various agents in detoxifying diseased root surfaces. J. Periodontol. **54**:77.

Seibert, J. 1978. Incorporating root planing and gingival curettage into a clinical practice. Continuing Dental Education, University of Pennsylvania School of Dental Medicine **1**: No. 8.

Silvertson, J.F., and Burgett, F.G. 1976. Probing of pockets related to the attachment level. J. Periodontol. **47**:281.

Spray, J.R., et al. 1978. Microscopic demonstration of the position of periodontal probes. J. Periodontol. **49**:148.

Stahl, S.S. 1977. Repair potential of the soft tissue–root interface. J. Periodontol. **48**:545.

Stahl, S.S., et al. 1971. Soft tissue healing following curettage and root planing. J. Periodontol. **42**:678.

Tagge, D.L., et al. 1975. The clinical and histological response of periodontal pockets to root planing and oral hygiene. J. Periodontol. **46**:527.

Theilade, E., et al. 1966. Experimental gingivitis in man. II. A longitudinal clinical and bacteriological investigation. J. Periodont. Res. **1**:1.

Volkinburg, J.W., et al. 1976. The nature of root surfaces after curette, cavitron and alpha-sonic instrumentation. J. Periodont. Res. **11**:374.

Waerhaug, J. 1976. The interdental brush and its place in operative crown and bridge dentistry. J. Oral Rehabil. **3**:107.

Waerhaug, J. 1978. Healing of the dento-epithelial junction following subgingival plaque control. I. As observed in human biopsy material. J. Periodontol. **49**:1. (a)

Waerhaug, J. 1978. Healing of the dento-epithelial junction following subgingival plaque control. II. As observed on extracted teeth. J. Periodontol. **49**:119. (b)

Waerhaug, J. 1977. Subgingival plaque and loss of attachment in periodontosis as evaluated on extracted teeth. J. Periodontol. **48**:125.

Waerhaug, J. 1981. Effect of toothbrushing on subgingival plaque formation. J. Periodontol. **52**:30.

Walker, S.L. March 1976. A study of root planing by scanning electron microscopy. Dent. Hyg. **50**:109.

Wilkinson, R.F., and Maybury, J.E. 1973. Scanning electron microscopy of the root surface following instrumentation. J. Periodontol. **42**:559.

24 SOFT TISSUE CURETTAGE

OBJECTIVES: *The reader will be able to*

1. Define soft tissue curettage.
2. Identify the objectives for soft tissue curettage.
3. Identify and recognize indications and contraindications for performing soft tissue curettage for a patient.
4. Discuss the role of patient self-care and root planing in the success of the soft tissue curettage treatment.
5. Describe the five steps of the curettage technique.
6. Describe techniques for tissue management after the curettage procedure.
7. Identify several factors that help provide the clinician with an evaluation of the completion and success of soft tissue curettage both at the time of the appointment and after healing.
8. Identify the need for placement of a periodontal dressing following curettage.
9. Describe the controversy surrounding the question of effectiveness of soft tissue curettage.
10. Compare the technique and effects of chemical curettage with soft tissue curettage.

Soft tissue curettage is the process of converting a chronic inflammatory wound to a surgical wound by removing the diseased soft tissue lining of a periodontal pocket (Goldman and Cohen, 1980). Whereas root planing is used to treat the hard tissue wall of the pocket, soft tissue curettage is used to treat the adjacent soft tissue wall. When indications for soft tissue curettage are present, a sharp curette is applied against the soft tissue to remove the inflamed sulcular epithelium and underlying diseased connective tissue. The goal of this procedure is to reduce inflammation and improve healing so that there is reduction of the clinical pocket depth, resulting in tissues that can be maintained in a healthy state by the patient.

The pocket depth can be reduced in one of four ways: (1) shrinkage of the marginal gingiva due to reduction of edema, (2) healing of apical soft tissues resulting in increased resistance to probing (see Chapter 14), (3) formation of a new long junctional epithelium that attaches to the tooth surface, and (4) new attachment of connective tissue fibers. Reduction of edema in the marginal gingiva and interdental papillae will result in shrinkage of these tissues following treatment. Healing within the pocket restores the soft tissues at the pocket base

to their normal firm consistency. When these tissues are inflamed, the periodontal probe can easily pass through the inflamed connective tissue fibers until it reaches intact, noninflamed tissues. Even though the actual attachment of these inflamed fibers is not severed, the clinical measurement indicates that their attachment to the tooth has been destroyed. Following healing, the probe can no longer penetrate through the restored tissue fibers, so that an apparent gain in attachment is observed, although there never actually is any alteration in the histologic attachment of the tissues.

Caton and Zander (1979) studied tissue healing following root planing and curettage and found that the most frequent means of attachment is the formation of a long junctional epithelium. Listgarten and Rosenberg (1979) reported that the length of this new long junctional epithelium ranged from 1.0 to 4.5 mm in patients who were studied, with an average length of 2.8 mm. This epithelium is impenetrable to a periodontal probe under healthy conditions, so that its presence would be likely to produce an apparent gain in clinical attachment and a decrease in the clinical probing depth. A long junctional epithelium forms as effective a barrier against further destruction by bacterial plaque as a normal-length junctional epithelium (Magnusson et al., 1983).

The least likely and least predictable cause of clinical pocket depth reduction is an actual gain in attachment (new attachment) of connective tissue fibers at a more coronal level. One reason cited for failure of this type of attachment to occur is that all the pocket epithelium must be removed to prevent reepithelialization from occurring over the new connective tissue before it has a chance to reestablish attachment to the root surface (Goldman and Cohen, 1980). Many investigators have found that complete removal of all pocket epithelium, including the junctional epithelium, sulcular epithelium, and marginal epithelium, is difficult if not impossible (Lopez and Belvederessi, 1977; Morris, 1954; Stahl et al., 1971).

The curettage procedure described in this chapter should not be confused with "coincidental curettage," which is described in earlier chapters. Soft tissue curettage refers to a definitive procedure designed for the intentional removal of soft tissues. The term *curettage* can be used in a number of different ways. Some clinicians use curettage to refer to the use of a curette against both hard (i.e., scaling, root planing) and soft tissues. Others use the term to describe the removal of soft tissues that occurs simultaneously with root planing. In this chapter soft tissue curettage is considered a procedure that is performed separately from root planing.

Hall (1983) has provided additional definitions to distinguish between *gingival curettage*, removal of the gingival lining of a shallow true pocket or pseudopocket with gingival shrinkage as the goal, and *subgingival curettage*, removal of the epithelial lining and some subjacent connective tissue in deep pockets with new connective tissue attachment as the goal. Although both gingival and subgingival curettage are discussed in this chapter, the emphasis is on gingival curettage.

The sequencing of soft tissue curettage as a part of the periodontal treatment may occur in different ways, depending on the preferences of the clinician. Some clinicians prefer to perform soft tissue curettage at the same appointment in which they do root planing as part of a final effort to create an environment within the pocket that is conducive to optimal wound healing. Their rationale is that much coincidental curettage has already occurred during the root planing procedure, and it will facilitate healing if the removal of remaining diseased tissue is completed. Advantages to this approach are that the patient is already prepared (i.e., anesthesia and root planing have been accomplished), so that less time is needed to perform curettage during this appointment (Ainslee and Caffesse, 1981; Barrington, 1981).

Other clinicians take a more conservative approach, stating that because soft tissue curettage is a type of surgical procedure, the indications for performing it must be evaluated after other methods of treatment, including plaque control, scaling, and root planing, have been performed. These clinicians prefer to evaluate the need for curettage only after these other treatments and the resultant healing can be studied. With this approach the indications and need for soft tissue curettage may have been resolved by one or all of the previous treatment modes (Goldman and Cohen, 1980; Wirthlin, 1981). An advantage of this approach is that the patient need not undergo the procedure unless it is necessary, and thus additional manipulation of the tissues is avoided. The decision regarding which approach to take depends on the preferences and attitudes that prevail in a given practice. Both approaches have been shown to improve the health of the periodontal tissues.

INDICATIONS AND CONTRAINDICATIONS

The *indications* for soft tissue curettage include:
1. Soft, boggy, edematous gingiva associated with chronically inflamed tissues
2. Gingival or supraboney pockets
3. Inflammation that persists in spite of plaque control or scaling and root planing

Contraindications include
1. Patients with deep infrabony pockets
2. Patients with insufficient attached gingiva and mucogingival involvement
3. Patients with systemic complications
4. Patients with acute gingival infections such as acute necrotizing ulcerative gingivitis (ANUG)
5. Patients whose gingiva is more fibrotic than edematous: areas where shrinkage is difficult to achieve, such as the palatal areas of maxillary anterior teeth and retromolar areas (Goldman and Cohen, 1980; Chace, 1974, 1983).

Soft tissue curettage is most effective on edematous tissues because shrinkage of the treated tissues resulting from a resolution of the inflammation is the desired goal. Shrinkage is unlikely in fibrotic gingiva because the bulk of the tissue is due to excess collagen fibers rather than edema produced by the inflammatory process. The same problem may exist on the palatal surfaces of maxillary anterior teeth and in retromolar areas. Although the clinician should be aware of these considerations, inflammatory conditions may exist within these areas. Curettage may still be considered in these cases if it is felt that there might be some tissue resolution.

The success of soft tissue curettage depends greatly on the ability of the clinician to remove as much of the soft tissues that are inflamed and beyond repair as possible. Adaptation of instruments in deep, narrow pockets without causing traumatic injury to the soft tissues is difficult. Removal of all the inflamed soft tissues without traumatizing the intact tissues is especially difficult in these areas. In these situations curettage may be completed more effectively in an open-flap environment rather than in the closed-flap procedure that is discussed later in this chapter. Probably the most important reason why soft tissue curettage is not the best treatment for deep infraboney pockets associated wtih moderate to severe periodontitis is that it cannot eliminate the need for surgical treatment of the pocket wall and underlying bone. Pockets displaying these characteristics would not be reduced to a maintainable level by soft tissue curettage alone, and the bone contours would still be nonphysiologic, resulting in a continuation of the disease.

A similar problem exists in cases in which there is inadequate attached gingiva and mucogingival involvement. Not only are these tissues much more delicate and likely to be perforated during curettage, but surgical intervention is required to solve the existing problems so that the patient can resume normal home care and maintenance procedures. Curettage alone will often not meet the patients' needs in these cases. A modification of soft tissue curettage called aggressive curettage has been described as an effective method for treating patients with infraboney pockets. This technique removes the entire col area, so that interproximal tooth surfaces are accessible for cleaning (Green and Green, 1979).

Patients with systemic complications, such as diabetes, or gingivitis caused by hormonal imbalances or nutritional deficiencies, may not be good candidates for soft tissue curettage. Healing is hindered in patients with diabetes, and any tissue manipulation will be more traumatic in these patients. When the inflammatory response is complicated by systemic disturbances, curettage is less likely to effect an acceptable clinical result. Patients who are suffering from medical disorders that limit their ability to withstand the physical or emotional stress of periodontal treatment may not be good candidates for soft tissue curettage. In some situations, however, curettage for these patients may be the treatment of choice in lieu of more demanding surgical interventions.

Acute periodontal infections such as ANUG or gingivostomatitis are also contraindications for soft tissue curettage. Manipulation of these very delicate tissues will not only be painful for the patient, but might also create unnecessary trauma in the tissues. Periodontal treatment for these patients should be postponed until the acute conditions have been resolved.

Patients who will not or cannot maintain optimal home care procedures to prevent the recurrence of periodontal disease are not good candidates for the curettage procedure. This treatment is aimed at elimination of the inflammation and at reduction of clinical pocket depths so that patients can maintain their mouths in a healthier state. If the patient will not or cannot maintain optimal plaque control, the purpose for performing this procedure is undermined and the curettage will have only short-term value to the patient.

A closer look at the disease process of gingival inflammation shows how soft tissue curettage contributes to the reduction of inflammation. A review of the incipient lesion of gingivitis shows that there is loss of integrity of the sulcular epithelium resulting from inflammation. The resultant ulceration of these tissues provides access for the inflammatory process into the underlying connective tissues, and the result is bleeding and breakdown of these subsulcular fibers. As the connective tissues become involved in the battle of inflammation, many of them are destroyed and lose their firm consistency. This allows the sulcular epithelium to proliferate in a rete peg formation deeper and deeper into the connective tissues because there is no longer sufficient "contact inhibition" to prevent overgrowth of epithelium. As the inflammation persists, there is continuing destruction of gingival fiber groups of the subsulcular connective tissue extending into the major fiber groups and down into the periodontal ligament, junctional epithelium, and bone. The goal of the curettage procedure is to remove the soft, mushy, diseased connective tissue and the affected sulcular epithelium so that the remaining tissues have a healthier environment to repair themselves during wound healing. This diseased tissue is often granular in nature and is called *granulomatous tissue*. It is connective tissue that has tried to repair itself but has failed in the unfavorable environment produced by the chronic inflammation. As a result of curettage, the chronic wound is converted to a surgical wound and an acceptable environment for healing is provided so

that the tissues can be restored to health (Figs. 24-1 to 24-6).

Frank (1980) and Saglie et al. (1982) have confirmed that gram-negative bacteria do penetrate the apical and lateral epithelial walls of deep pockets in cases of advanced chronic periodontitis. Evidence of bacterial invasion into the adjacent connective tissues was also found. These findings suggest that even after thorough removal of the major source of the bacteria in attached and unattached plaque in periodontal pockets following scaling and root planing, the bacteria that have invaded the epithelial walls could recolonize the pocket and reinstate the inflammatory conditions. The results of these studies strengthen the rationale for performing soft tissue curettage of the infected pocket wall to assist in the removal of these invasive bacteria.

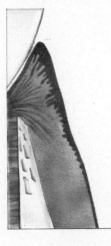

Fig. 24-1. Cross-sectional diagram of normal healthy sulcus. Appearance of sulcular epithelium and underlying connective tissues is normal .There is a slight inflammatory infiltration in subsulcular areas. (Adapted from Seibert, J.S. 1978. Continuing Dental Education, University of Pennsylvania School of Dental Medicine **1:** No. 8.)

Fig. 24-2. Number of inflammatory cells increases significantly with presence of plaque and calculus in sulcus. (Adapted from Seibert, J.S. 1978. Continuing Dental Education, University of Pennsylvania School of Dental Medicine **1:** No. 8.)

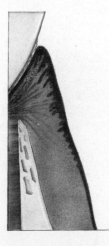

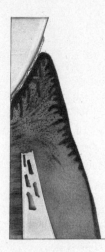

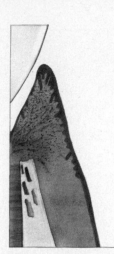

Fig. 24-3. As inflammatory process continues to affect tissues, there is weakening of subsulcular connective tissues, which allows epithelium to proliferate into connective tissue spaces, producing rete peg appearance of these tissues. There is further breakdown of gingival fiber groups, allowing apical migration of junctional epithelium along root surface. Loss of crestal bone is also apparent. (Adapted from Seibert, J.S. 1978. Continuing Dental Education, University of Pennsylvania School of Dental Medicine **1:** No. 8.)

Fig. 24-4. It is difficult to remove all rete peg extensions of epithelium into connective tissue. Coincidental curettage or light curettage might produce a wound site similar to this in tissues. (Adapted from Seibert, J.S. 1978. Continuing Dental Education, University of Pennsylvania School of Dental Medicine **1:** No. 8.)

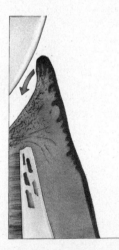

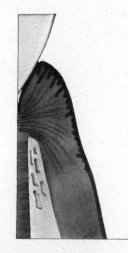

Fig. 24-5. Complete curettage involves removal of all sulcular epithelium and junctional epithelium as is shown here. (Adapted from Seibert, J.S. 1978. Continuing Dental Education, University of Pennsylvania School of Dental Medicine **1:** No. 8.)

Fig. 24-6. Healing following soft tissue curettage reveals that healthy epithelium has again been restored to sulcus and that subsulcular connective tissues have regenerated to their normal form and function. Although attachment is now slightly apical to where it existed normally, adherence of gingival tissues to tooth is favorable. (Adapted from Seibert, J.S. 1978. Continuing Dental Education, University of Pennsylvania School of Dental Medicine **1:** No. 8.)

PATIENT PREPARATION

For the goals of treatment to be realized, the new surgical wound must be able to repair itself in an environment that is favorable for healing. There are several requirements in patient preparation for curettage that should be completed before the curettage is performed. First, the patient should be educated and motivated to practice optimal plaque control procedures. Effective plaque control will accomplish two things: the tissue will undergo some healing and improvement from the plaque control alone, so that the indications for curettage can be more carefully evaluated, and the increased health of the tissue and decreased inflammation brought on by plaque control will improve conditions for performing the soft tissue curettage procedure. A reduction in inflammation will result in a reduction in tissue sensitivity, bleeding, and better tissue tonus, or firmness. The firmer the soft tissues are, the easier they will be to manipulate during curettage. Conversely, tissues that are friable and spongy require more careful instrumentation technique and tissue support in order to prevent excessive tissue trauma during curettage. The second reason for the patient to establish good plaque control habits before the curettage is to ensure that the treated areas will be maintained after the procedure. If the patient's home care is less than adequate, it may be advisable to postpone the curettage until there is evidence of the patient's ability to maintain plaque control.

Another prerequisite for the success of curettage is the complete preparation of adjacent root surfaces. This preparation should include removal of all plaque, its associated endotoxins, plaque-retentive surfaces, and calculus. The soft tissue wall of the pocket cannot heal if it constantly encounters the diseased hard tissue wall that was a source of inflammation from the start (Aleo, et al., 1974, 1975). Therefore, complete, definitive root planing must be performed to prepare the root surface and provide submarginal plaque control before the curettage procedure can be performed (Jones and O'Leary, 1978). If root planing was done at a previous appointment, the results should be reevaluated and the root reprepared as necessary immediately before the curettage.

The patient's assessment data for periodontal treatment should be reviewed before treatment begins. These data should include an updated medical history and the periodontal chart so that information regarding pocket morphologies and the degree of periodontal involvement can be examined. This information in conjunction with clinical signs and symptoms will help the clinician determine current indications and contraindications for performing soft tissue curettage. The patient must be informed of the purpose of this treatment procedure and provided with a description of what the treatment involves. Patient consent and cooperation are as important for the success of curettage as for any dental procedure. The patient should be encouraged to ask questions, and potential results should be discussed. This dialogue reinforces the importance of the patient's role as a partner in care and encourages self-evaluation of progress through treatment.

Anesthesia is recommended for the soft tissue curettage procedure. Even though there are some patients who feel that they could tolerate the curettage without anesthesia, most patients will be more comfortable if they are anesthetized. An exception to this recommendation may be a case in which only one papilla or localized area is being treated rather than a whole segment of the mouth. In such an instance administering appropriate anesthetic may be just as painful for the patient as is quickly doing the curettage procedure. Another exception is the patient who is allergic to anesthetic solutions or who refuses anesthesia for reasons that cannot be negotiated. In many cases, however, the patient may already have been anesthetized for root planing and thus is prepared for soft tissue curettage.

Infiltration anesthesia supplemented with interpapillary injections is best for this procedure (see Plate 4, *D*). A long-lasting injection such as a block is unnecessary for curettage, since the procedure can be performed in a relatively short period of time and certainly does not require the same extent of anesthesia as root planing. Interpapillary injections are especially helpful for curettage because in addition to providing local anesthesia to the area, the solution improves tissue tonus, which makes handling of the tissue easier during the curettage. The vasoconstrictor available in most anesthetic solutions will also provide local hemostasis or control of bleeding to the area, which makes the procedure easier for the clinician and the patient. Patients for whom the use of a vasoconstrictor is contraindicated should be given an anesthetic agent that does not contain a vasoconstrictor, even though this will diminish the hemostatic effect.

ARMAMENTARIUM

The instruments and supplies needed for the curettage procedure are essentially the same as those used for root planing. An explorer is used to evaluate the root surfaces for any deposits that are still remaining. The curettes must be extremely sharp so that they will cut the soft tissue easily. Dull curettes will tear and pull on the tissues rather than cut out the inflamed tissues smoothly. The wound that is created during curettage will heal much faster if the surface is smooth and free of tears, cuts, or tissue tags. Much of the technique for curettage that will be described is aimed at producing a wound that will heal easily and quickly. For this reason, the clinician is advised to keep a separate set of curettes for curettage so that the blades can be maintained in a surgically sharp condition. Curettes that have just been used for root planing are likely to be dull and worn from that procedure and should not be used for the curettage procedure. Any sharp curette can be used for this procedure as long as it has adequate access to all areas that need to be treated. Gracey curettes are illustrated because they have excellent access to any area or pocket morphology because of their varied shank designs and small blade size. When Gracey curettes are selected, any combination of designs that will serve all areas may be used. A suggested combination is 1/2, 7/8, 11/12, and 13/14. The basic instrumentation principles are the same in soft tissue curettage as they are in scaling and root planing except that the cutting edge is directed toward the soft tissue rather than toward the tooth. When Gracey curettes are used, the lower cutting edge should be turned toward the soft tissue. The working angulation will vary between 45 and 90 degrees to the soft tissue.

Other supplies needed for the curettage procedure include an anesthesia setup, a periodontal probe to record pretreatment pocket depths, a mouth mirror, and gauze sponges. In addition, normal saline and an aspirating syringe should be used for cleansing the area during the procedure to reduce the chances of introducing microorganisms into the surgical site.

Referral to the information in Chapter 3 will remind the clinician that there is the potential for large numbers of bacterial colonies to grow in the water supply of the dental unit. The water syringe must be thoroughly flushed before daily use. This is especially important if the unit water supply will be used for a procedure such as curettage. Irrigation of the surgical site is an important factor in providing optimal conditions for wound healing. Inflamed tissue, plaque, calculus, and other debris that the curette may not have carried out of the pocket should be flushed out of the pocket area to cleanse the wound. An oxygenating agent may also be included on the tray setup to cleanse the postoperative site further of remaining debris and to facilitate healing.

CURETTAGE PROCEDURE

When the patient has been prepared and the tray setups are ready, the curettage procedure can begin. There are five basic steps that should be followed to ensure that all the inflamed granulomatous tissue is removed from the site and to obtain a clean wound. These steps are described in detail.

1. *Buccal and lingual pocket walls* should be curetted by placing the instrument with the cutting edge against the soft tissues at a 45- to 90-degree angle and positioning the blade for a horizontal or circumferential stroke (Fig. 24-7; see also Plate 4, *E*). The toe should be positioned near the base of the pocket and moved gently across the bottom part of the pocket. The geography of the pocket bases should have already been plotted on the periodontal chart so that the clinician can estimate the location of the junctional epithelium and avoid tearing the underlying gingival connective fibers. The stroke should move in a horizontal direction across the buccal or lingual wall of the pocket from distal line angle to mesial line angle. A smoother incision will be made if the strokes are long and light rather than short and irregular. A parallel to this comparison is the difference between cutting a piece of paper with scissors using a long stroke or a series of shorter strokes. The more often the hand stops and starts another stroke, the more jagged the edge of the paper will appear. The same is true in curettage along the soft tissue wall. Because tissue tags or even minute tears will hinder the healing of the pocket wall, they should be avoided as much as possible.

The length of the stroke must be guided by the ability of the clinician to control the adaptation and

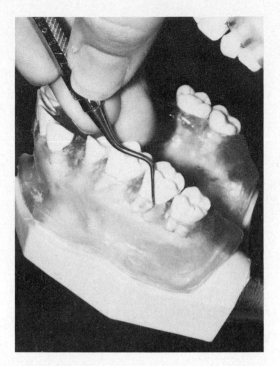

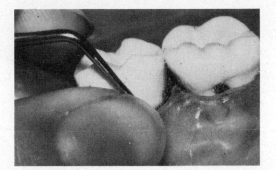

Fig. 24-8. When initiating curettage stroke against buccal or lingual walls, it is important that soft tissue wall be supported against cutting edge with index finger as shown. Finger should follow strokes as they move across buccal or lingual surfaces.

Fig. 24-7. Adaptation of Gracey 7/8 curette is shown on typodont, demonstrating proper adaptation and angulation for soft tissue curettage of buccal wall of this tooth. Transparent "gingiva" allows visibility of curette blade so that reader can see that lower cutting edge is being adapted to soft tissue rather than to root surface.

angulation of the curette. Neither of these two factors should be compromised by the length of the stroke, since they will affect the quality of the wound that is created. It is important to support the soft tissue with a finger of the other hand during each stroke (Fig. 24-8; see also Plate 4, *G*). Unless gentle external pressure against the instrument blade is supplied, the curette will simply displace the soft tissue rather than cut it. The finger support should be directly opposite the cutting edge at all times. It is therefore necessary to rely on tactile sensations through the curette and the supporting finger and on visualization of the proper orientation of the shank of the curette to monitor instrument application. If the angulation is optimal, the clinician will feel the resistance of the tissues to the sharp cutting edge and the sensation of peeling away diseased tissue from healthy tissue. Another evaluation of angulation is whether or not the cli-

nician is actually removing the granulomatous tissue from the pocket. If not, angulation may be at fault, as may be the amount of pressure being applied against the tissue from either the curette or the supporting finger. Incorrect adaptation of the toe of the curette may be felt by the supporting finger if the toe is directed into the soft tissue or by the operating hand if the toe is being directed against adjacent tooth surface. A light and perceptive operating grasp is as necessary for this procedure as for any other instrumentation technique.

The buccal or lingual pocket walls may require several well-executed strokes over the same area to remove all inflamed tissue (see Plate 4, *H*). When the base portion of the wall is curetted, the blade should be moved somewhat coronally. If the length of the curette blade cannot accommodate the entire pocket wall, several strokes may be performed at different levels to complete the curettage of this area. The curettage is complete when the inner pocket wall feels firm to the curette blade, indicating that the inflamed mushy tissue has been removed, and when no more granulomatous tissue is being brought out of the area by the curette.

2. *Interdental papillae* are curetted by placing the curette so that the cutting edge is against one or the other of the papilla walls and executing a series of short, vertical strokes that extend from the base of the interdental pocket area up to the free margin of the papilla (see Plate 4, *F*). These strokes should extend from the buccal or lingual angles of the tooth and into its midline. While the

papilla is being curetted, there should be support from both of its sides by a finger and thumb of the opposite hand. The clinician will not be able to see the curettage in these areas because of the finger support (Figs. 24-9 and 24-10). Tactile information must be used.

3. *Marginal gingiva,* specifically the free gingival margin, is one area that is often curetted inadequately during the procedure. To overcome this problem, a special stroke is warranted. The curette blade should be placed about 80 degrees from the free margin of the gingiva and moved circumferentially along the margin so that the free gingival crest is retracted away from the tooth. This stroke should remove epithelium and inflamed tissue that still remains at the crest of the gingiva. The presence of any remaining tissue tags that might have been produced by earlier strokes should be detected. These tissue tags will be removed in step 5.

4. *Junctional epithelium* does not usually require a separate step, because the other steps of the procedure will have removed all or most of this tissue already. Submarginal scaling and root planing procedures will often remove this epithelium at the pocket base. When shrinkage of the tissue is the goal, total removal of this epithelium is unnecessary. If, however, the goal is for a more coronal reattachment of tissues after healing, then it is necessary to perform a separate step that will guarantee that all sulcular epithelium is removed. This removal can be accomplished by placing the toe of the curette along the base of the pocket and performing light, circumferential strokes along the pocket base. The clinician must also consider that a definitive, cutting stroke at the base of the pocket might also cut into the 1 to 2 mm of gingival attachment fibers that exist below the junctional epithelium. There is a chance that a deeper pocket may be produced in this manner as evidenced by a loss of clinical attachment.

5. *Tissue tags* should be removed as a final step in the curettage procedure so that the free gingival margin is smooth and clear of tears or excess pieces of tissue that will hinder the healing process. These tissue tags should be detected during the stroke involving the marginal free gingiva or by close inspection of the margin. They are excised by placing the cutting edge against the tissue and pressing it laterally against the tooth surface. When all steps

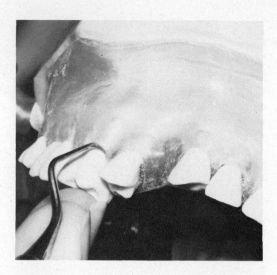

Fig. 24-9. Gracey 7/8 curette is shown being inserted into sulcus for interproximal strokes. Lower cutting edge is directed against soft tissue, and terminal shank of instrument is maintained nearly parallel to long axis of tooth.

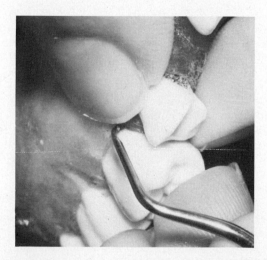

Fig. 24-10. Close-up view of curettage being simulated on interdental papilla, showing that tissue support should come from both sides of papilla with thumb and index finger of other hand. Blade of instrument often will be completely covered from view while these strokes are being implemented.

have been accomplished, the wound should be free of all inflamed tissues, and the gingival margins should be smooth and free of tags, tears, or gouges.

POSTTREATMENT TISSUE MANAGEMENT

After the tissues have been inspected, the pockets should be irrigated thoroughly to remove any tissue remnants (Moskow, 1962). A wound that is clean and smooth will heal more quickly. After irrigation of the pocket, the tissues should be readapted to the teeth by applying gentle lateral pressure for several minutes with a sterile gauze square that has been soaked in warm normal saline. The pressure will stop bleeding, readapt tissue, and help in the formation of a thin blood clot. If this compression is sufficient to control bleeding and the tissue remains in close contact with the tooth, then no other postoperative treatment is necessary. If, instead, there is incessant bleeding and/or the tissues tend to stand away from the tooth, placement of a periodontal dressing is indicated. The pressure of the dressing against the wound site will help control the bleeding and assist in the formation of the blood clot. The protective coverage provided by the dressing will also help keep the wound site free of food debris, plaque, and other material that would retard healing. A periodontal dressing is recommended for best results if the goal of the curettage is for reattachment instead of shrinkage. If this is the case, the pack should remain on the wound site for 7 to 10 days. When only shrinkage is expected, the pack can be removed in 3 or 4 days (Chace, 1974). More detailed information regarding periodontal dressings is given in Chapter 25.

The patient should be instructed to perform gentle home care of the curettage site on the first day. This includes rinsing with mild salt water and plaque control with a soft brush or gauze. The patient should be warned not to rinse vigorously for 1 to 2 hours after the procedure to avoid dislodging blood clots. Extreme temperatures and spicy foods should also be avoided to minimize sensitivity in the area. Usually, regular home care procedures can be instituted on the day following the procedure. When a periodontal dressing is placed, special instructions regarding its care should be given (see Chapter 25).

WOUND HEALING

Immediately after curettage is performed, the gingiva will show evidence of bleeding and blood clots and will appear red or blue-red colors. (see Plate 4, *I*). A day later the gingiva will show signs of edema and a red or blue-red color. There may still be evidence of sloughing tissue and clotted blood. By the fourth day the intensity of red in the gingiva will have diminished, as well as the edema and swelling. By the sixth day the gingiva may appear light red with a further reduction of edema, and marginal gingiva may show constriction and some recession. Healing should be complete in 7 to 10 days unless it has been interrupted by incomplete curettage or root planing, poor plaque control, or systemic complications (Goldman and Cohen, 1980) (see Plate 4, *J*).

EVALUATION OF CURETTAGE

After 1 week or more of healing, the patient should be recalled for an evaluation of the tissue response to curettage. This examination should include evaluation of tissue color, contour, and consistency, reduction of pocket depth, and status of the sulcular epithelial lining. The appearance of the gingiva should be compared with its precurettage characteristics and expectations of normal, healthy gingiva. Reexamination and comparison with precurettage periodontal charts will indicate the areas and extent of pocket reduction. Probing will also indicate the status of the pocket lining according to the presence or absence of bleeding.

Any area where signs of inflammation still exist should be carefully reexplored for the presence of plaque or calculus. The possibility of incomplete curettage or residual debris should also be considered. If local factors are at fault, they should be eliminated and additional curettage should be performed if necessary.

Soft tissue curettage is a procedure that can be performed successfully by the clinician who develops an appreciation for its indications and limitations. Many of the principles of instrumentation are similar to those already used during scaling and root planing procedures, so that transference of those skills to the treatment of diseased soft tissue lining of the pocket is easily made. A thorough background in the nature of healthy and diseased periodontal tissue will enhance the clinical skills of the clinician in assessment, planning, implementation, and evaluation of soft tissue curettage.

EFFECTIVENESS OF CURETTAGE

There is no doubt that scaling, root planing, and curettage are effective means for reducing gingival inflammation due to chronic gingivitis and periodontitis. An interesting controversy exists, however, as to whether or not curettage is a necessary component of initial therapy. It has been described as the oldest therapeutic procedure in the practice of periodontics and as indispensable for the maintenance of all treated cases (Chace, 1983). Ramfjord et al. (1968) compared the use of curettage with other surgical techniques during a longitudinal study that began in 1963. Their first conclusions, after 5 years, were that curettage was able to produce more favorable results in pocket depth reduction than surgical elimination of pockets, and that the surgical techniques resulted in a slight loss of attachment that was not seen following curettage. Ten years after treatment, however, results indicated that both experimental groups (surgical pocket elimination and curettage) showed a significant loss of attachment and that pocket reduction was greater and better sustained in the patients who had undergone pocket elimination surgery (Ramfjord et al., 1973). More recent reports of this longitudinal study included those patients who had completed 8 years of recall treatment and scoring. The findings at this point demonstrated that soft tissue curettage had resulted in sustained pocket reduction and gains of attachment levels for both moderately deep pockets (4 to 6 mm) and deep pockets (7 to 12 mm). The differences between the treatment results obtained by soft tissue curettage as compared with the two surgical techniques used were not statistically significant. These data indicate that not only is soft tissue curettage an effective method for treatment of moderate to severe cases of periodontitis, but also that during the length of this study, soft tissue curettage was just as effective as pocket elimination surgery or modified Widman flap surgery in most cases (Knowles et al. 1979).

Zamet (1975) compared the clinical results after curettage, replaced flap, and apically repositioned flap procedures. After 4 months, results in all three treatment groups were comparable for plaque, gingival inflammation, pocket depth, attachment, and contour with no significant differences between groups, and all procedures reduced pocket depths. This study would seem to confirm the value of curettage as a method of producing pocket depth reduction.

Several other investigators, however, have attempted to determine whether or not curettage following scaling and root planing is any more effective in treating inflamed tissues than scaling and root planing alone. Ainslie and Caffesse (1981) evaluated this question by comparing scaling and root planing in one treatment group with scaling, root planing, and immediate soft tissue curettage in another group. Although both treatment combinations were successful in reducing inflammation, they concluded that there was not a statistical difference in the results obtained by the two treatment groups. They stated further that scaling and root planing alone resulted in a tendency for greater clinical gain of attachment than if curettage was performed. The implications of this study are that soft tissue curettage requires extra effort on the part of both the patient and the clinician without demonstrating additional benefits.

Echeverria and Caffesse (1983) performed a similar evaluation, but they instituted curettage 4 weeks after scaling and root planing rather than performing it concurrently with scaling and root planing. Their findings indicate that although the combination of scaling, root planing, and curettage is an effective treatment to reduce gingival inflammation and pocket depth, it was no more effective than scaling and root planing alone. They concluded that gingival curettage is not necessary in routine treatment of shallow, supraboney pockets.

Many clinicians are convinced of the value of soft tissue curettage as a means of treating and maintaining patients suffering from chronic inflammation of periodontal tissues (Barrington, 1981; Chace, 1974, 1983; Deasy and Vogel, 1978; Hirschfeld, 1962). Current research, however, casts some doubt on the necessity of performing curettage as a separate procedure in addition to scaling and root planing. Each professional has a responsibility to continue to evaluate the current research in the literature and to determine which clinical measures will provide optimal care for each patient.

CHEMICAL CURETTAGE

Chemical solutions have been studied as a means of accomplishing the effective removal of inflamed soft tissues within a chronically inflamed pocket. Kalkwarf et al. (1982) described a technique for using sodium hypochlorite solution for this purpose and described its effect on the soft tissues. Sodium hypochlorite solution was applied to the soft tissue lining of the treated pockets for 1 minute, with care taken not to spill it on any of the adjacent tissues. Several drops of 5% citric acid were then introduced into the pocket to neutralize the environment. The area was thoroughly irrigated with water prior to instrumentation against the soft tissue wall with a sharp curette. The chemical treatment of the pocket produced chemolysis of the inflamed epithelium and connective tissue, so that it was removed from the pocket with fewer strokes and more completely than by hand curettage alone. Chemical curettage had the additional advantages of not requiring anesthesia, of producing a more predictable and uniform removal of the pocket lining, and of reducing hemorrhage. Healing was similar to that which follows hand instrumentation for curettage. Both root planing and effective plaque control are prerequisites for the chemical treatment, as they are for traditional soft tissue curettage techniques. Vieira et al. (1982) confirmed that the effects of chemical curettage using sodium hypochlorite and citric acid (antiformin) were similar to those found after soft tissue curettage in a study done on beagle dogs. They concluded that healing following chemical curettage involved the formation of a long junctional epithelium, and that the healing response to chemical curettage was similar to, although not improved over, healing following soft tissue curettage.

ACTIVITIES

1. Practice the adaptation of instruments and steps in tissue removal in a laboratory situation using the jaws of freshly killed hogs. Make arrangements with a local slaughterhouse to secure one-half jaw per student. Wearing disposable gloves, create pockets or sulci around each tooth by cutting the tissues away from the teeth using the toe of a large curette. Experiment with the curettage technique, simulating all steps as closely as possible. At the conclusion of the lab, cut a flap at either end of the area worked on and retract the tissue down to check for remaining tissue tags or gouges. This is a useful way to practice curettage on something other than another human being.

2. A useful analogy can be drawn between a bruised apple and the principles of curettage that is helpful in planning an inquiry approach to learning. All that is needed is a bruised apple floating in a pan of water and a spoon.

Pose the situation of an apple-bobbing contest with a huge bruise visible on the only available apple. What is wrong with the apple? How can you tell? What could be done about the problem? What kind of tool would be most helpful in removing the bruised area? What technique would you use to implement the tool? How could you tell that all of the bruise was removed? How would you keep the apple from bobbing away from you as you tried to remove the bruise?

Use answers to illustrate the indications, armamentarium, technique, and evaluation of the soft tissue curettage procedure. It is important that all answers be valued and discussed as to their implications and consequences to help the students develop skills in critical problem solving.

3. Observe a faculty member or more advanced student performing soft tissue curettage for a clinic patient.
4. Observe an open-flap curettage in progress.
5. View a videotaped close-up demonstration of soft tissue curettage being performed for a patient.

REVIEW QUESTIONS

1. Define the following terms:
   a. Soft tissue curettage
   b. Coincidental curettage
2. Of the two methods of achieving pocket elimination—shrinkage and reattachment—which is most likely to occur as a result of soft tissue curettage?
3. True or false. The only tissue that is likely to be removed during the curettage procedure is the epithelial lining of the sulcus or pocket wall.
4. You performed curettage for a patient 2 weeks ago, and when he returns, you find that the tissue has not healed completely and there is still bleeding on examination, edema, and redness of the treated areas. Plaque control has been maintained, and no systemic disturbances are present. List three possible causes of this failure of the tissues to heal that could be traced to poor clinician technique.
5. Identify each of the following statements as to whether they are indications or contraindications for you to begin soft tissue curettage:
   a. Area has primarily gingival pockets or pseudo-pockets
   b. Presence of boney defects in the underlying bone

   c. Bleeding on probing

   d. Recent history of cardiac disease and valve damage

   e. Boggy, edematous tissues

   f. Rough root surfaces

   g. Ineffective plaque control

   h. Mucogingival or frenum involvement

6. Which of the following situations would indicate the necessity of placing a periodontal dressing following the soft tissue curettage procedure?

   a. Profuse bleeding follows curettage.

   b. Free gingiva adheres closely to the tooth surfaces.

   c. Free gingiva stands away from the tooth surfaces.

   d. Goal of the procedure is reattachment.

REFERENCES

Ainslie, P.T., and Caffesse, R.G. 1981. A biometric evaluation of gingival curettage. Quintessence Int. **12**:519.

Aleo, J.J., et al. 1974. The presence and biologic activity of cementum-bound endotoxin. J. Periodontol. **45**:672.

Aleo, J.J., et al. 1975. In vitro attachment of human gingival fibroblasts to root surfaces. J. Periodontol. **46**:639.

Barrington, E.P. 1981. An overview of periodontal surgical procedures. J. Periodontol. **52**:518.

Caton, J.G., and Zander, H.A. 1979. The attachment between tooth and gingival tissues after periodic root planing and soft tissue curettage. J. Periodontol. **50**:462.

Chace, R. 1974. Subgingival curettage in periodontal therapy. J. Periodontol. **45**:107.

Chace, R. 1983. Subgingival curettage. In Clark, J.W., editor. Clinical dentistry. New York: Harper & Row, Publishers, Inc.

Deasy, M.J., and Vogel, R.I. 1978. The relevance of curettage in periodontal therapy. Ann. Dent. **37**:70.

Echeverria, J.J., and Caffesse, R.G. 1983. Effects of gingival curettage when performed 1 month after root instrumentation. J. Clin. Periodontol. **10**:277.

Frank, R.M. 1980. Bacterial penetration in the apical pocket wall of advanced human periodontitis. J. Periodont. Res. **15**:563.

Goldman, H., and Cohen, D.W. 1980. Periodontal therapy, ed. 6. St. Louis: The C.V. Mosby Co.

Green, M.L., and Green, B.L. 1979. Aggressive curettage. Dent. Hyg. **53**:409.

Hall, W.B. 1983. Procedure code 452: eliminating the confusion. CDA J. **11**:33.

Hirschfeld, L. 1952. Subgingival curettage in periodontal treatment. J. Am. Dent. Assoc. **44**:301.

Hirschfeld, L. April 1962. The role of subgingival curettage in periodontal therapy. Alpha Omegan, p. 115.

Jones, W.A., and O'Leary, T.J. 1978. The effectiveness of *in vivo* root planing in removing bacterial endotoxin from the roots of periodontally involved teeth. J. Periodontol. **49**:337.

Kalkwarf, K.L., et a. 1973. Longitudinal study of periodontal therapy. J. Periodontol. **44**:66.

Kalkwarf, K.L., et al. 1982. Histologic evaluation of gingival curettage facilitated by sodium hypochlorite solution. J. Periodontol. **53**:63.

Knowles, J.W., et al. 1979. Results of periodontal treatment related to pocket depth and attachment level: eight years. J. Periodontol. **50**:225.

Kon, S., et al. 1969. Visualization of microvascularization of the healing periodontal wound. II. Curettage. J. Periodontol. **40**:96.

Listgarten, M.A., and Rosenberg, M.M. 1979. Histological study of repair following new attachment procedures in human periodontal lesions. J. Periodontol. **50**:333.

Lopez, N.J., and Belvederessi, M. 1977. Subgingival scaling with root planing and curettage: effects upon gingival inflammation—a comparative study. J. Periodontol. **48**:354.

Magnusson, I., et al. 1983. A long junctional epithelium—a locus minoris resistentiae in plaque infection? J. Clin. Periodontol. **10**:333.

Morris, M. 1954. The removal of pocket and attachment epithelium in humans: a histological study. J. Periodontol **25**:7.

Moskow, B. 1962. The response of the gingival sulcus to instrumentation: a histological investigation. J. Periodontol. **33**:282.

Ramfjord, S.P., et al. 1968. Subgingival curettage versus surgical elimination of periodontal pockets. J. Periodontol. **39**:167.

Saglie, R., et al. 1982. Bacterial invasion of gingiva in advanced periodontitis in humans. J. Periodontol. **53**:217.

Seiberg, J. 1978. Incorporating root planing and gingival curettage into a clinical practice. Continuing Dental Education, University of Pennsylvania School of Dental Medicine **1**: No. 8.

Stahl, S.S., et al. 1971. Soft tissue healing following curettage and root planing. J. Periodontol. **42**:678.

Valentine, R. 1977. Periodontal documentation and therapy: a laboratory program for dental students and expanded duty auxiliaries, ed. 3. Philadelphia: University of Pennsylvania School of Dental Medicine.

Vieira, E.M., et al. 1982. The effect of sodium hypochlorite and citric acid solutions on healing of periodontal pockets. J. Periodontol. **53**:71.

Wirthlin, M.R. 1981. The current status of new attachment therapy. J. Periodontol. **52**:529.

Zamet, J.S. 1975. A comparative clinical study of three periodontal surgical techniques. J. Clin. Periodontol. **2**:87.

Plate 4

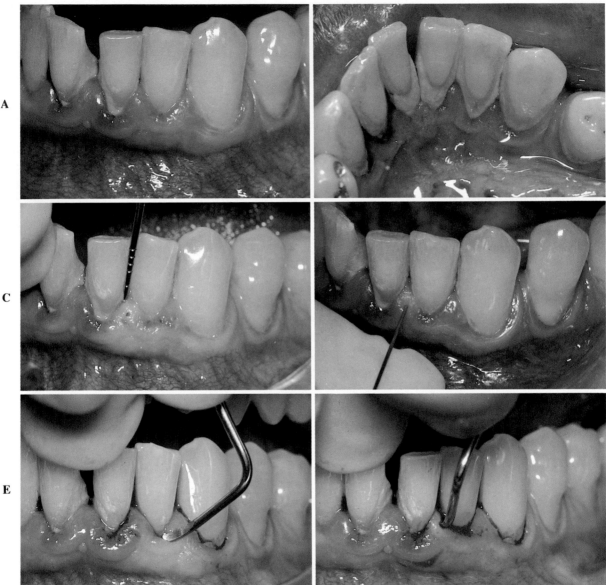

Plate 4. Series depicting steps involved in treatment of selected teeth by scaling and soft tissue curettage. **A,** Pretreatment condition of patient prior to scaling and soft tissue curettage. Clinical examination reveals signs of marginal gingivitis. Gingival tissues are red and edematous. Plaque and calculus are clearly visible. **B,** Lingual view of mandibular incisors shows heavy calculus deposits. Removal of these deposits must precede soft tissue curettage procedure. For this patient scaling and curettage were performed during same appointment. **C,** Clinical pocket depth of 3 mm is measured on distal surface of tooth No. 24 prior to treatment. **D,** Interpapillary injection is given to each interdental papilla. Blanching of tissues can be seen. Local anesthetic will not only make curettage procedure more comfortable for patient but will also provide control of bleeding (hemostasis). **E,** Close-up view of Gracey curette as it is inserted shows that lower cutting edge will be adapted against soft tissues during curettage. **F,** Gracey curette is shown correctly positioned to perform vertical curettage strokes against distal aspect of interdental papilla on tooth No. 23.

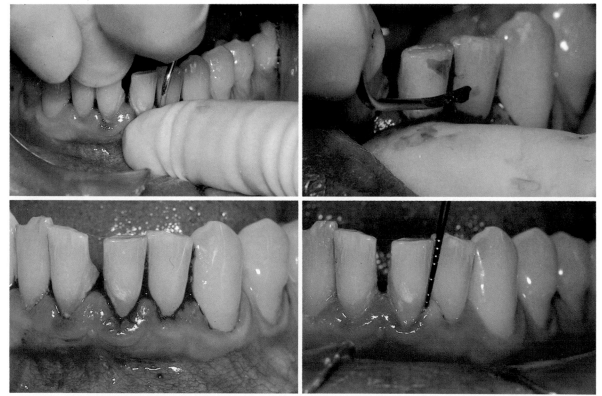

Plate 4, cont'd. **G,** External finger support against gingiva should be applied opposite cutting edge of curette for all strokes. This position stabilizes soft tissues and prevents them from being deflected away from cutting edge so that strokes will be more effective. Gloves are worn to protect both clinician and patient from disease transmission. **H,** Sample of inflamed epithelial lining and connective tissue that was removed during curettage procedure. **I,** Appearance of soft tissues immediately after scaling and curettage can be seen on teeth No. 22 to No. 24. **J,** After only 1 week of healing, reduction of gingival inflammation can be seen. Gentle probing reveals clinical pocket depth reduction of more than 1 mm on distal aspect of tooth No. 24. (Courtesy Catherine Shifter, R.D.H., M.Ed., and Robert Benedon, D.M.D.)

25 PERIODONTAL DRESSINGS AND SUTURE REMOVAL

OBJECTIVES: *The reader will be able to*

1. List and explain the functions of a periodontal pack.
2. Compare and contrast the properties of a pack that contains eugenol with a pack that does not contain eugenol.
3. Describe the placement of a periodontal pack on a surgical area with no missing teeth and on an area with several missing teeth.
4. Describe the removal of sutures and of a periodontal pack.
5. Place and remove a periodontal pack on a typodont and/or a partner.
6. Remove sutures.
7. Instruct a patient in caring for a periodontal pack.

With the hygienist's increasing role in the area of periodontics including root planing and soft tissue curettage, the hygienist's knowledge must fully expand to include placement and removal of periodontal dressings and suture removal. The hygienist may place packs for patients after soft tissue curettage or periodontal surgery has been performed. In addition, the hygienist must be able to remove the pack and any sutures that may have been placed. In this chapter basic information is presented about the types of periodontal dressings as well as the techniques for the placement and removal of packs and the removal of sutures.

Initially, the periodontal dressing is a puttylike material that is gently molded over the surgical area; over a period of several hours the pack hardens into a hard, brittle material. The primary functions of the dressing are to protect the area and thus promote healing, and to make the patient more comfortable. The dressing does not directly stimulate healing. It indirectly protects the area from irritants such as hot or spicy foods, sharp pieces of food, and other oral debris. In addition, a periodontal dressing protects newly exposed root surfaces from temperature changes, stabilizes mobile teeth, protects sutures, helps maintain the position of repositioned soft tissues, and helps control bleeding, although bleeding should be controlled before pack placement (Baer et al., 1969; Blanque, 1962; Carranza, 1979; Goldman and Cohen, 1980;

Levin, 1980; Valentine, 1976; Watts and Combe, 1979).

Periodontal dressings are indicated for most periodontal surgery procedures, such as flaps, gingivectomy, gingivoplasty, or mucogingival surgery, and for some soft tissue curettage procedures (Carranza, 1979; Goldman and Cohen, 1980; Valentine, 1976; Watts and Combe, 1979). The routine use of periodontal dressings for all periodontal surgery procedures has been questioned (Jones and Cassingham, 1979; Levin, 1980; Pihlstrom et al., 1977; Stahl et al., 1969; Watts and Combe, 1979). Periodontal dressings, by virtue of being in place for 7 to 10 days, promote plaque and food debris buildup because the patient cannot cleanse the area thoroughly. Since plaque and its by-products are the primary etiologic factors in periodontal disease, thorough cleansing of an area after surgery is essential to prevent a renewed inflammatory process. Therefore if healing and patient comfort were acceptable without the use of a periodontal dressing, the plaque and food debris would be greatly reduced and chances of a renewed inflammation decreased.

Stahl et al. (1969) found that healing was the same for packed and unpacked areas after gingivectomies. Jones and Cassingham (1979) found no difference in healing between packed and unpacked areas after periodontal flap surgery, but did find greater patient pain and discomfort in the unpacked areas. Even though healing was acceptable in the packed and unpacked areas in both of these studies, the patient discomfort without a pack indicates the need for one. Pihlstrom et al. (1977) found that a tight-fitting periodontal dressing used after subgingival curettage led to a decrease in the viable microorganisms as compared with areas that received no dressing or curettage. In this instance the pack was advantageous to the healing process. Thus far, it is safe to say that the use of dressings is being questioned, but there is no conclusive evidence to contraindicate their use (Watts and Combe, 1979). There are indications (e.g., patient comfort, protection, healing, and others previously mentioned) for the use of periodontal dressings. Presently the majority of clinicians use periodontal dressings after periodontal surgery; yet their use should continue to be evaluated.

TYPES OF PERIODONTAL DRESSINGS

There are a variety of materials that can be used as periodontal dressings. The two most widely used materials are zinc oxide–eugenol and zinc oxide–noneugenol dressings (Baer et al., 1969; Carranza, 1979; Goldman and Cohen, 1980; Levin, 1980; Watts and Combe, 1979). Cyanoacrylates are used in other countries and in the United States experimentally, but they have not yet been approved for routine use in the United States (Baer et al., 1969; Forrest, 1974; Levin, 1980; Levin et al., 1975; Watts and Combe, 1979). Methacrylic gels, tissue conditioners, have also been used as periodontal dressings (Addy et al., 1975; Levins, 1980; Watts and Combe, 1979).

The inclusion of eugenol in periodontal packs is somewhat controversial and continues to be investigated and analyzed by many researchers and clinicians (Baer et al., 1969; Carranza, 1979; Frisch and Bhaskar, 1967; Goldman and Cohen, 1980; Haugen and Gjermo, 1978; Haugen, 1980; Haugen and Mjör, 1979; Levin, 1980). Eugenol is considered to be an *obtundent* material, a material that is soothing to tissues. Some investigators believe that eugenol is an obtundent to all tissues, including bone, and that it should be included in a dressing to promote healing and patient comfort. Other investigators believe that eugenol is irritating to bone and that it may even stimulate destruction of the bone and therefore should not be included in the

pack. Reports of animal studies in which a zinc oxide–eugenol dressing was placed against exposed bone indicate there is incomplete healing, or destruction, of the bone (Carranza, 1979; Goldman and Cohen, 1980; Haugen and Mjör, 1979; Levin, 1980). Studies done with animals and humans to compare the wound healing in areas packed with zinc oxide–eugenol versus zinc oxide–noneugenol dressings have shown there is no difference in the epithelialization and wound healing (Frisch and Bhaskar, 1967; Haugen and Gjermo, 1978; Haugen, 1980; Levin, 1980) in spite of the previously mentioned reports of bone destruction. There is no conclusive research to direct the clinician to choose either pack. It seems that clinicians select the type of periodontal pack to use on the basis of several factors, such as ease of manipulation, consistency of the pack, and storage, besides the absence or presence of eugenol.

Patient sensitivity to ingredients in the dressing is also a consideration when one is being selected. A case of anaphylaxis seemingly related to the presence of eugenol, has been reported (Poulson, 1974). In addition, a case of an allergic response to rosin has been described (Lysell, 1976). It is important to take a thorough medical history to detect allergies, determine the ingredients in a dressing, and ensure that the patient is not allergic to any of them. Determining the ingredients of a periodontal dressing can sometimes be a challenge, since the formulations are copyrighted. If the material being used is an accepted material by the American Dental Association, its ingredients will be listed in the most recent *Accepted Dental Therapeutics* (ADA, 1982). If the material is not listed, the manufacturer can be contacted or the research literature can be consulted. Research articles usually list the ingredients of th periodontal dressings used in the study.

Zinc oxide–eugenol dressings

Dressings with eugenol are supplied in powder and liquid forms. The powder contains zinc oxide, tannic acid, and rosin. Some powders also contain ingredients such as kaolin, zinc stearate, or asbestos. Asbestos fibers have been associated with lung disease (Bakdash, 1976) and are considered a health hazard. Therefore most products no longer contain asbestos. Tannic acid is also deleted by some manufacturers because its absorption has been associated with liver disease (Baer et al., 1969; Watts and Combe, 1979). The liquid contains eugenol and an oil such as mineral or peanut oil, and some liquids contain ingredients to modify or improve the color and flavor (ADA, 1982; Carranza, 1979; Watts and Combe, 1979). Table 25-1 lists the ingredients and their functions in one of the packs with eugenol.

The setting reaction of a zinc oxide–eugenol dressing is between the zinc oxide and the eugenol (forming zinc eugenolate). It is a slow-setting reaction, which allows sufficient working time. There is always free, unreacted eugenol; it is this free eugenol (and its effects on the tissues) that is controversial.

Zinc oxide–eugenol dressings can be mixed in a large quantity, divided into smaller amounts, wrapped tightly, and frozen. The frozen pack must be defrosted and at room temperature to be used. Mixing in advance is advantageous, since the initial mixing of these dressings is somewhat time consuming.

The packs with eugenol are firm, heavy packs that are easily manipulated by the clinician, since they do not stick to the clinician's fingers as much as the noneugenol packs do. A disadvantage of this firmness is that the clinician must use more pressure to adapt these packs, and the pressure can displace repositioned flaps; a softer pack may be indicated in those situations.

Zinc oxide–noneugenol dressings

The most common noneugenol periodontal dressing (Coe-Pack*) is supplied in two pastes that contain zinc oxide, magnesium oxide, and hexachlorophene in one paste and hydrogenated rosin, chlorothymol, and benzyl alcohol in the other paste (ADA, 1982; Carranza, 1979; Goldman and Cohen, 1980; Watts and Combe, 1979). (Table 25-2 lists the ingredients and functions of each component.) The setting reaction of Coe-Pack is between a metallic oxide and fatty acids.

The noneugenol pack is a very pliable pack that is mixed when the clinician is ready to use the pack. The pliability of the material is ideal for a

*Coe Laboratories, Inc., Chicago.

Table 25-1. Ingredients and some of the functions of a zinc oxide–eugenol dressing*

Ingredient	Amount		Function
Powder (each 100 g)			
Zinc oxide	40	g	Setting reaction; slightly antiseptic and astringent
Rosin	40	g	Filler to increase strength
Tannic acid	20	g	Slightly hemostatic
Liquid (each 100 ml)			
Eugenol	46.5	ml	Setting reaction; slightly anesthetic; obtundent
Peanut oil	46.5	ml	Regulates setting time
Rosin	7.5	ml	Filler to increase strength

From ADA Council on Dental Therapeutics 1982. Accepted dental therapeutics. ed. 39. Chicago: American Dental Association.
*Kirkland Pack, Pulpdent Corporation of America, Brookline, Mass.

Table 25-2. Ingredients and some of the functions of a zinc oxide–noneugenol dressing*

Ingredient	Percentage	Function
Paste 1 (pink)		
Zinc oxide	45	Slightly antiseptic and astringent
Magnesium oxide	32	Setting reaction
Peanut oil	11	
Mineral oil	6	Regulate setting time
Rosin oil	3	
Other formulating and bacteriostatic agents	3	Bacteriostatic
Paste 2 (amber)		
Polymerized rosin	53	Increases strength
Coconut fatty acid	30	Setting reaction
Chlorothymol	3	Bacteriostatic
Peruvian balsam	3	Unspecified
Other formulating agents	3	Unspecified

From ADA Council on Dental Therapeutics. 1982. Accepted dental therapeutics, ed. 39. Chicago: American Dental Association.
*Coe-Pack, Coe Laboratories, Inc.

pack being placed over a repositioned flap or over very fragile tissue. The noneugenol pack is usually more pleasant tasting than the packs containing eugenol. The noneugenol pack can be made firmer by adding powder, which is usually mixed with a eugenol liquid; the addition of the powder gives the noneugenol pack more body and makes the pack less sticky (Valentine, 1976). The noneugenol pack can also be placed in a cup of cold water for several minutes after it is mixed to be made firmer and possibly less sticky.

The manufactures of Coe-Pack have recently introduced another noneugenol dressing, Coe-Pack Hard and Fast Set, which sets in a shorter period of time, is less sticky, and is harder.

Another type of zinc oxide–noneugenol dressing available is the premixed dressing. One such dressing, Peripac,* contains calcium phosphate, zinc oxide, acrylate, organic solvent, and flavoring and coloring agents (Haugen and Gjermo, 1978). When this material is exposed to air or moisture, it sets by the loss of organic solvent (Watts and Combe, 1979). Peripac is a brittle dressing and is not as popular as the previously mentioned zinc oxide–noneugenol dressing. Peripac has been associated with greater patient pain and swelling than other dressings (Haugen and Gjermo, 1978).

Cyanoacrylate dressings

Cyanoacrylate dressings are rather experimental at this time. These packs do not require mixing; the plastic is applied either in drops or is sprayed on the tissue. The application is considered to be timesaving and relatively easy, once the clinician has had experience with the material. The material is much less bulky than that of the other packs, adapts well to the tissues, and helps control bleeding (Forrest, 1974; Levin, 1980; Levin et al., 1975; Watts and Combe, 1979). As mentioned earlier in the chapter, the cyanoacrylate dressings have not yet been approved for use in the United States other than for research.

Methacrylic gel dressings

Methacrylic gels are used in prosthetics as tissue conditioners or denture liners. The gels adapt

*de Trey Freres S.A., Zurich, Switzerland.

closely to the tissues and are very compatible with the wound site. But tissue conditioners cannot be used alone because of their poor retention; they have been used in conjunction with a zinc oxide–noneugenol dressing (Addy et al., 1975; Levin, 1980; Watts and Combe, 1979). Addy et al. (1975) reported the application of an antibacterial agent via a methacrylic gel and zinc oxide–noneugenol dressing. This type of dressing is not widely used.

Antibacterial and other agents

Agents to promote healing such as antibacterial or antibiotic agents have been added to periodontal dressings. Presently the addition of antibacterial agents to dressings is an accepted practice, although their effectiveness is yet to be proved conclusively (Haugen et al., 1977; O'Neil, 1975). The addition of antibiotic agents is unacceptable because of the chance of sensitizing a patient to the agent and also because the ingredients in the dressings inactivate the antibiotic (Levin, 1980; Watts and Combe, 1979). The addition of other antibacterial agents such as chlorhexidine gluconate (Addy et al., 1975) has been experimented with but has not yet been approved.

MIXING AND APPLICATION OF A PERIODONTAL DRESSING

The mixing of a noneugenol dressing is first. Subsequently, the mixing of a zinc oxide–noneugenol dressing is described. The application of the dressing is the same for both types.

The materials needed to place a periodontal pack are pictured in Fig. 25-1. Petroleum jelly is used to coat the patient's lips and the clinician's hands; the coating should be thin so that the petroleum does not become incorporated into the pack. The second tongue blade is used to mix the pack. The curette and/or the college pliers are used to adapt the pack into the interproximal areas. The dry foil is used to protect the pack while it hardens.

Preparing the patient

The purpose and appearance of the periodontal pack should be explained to the patient before it is placed. The procedure for placing the pack and the taste and feel of the pack should also be explained

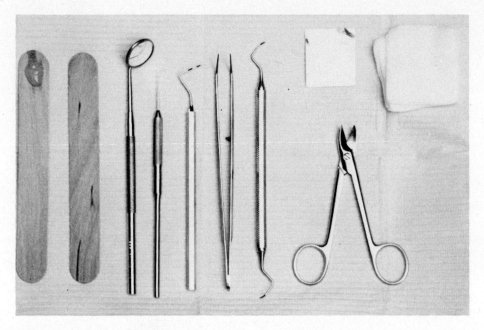

Fig. 25-1. Tray setup for placement of periodontal dressing: petroleum jelly, tongue blade, mirror, explorer, probe, college pliers, curette, dry foil, scissors, and gauze.

to the patient. Then the patient's lips should be lightly coated with petroleum jelly to prevent the pack from sticking to the patient's lips and cheeks.

Mixing a noneugenol dressing

The pack should be mixed according to the manufacturer's directions. In this instance, equal lengths of the material are expressed from each of the tubes and mixed until the color is homogeneous (Figs. 25-2 and 25-3). The particular stroke used for mixing is not important as long as the material is homogeneous in color. A zinc oxide powder may be added to the mix to make the material stronger and less sticky (Figs. 25-4 and 25-5). Once the material is mixed, it should be formed into rolls about the length of the area to be packed and about two thirds the diameter of a pencil (Fig. 25-6).

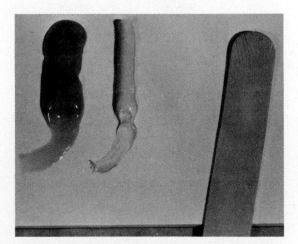

Fig. 25-2. Equal lengths of noneugenol pastes expressed onto pad to be mixed.

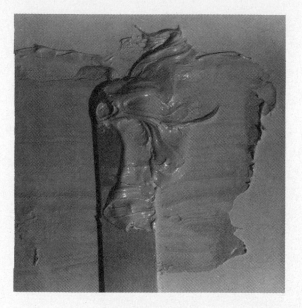

Fig. 25-3. Pastes are mixed until color is homogeneous.

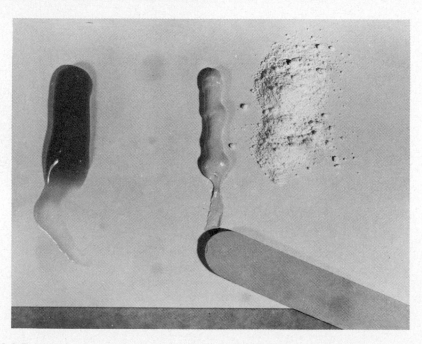

Fig. 25-4. To improve strength and workability, zinc oxide powder is incorporated into paste 1 and then mixed with paste 2.

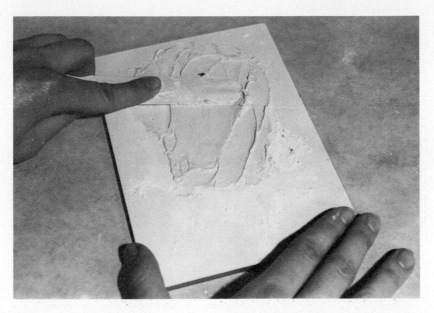

Fig. 25-5. Paste 1, with zinc oxide powder, is being mixed with paste 2 until color is homogeneous.

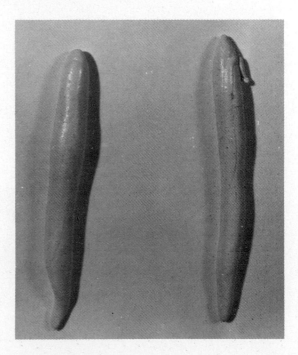

Fig. 25-6. After complete and proper mixing, two rolls, approximating length of wound, are formed.

Placing the pack

The area to be packed should be gently dried with gauze, and the bleeding should be controlled. The pack can help control the bleeding, but it is not the primary means of controlling bleeding. If an area is bleeding, pressure can be applied to the area or the supervising dentist can be asked to assess the situation if the bleeding is profuse (Carranzo, 1979). Once the bleeding is controlled and the area has been dried, the pack is wrapped around the most distal tooth in the area being packed. The pack is gently adapted to the area by pressing the pack against the wound site and spreading it up along the teeth. The entire wound is covered, and

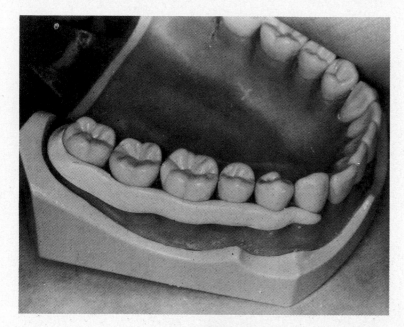

Fig. 25-7. One roll is applied to buccal surface, being wrapped around distal-most tooth and extending to most anterior tooth.

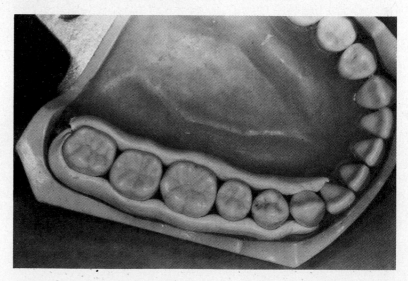

Fig. 25-8. Other roll is applied to lingual surface but is not yet adapted into interproximal areas.

the pack is extended to the most anterior tooth involved (Fig. 25-7). The other roll is applied to the opposite side of the involved area (Fig. 25-8). Once the pack has been gently applied to the area, wet gauze can be wrapped around one of the clinician's fingers and the pack can be adapted to the area more completely (Fig. 25-9). The pack is then pressed into the interproximal areas with the back of a curette or the back of the beaks of a pair of college pliers (Fig. 25-10). When the pack is adapted into the interproximal areas, the pack from the facial and lingual surfaces should join and a mechanical lock will be formed between the pack and the teeth. Even if the facial and lingual packs do not join, the pack will still form a mechanical lock in the embrasure areas between the teeth. This lock is important for retention of the pack.

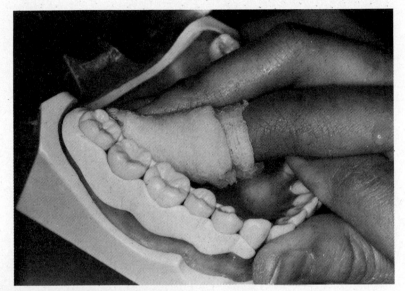

Fig. 25-9. Dressing is being adapted with damp gauze wrapped around clinician's finger.

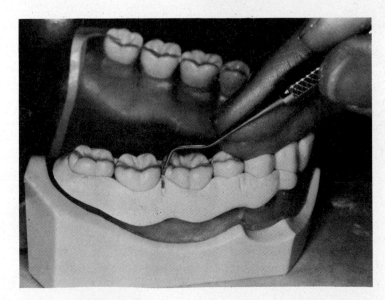

Fig. 25-10. Dressing is being pressed into interproximal areas with back of a curette.

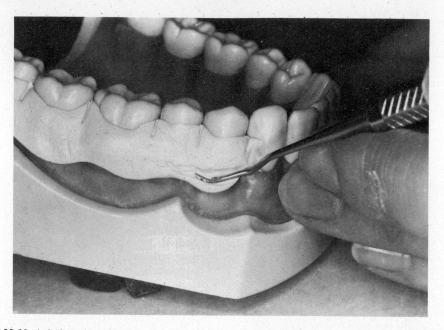

Fig. 25-11. Apical portion of pack is being trimmed by gently and firmly pressing curette into material and peeling it away.

Muscle trimming and removing excess

The periodontal dressing must be molded to the shape of the oral structures so that it does not interfere with the patient's normal activities any more than is necessary. One way of ensuring this is to muscle trim the pack by pulling the patients lips and cheeks over the pack to help identify where the pack may be impinging on muscle attachments. Grooves or inverted Vs will be created in the apical margin of the pack in areas where the pack is impinging on the attachments; any of these identified areas should be trimmed away with a curette. Excess pack material in the apical (Fig. 25-11) and/ or occlusal areas should also be trimmed away. The apical area will fold over if it is extended too far into the mucobuccal fold area. The pack should not extend any further occlusally than the middle third of the teeth; under no circumstances should the pack interfere with the patient's occlusion. This means that the pack should be cleared away from the occlusal surfaces and from any surfaces of anterior teeth that may be involved in the patient's occlusion. Excess pack should be removed from the teeth with a curette. It must be remembered

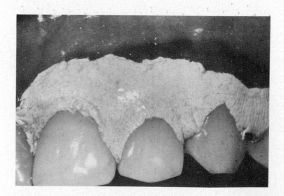

Fig. 25-12. Properly placed, adapted, and smoothed periodontal dressing. It has been muscle molded and trimmed so that none of the material impinges on soft tissue.

that the pack hardens into a very brittle material, which can be irritating to the patient's soft tissue; therefore every effort must be made to provide the patient with a well-contoured, smooth periodontal dressing that is as unobtrusive as possible (Fig. 25-12).

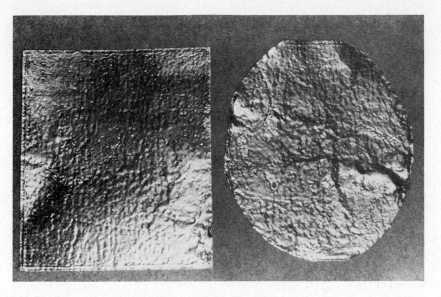

Fig. 25-13. Dry foil on left is as manufacturer supplies it. The foil on right is trimmed and ready to be applied.

Applying dry foil

Dry foil is a specially treated and manufactured paper that looks like a small rectangle of aluminum foil (Fig. 25-13). The dry foil has an adhesive on the nonshiny side, which can adhere to the periodontal pack and teeth. The dry foil acts to protect the pack while it hardens (Valentine, 1976). The foil prevents food and other debris from becoming impregnated into the soft periodontal pack (Fig. 25-14). The dry foil can be removed from the pack several hours after it has been placed; the clinician can instruct the patient to remove the foil and show the patient how to peel the foil away from the hardened pack. Placing the dry foil over the soft pack is not essential or crucial; a pack will harden and remain on the teeth as long as necessary without dry foil being applied.

Evaluating the pack

The pack should be evaluated according to the criteria presented and summarized in the check-off sheet at the end of this chapter. If any of the criteria are not met, the clinician should modify the pack

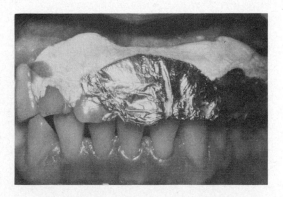

Fig. 25-14. This dry foil had been properly applied; use of foil in anterior is unusual, since it is not esthetically pleasing.

to meet these criteria. In most instances there is ample working time to modify, and even add to, the dressing as needed. The exception to this is with Peripac, since it sets on exposure to air and moisture and becomes very brittle.

Date <u>July 2, 1984</u>

Dear <u>Mr. Jones</u>,

    A periodontal pack has been placed to protect your gums while they heal. The pack should remain in place for about 5 to 7 days. A few instructions are listed below to help you care for your mouth while the pack is in place.

1. Avoid eating or drinking for 1 hour while the pack is hardening.

2. Avoid the following kinds of foods:
   Hard foods such as hard pretzels
   Sharp foods such as potato chips
   Sticky foods such as toffee
   Spicy foods such as pizza

3. Do not brush the area covered by the pack. The pack can be gently wiped with moist gauze or cotton.

4. The rest of the areas of your mouth can be brushed and flossed as usual; just be careful not to dislodge the pack.

5. You can rinse your mouth with warm water or warm salt water four or more times a day.

6. If there is any bleeding from the area, apply pressure to the area for 15 minutes. DO NOT RINSE. If the bleeding persists or is very heavy, call the office for instructions.

7. If the pack becomes dislodged from the area, please call the office.

8. Be sure to return to the office for your follow-up appointment in 5 to 7 days so the pack can be removed.

If you have any questions, please call the office.

Fig. 25-15. Sample patient instruction sheet.

Patient instructions

The patient should be instructed in care of the mouth with a periodontal dressing in place (Carranza, 1979; Goldman and Cohen, 1980; Valentine, 1976). It is helpful to supply the patient with a list of written instructions to be referred to at home (Fig. 25-15). The patient should be cautioned that the dressing will gradually harden and that care should be taken so that it is not dislodged within the first few hours. The dressing cannot be brushed, but the patient can rinse, brush, and floss the other areas of the mouth. There may be some slight oozing of blood from the surgical area. Oozing is considered normal, but profuse bleeding should be reported.

The patient should be given an appointment to return to the office in 5 to 7 days to have the dressing removed. The dressing will be removed and the tissue evaluated. In some instances the dressing may be replaced for an additional week if healing is slow.

Alternative packing procedures

In some cases the patient will have an area of missing teeth or isolated teeth, which requires the packing technique to be modified. If a few teeth are missing and the pack cannot be held onto the area, dental floss can be tied around the teeth to bridge the area and the pack can be applied around the floss. Some patients have only a few teeth in a quadrant, and these teeth are spread far apart; these teeth can be packed individually rather than trying to tie dental floss around several teeth in a quadrant. If the pack will not remain around an isolated tooth, a strip of gauze can be tied around the cervical area of the tooth and the pack can then be applied (Carranza, 1979).

Mixing a zinc oxide–eugenol dressing

The technique for mixing a zinc oxide–eugenol dressing is shown in Figs. 25-16 and 25-17. The material is mixed on a waxed pad with a tongue blade. If a large amount of material is to be mixed, a piece of waxed paper, taped to a counter, can be used. The manufacturer's directions should be followed; usually the powder is gradually incorporated into the liquid to form a thick paste. The consistency must be very thick, so additional powder is added by kneading it into the paste with the fingers. The fingers can be cleaned with orange solvent or tincture of green soap; rubber gloves can

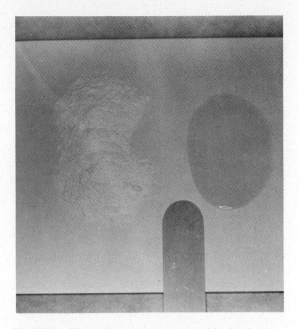

Fig. 25-16. Zinc oxide–eugenol powder and liquid placed on pad prior to mixing.

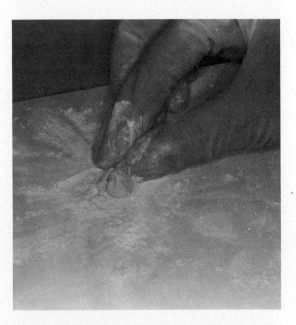

Fig. 25-17. Material is being kneaded to incorporate more powder, after being mixed with tongue blade.

be worn during the mixing (Carranza, 1979). Once the mix has been completed, placement of the dressing is done as previously described.

Manipulation of a premixed dressing

Manipulation of the dressing should be according to the manufacturer's directions. Usually the desired amount of material is removed from the container with a sterile tongue blade and placed on a waxed mixing pad. The material can be formed into two strips of the desired diameter and length and applied as described previously.

REMOVAL OF A PERIODONTAL DRESSING

The patient should return in 5 to 7 days to have the pack removed (Fig. 25-18). When the dressing is removed, the clinician will inspect the area to evaluate the healing. The area will be covered with plaque and other visible debris, which can be gently rinsed away; visible calculus should also be re-

moved. At the end of 5 to 7 days, the tissue should begin to look as if epithelialization is occurring. If the area is very red, inflamed, or an exudate is present, the area may need to be explored for the presence of plaque and calculus. The supervising dentist should be consulted and another dressing placed. If tissue shrinkage has occurred, the newly exposed root surfaces may be sensitive; therefore compressed air should be used with great care (Carranza, 1979; Goldman and Cohen, 1980).

Loosening the pack

The dry foil is loosened with an explorer and removed (Fig. 25-19). The pack is gently loosened from the site with a pair of college pliers and a curette (Figs. 25-20 and 25-21). After the pack has been sufficiently loosened, it can be lifted away from the wound site (Fig. 25-22); many times the pack will come off in one solid strip (Fig. 25-23). Both the facial and lingual portions of the pack are removed. The large pieces of excess pack can be

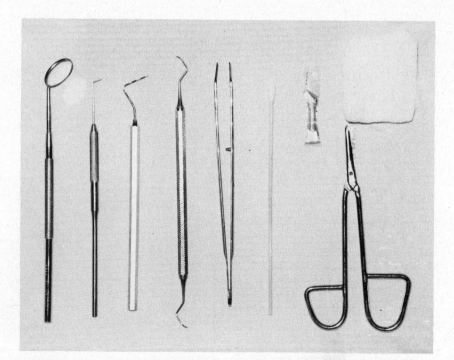

Fig. 25-18. Tray setup for removal of periodontal pack and sutures. Note that suture scissors have a curved blade to reach suture without harming tissue.

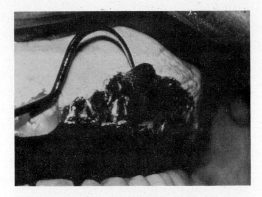

Fig. 25-19. Dry foil is loosened with an explorer and removed.

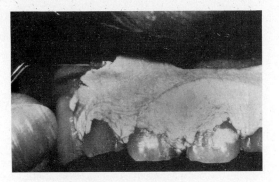

Fig. 25-20. Pack is loosened with a curette.

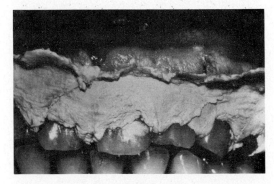

Fig. 25-21. Loosened dressing.

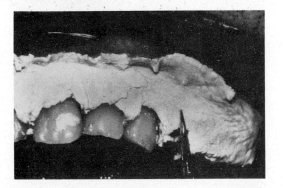

Fig. 25-22. Pack is lifted off wound with college pliers.

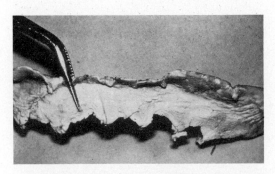

Fig. 25-23. Pack in one piece after removal.

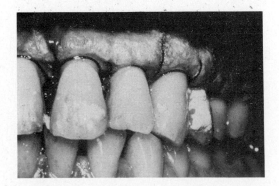

Fig. 25-24. Some large pieces of dressing remain on teeth. Pieces should be removed gently with a curette.

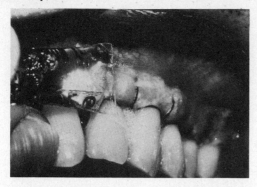

Fig. 25-25. Area is rinsed with oxygenating agent.

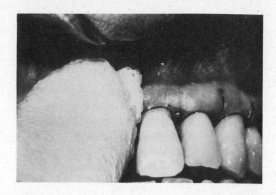

Fig. 25-26. Damp gauze can be used to gently cleanse area of small pieces of dressing and debris.

Placement and removal of periodontal packs

Suggested check-off sheet

Mark **S** for satisfactory completion or **U** for unsatisfactory completion of each criterion in the appropriate space.

PERFORMANCE CRITERIA: Does the student	Faculty	Student
1. Assemble the necessary armamentarium		
2. Mix the pack according to the manufacturer's direction		
3. Shape the pack into two rolls, each the length of the site and two thirds the diameter of a pencil		
Placement of the pack		
4. Gently adapt the pack to the area with damp fingers and damp gauze		
5. Adapt the pack interproximally with a curette or cotton pliers		
6. Muscle mold and trim the pack		
7. Smooth the pack		
8. Produce a pack that		
a. Extends to the middle third of the tooth but not onto the occluding surfaces		
b. Extends beyond all margins of the wound		
c. Does not interfere with normal function		
Removing the pack		
9. Remove the dry foil if still present		
10. Loosen the lingual and buccal packs		
11. Remove the lingual pack		
12. Cut sutures from the lingual portion if necessary		
13. Remove the buccal pack		
14. Cleanse the area with an oxygenating agent		
15. Remove remaining sutures if necessary		
16. Recleanse the area		
17. Gently remove any calculus or granulation tissue		
18. Evaluate healing of the wound site		

removed from the teeth with a curette, being careful of the tender soft tissues and newly exposed root surfaces (Fig. 25-24). The area is then gently rinsed with an oxygenating liquid such as Glyoxide. The oxygenating agent helps to gently cleanse the area of surface debris (Figs. 25-25 and 25-26) (Valentine, 1976). Removal of a dressing placed over an area with sutures is described further in the following section.

REMOVAL OF SUTURES

Sutures are placed after most surgical procedures to reapproximate the soft tissues and promote healing. A variety of absorbable and nonabsorbable suture materials are available. The absorbable sutures include surgical gut, collagen, polyglycolic acid, and polyglactin acid; the nonabsorbable materials are silk, nylon, polypropylene, silver wire, and mersilene (Chung and Weinberg, 1978; Goldman and Cohen, 1980). Black silk suture material is the most popular for periodontal surgery because of its easy manipulation, durability, and strength.

The suture material can be threaded through a needle or attached, swaged, to the needle by the manufacturer (Fig. 25-27); swaged needles are more popular. Most of the needles used in dentistry are curved to allow safe, easy manipulation.

Types of sutures

There are a variety of suture patterns, such as interrupted, sling, continuous sling, and simple mattress, that are used to reapproximate tissues. The surgeon selects the type of suture based on the surgery, healing, and desired outcome. When removing sutures, it is important to know the type of suture placed, the number of knots, and the location of the knots. Figs. 25-27 through 25-29 illustrate and describe three types of commonly used sutures: interrupted, sling, and continuous sling. Note the pattern of the sutures and the lo-

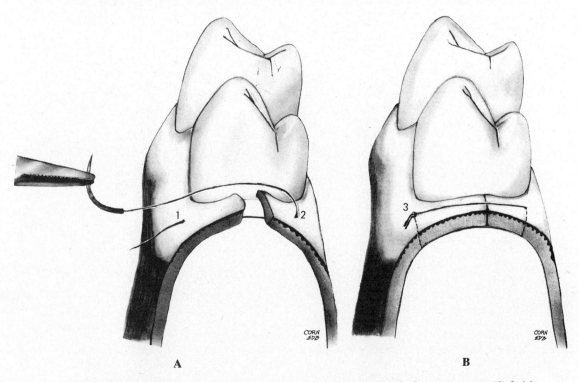

A   **B**

Fig. 25-27. Placement of interrupted suture with a curved, swaged needle. **A,** Suture penetrates *(1)* facial aspect of buccal flap, enters connective tissue of lingual flap, and *(2)* exits lingual flap. **B,** Suture is carried to facial aspect and tied *(3)*. (From Goldman, H.C., and Cohen, D.W. 1980. Periodontal therapy, ed. 6. St. Louis: The C.V. Mosby Co.)

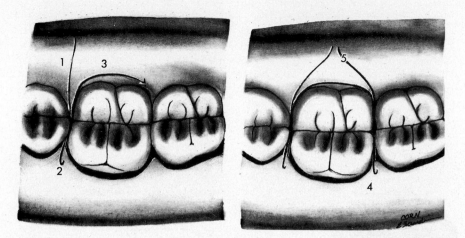

Fig. 25-28. Placement of continuous sling suture to reapproximate buccal tissue. *1,* Needle passes through interdental space from lingual aspect without penetrating tissue and leaves a tail of suture; *2,* buccal tissue is penetrated, and needle passes under contact without entering lingual tissue; *3,* suture is carried around lingual aspect of tooth; *4,* needle penetrates buccal tissue; *5,* suture is knotted on lingual aspect. (From Goldman, H.C., and Cohen, D.W. 1980. Periodontal therapy, ed. 6. St. Louis: The C.V. Mosby Co.)

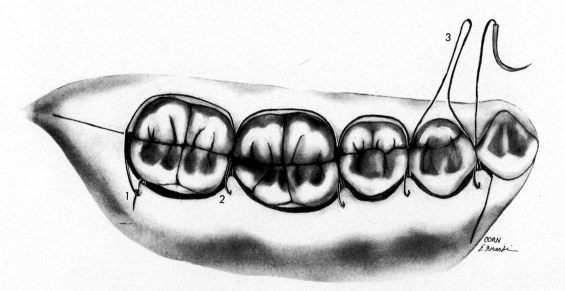

Fig. 25-29. Placement of continuous sling suture to reapproximate lingual tissue. *1,* Loose loop of suture material is tied to ease suture removal; *2,* sling sutures are placed as in Fig. 25-28; *3,* final knot is tied with loop of lingual suture material. (From Goldman, H.C., and Cohen, D.W. 1980. Periodontal therapy, ed. 6. St. Louis: The C.V. Mosby Co.)

cation of the knot. Additional suture patterns (Goldman and Cohen, 1980) are used; however, only the more common ones are presented here. It is helpful if the clinician who places the sutures indicates in the chart the type of suture placed and the number of knots.

Principles for removing sutures

Removing sutures is a relatively simple procedure, but a few basic principles must be observed.

The knot must *never* be pulled through the tissue. The suture is cut so that the knot is pulled away from the tissue (see Fig. 25-31). As little of the suture exposed to the oral cavity as possible is carried through the tissue while the suture is being removed. This is done to decrease the amount of debris and bacteria introduced into the tissue. Finally, all of the suture material and knots must be accounted for after the removal procedure. Figs. 25-30 through 25-32 illustrate and describe the re-

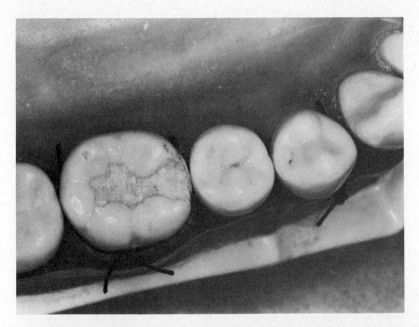

Fig. 25-30. Sling suture to reapproximate lingual tissue around molar and interrupted suture mesial to premolar are ready to be removed.

A

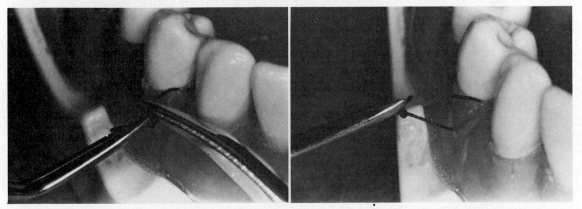

B

Fig. 25-31. Removal of interrupted suture. **A,** Knot is grasped with cotton pliers, pulled away from tissue, and cut with scissors. **B,** Suture is pulled out of tissue.

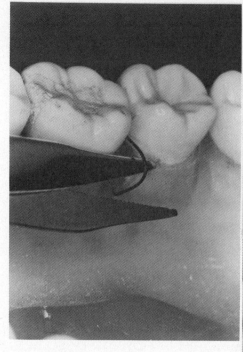

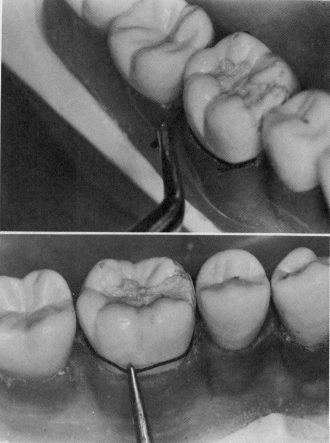

A

B

C

Fig. 25-32. Removal of sling suture. Buccal knot was cut first. **A,** Lingual portions of suture entering tissue are cut. **B,** Loose interproximal suture is removed. **C,** Lingual loop is removed.

moval of interrupted and sling, sutures from a ty-podont. The general principles discussed are followed during the removal procedure.

Sometimes the sutures will become incorporated in the pack. Most practitioners tie sutures on the facial surface so it is best to remove the lingual portion of the pack first, since the knots could not be incorporated in the lingual pack. The facial portion of the pack is gently loosened and removed; if a suture is incorporated in the pack, the suture can be cut from the lingual surface and the suture will be removed along with the pack.

Once the dressing and sutures are removed, the area is cleansed and the tissue is evaluated as previously described.

ACTIVITIES

1. Place and remove a periodontal dressing in one or more of the following situations:
   a. For a partner
   b. On a typodont with missing teeth
   c. On a typodont with sutures placed
2. Conduct a panel discussion with periodontists and/or dentists from your area on the subject "Eugenol versus noneugenol periodontal dressings."
3. Prepare a table clinic on how to place and remove a periodontal pack.
4. Prepare a review of the literature for any of the four types of periodontal dressings.
5. Prepare a presentation about the various suture techniques and the techniques for removing each type.

REVIEW QUESTIONS

1. List the purposes of periodontal dressings.
2. If a choice were given, which type of periodontal dressing, eugenol or noneugenol, would be placed after a soft tissue curettage procedure?
3. After a pack has been placed on a surgical site, the patient asks how to care for the pack. Briefly outline the directions to be given to the patient.
4. Describe how to remove sutures that have become embedded in the pack.

REFERENCES

ADA Council on Dental Therapeutics. 1982. Accepted dental therapeutics, ed. 39. Chicago: American Dental Association.

Addy, et al. 1975. A chlorhexidine-containing methacrylic gel as a periodontal dressing. J. Periodontol. **46**:465.

Baer, P.N., et al. 1969. Periodontal dressings. Dent. Clin. North Am. **13**:181.

Bakdash, M.B. 1976. Asbestos in periodontal dressings, a possible health hazard. Quintessence Int. **7**:61.

Blanque, R.H. 1962. Fundamentals and technique of surgical periodontal packing. J. Periodontol. **33**:346.

Carranza, F.A. 1979. Glickman's clinical periodontology. Philadelphia: W.B. Saunders Co.

Chung, H., and Weinberg, S. 1978. Suture materials in oral surgery: a review. Oral Health **68**(10):31.

Dahlberg, W.H. 1969. Incisions and suturing: some basic considerations about each in periodontal flap surgery. Dent. Clin. North Am. **13**:149.

Forrest, J.O. 1974. The use of cyanoacrylates in periodontal surgery. J. Periodontol. **45**:225.

Frisch, L., and Bhaskar, S.N. 1967. Tissue response to eugenol containing periodontal dressings. J. Periodontol. **38**:402.

Geiger, B., et al. 1981. Periodontal dressings: rationale and procedures. Dent. Hyg. **55**(9):21.

Goldman, H.C., and Cohen, D.W. 1980. Periodontal therapy, ed. 6. St. Louis: The C.V. Mosby Co.

Grant, D.A., Stern, I.V., and Everett, F.G. 1979. Periodontics in the tradition of Orban and Gottlieb. St. Louis: The C.V. Mosby Co.

Haugen, E. 1980. The effect of periodontal dressings on intact mucous membrane and on wound healing. Acta Odontol. Scand. **38**:363.

Haugen, E., and Gjermo, P. 1978. Clinical assessment of periodontal dressings. J. Clin. Periodontol. **5**:50.

Haugen, E., and Mjör, I. 1979. Bone tissue reactions to periodontal dressings. J. Periodont. Res. **14**:76.

Haugen, E., et al. 1977. Some antibacterial properties of periodontal dressings. J. Clin. Periodontol. **4**:62.

Haugen, E., et al. 1978. The sensitizing potential of periodontal dressings. J. Dent. Res. **57**:950.

Jones, T.M., and Cassingham, R.J. 1979. Comparison of healing following periodontal surgery with and without dressings in humans. J. Periodontol. **50**:387.

Levin, M.P. 1980. Periodontal suture materials and surgical dressings. Dent. Clin. North Am. **24**:767.

Levin, M.P., et al. 1975. Cyanoacrylate as a periodontal dressing. J. Oral Med. **30**:40.

Lysell, L. 1976. Contact allergy to rosin in a periodontal dressing. J. Oral Med. **31**:24.

Macht, S.D., and Krizek, T.J. 1978. Sutures and suturing—current concepts. J. Oral Surg. **36**:710.

Manor, A., et al. 1982. Unusual foreign body reaction to a braided silk suture: a case report. J. Periodontol. **53**:868.

Nelson, E.H., et al. 1977. A comparison of the continuous and interrupted suturing techniques. J. Periodontol. **48**:273.

O'Neil, T.C. 1975. Antibacterial properties of periodontal dressings. J. Periodontol. **46**:469.

Pihlstrom, B.L., et al. 1977. The effect of periodontal dressing on supragingival microorganisms. J. Periodontol. **48**:440.

Poulson, R.C. 1974. An anaphylactoid reaction to periodontal surgical dressing: report of case. J. Am. Dent. Assoc. **89**:895.

Stahl, S.S., et al. 1969. The effects of periodontal dressings on gingival repair. J. Periodontol. **40**:34.

Stroh, C., and Chinn, S.A. 1976. Periodontal dressings. Seattle: University of Washington.

Valentine, R.M. 1976. Expanded duties: a self-determined pace laboratory program. Philadelphia: University of Pennsylvania.

Wampole, H.S., et al. 1978. The incidence of transient bacteremia during periodontal dressing change. J. Periodontol. **49**:462.

Watts, T.L.P., and Combe, E.C. 1979. Periodontal dressing materials. J. Clin. Periodontol. **6**:3.

Watts, T.L.P., and Combe, E.C. 1981. Effects of noneugenol periodontal dressing materials upon the surface hardness of anterior restorative materials in vitro. Br. Dent. J. **151**:423.

26 POLISHING THE TEETH

OBJECTIVES: *The reader will be able to*

1. Recognize the categories of tooth discolorations or stains.
2. Educate the patient to recognize the problem of tooth discoloration and how to prevent recurrence.
3. Explain to the patient how discolorations are formed and the three levels of procedures that can be done to prevent, remove, or cover these tooth discolorations:
   a. Patient—prevention
   b. Hygienist—oral prophylaxis
   c. Dentist—selected grinding, bleaching, the use of composite resins, or tooth crowning
4. Recommend proper home care, including types of dentifrice for the patient to use.
5. Select the proper abrasives and procedures to remove extrinsic stain in the dental office.
6. Polish stains from the teeth using light, intermittent pressure and adaptation to gain access to cervical and proximal areas.
7. Identify when to use a brush for polishing.
8. Describe ways to minimize frictional heat.

Following scaling, root planing, and other necessary periodontal procedures, the teeth should be evaluated for stain. If the dental hygienist involves the patient in removing plaque and food debris with a brush and floss at the beginning of each appointment, it should not be necessary to polish the teeth to remove plaque. Stain that cannot be removed by the patient is the primary factor that determines the need for polishing.

In deciding which teeth to polish and the necessary materials for the polishing procedure, it is important to evaluate the stains present on the teeth and the abrasives and mechanical devices available for optimum use.

The important aspect of dental staining to the patient is the appearance of the teeth. While the patient tends to focus on the color and appearance of the teeth, the dental professional is more concerned with the health of the tissues and teeth as affected by stains and deposits. Dental stains are associated with and/or embedded in deposits that, if not removed, are an important factor in the initiation of caries and gingival problems. Therefore it is beneficial to both the patient and the professional to use tooth discoloration as a means of encouraging better home care procedures. In an attempt to achieve a whiter and brighter appearance of the teeth, the patient may practice better toothbrushing and, with this, the cleaning of critical gingival areas.

Most dental hygienists have learned to polish all tooth surfaces after a scaling procedure, regardless of the presence of plaque or stain. It has traditionally been viewed as the finishing procedure of the oral prophylaxis, receiving good acceptance among patients, since it makes the teeth feel uniformly smooth and clean (Hunter et al., 1981).

Over the past several years the concept of "selective polishing" has been discussed as a logical alternative to polishing all teeth (Primosch, 1980; Rohleder and Slim, 1981). The rationale is partly to ensure that the patient realizes his/her role in maintaining oral cleanliness and partly to minimize polishing away the fluoride-rich outer layer of enamel (Mellberg, 1977; Retief et al, 1980; Shern et al, 1977). Since studies have shown that polishing does not improve the uptake of professionally applied fluoride in enamel, the prime clinical reason for polishing all surfaces has been cast in doubt (Tinanoff et al., 1974; Steele et al., 1982). In addition, polishing and hand planing over years of routine care changes the morphology of the teeth

(Swan, 1970). This makes the assumption of a complete polish of all teeth at every recall even more questionable.

A recent study has shown, however, that there are significantly different accumulations of plaque after 3 days on teeth that were professionally polished as opposed to those that were self-polished with a toothbrush (Waring et al., 1982). A split-mouth technique was used. Half of the teeth in each of 15 persons' mouths were polished, and half were self-brushed. After 3 days of no-oral-hygiene procedures, the polished teeth had less plaque.

A clinician is therefore faced with a dilemma: should all teeth be polished to remove deposits and retard buildup, or should only selective polishing be performed in order to avoid stripping enamel (and its greatest fluoride concentrations) from the teeth and to enhance patients' awareness of their role in deposit removal? The decision should involve the patient and his/her preferences and the judgment of the clinician regarding what is best for the individual patient. Is the patient a heavy plaque former? What is the patient's caries rate or susceptibility to caries? What is the patient's periodontal index? What is the purpose of the polish for this patient? How will the outcome of polishing or not polishing likely affect the patient's primary oral problem?

The following information about deposits should aid in assessing whether polishing should be selective or universal for a patient and what procedures should be followed.

DENTAL STAINS
Definitions and classifications

Staining or discoloration can occur in three ways: (1) it can adhere directly to tooth surfaces; (2) it can be contained within calculus and soft deposits; and (3) it can be incorporated in the tooth structure.

Discolorations are classified as either endogenous or exogenous (Corranza, 1979; Shaw and Murray, 1977; Vogel, 1975; Winter, Murray, and Shaw, 1978). *Endogenous* is the term used for stains that develop within the tooth. Usually these are dentin discolorations showing through enamel. *Exogenous* stains originate outside of the tooth or the oral cavity. Within this classification, exogenous stains are further categorized on the basis of their ability to be removed. *Extrinsic* stains are on the exterior of the tooth and are removable by the individual or the dental professional. *Intrinsic* stains are of exogenous origin but become incorporated into the tooth structure and are not removable by the patient or by polishing and scaling.

The essentials of a classification that is prevention oriented are shown in the following outline:*

  I. Hereditary
 II. Congenital
    A. During development or maturation
    B. Drug related
III. Environmental
    A. Developing permanent dentition
    B. Normal expectancy
      1. Aging
      2. Fracture lines
      3. Attrition
      4. Abrasion
      5. Erosion
    C. Pathologic incursions
      1. Caries
      2. Pulpal changes
    D. Stains
      1. Foods
      2. Drugs
      3. Pigment forming bacteria, including green, black etc.
      4. Metals
      5. Iatrogenic

This classification was developed to enable the dental professional, along with the medical professional, to more readily understand those areas where preventing tooth abnormalities and discolorations might be aided. The primary categories of this classification—genetic, congenital or developmental, and environmental—are briefly described.

Hereditary or *genetic factors* can affect both the primary and the permanent dentition and the developing sequences in the formation of the tooth structure itself. There is little if anything that members of the health profession can do to prevent these hereditary defects.

Developmental or *congenital defects* are associated with several disease processes wherein the dental professional can be of value in consulting with the physician; however, little can be done by members of either profession to alleviate these den-

*Modified from Rakow, B., and Light, E.I. (1976). J. Prevent. Dent. **3:**13.

Table 26-1. Extrinsic stains

Stain category	Primary tooth sites	Composition	Associated with
Green	Cervical one third to one half of labial surfaces of maxillary anterior teeth	Inorganic elements, chromogenic bacteria	Poor oral hygiene; surface irregularities; highest in children
Black-line	Thin band along gingival margin of lingual and buccal surfaces	Ferric sulfide	Iron in saliva, gingival fluid; plaque or bacteria; all ages
Orange	Thin line; cervical one third of incisors	Chromogenic bacteria	Poor oral hygiene; highest in children
Tobacco	Cervical one third to one half of lingual surfaces; pits and fissures	Tars, pigments	Smoking; chewing tobacco
Food	Same as above	Food colors	Consumption of tea, coffee, cola drinks, berries, spices, colored candies
Metallic	Cervical one third; random surfaces	Associated with particular metals	Environmental, food, water
Drug, therapeutic	Plaque-associated areas	Plaque bacteria; tin; reactions with food colors	Extended antibiotic use, stannous fluoride, chlorhexidine

tal defects. Another phase of problems in the developmental or congenital area deal with medications that are delivered to the mother and that affect the developing teeth in utero, or that are given to children during the formation of their primary or permanent dentition. Here the dental professional can be of much value when consulted for information, especially about compounds such as tetracyclines and fluorides. In this regard it is interesting to note the article on prevention of dental problems in the *Journal of the American Medical Association* in which specific recommendations for the administration of tetracycline are presented (Rall, 1977).

The third category in this preventive classification are the areas focused on in this chapter. These are *environmental* and include what are termed *pathologic incursions,* such as caries, pulpal changes, and stains due to foods, drugs, pigments, and metals and iatrogenic stains or those stains resulting from procedures or drug therapy used in the dental or medical office or from professionally prescribed drugs.

The primary tooth discolorations for patient prevention and/or professional removal by the prophylaxis are described in Table 26-1. Individuals vary widely in the rate and amount of extrinsic stain accumulation. Certain factors predispose a person to the accumulation of both dental deposits and stains; these include enamel roughness, salivary composition, salivary flow rates, and poor oral hygiene.

Extrinsic stains can be identified by color, distribution, and tenaciousness and by age, sex, home care, and other factors in which the preventive classification and the standard classification agree (Reid, Beeley, and MacDonald, 1977). The major colored stains are:

Green stain. This occurs primarily in the cervical areas of the maxillary anterior and is associated with the primary dental cuticle. It usually is crescent shaped, close to the gingiva, and ranges in color from light green to yellow green to dark green. Usually green stain occurs when an individual practices poor oral hygiene, and it tends to recur after removal.

Black-line stain. This usually occurs as a continuous thin band along the gingival margin and follows the crestal contour on lingual or proximal surfaces. It occurs at all ages and if found more often in females. The primary cause of this deposit is iron compounds in saliva or gingival fluid that become embedded in plaque and/or plaque bacteria. This stain is a ferric sulfide compound (Reid, Berley, and MacDonald, 1977).

Orange stain. This is fairly rare, occurring in approximately 3% of the population. It occurs usually at the cervical third of incisor teeth and is attributed to chromogenic bacteria.

All of the aforementioned colored stains occur more extensively if home care is inadequate. Professional scaling and prophylaxis will remove these stains easily, but there is a tendency for recurrence.

Table 26-2. Effect of smoking on extrinsic stain

Number of cigarettes per day	Percent with moderate to severe stain
0	18
1 to 10	35
11 to 20	51
>20	78

Modified from Ness, L., Rosekrans, D. de L., and Welford, J.F. 1977. Community Dent. Oral Epidemiol. **5**:55.

Tobacco stain. This tooth discoloration ranges in appearance from tan to dark brown or black and covers approximately the cervical one third to one half of most teeth. It occurs mostly on lingual surfaces. It is also commonly found in pits and fissures and other irregularities of enamel. Tobacco staining is directly proportional to the number of cigarettes smoked per day (Ness, Rosekrans, and Welford, 1977) (Table 26-2). Staining is also high in individuals who chew tobacco. Tobacco stains may penetrate enamel and become intrinsic.

Food stain. This is a common stain in individuals consuming large quantities of coffee and tea. Other categories of colored food that may contribute to stain include cola drinks, berries such as raspberries and blueberries, spices, and licorice and other colored candies. Stains resulting from ingestion of these foods range from tan to dark brown in color and occur over broad tooth surfaces and in pits and fissures.

Metallic stains. These vary in color depending on the metal or metallic salt ingested. Green or blue-green colors result from copper or brass, whereas brown colors may result from an ingestion of materials or dust particles containing iron. While the majority of these stains have been attributed to industrial dust, it is possible to ingest high quantities of metals in various foods and/or water.

Stains due to drug and/or therapeutic agents. These stains can originate from many sources, only a few of which are described here. After extended topical or systemic antibiotic use, or in studies of antibacterial agents with antiplaque activity, surface discolorations and staining have occurred (Moffit et al., 1974; Solheim, Erikson, and Nordbo, 1980). These have been attributed to direct effects of the agents on plaque bacteria, as well as an enhanced affinity for food colorants. A brown to black pigmented stain in plaque-associated areas has also been reported in several clinical studies and is attributed to dentifrices containing stannous fluoride (Yankell and Emling, 1978).

Two other tooth discolorations are discussed here from the professional's point of view. The first of these is caries. Initial or incipient carious lesions will appear slightly whiter and chalky and dull in comparison with unaffected enamel. Often these are not observed by the patient but should be pointed out at a dental examination. Recurring caries will appear as a grey area adjacent to the margin of a defective restoration. With increased caries development or lesion size, the decalcified areas will become stained with food and bacterial debris, and the amount of discoloration will depend on the time period of the active decay process. The second area of importance includes stains due to defective restorations. These stains occur around the restoration usually because of leakage at the site. This stain indicates that the amalgam should be replaced.

Prevention (home care)

Toothbrushing is the most common means of home care in this country. Although proper toothbrushing with a toothbrush alone or with water can remove all dental deposits, this does result in pellicle stains (Manly, 1943). Toothpastes are formulated to aid in the removal of debris and discoloration from tooth surfaces and to impart a gloss or luster (polish). Toothpastes are composed of many ingredients, each with a specific function (Gershon and Pader, 1972; Goldstein, 1976; Yankell and Emling, 1978) (Table 26-3). Following is a summary of abrasives in toothpastes:

Calcium carbonate (CaCO₃ [Macleans, Phillips, Aquafresh]). Precipitated calcium carbonate (chalk) was widely used in dentifrice products until the mid 1950s. This material is decomposed in an acid pH.

Dibasic calcium phosphate (CaHPO₄ [Colgate, Listerine, Pearl Drops]). The anhydrous or the dihydrate forms of dibasic calcium phosphate are used. The anhydrous form is much more abrasive than the dihydrate form. Although dicalcium phosphate dihydrate is not compatible with sodium fluoride or stannous fluoride, sodium monofluorophosphate can be maintained in soluble form in the presence of this agent for relatively long periods of time.

Tribasic calcium phosphate (Ca₃[PO₄]₂ [Craig-Martin]). The abrasiveness of tribasic calcium phosphate (TCP) is similar to medium-grade dibasic calcium phosphate dihydrate. TCP is used primarily in ammoniated toothpaste, since it is highly compatible with diammonium phosphate.

Table 26-3. Toothpaste composition

Ingredient	Approximate composition (%)	Function
Abrasive(s)	20 to 60	Clean; polish
Water	20 to 50	Provide a vehicle
Humectant(s)	10 to 40	Prevent caking or hardening; retain moisture
Binding agent(s)	1 to 5	Prevent separation; add thickness
Surface active agent(s), detergent(s)	1 to 2	Remove surface deposits, debris; provide foam
Flavor(s), sweetening agent(s)	1 to 5	Add taste
Therapeutic agent(s)	0.01 to 10	Prevent and/or reduce caries, sensitivity, etc.
Miscellaneous	0.1 to 5	Color; preserve; stabilize

Modified from Yankell, S., and Emling, R.C. 1978. Continuing dental education, University of Pennsylvania School of Dental Medicine **1**: No. 7.

Calcium pyrophosphate (Ca$_2$P$_2$O$_7$ [Gleem]). Calcium pyrophosphate is more abrasive than dicalcium phosphate dihydrate and more compatible with fluoride compounds because it is one of the most inert calcium phosphate salts.

Alumina compounds (Ultra-Brite). Hydrated alumina compounds are available in various particle sizes and thus various degrees of abrasiveness. These compounds do not contain calcium and do not appear to react with fluorides.

Silicates and silicas (Sensodyne, Close-up, Crest, Macleans, Aim, Aquafresh). Silica compounds are available in various molecular weights and grades of abrasiveness. Dehydrated silica gels prepared to yield an amorphous granular xerogel with a microporous structure of specific particle sizes are also transparent. When coupled with the proper humectant systems, silicates and silicas can be used to produce translucent or transparent clear gel products.

With scanning electron microscopy, changes on the tooth surface have been studied after the use of toothpastes that varied considerably in abrasive composition. Pellicle was present within 24 hours after cleaning the tooth completely, and pellicle thickness increased with time. Thicker pellicles formed during the use of nonabrasive toothpastes. It was concluded that abrasives were necessary to control pellicle thickness and prevent stain buildup. If pellicle was allowed to remain undisturbed, it became more difficult to remove because of changes in physical properties (Saxton, 1976). This study emphasizes the importance of suggesting products with good abrasives to be used properly by the individual on a consistent basis. For patients with exposed dentin or cementum, it is imperative to stress proper brushing procedures. Since these

tooth structures are softer than enamel, they are more prone to the abrasives in dentifrices if improperly used. Unfortunately, no standards have been established as to the optimal amount of abrasiveness in toothpastes (ADA Council, 1982).

Professional treatment

Extrinsic stains. After the teeth are scaled and prepared, they should be cleaned with a professional prophylaxis paste. Although there are many prophylaxis pastes available, these vary considerably in the abrasives they contain and in their relative abrasiveness. The abrasives contained in these products essentially are similar to those in dentifrice products (Craig, O'Brien, and Powers, 1983; Davis, 1978; O'Brien and Ryge, 1978); the major difference is that the levels in professional products are much higher.

Abrasive agents are incorporated into professional products for the purpose of cleaning and polishing. These factors are significantly interrelated (Fig. 26-1), and the terms can be confusing. A dental abrasive changes the surface of the tooth by frictional grinding, rubbing, scraping, scratching, etc., to remove irregularities. As this process proceeds from coarse abrasion (cleaning) to polishing, the surface of the tooth passes through various stages: from an irregular surface, to a grooved surface, to a finely scratched surface, which is increased in smoothness and light reflectance. The last state is regarded as the polished surface.

Factors determining the abrasiveness or polishing potential of an agent include its hardness, shape, size, and concentration. Different abrasives commonly used vary markedly in their inherent

ABRASION		POLISHING
Large	Particle size	Small
Irregular	Shape	Regular
High	Concentration	Low
Increased	Hardness	Decreased
Firm	Pressure	Mild
Rapid	Speed	Slow
Soft (dentin and cementum)	Tooth surface texture	Hard (enamel)

Fig. 26-1. Factors influencing tooth cleaning.

hardness and shape. Within the same abrasive, sizes are graded from fine to coarse. With abrasive compounds that are harder, of rougher shape, increased particle size, or high concentration, abrasiveness is maximized. As each of these factors decreases, less surface abrasion occurs and the surface becomes smooth, or polished.

Additional factors related to the method(s) of applying the prophylaxis product must be considered in the polishing and cleaning procedure. These include the pressure and speed used to apply the product and the surface (enamel, restorative material, etc.) being treated. With greater pressure or speed, increased friction occurs, resulting in the generation of heat and discomfort to the patient. As a general rule, it is imperative to maintain a slow, steady rate of abrasiveness to minimize the potential damage to denuded enamel and gingival areas and to sustain patient comfort.

Two abrasive agents used in prophylaxis products or available as chemical compounds are pumice and calcium carbonate (chalk, whiting). Pumice is manufactured in a wide variety of particle sizes, and its use ranges from an abrasive stain removal agent to fine polishing of acrylic dentures. Calcium carbonate is also manufactured in several particle shapes and sizes. This compound has more of a polishing action, since it produces minimal scratching and results in a smooth surface that reflects light. Although professional products have been categorized as fine, medium, or coarse, there are no standards to define exactly what these terms mean. One manufacturer's fine prophylaxis paste may be more abrasive than another manufacturer's medium paste, since they may contain different abrasives. The limitations within these gradings must be confined to products made by the same manufacturer and containing the same abrasive ingredient. No attempt should be made to match one manufacturer's fine abrasive product with another manufacturer's product labeled as being in the same category even if they contain the same abrasive(s). The dental professional must learn how to use each manufacturer's products in his/her own practice. It is important to evaluate different manufacturers' products to become familiar with the polishing and abrasive characteristics first in laboratory experiments, if possible, prior to using them on patients.

Since prophylaxis pastes are more abrasive than toothpastes, it is important to be selective in the teeth that are polished. With a professional prophylaxis and the use of highly abrasive materials, a thin surface of enamel is removed. This is reformed fairly quickly and mineralized in the mouth as a result of the high calcium phosphate content of saliva and enamel remineralization can be enhanced by the use of fluoride toothpaste. Therefore it is also recommended that prophylaxis paste contain a fluoride compound (ADA Council, 1982). This has the advantage of providing high levels of fluoride during the prophylaxis period and enabling fluoride to be associated with the enamel subsurface after the abrasive procedure. It is also recommended that abrasive procedures be followed by professional fluoride treatments, as discussed in Chapter 29.

Intrinsic stains. Although this area is not of major concern to the dental hygienist in the activities that he/she will be performing, it is important to be aware of the background of intrinsic stains and their care so that they may be described to patients. In the case of caries, there are several types of restorative materials available, and it would be helpful for some of these differences to be explained to patients. The most common restorative materials are dental amalgams or the common silver fillings. These materials are placed primarily on the occlusal surfaces or on other surfaces of premolar and molar teeth. They have high density and are long lasting. They must be placed with proper cavity liners to prevent leaching of tin or other metals from the amalgam into the dentin and causing or enhancing intrinsic staining.

Two materials are used to restore anterior teeth. The most common material until recently has been a silicate cement, which can be mixed to various shades to match the color of the teeth. This material is softer than enamel and has the capacity to take on colorations and become stained; over a period of time silicates will deteriorate and have to be replaced. New composite materials have been developed that are much harder and longer lasting than silicate cement. These composites, when bonded to the enamel with an acid-etch procedure, have been a major factor in improving the cosmetic properties of anterior restorations.

Professional methods for improving intrinsic stain appearance include such procedures as bleaching the teeth (Heringer, 1976), using composite restoration materials as overlays, and, if significant intrinsic staining has occurred, using crown(s) to completely cover the affected tooth or teeth. Although bleaching has often been attempted and is satisfactory for relatively minor intrinsic stain(s), a number of concerns have recently been itemized (Cooley, 1976). These include the need to know more about the histologic effects after bleaching and the chemical reactions during the application of concentrated peroxides. Effects on the pulp after bleaching are unknown, as are potential dehydration effects on the enamel.

Several researchers have used resin veneers or composite materials in 6- to 12-month evaluations (Cooley, 1976; Spencer, 1972; Stuart, 1975). Results have been encouraging, particularly in matching color with other teeth in the mouth, in the relatively short time required to do invidividual teeth (ranging from 15 to 30 minutes per tooth), and in the excellent patient acceptance after completion of treatments. Difficulties with these materials include flaking or cracking, especially when fibrous or hard-consistency foods are eaten. Tooth capping or full porcelain or acrylic crowns are used when major intrinsic staining has occurred; however, this should not be done on deciduous or young permanent dentition. It is desirable to have complete development of the pulp prior to crowning. A second drawback of this treatment is the expense and time incurred in having the procedure performed. A third difficulty is the creation of an artificial margin between the tooth crown and root, which can be a primary site for plaque adherence. Many dental professionals are reluctant to sacrifice large areas of healthy tooth structure for purely cosmetic purposes.

Stain evaluation

Attempts have been made to develop scoring procedures to evaluate intrinsic and extrinsic staining. One of the first attempts to evaluate stain clinically was the categorization of both the intensity and severity of the stain and the tooth area covered (Lobene, 1968). This scoring system is shown in Table 26-4. This scoring procedure was used to study the effects of dentifrices on tooth stains after controlled brushing times. The products evaluated differed significantly in their ability to remove stains. Another approach to quantitation of tooth stain has been the use of chips of various colors combined with a tooth surface scoring area to evaluate new antiplaque materials (Yankell et al., 1982). A stain index has been proposed to detect small changes in staining levels between different groups. In this procedure, stained areas are drawn on a reproduced grid system to determine the area of the tooth covered. No attempt has been made in this system to quantitate the intensity of tooth stain; rather, staining is graded on a stain, no stain basis (Shaw and Murray, 1977).

Table 26-4. Scoring tooth stains*

Stain characteristic	Score	Description of stain
Intensity	0	None
	1	Light
	2	Moderate
	3	Heavy
Extent	0	None detected
	1	One third of region
	2	Two thirds of region
	3	>Two thirds of region

Modified from Lobene, R.R. 1968. J. Am. Dent. Assoc. 77:844.
*The facial surfaces of the eight incisors are scored. Each incisor is divided into the gingival and body regions. Each region is scored for both intensity and extent.

What is recommended for the professional office? Staining records should be maintained for individuals who present this problem, whether this symptom is recognized by the patient or evaluated by the professional. The scoring system shown in Table 26-4 offers criteria for analyzing intensity and tooth area and for recording the maximum amount of information to be used for planning treatment and for review of conditions at recall.

MECHANICAL DEVICES FOR POLISHING

The simplest device for polishing stains from the teeth is a *porte polisher* (Fig. 26-2). This hand instrument is designed to hold wooden points, which can then be thoroughly adapted to the various aspects of the teeth to rub the abrasive against the tooth surface. Each stroke generated by the wrist rock moves the wedge-shaped, tapered, or pointed wooden point over the tooth surface (Fig. 26-3). This procedure requires considerable hand strength and control and is a slow, tedious process. It does, however, have several advantages, including (1) its portability (since it can be used when electricity is not available, at the bedside, or in other settings where engine-driven equipment cannot be used); (2) the gentle massage provided to the soft tissues as long as strokes are carefully controlled and approximate the gingival margins; (3) ready access to selected tooth surfaces that are obscured by tooth malpositions; (4) generation of minimal frictional heat; (5) lack of engine noise

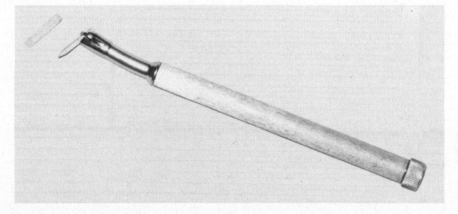

Fig. 26-2. Porte polisher is a hand instrument into which variously shaped orangewood points may be inserted and used to polish teeth with an abrasive.

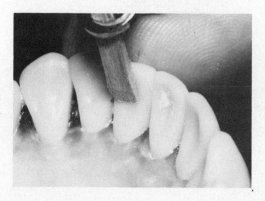

Fig. 26-3. Wooden point is closely adapted to tooth to rub the abrasive against stained areas. Short strokes are used in gingival, middle, and incisal or occlusal thirds of tooth to ensure a clean, well-polished surface.

(and thus its greater acceptance by patients; and (6) the simple procedures for cleaning and sterilizing as compared with those required for cleaning and sterilizing engine-driven handpieces and prophylaxis angles.

In the early days of dental hygiene, porte polishing was one of the first procedures learned in educational programs because it developed hand strength, control, and a functional wrist rock. Motor-driven polishing has become more common in educational programs in recent decades, since it requires less time to complete and is the method of choice in clinical practice. Despite the predominant use of motor-driven polishing, the porte polisher is a valuable adjunct instrument that should be the method of choice for some patients and in some clinical settings. An activity at the conclusion of this chapter provides students with an opportunity to use the porte polisher.

Engine-driven polishing is more widely used in clinical practice because of its efficiency and the lesser amount of effort required to polish a complete dentition. The power is derived in most instances from (1) an electric motor, which drives a belt over a series of pulleys to turn the handpiece gears (the familiar slow-speed "drill"); (2) a small electric motor that attaches to the base of the handpiece and to electric supply hosing; or (3) compressed air supplied by hosing to an air turbine handpiece. Whatever mechanism or power source is used in any given clinical setting, it is extremely important for the dental hygienist to become familiar with (1) the kind of system used, (2) the specific procedures necessary for operating and maintaining the system, and (3) the checklist of what to inspect if the system fails to rotate the polishing instrument.

The handpiece and the prophylaxis angle (which holds the rubber cup and brush attachments that polish the teeth) require proper care and maintenance. A nonfunctional handpiece, prophylaxis angle, or power line makes motordriven polishing impossible. Identifying and correcting the reason for the malfunction require the hygienist's mechanical abilities. A sterile porte polisher should be kept close at hand for those times when basic cleaning and oiling do not restore function to the modern convenience.

The handpiece selected for use should be specifically designed for the system being used. The handpiece may screw, snap, lock, or clip onto the power source. Attached to the handpiece is the prophylaxis angle, which, as mentioned before, holds the rubber cup or brush (Fig. 26-4). The cup or brush may attach by means of a metal mandrel that is latched into place. The metal mandrel slides

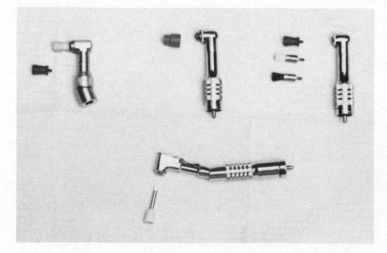

Fig. 26-4. Prophylaxis angles vary in design to accommodate handpiece systems and vary in mechanism used to attach polishing cups or brushes. Attachment may screw in, snap on over a knob, or fit into angle with a mandrel and latching mechanism.

through the head of the angle to the latch at the back of the angle head. Other styles of cups and angles enable the rubber cup to screw into the head of the angle. Reverse threads are used so that the rubber cup will not unscrew while running in a clockwise rotation against the tooth. Yet another style allows the cup or brush to snap over a knob on the face of the angle head. The cup and knob must be dry and oil-free, or the cup will slip against the knob instead of gripping it firmly.

Some cups are impregnated with fluoride. They have been shown to increase enamel fluoride content by 400 to 700 ppm and to reduce enamel solubility by 20% to 28%. They also remove stained pellicle more efficiently and with less abrasion of the enamel than the other cups tested. The cups are made of thermoplastic resins and a 6% mixture of sodium fluoride and stannous fluoride. In instances where stains require polishing, the use of fluoride-impregnated cups is indicated (Stookey and Schemehorn, 1976; Stookey and Stahlman, 1976).

Prophy-Jet

A third method for polishing the teeth has been introduced that requires no hand pressure against the tooth. The Dentsply/Cavitron Prophy-Jet (Fig. 26-5) projects a slurry of water and sodium bicarbonate against the tooth surface, cleaning away the stain and polishing the teeth. It uses air pressure of 50 to 100 pounds per square inch (psi) and water pressure of 10 to 50 psi. The water temperature is thermostatically controlled at approximately 37.7°

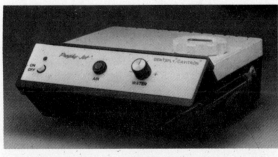

Fig. 26-5. Dentsply/Cavitron Prophy-Jet uses a slurry of sodium bicarbonate and water under air pressure to clean stain and polish teeth.

C (100° F). The handpiece has a nozzle through which the slurry is propelled when a foot control is activated. The nozzle should be held 1 cm from the tooth and be angled diagonally toward the tooth and not at right angles to it. The stream should not be aimed at the soft tissue.

The instrument removes stain rapidly and thoroughly. One study compared it with the rubber cup and with the ultrasonic scaler for its ability to remove stain and the surface roughness it produced. The rubber cup produced shallow, curved scratches on enamel; the ultrasonic scaler produced linear scratches that were deeper and broader than those left by the rubber cup; and the Prophy-Jet left a nonuniformly roughened surface with ridges on the enamel. The greatest variance from smoothest surface to roughest surface was observed with the Prophy-Jet. That is, in comparisons with the other two methods, the Prophy-Jet produced the smoothest polish among all the teeth that were judged to be smooth, but also the roughest result among all the teeth that were judged to be rough. Overall, however, it created no greater abrasion than the other devices (Willmann et al., 1980).

Given the comparative newness of the device, clinicians should be alert to forthcoming evaluations. Used carefully and according to the manufacturer's instructions, it can serve a useful role in removing heavy stain that would require extensive pressure and time to remove with conventional methods.

POLISHING PROCEDURE

All parts of the handpiece and angle must ensure that adequate torque is maintained to move the abrasive against the tooth for polishing. The abrasive is carried to the tooth by dipping the rubber cup or brush into the abrasive, placing the cup or brush against the tooth, and activating the rheostat so that the applicator rotates, thus polishing the tooth with the abrasive.

The abrasive can be held in a dappen dish or in a small cup held by a finger on the mirror-holding hand for ready access. Or the chairside assistant can apply the abrasive directly to the teeth with a plastic syringe just ahead of the path of the rubber cup or brush. Regardless of how the abrasive is to be placed on the tooth, it is important that adequate amounts be used. Usually a full rubber cup of abrasive will be sufficient for one or two teeth. A bare

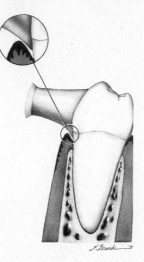

Fig. 26-6. Rubber cup should be adapted so that it slides slightly subgingivally in cervical area.

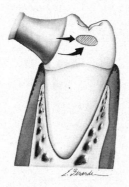

Fig. 26-7. Rubber cup should be adapted so that it has as much access to proximal surface as possible and so that it slides up under contact point.

or salivaladen cup devoid of polishing agent does not polish the teeth and generates heat. Cups are available with webbing inside the cup to retain the agent more readily.

The rubber cup can be adapted to all exposed tooth surfaces. It can and should be slipped slightly subgingivally so that the lip of the cup cleans the most coronal aspects of the sulcus (Fig. 26-6). It should be applied to proximal surfaces by sliding the lip of the cup as far proximally as possible and slightly under the contact point area (Fig. 26-7).

Adapting the lip of the cup into the occlusal grooves will often suffice for stain removal from those difficult areas.

When the rubber cup does not remove occlusal stain adequately, a small brush may be attached for use on the occlusal surfaces. Brushes *should not* be used on any other tooth surfaces, since they are highly abrasive (Thompson and Way, 1981), are difficult to control, and may easily abrade the soft tissues. Brushes are available with soft or firm bristles. The softer bristles are usually adequate for stain removal, and they hold abrasive more readily.

Whether a cup or brush is being used, the attachment and abrasive should be used with *light intermittent pressure*. This on-and-off application on the tooth allows the heat that is generated by the process to dissipate between each stroke. Constant pressure between the rubber cup or brush and the tooth builds up frictional heat, causing first discomfort, then pain, and finally possible pulp damage. The rule is to apply the cup on and off the tooth with light pressure. This is especially critical for anterior teeth, which provide minimal insulation for the pulp because of the comparative lack of bulk of dentin and enamel.

Clinicians should observe the patient's facial expression carefully to detect signs of discomfort from heat being felt. If the clinician suspects that the patient is in pain, the patient should be asked if he/she feels heat, and if so, the polishing procedure should be altered to reduce heat, usually by lessening the duration of each application of the cup or brush to the tooth.

The speed of the cup is critical in both minimizing frictional heat and in ensuring effective polishing. A speeding cup is both harmful and ineffective. Since it is rarely possible to determine the exact revolutions per minute (rpm) at which the handpiece is operating, most clinicians operate the handpiece at the *lowest possible speed* that moves the cup or brush against the tooth without stalling. Sound also provides a clue for determining whether the cup is rotating too rapidly. A high whine or whistle in the handpiece usually indicates excessive speed. To achieve the lowest possible speed, the rheostat may need to be activated to a high or medium speed and then backed down to a low speed before touching the tooth with the attachment.

The order or sequence of polishing can follow the one outlined for instrumentation in Chapter 5. Positioning of the patient, clinician, and assistant is basically unchanged. The procedure will require adequate evacuation, since the polishing agent and the mechanical stimulation usually increase salivary secretions. The tri-syringe can be used to flush the areas with a water stream as each arch segment is completed. At the completion of the procedure, the patient should be encouraged to rinse thoroughly to remove all residual polishing agent. Proximal areas should be flossed.

Inspection for remaining stain should be performed with good intraoral light, compressed air, and the mouth mirror. Final inspection for plaque should be accomplished with a disclosant as described in previous chapters.

Any remaining stain should be removed by the clinician, and plaque should be removed by the patient.

One area that tends to cause frustration is the mandibular anterior lingual area. Frequently a light pink staining will reappear with each disclosing and will not disappear with repeated polishing and brushing. In almost all cases the disclosant is adherent to a thin sheet of calculus, otherwise not visible on the lingual surfaces. Instrumentation with a scaler or curette is necessary to remove it. Then the area can be repolished.

THE ROLE OF POLISHING IN DENTAL HYGIENE CARE

Polishing for stain removal rather than for removing all soft deposits may be a new experience for some patients. Many patients may have learned to treat the professional oral prophylaxis as a cosmetic procedure or as the key to "healthy gums." Accepting a portion of the responsibility may be an unfamiliar role for the patient. Therefore, it is wise to share with the patient the purpose of polishing, the effect of repeated polishing on the teeth, the rate of reformation of plaque on the teeth after polishing, and how the patient can participate in ongoing "prophylaxis" (i.e., *prevention*). This explanation may make it easier for the patient to accept the change and to reinforce the concomitant plaque control messages he/she has been offered throughout care.

ACTIVITIES

1. Go without brushing your teeth in the AM. Rinse your mouth with grape juice (swallow or spit out), and describe how your mouth feels and the appearance of your teeth and deposits. Which deposits do you think are "colored"? How do you think this relates to not brushing after meals and eating colored foods? How can you "feel" the grape juice remaining in your mouth? What do you think is happening with the grape juice and the dental deposits allowed to form overnight? Evaluate the ease of removal of the colored deposits.
2. Examine a series of student partners. If intrinsic stains are found, can you relate this to childhood diseases, medications (antibiotics), fluorides, silicate filing materials, etc.? If extrinsic stains are found, can you relate this to tea, coffee, and/or tobacco consumption; use of poorly abrasive toothpastes; etc.?
3. Polish stain from a partner's teeth using a porte polisher and engine polishing. Compare the results, the effort involved, and your partner's preference.
4. Examine the variety of tips available for use in the porte polisher.
5. Perform routine maintenance on the handpiece and contra-angle to be used for engine polishing.
6. Given a variety of nonfunctioning engine polishers, determine why each is not working and correct the problem.
7. Change a belt on a belt-driven engine.
8. Use the Prophy-Jet to polish a quadrant of teeth heavily laden with stain. Polish a second quadrant with an engine-driven rubber cup. Compare results regarding (1) cleanliness of the teeth, (2) time, (3) patient acceptance, and (4) amount of recurrent stain at the recall visit.
9. Role play an encounter with a patient who wishes to have all of his/her teeth polished regardless of the presence of stain.

REVIEW QUESTIONS

1. Why are dental stains important:
   a. To the patient?
   b. To the dental professional?
2. Define the following stain classifications:
   a. Exogenous
   b. Endogenous
   c. Extrinsic
   d. Intrinsic
3. How is prevention-oriented classification of stains:
   a. Different from the standard textbook classifications?
   b. Similar to the standard textbook classifications?
4. What is the primary importance of the abrasive in toothpaste?

5. Compare abrasives in toothpastes and professional products.
6. What factors affect abrasiveness and polishing?
7. How can frictional heat be minimized during engine polishing?
8. What are six advantages of a porte polisher?
9. What is the primary disadvantage of a porte polisher?
10. What is the primary indication for polishing teeth?
11. How does the Prophy-Jet polish teeth?

REFERENCES

ADA Council on Dental Therapeutics. 1982. Accepted dental therapeutics, ed. 39. Chicago: American Dental Association.

Cooley, R.O. 1976. Resin veneer ends discoloration problem. Dent. Stud. **54**:28.

Corranza, F.A., Jr. 1979. Glickman's clinical periodontology, ed. 5. Philadelphia: W.B. Saunders Co.

Craig, R.G., O'Brien, W.J., and Powers, J.M. 1983. Dental materials: properties and manipulation, ed. 3. St. Louis: The C.V. Mosby Co.

Davis, W.B. 1978. Cleaning, polishing and abrasion of teeth by dental products. Cosmet. Sci. **1**:38.

Gershon, S.D., and Pader, M. 1972. Dentrifices. In Balsam, M.S., and Sangarin, E., editors. Cosmetics: sciences and technology, vol. 1. New York: Wiley-Interscience.

Goldstein, R.E. 1976. Esthetics in dentistry. Philadelphia: J.B. Lippincott Co.

Heringer, E. 1976. Bleaching removes some discoloration. Dent. Stud. **54**:31.

Hunter, E.L., et al. 1981. The prophylaxis polish—a review of the literature. Dent. Hyg. **55**(9):36.

Lobene, R.R. 1968. Effect of dentrifices on tooth stains with controlled brushing. J. Am. Dent. Assoc. **77**:849.

Manly, R.S. 1943. A structureless recurrent deposit on teeth. J. Dent. Res. **22**:479.

Mellberg, J.R. 1977. Enamel fluoride and its anti-caries effects. J. Prevent. Dent. **4**:8.

Moffitt, J.M., et al. 1974. Prediction of tetracycline-induced tooth discoloration. J. Am. Dent. Assoc. **88**:547.

Ness, L., Rosekrans, D. de L., and Welford, J.F. 1977. An epidemiologic study of factors affecting extrinsic staining of teeth in an English population. Community Dent. Oral Epidemiol. **5**:55.

O'Brien, W.J., and Ryge, G. 1978. An outline of dental materials and their selection. Philadelphia: W.B. Saunders Co.

Primosch, R.E. 1980. Rubber cup prophylaxis: a reevaluation of its use in pediatric dental patients. Dent. Hyg. **54**:525.

Rall, D. 1977. From the NIH: research findings of potential value to the practitioner. JAMA **237**:635.

Reid, J.S., Beeley, J.A., and MacDonald, D.G. 1977. Investigations into black extrinsic tooth stain. J. Dent. Res. **56**:895.

Retief, D.H., et al. 1980. In vitro fluoride uptake distribution and retention by human enamel after 1- and 24-hour application of various topical fluoride agents. J. Dent. Res. **59**:573.

Rohleder, P.V., and Slim, L.H. 1981. Alternatives to rubber cup polishing. Dent. Hyg. **55**(9):16.

Saxton, C.A. 1976. The effects of dentrifices on the appearance of the tooth surface observed with the scanning electron microscope. J. Periodont. Res. **11**:74.

Shaw, L., and Murray, J.J. 1977. A new index for measuring extrinsic stain in clinical trials. Community Dent. Epidemiol. **5**:116.

Shern, R.J., et al. 1977. Enamel biopsy results of children receiving fluoride tablets. J. Am. Dent. Assoc. **95**:310.

Solheim, H., Eriksen, H.M., and Nordbo, H. 1980. Chemical plaque control and extrinsic discoloration of teeth. Acta. Odontol. Scand. **38**:303.

Spencer, D.E. 1972. A conservative method of treating tetracycline stained teeth. J. Dent. Child. **39**:443.

Steele, R.C., et al. 1982. The effect of tooth cleaning procedures on fluoride uptake in enamel. Pediatr. Dent. **4**:228.

Stookey, G.K., and Schemehorn, B.R. 1976. Studies evaluating a fluoride-containing prophylactic cup. Dent. Hyg. **50**:253.

Stookey, G.K., and Stahlman, D.B. 1976. Enhanced fluoride uptake in enamel with a fluoride-impregnated prophylactic cup. J. Dent. Res. **55**:333.

Stuart, R. 1975. Treatment of anterior teeth for aesthetic problems. Quintessence Int. **6**(6):31.

Swan, R.W. 1979. Dimensional changes in a tooth root incident to various polishing and root planing procedures. Dent. Hyg. **53**(1):17.

Thompson, R.E., and Way, D.C. 1981. Enamel loss due to prophylaxis and multiple bonding/debonding of orthodontic attachments. Am. J. Orthod. **79**:282.

Tinanoff, N., et al. 1974. Effect of a pumice prophylaxis on fluoride uptake in tooth enamel. J. Am. Dent. Assoc. **88**:384.

Vogel, R.I. 1975. Intrinsic and extrinsic discoloration of the dentition (a literature review). J. Oral Med. **30**(4):99.

Waring, M.B., et al. 1982. A comparison of engine polishing and toothbrushing in minimizing dental plaque reaccumulation. Dent. Hyg. **56**(12):25.

Willman, D.E., et al. 1980. A new prophylaxis instrument: effect on enamel alterations. J. Am. Dent. Assoc. **101**:923.

Winter, G.B., Murray, J.J., and Shaw, L. 1978. Cosmetics and dental history. Cosmet. Sci. **1**:1.

Yankell, S., and Emling, R.C. 1978. Understanding dental products: what you should know and what your patient should know. Continuing Dental Education, University of Pennsylvania School of Dental Medicine **1**:No. 7.

Yankell, S.L., et al. 1982. Effects of chlorhexidine and four antimicrobial compounds on plaque, gingivitis, and staining in beagle dogs. J. Dent. Res. **61**:1089.

27 CARE OF REMOVABLE DENTAL APPLIANCES

OBJECTIVES: *The reader will be able to*

1. Articulate a rationale for cleaning removable dental appliances.
2. Explain to patients why cleaning removable appliances is necessary.
3. Describe the commercial and noncommercial agents available for cleaning dentures.
4. Describe the method for cleaning the following removable appliances:
   a. Full denture
   b. Overdenture
   c. Partial denture
   d. Orthodontic appliance
5. Instruct patients on how to properly clean removable appliances.

Throughout this book the patient as a partner in care has been emphasized. Once again, the importance of entrusting the patient as a partner is essential in order to prepare the patient to properly care for removable appliances at home. Care of several appliances—full dentures, partial dentures, overdentures, and orthodontic appliances—is discussed in this chapter. Some of these appliances replace some or all of the patient's teeth, and care for them may be another procedure in addition to daily brushing and flossing. The full dentures replace all of the patient's teeth, so care of natural teeth is not a concern. Care of the patient's gingival and other soft tissues is still a concern. Patients with partial dentures, overdentures, and orthodontic appliances must care for natural teeth, their soft tissues, and the appliance. Thus patient motivation is a primary concern, just as it was in Chapter 17; the principles learned in that chapter should be applied when teaching a patient to care for a removable appliance.

When teaching a patient to care for the appliance, the clinician must be sensitive to the patient's emotional reactions to removing the appliance. For example, some patients will not remove dentures if they will be seen by someone. Such a patient may need some reassurance regarding the clinician's reaction to seeing the patient without the denture. Ultimately, the patient must realize that removal and cleaning of the denture is essential to his/her well-being.

RATIONALE FOR CLEANING REMOVABLE APPLIANCES

Just as plaque accumulates on natural teeth, it accumulates on appliances. The plaque is referred to as *denture plaque*. The plaque is irritating to the soft tissues. In addition, materia alba and food debris collect on the appliances and must be removed.

Oral lesions have been associated with removable appliances, primarily denture stomatitis and *Candida albicans* infections (Budtz-Jorgensen, 1978, 1981; Budtz-Jorgensen and Bertram, 1970). *Denture stomatitis* is the term used to describe the red, inflamed mucous membrane under the appliance. *C. albicans* seems to be the primary factor in denture stomatitis. Cleaning the denture reduces the *C. albicans* and lessens the denture stomatitis.

Lesions have also been associated with allergic reactions and trauma from the denture (Budtz-Jorgensen, 1981). Allergic reactions are rare, but the clinician should be aware of the possibility. Trauma from an ill-fitting denture is rather common. The patient's tissues should be inspected for traumatic ulcers, and the patient encouraged to seek professional care to modify the appliance. Sometimes patients try to repair dentures or other appliances at home; such procedures should be discouraged.

CLEANING FULL DENTURES

A set of full dentures is shown in Fig. 27-1. The dentures are made of an acrylic base and usually acrylic teeth. There are no metal components in a full denture. A full denture replaces all of the teeth in an arch, so the patient has no natural teeth in that arch. A patient will have either an upper or a lower denture or both.

There are several methods and agents available to clean full dentures. Dentures can be cleaned by mechanical or chemical means (Budtz-Jorgensen, 1979). The various methods are described below.

The *mechanical methods* of cleaning dentures include a brush, pastes and powders, and ultrasonic agitation. The most common method of cleaning a denture is with a brush and either soap or toothpaste. This is an effective means of cleaning the denture, but overly vigorous cleaners can wear away the acrylic. If too much pressure is applied while brushing the denture over a long period of time, the acrylic will be damaged (Budtz-Jorgensen, 1979). Pastes and powders such as regular toothpaste increase the wear on the acrylic because of the abrasive agents contained in the materials. Thus the use of such highly abrasive agents is not recommended.

Ultrasonic agitation of dentures in a disinfectant solution decreases the amount of microorganisms present on the dentures (Butz-Jorgensen, 1979). However, ultrasonic agitation is not very effective in removing stains. Ultrasonic cleaners are used most often in dental offices, rather than by denture wearers in their homes.

The *chemical denture cleaners* available are oxidizing-type cleaners, acids, or enzymes (ADA Council, 1983; Budtz-Jorgensen, 1979). These agents are commercially produced.

The *oxidizing-type cleaners* are either hypochlorites or peroxides and monopersulfates (ADA Council, 1983). The *hypochlorites* dissolve the organic matrix that calculus forms on. The denture is soaked in the agents; then the calcium phosphate is rinsed or washed away. These agents are corrosive to metal, which is not a concern with full dentures but is with partial dentures. These agents will remove some stains but not all of them. The *peroxides and monopersulfates* are supplied as either powders or tablets to which water is added. These are oxidizing agents containing peroxide, and they remove some stains, materia alba, and plaque (ADA Council, 1983). It is believed that they have an antibacterial effect, reducing the chances of denture stomatitis. These agents may whiten the plastic. Although they remove some stain, they do not remove all the stain.

A   B

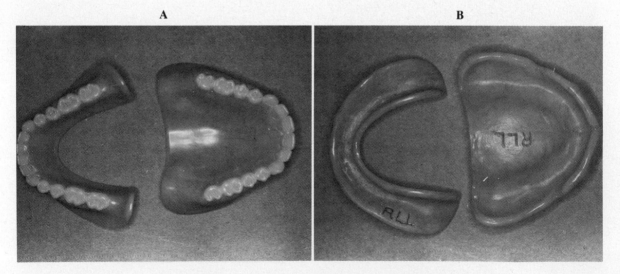

Fig. 27-1. Full dentures. **A,** Tooth surface. **B,** Soft tissue surface.

Dilute acids, such as 3% to 5% hydrochloric acid, are available (ADA Council, 1983). These are dilute acids, but they can stain clothes and cause damage to metal components. These agents dissolve the calcium phosphate present on the denture. Hydrochloric acids are available for professional use with ultrasonic cleaners, but they are of a higher concentration, such as 30%.

Enzymes used for cleaning dentures contain protease and mutase and work by breaking down the proteins and polysaccharides in the denture plaque (ADA Council, 1983). These are not very effective in stain removal.

EVALUATING THE EFFECTIVENESS OF DENTURE CLEANERS

The effectiveness of the cleaners is somewhat difficult to establish because the agents are commercially produced and have not been compared with each other in many studies. The American Dental Association (ADA Council, 1983) recently published a report in which they concluded that plaque ". . . could not be effectively removed by most of the commercial products, and no product tested was able to consistently remove mature plaque." The manufacturer's recommended soaking time is usually about 15 minutes, during which time the plaque cannot be soaked off the denture. This finding is contrary to most of the advertised claims. However, the agents do provide some cleaning if used for longer periods of time.

The denture cleaners are fairly safe, but they can cause eye irritation or be dangerous if ingested by children. Thus it is important to advise patients to keep the agents out of the reach of children and to read the labels carefully.

DENTURE CLEANING RECOMMENDATIONS

Mechanical brushing of the denture (Fig. 27-2) with a mild abrasive paste, powder, or soap is the most effective means of cleaning a denture (Budtz-Jorgensen, 1979). A denture brush can be used, and the patient should be advised to brush all areas of the denture. The surface closest to the tissue as well as the tooth-bearing surfaces should be brushed.

If the patient prefers, a chemical agent can be used. The daily, overnight soaking in a commercially available peroxide solution is recommended (Budtz-Jorgensen, 1979). A 15- to 30-minute soaking will not be sufficient. Daily, overnight soaking in the hypochlorite cleaners is not recommended because of the bleaching effect.

A   **B**

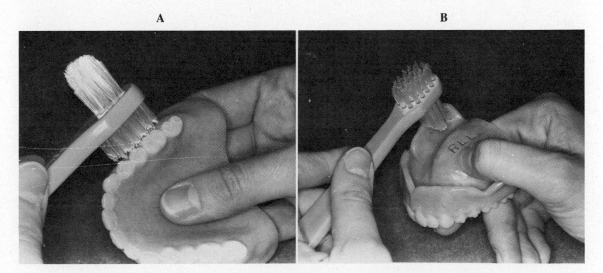

Fig. 27-2. Mechanical brushing of full denture. **A,** Teeth are brushed with large brush of a denture brush, and, **B,** inner surface is brushed with small rounded brush. It is suggested that this be done over a sink partially filled with water to cushion impact if denture is dropped.

Further instructions to the patient should include a soft tissue self-examination and to keep the denture out of the mouth at least several hours a day. Keeping the dentures out overnight is suggested (McDermott et al., 1981). Removal of the dentures has been shown to reduce denture stomatitis.

In addition to the commercially available cleaners, a solution of 1 tablespoon of Clorox and 1 tablespoon of Calgonite can be used for an *occasional* 15-minute soak (McDermott et al., 1981). This is a strong solution. It should not be used with metal-containing appliances and should be used sparingly with full dentures because of its bleaching effect.

Stains and calculus on dentures should be professionally removed with hand or mechanical scaling devices.

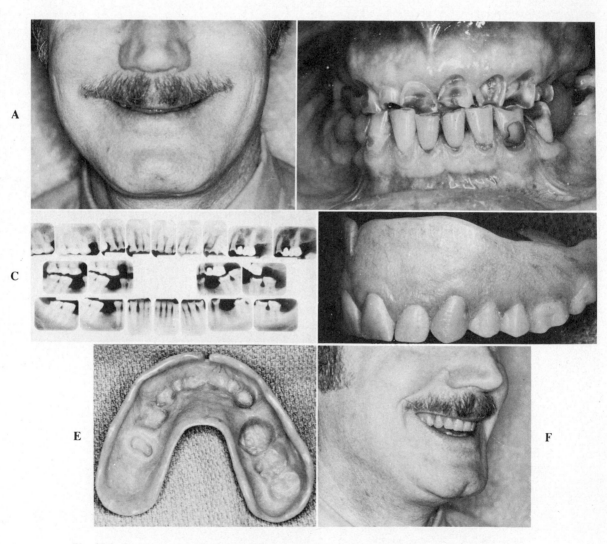

Fig. 27-3. Overdenture. **A,** Patient is shown. **B,** Patient's teeth are eroded. **C,** Radiographic series of the patient's teeth. **D,** View of tooth surface of overdenture. **E,** Inner surface of denture with indentations for natural teeth. **F,** Patient with denture inserted. (From Brewer, A.A. and Morrow, R.M. 1980. Overdentures. St. Louis: The C.V. Mosby Co.)

CLEANING OVERDENTURES

An overdenture is pictured in Fig. 27-3. Overdentures differ from full dentures in that there are natural teeth present in the person's mouth and the denture fits over them. Overdentures must be cleaned like full dentures, with an addition. The indentations for natural teeth must be cleaned thoroughly. The indentations can be cleaned with a cotton-tipped applicator.

In addition to cleaning the dentures, these patients must also receive instructions on how to care for their natural teeth. The maintenance of the natural teeth is essential to the retention of the overdenture.

CLEANING PARTIAL DENTURES

Partial dentures should not be soaked in commercially available agents or in a solution of Clorox and Calgonite. A partial denture is shown in Fig. 27-4. Partial dentures are characterized by having metal brackets that fit around the natural teeth. These metal components can be damaged by the above-mentioned agents.

Cleaning partial dentures is done by mechanical brushing with a lowly abrasive paste or powder.

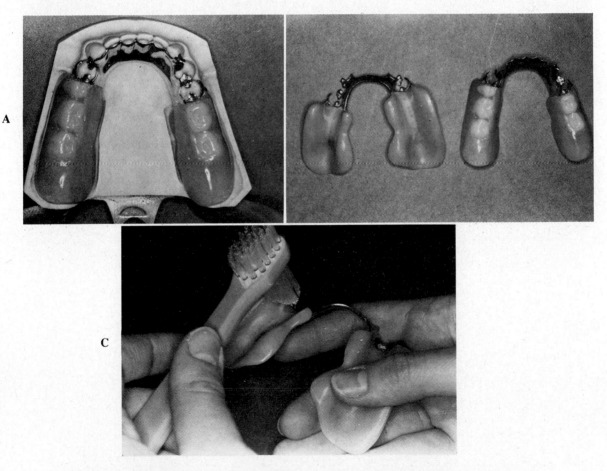

Fig. 27-4. Partial denture. **A,** Partial denture on typodont model. **B,** Partial denture, teeth and soft tissue sides. **C,** Cleaning soft tissue side with a denture brush.

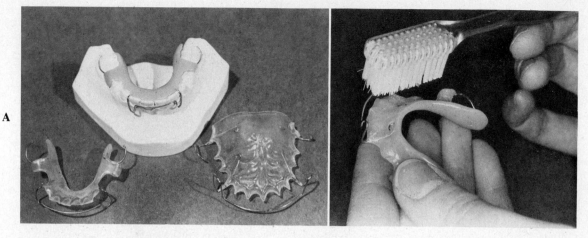

A

B

Fig. 27-5. Orthodontic Hawley appliance. **A,** Appliance placed on model and on table surface. **B,** Brushing appliance with a toothbrush.

CLEANING ORTHODONTIC APPLIANCES

A removable orthodontic Hawley appliance is shown in Fig. 27-5. This type of appliance is usually used after orthodontic treatment to maintain the teeth in their new positions. It is also sometimes used for minor tooth movement. The appliance is composed of shaped pieces of wire imbedded into acrylic. Since the appliance has metal wire, it cannot be soaked in commercial agents or in Clorox and Calgonite. The preferred method of cleaning the appliances is with a toothbrush and toothpaste.

Usually persons wearing orthodontic appliances are young persons in their teenage years. Again, it is important to instruct these patients in care of their natural dentitions.

SUMMARY

Cleaning removable appliances is an important part of routine home care procedures. Just as plaque accumulates on the natural teeth, it also accumulates on the appliances and must be removed.

SUGGESTED ACTIVITIES

1. Secure full and partial dentures from a dental laboratory and practice cleaning them.
2. Review the most recent American Dental Association catalog and send for a complimentary copy of any pamphlet pertaining to care of removable appliances.
3. Read the labels of several commercially available cleaning agents to determine their types.

4. Full dentures, particularly those worn by persons living in a community setting such as a nursing home, should be marked with the individuals' names (Pierce and Olsen, 1981; Woodward, 1979). Arrange for a demonstration of how to mark dentures.

REVIEW QUESTIONS

1. State the rationale for cleaning removable appliances.
2. Describe how to clean a full denture, overdenture, and orthodontic appliance.
3. A patient asks if soaking her denture in a commercially available agent is enough. How do you respond?

REFERENCES

ADA Council on Dental Materials, Instruments, and Equipment. 1983. Denture cleansers. J. Am. Dent. Assoc. **106:**77.

American Dental Association. 1981. Dentists' desk reference: materials, instruments, and equipment. Chicago: American Dental Association.

Brewer, A.A., and Morrow, R.M. 1980. Overdentures. St. Louis: The C.V. Mosby Co.

Budtz-Jorgensen, E. 1978. Clinical aspects of Candida infection in denture wearers. J. Am. Dent. Assoc. **96:**474.

Budtz-Jorgensen, E. 1979. Materials and methods for cleaning dentures. J. Prosthet. Dent. **42:**619.

Budtz-Jorgensen, E. 1981. Oral mucosal lesions associated with the wearing of removable dentures. J. Oral Pathol. **10:**65.

Budtz-Jorgensen, E., and Bertram, U. 1970. Denture stomatitis. Acta Odontol. Scand. **28:**71.

McDermott, I.G., et al. 1981. Suggestions to patients: learning to wear and care for new dentures. Iowa Dent. J. **67:**39.

Pierce, S.F., and Olsan, K.E. 1981. Denture identification for nursing home patients. Ill. Dent. J. **50:**243.

Woodward, J.D. 1979. Denture marking for identification. J. Am. Dent. Assoc. **99:**59.

28 THE ROLE OF OCCLUSION IN DENTAL HEALTH AND DISEASE

OBJECTIVES: *The reader will be able to*

1. Discuss the three approaches to the study of occlusion.
2. Describe Angle's classification system.
3. Define overbite and overjet and demonstrate how to measure each one.
4. Explain why it is important to examine the occlusion of a child with primary or mixed dentition.
5. Define the following terms:
   a. Occlusal trauma
   b. Occlusal traumatism
   c. Primary occlusal trauma
   d. Secondary occlusal trauma
   e. Centric stops
   f. Centric relation
   g. Centric occlusion
   h. Lateral and protrusive excursions
   i. Working and nonworking interferences
6. Recognize the differences between periodontitis and occlusal traumatism.
7. List, recognize, and record etiologic factors of occlusal trauma.
8. List, recognize, and record the subjective, clinical and radiographic signs and symptoms of occlusal trauma.
9. Complete an occlusal screening for a partner.

The study of occlusion requires the student to examine the tooth anatomy, supporting structures, temporomandibular joint (TMJ), muscles of mastication, and blood and nerve supply to those areas. Many common complaints such as headaches, sore muscles, toothaches, and sensitivity to temperature changes can be traced to occlusal or TMJ problems.

Occlusion is important throughout the patient's life. Even a newborn has an occlusal relationship. When the infant closes his/her mouth, occlusion is obtained by placing the tongue between the maxillary and mandibular gum pads (Borell, 1980). From infancy onward, the patient's occlusion is important to necessary functions such as suckling, swallowing, chewing, speaking, and even smiling. The patient's occlusion contributes to oral health and disease.

It is no wonder that occlusal relationships are important in each dental specialty: pedodontics,

orthodontics, periodontics, prosthodontics, restorations, oral surgery, and endodontics. Pedodontists examine children's occlusion and growth patterns. If a primary tooth is lost prematurely, the pedodontist will recommend placement of a space maintainer to preserve the needed room for the succeeding permanent tooth. Through such use of space maintainers (see Fig. 27-5), normal occlusal relationships are encouraged. Pedodontists and orthodontists evaluate the growing child's occlusion. Pedodontists examine children's occlusions during their development to detect early signs of malocclusions. If a malocclusion is detected early, treatment may be possible with a minimal amount of therapy. More severe malocclusions must be treated by orthodontists who have additional education in this area. Periodontists are interested in occlusion because some patients' occlusions can exacerbate the damage to supporting structures of the teeth,

483

which complicates periodontal treatment. Dentists performing prosthetic and restorative dentistry are concerned with occlusion, since each restoration placed in a patient's mouth will affect the patient's occlusion in either a positive or negative manner. Prosthodontists are especially concerned with occlusion, since they replace missing teeth and must reproduce occlusal relationships. For example, a prosthodontist making full maxillary and mandibular dentures must recreate occlusal relationships that are compatible with the patient's TMJ and neuromusculature and ensure the patient's comfort and function. Oral surgeons are particularly aware of occlusion when performing facial reconstruction procedures. Endodontists are concerned with occlusion because an endodontically involved tooth can be adversely affected by occlusal trauma (Stallard, 1968).

With the increasing responsibilities of dental hygienists in all of the specialties, the hygienists' awareness and knowledge of occlusion must also increase. The hygienist performing advanced periodontal skills should have an understanding of the possible effects a patient's occlusion may have on the periodontal treatment provided. A hygienist performing restorative or prosthetic procedures should understand how the restorations he/she placed may affect the patient's occlusion.

The purpose of this chapter is to provide the dental hygiene student with some basic information about occlusion and some methods for detecting occlusal conditions that may be problematic for some patients. The primary role of the dental hygienist in the area of occlusion is to detect potential or current occlusal problems and to alert the supervising dentist to those findings.

APPROACHES TO OCCLUSION

The study of occlusion can be confusing because it is complex and there are various approaches to its study. Presently, there are three commonly accepted approaches to the study of occlusion and treatment of occlusal problems: the prosthetic concept, the orthodontic concept, and the concept of dynamic individual occlusion (Mosteller, 1980; Ramfjord and Ash, 1971). Each of these approaches, or concepts of occlusion, has a particular set of understandings to guide occlusal treatment.

The *prosthetic concept* of balanced occlusion was developed to guide the construction of full dentures. The word *balanced* is very crucial to this approach. The underlying principle is that the occlusion should be balanced: there should be simultaneous, bilateral contact of the teeth during mandibular lateral and protrusive movements. This balance is necessary to prevent full dentures from tilting or becoming dislodged. The prosthetic approach is applicable to persons with full dentures, rather than to persons with natural dentitions (Mosteller, 1980; Ramfjord and Ash, 1971; Weisgold, 1975).

The *orthodontic concept* of occlusion is most concerned with tooth-to-tooth, particularly the cusp-to-fossa, relationships between the teeth. Angle's classification and the positions of supporting cusps, discussed later in this chapter, are elements of the orthodontic concept. When orthodontia is performed, teeth are moved to approximate pre-established concepts of ideal occlusal relationships, such as a Class I molar relationship (Mosteller, 1980; Perry, 1976; Ramfjord and Ash, 1971). The issue of orthodontists being overly concerned with cusp-to-fossa relationships, without enough regard for the neuromuscular and vascular components of occlusion and the TMJ, has been raised (Perry, 1976).

The concept of *dynamic individual occlusion*, as reflected by its name, considers each person's particular occlusion and recognizes that the systems affecting occlusion are in a continual state of flux. Dynamic individual occlusion considers all factors, such as the neuromusculature and vascular systems associated with the TMJ and occlusion; stress and other psychologic conditions; tooth-to-tooth relationships; and other oral conditions such as restorative, periodontal, and endodontic health (Mosteller, 1980; Ramfjord and Ash, 1971).

In general, the approach to occlusion presented in this chapter follows the dynamic individual concept of occlusion. The discussion of the relationship between occlusal and periodontal health, the occlusal screening, and the occlusal analysis are all drawn from this approach. In fact, an occlusal screening and analysis are the beginning steps in the approach, namely to evaluate the person's individual and dynamic occlusion. Elements of the orthodontic approach such as Angle's classification, overjet, overbite, and positions of supporting cusps are presented because they are widely accepted and used measures of occlusion.

ANGLE'S CLASSIFICATION: IDEAL OCCLUSION

In 1899 Dr. E.H. Angle proposed a classification system of malocclusion that was designed to help identify occlusions that needed treatment (Jago, 1974). Angle's classification evaluates the mesiodistal relationship between the first molars (Thurow, 1977). Currently, practitioners evaluate the cuspid relationship as well. There are three classifications in this system—I, II, and III—and Class II is subdivided into division 1 and division 2. (See Figs. 28-1 to 28-3 for a description of the classifications.) According to this classification, only Class I is the ideal occlusion, and any other type of occlusion is considered a malocclusion or a "bad" occlusion that could require treatment to become normal. The terms *occlusion* and *malocclusion* are used synonymously for Class II, division 1; Class II, division 2; and Class III. So a Class III occlusion may be the same as a Class III malocclusion. The terms can also be used synonymously, although they usually are not, for Class I. It is possible for a patient to exhibit ideal first molar and cuspid relationship and to have crowded anterior teeth. Many practitioners would call that type of condition a *Class I malocclusion,* although calling it *Class I occlusion with anterior crowding* would also be acceptable.

It becomes obvious from the example given that Angle's classification has a limited meaning, since it uses information about only a few teeth to determine the type of occlusion for the entire dentition. The meaning of Angle's classification is further clouded by the clinician's subjectivity (Jago, 1974). If the first molars are more than half a cusp from the ideal Class I, the occlusion is considered a Class II or III. Practitioners vary in their interpretation of *half a cusp.* Several dental personnel, especially orthodontists, have tried to develop new classification systems to overcome the shortcomings of Angle's system. However, none of the other systems has received the universal acceptance of Angle's classification (Thurow, 1977). Hence, in spite of its shortcoming, Angle's classification is used by practitioners throughout dentistry because it is a widely accepted, efficient system. However, a more precise and descriptive system may be developed in the future.

Angle's classification can also be used to evaluate the molar relationship in the primary and mixed dentition. The primary second molars are used to determine the relationship in the primary dentition and in the mixed dentition until the permanent first molars are sufficiently erupted.

During the clinical examination, Angle's classification should be noted and the patient's overjet and overbite should be measured with a periodontal probe.

The *overjet* is the distance between the labial or lingual surface of the maxillary incisors and the facial surface of the lower incisors (Thurow, 1977). The overjet is measured while the patient's teeth are fully occluded. The probe is placed perpendicular to the long axis of the teeth with the point against the facial surface of the lower incisor and the side resting against the incisal edge of the maxillary incisor. The amount of overjet is the measure from the facial surface of the lower incisor to the labial or lingual surface of the maxillary incisor, depending on the particular clinic's or office's preference. If the measurement is to the labial surface of the maxillary incisor, the labiolingual width of the incisal edge is included; it would seem that measuring to the lingual surface would provide a more meaningful measure. It is important to be aware of which method is being used (Fig. 28-4, *A*).

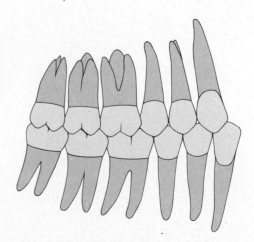

Fig. 28-1. Class I occlusal relationship. Mesiobuccal cusp of maxillary molar aligns with buccal groove of mandibular molar; maxillary cuspid rests between mandibular cuspid and first premolar. (From Thurow, R.C. 1977. Atlas of orthodontic principles, ed. 2. St. Louis: The C.V. Mosby Co.)

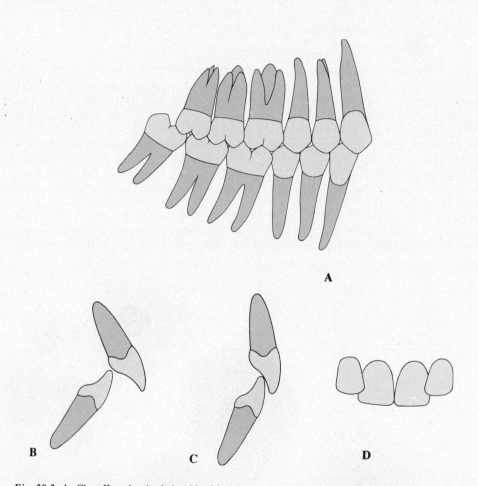

A

B   **C**   **D**

***Fig. 28-2.* A,** Class II occlusal relationship. Mesiobuccal cusp and maxillary cuspid are mesial to mandibular landmarks. **B,** Class II, division 1. Anterior teeth are flared. **C** and **D,** Class II, division 2. Anterior central teeth are verted lingually. (From Thurow, R.C. 1977. Atlas of orthodontic principles, ed. 2. St. Louis: The C.V. Mosby Co.)

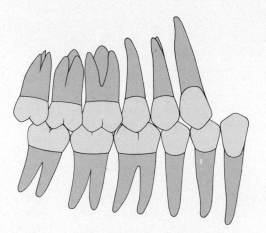

Fig. 28-3. Class III occlusal relationship. Mesiobuccal cusp and maxillary cuspid are distal to mandibular landmarks. (From Thurow, R.C. 1977. Atlas or orthodontic principles, ed. 2. St. Louis: The C.V. Mosby Co.)

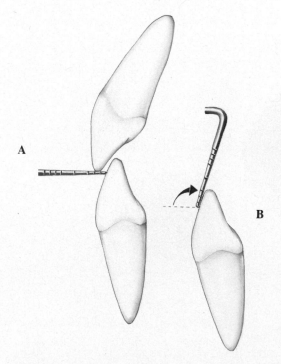

Fig. 28-4. **A,** Overjet is measured. **B,** Overbite is measured.

The *overbite* is the amount that the maxillary anterior teeth overlap the mandibular anterior teeth in a vertical plane (Thurow, 1977). If a patient has an edge-to-edge relationship between the maxillary and mandibular teeth, the amount of overbite is 0 mm. Usually the overbite is 2 to 3 mm. In a severe overbite the incisal edge of the mandibular teeth may occlude with the soft tissue of the hard palate. The overbite is measured in two steps. First, the probe is placed as if the overjet were being measured. Then the probe is held in that position as the patient slowly opens the mouth. When the patient's mouth is open, the probe is placed upright. The distance from the tip of the probe to the incisal edge of the lower anterior tooth is the amount of overbite (Fig. 28-4, *B*). If the teeth are out of alignment, the overjet and overbite may vary; more than one measurement may be taken and recorded.

An alternative method for measuring an overbite involves placing a pencil, instead of the probe, against the tooth. A pencil mark is made, the pencil is removed, and the patient is asked to open his/her mouth. Then the clinician can measure the amount of overbite by placing the probe upright against the mandibular tooth with the point at the level of the pencilmark.

Overjets and overbites are measured the same way for the primary and mixed dentitions. Severe overbite are more common in the primary dentition than in the permanent dentition.

DEVELOPMENT OF OCCLUSION

As mentioned earlier in the chapter, even the infant has an occlusal relationship. From the start of life until its end, occlusion is important to people's well-being. This section briefly describes the development of occlusion from birth through the primary, mixed, and permanent dentitions. The characteristic occlusal relationships during each of these periods are discussed. However, several influences on the development of occlusion must be mentioned and kept in mind. The influences are biologic, anatomic, physiologic, pathologic, and environmental (Levine and Pulver, 1979).

Biologically, jaw size, tooth size, and the pattern of growth are believed to be inherited. Thus the development of a person's occlusion will be affected by his/her genetic endowment. The development is not solely determined by genetics, though; environmental and other factors play an important role (Levine and Pulver, 1979).

Anatomic influences include the craniofacial, vascular, muscular, neural, and endocrine structures and systems of the person. In particular, the systems composing the head, neck, face, and TMJ are of concern.

The *physiologic* influences include differential growth patterns and recognition that chronologic and physiologic ages do not always coincide. Differential growth is a concern in evaluating the development, because the maxilla and mandible grow at different rates. Thus at birth it is normal for a child to have a retrognathic mandible because its growth is slower in utero. The coincidence of chronologic and physiologic age is to be considered in evaluating eruption of the teeth. The eruption charts have estimated a physiologic process—tooth eruption—which varies for each person according to chronologic age. So, even though permanent first molars are "6-year" molars, very few children's molars erupt on schedule. Thus it is necessary to consider the child's overall physiologic development when assessing occlusal development (Levine and Pulver, 1979).

Pathologic influences include physical and developmental disabilities or abnormalities that may interrupt, accelerate, or delay a person's growth and development. These can range from very minor problems such as a congenitally missing tooth to more complex problems such as a cleft lip and palate. Both of these problems would affect the person's occlusion, but to much different extents (Levine and Pulver, 1979).

The final influence is *environmental*, which includes such factors as habits, carious lesions, traumatic injuries, iatrogenic dental treatment, and systemic disease. Habits such as finger or thumb sucking, improper swallowing, mouth breathing, bruxism, or tongue thrusting can affect the alignment of the teeth and growth of the jaws. Carious lesions, if left untreated, can cause tooth breakdown, which in turn can encourage tooth migration and loss of adequate space for the succeeding teeth. In the permanent dentition the teeth can drift and tilt, which would contribute to abnormally directed forces on the teeth. Traumatic injuries can cause tooth fracture or loss with sequelae similar to those of carious lesions. Iatrogenic dentistry, improperly placed restorations, or never-placed space main-

tainers, can damage or interfere with the occlusion. Finally, systemic diseases can retard the growth and development of the jaws, teeth, or the entire skeletal system (Levine and Pulver, 1979).

In summary, these influences should be considered in assessing a child's or adult's occlusion. Once again, the importance of a thorough medical history in order to fully understand a patient's condition is evident.

Primary dentition and occlusion

By the time the child is 2½ years old, a full set of primary teeth should be erupted. The teeth usually begin to erupt from the age of 4 to 6 months, and a deep overbite and overjet are common (Borell, 1980). The deep overbite and overjet are due to the slower growth rate of the mandible. The growth of the mandible should be sufficient, by the time the primary second molars erupt, that the overbite and overjet can approximate normal ranges. If not, the Class II molar relationship, if present, is likely to persist into the permanent dentition (Borell, 1980). The characteristics of the primary dentition include spaces between the teeth, upright teeth, and either a straight or mesial-step terminal plane between the opposing second molars (Borell, 1980; McDonald and Avery, 1983). Fig. 28-5 illustrates the difference between a straight and a

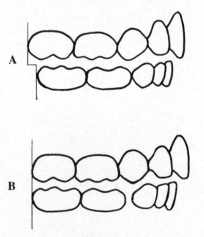

Fig. 28-5. Terminal plane is relationship between distal surfaces of maxillary and mandibular primary second molars. **A,** Mesial-step terminal plane: mandibular molar is mesial to maxillary molar. **B,** Straight terminal plane: molars are even. (From McDonald, R.E., and Avery, D.A. 1983. Dentistry for the child and adolescent. St. Louis: The C.V. Mosby Co.)

mesial-step terminal plane. The planes are important because the permanent first molars are guided into position by the distal surfaces of the second primary molars. The configuration of the plane, in conjunction with the presence or absence of the primate space, the space between the primary cuspids and the first molars, influences the likelihood of the development of a Class I molar relationship in the permanent dentition (Borell, 1980; McDonald and Avery, 1983). The development of a Class I relationship is possible with any combination of terminal plane and absence or presence of the primate space, but it is most likely if there is a mesial-step plane and a primate space (McDonald and Avery, 1983).

Mixed dentition and occlusion

The mixed dentition is characterized by the presence of both primary and secondary teeth. Permanent teeth are either *successional* (replacements for primary teeth) or *accessional* (new additions to the posterior portions of the dental arches) (Borell, 1980). The age span of the mixed dentition is usually 6 to 12 years. This period of time during the mixed dentition is of great importance to the development of normal occlusion. It is important for children to have their dentitions and occlusions evaluated and steps taken to enhance normal development. Eruption patterns should be assessed by the dentist and timely extraction of primary teeth performed. Evaluation of the *leeway space*, the sum of the mesiodistal widths of primary teeth from the cuspid to the second molar, should be done. The leeway space is usually wider than the widths of the successional teeth, and the maxillary leeway space is greater than the mandibular space. This enhances the development of a normal molar relationship in the permanent dentition (Borell, 1980).

The path of closure, lateral, and protrusive movements of the mandible should also be evaluated. These characteristic movements of the mandible are likely to continue into the permanent dentition. If problems or interferences are present in the mixed dentition, it is important that they be detected and treated (Borell, 1980). Evaluation of the path of closure and movements of the mandible were described in the section on occlusal analysis.

Permanent dentition and occlusion

By the time a person has reached the age of 12, the permanent dentition, excluding the third mo-

lars, is usually present. In a normal permanent dentition there are usually no interproximal spaces; there are axial tilts to the teeth to foster a trituration chewing stroke (Borell, 1980); and there is a Class I molar relationship. It can be emphasized again that "normal" does not equal "ideal" as far as occlusion is concerned. The previous description of normal is close to ideal, but there is a wide range of normal. One of the purposes of performing occlusal screenings and analyses is to determine if a particular patient's occlusion can be considered normal (i.e., not causing damage to the supporting structures). Many practitioners refer to an occlusion that is not causing harm, but is not ideal, as being a physiologic occlusion.

As part of the discussion of the permanent dentition, it is necessary to define some terminology, including centric occlusion, centric relation, lateral and protrusive excursions, working and nonworking sides, interferences, and, finally, to describe in greater detail the cusp-to-fossa relationships.

Centric occlusion, or maximum intercuspation, is the position of the mandible that is guided by the teeth (Ramfjord and Ash, 1971). Centric occlusion is the position assumed when a person is asked to close his/her mouth "as usual"; it is the position of the mandible during the last stages of chewing and swallowing. During centric occlusion the teeth have a characteristic pattern of occlusion. The *supporting cusps,* the buccal cusps of the mandibular posterior teeth and the lingual cusps of the maxillary posterior teeth, occlude with either the opposing marginal ridges or fossae. These cusp tips, marginal ridges, and fossae are referred to as *centric stops* (Ramfjord and Ash, 1971). Table 28-1 lists the centric stops. In order to visualize the relationships among the centric stops, the reader is encouraged to look at a set of study models of a normal occlusion while studying the table.

Centric relation is the most retruded position of the mandible (i.e., of the condyles) (Mostellar, 1980; Ramfjord and Ash, 1971). It is guided by ligaments and the structure of the condyles, articular disks, and glenoid fossae. Since centric relation is guided by anatomic structures other than the teeth, it is said to be a reproducible relationship between the jaws. Centric relation is used to determine the occlusion when full dentures are constructed. For most persons with natural dentitions, centric relation and centric occlusion are not the

Table 28-1. Centric stops during centric occlusion

Supporting cusps	Contact with	Fossae or marginal ridges
Maxillary lingual cusps		**Mandibular ridges or fossae**
Lingual cusps of premolars		Marginal ridges of second premolar and first molar
Mesiolingual cusps of molars		Central fossae of mandibular molars
Distolingual cusps of molars		Marginal ridges of mandibular molars
Mandibular incisal edges and buccal cusps		**Maxillary ridges or fossae**
Incisal edges		Lingual fossae of incisors
Cusp of canine		Mesial marginal ridge of first premolar
Buccal cusps of premolars		Marginal ridges of premolars
Mesiobuccal cusps of molars		Distal marginal ridge of second premolar and marginal ridges of molars
Distobuccal cusps of molars		Central fossae of maxillary molars

From Ramfjord, S.P., and Ash, M.M. 1971. Occlusion. Philadelphia: W.B. Saunders Co.

same; rather, centric occlusion is about 1 to 2 mm anterior to centric relation (Mostellar, 1980; Ramfjord and Ash, 1971). A discrepancy between centric relation and centric occlusion is noteworthy for the patient's chart, but it does not denote occlusal problems in and of itself (Mostellar, 1980; Ramfjord and Ash, 1971).

Protrusive excursion is the forward movement of the mandible from centric relation or centric occlusion until the anterior teeth are in an edge-to-edge relationship. During a protrusive excursion (i.e., once the anterior teeth are edge to edge, there should be no contact between the posterior teeth (Mosteller, 1980).

Lateral excursion is the movement of the mandible from centric occlusion or centric relation to the right or left until the cuspids on that side are in a cusp-to-cusp relationship. Some persons will not be able to achieve contact between the cuspids only; rather, they will have cusp-to-cusp contact with the premolars or molars as well. When the lateral excursion is done, the teeth on the opposite side, the *nonworking side*, should be out of occlusion. For example, if the patient moves the jaw to the right, he/she has performed a right lateral excursion. The right side is the *working side*, and the left side is the *nonworking* side. If any of the teeth, other than the right cuspids, are occluding, they are called *interferences: working interferences* if on the right side and *nonworking interferences* if on the left side. Nonworking interferences are much more likely to cause destruction to the supporting structures than are working interferences.

In fact, working interferences, if more than one tooth other than the cuspid, are many times beneficial (Mosteller, 1980; Ramfjord and Ash, 1971).

• • •

Thus far in the chapter, the development of normal occlusion has been described and its characteristics discussed. Many of the patients seen have occlusal problems that cause them great pain, discomfort, and tooth loss. The remainder of the chapter addresses occlusal trauma and assessment of occlusion.

TRAUMA FROM OCCLUSION

Ideally, the teeth are well aligned within each arch; contacts are present between adjacent teeth; marginal ridges of adjacent teeth are even; there are no rotated or malposed teeth (Krauss et al., 1969); and the teeth occlude in a Class I relationship (Thurow, 1977). This ideal arrangement of teeth permits the occlusal forces to be directed along the long axis of the teeth and permits forces to be shared by adjacent teeth (Carranza, 1979; Goldman and Cohen, 1980; Krauss et al., 1969; Ramfjord and Ash, 1971; Thurow, 1977). The supporting structures of the teeth—the periodontal ligament, cementum, and bone—accept and absorb the forces directed along the long axis of the tooth. The supporting structures can be damaged from forces that are in an oblique or horizontal direction to the long axis. In addition to permitting the forces to be directed along the long axis, this ideal arrangement also reflects a balance between the forces applied to the teeth by the tongue with the forces applied by the lips and cheeks (Carranza, 1979; Goldman and Cohen, 1980; Krauss et al., 1969; Ramfjord and Ash, 1971; Thurow, 1977). When forces are not directed through a normal arrangement, the supporting structures may be damaged; this damage is called *occlusal traumatism* ("Glossary of Terms," 1977). *Occlusal trauma* "is defined as that force or forces . . . capable of producing pathologic changes in the periodontium" ("Glossary of Terms," 1977).

There are two types of occlusal trauma: primary and secondary. *Primary occlusal trauma* is defined as excessive occlusal force applied to a tooth with normal supporting structures ("Glossary of Terms," 1977); and *secondary occlusal trauma* is defined as "normal occlusal forces causing trauma to the attachment apparatus of a tooth or teeth because of inadequate support structure" ("Glossary of Terms," 1977).

Occlusal trauma is a noninflammatory, destructive disease that affects the supporting structures; it is independent from periodontitis. In other words, occlusal trauma does not cause periodontal pockets (Carranza, 1979; Goldman and Cohen, 1980; Zander and Polson, 1977). However, a tooth that is periodontally involved may also be additionally adversely affected by occlusal trauma. Occlusal traumatism is reversible if the etiologic factor is removed or if the tooth moves away from the forces (Ramfjord and Ash, 1981). Therefore it is important to recognize and record the possible etiologic factors of occlusal trauma.

There are many possible *etiologic factors* of occlusal trauma. Any disturbance that interferes with the occlusal forces being directed normally or frequent, continuous, excessive forces exerted on one or a few teeth can cause destruction of the supporting structures and occlusal traumatism (Carranza, 1979; Goldman and Cohen, 1980). The possible etiologic factors can be divided into several categories: tooth position, tooth-to-tooth habits, foreign object–to–teeth habits, oral musculature habits, and iatrogenic factors (Carranza, 1979; Goldman and Cohen, 1980; Krauss et al., 1969). Following is a summary of the etiologic factors that may affect occlusion.

1. Tooth position
   a. Rotated teeth
   b. Malposed teeth
   c. Extruded or submerged teeth
   d. Drifted teeth
   e. Missing teeth
   f. Other malocclusion
2. Tooth-to-tooth habit
   a. Clenching
   b. Grinding
3. Foreign object–to–teeth habit
   a. Biting pipe, pen, pencil, or other objects
   b. Biting or chewing fingernails
   c. Sucking thumb or fingers
4. Oral musculature habits
   a. Tongue thrust
   b. Tongue resting position
   c. Lip or cheek biting or sucking
   d. Mouth breathing
5. Iatrogenic factors
   a. Improperly carved or contoured restorations
   b. Improperly fitted removable appliances

Etiologic factors that are causing occlusal traumatism or have the potential to cause occlusal traumatism should be noted in the patient's record during the various phases of the patient's oral examination.

In addition to etiologic factors being recorded, specific subjective, clinical, and radiographic signs and symptoms of occlusal traumatism should be detected and recorded by the clinician.

OCCLUSAL SCREENING

The subjective signs and symptoms reported by the patient are important in detecting occlusal traumatism. The patient will notice aching muscles, teeth that move, pain when biting, or pain with temperature changes. It is important to question the patient about habits he/she may have such as grinding or clenching the teeth, holding a pipe in the same area, chewing pens in the same area, biting the lip, sucking his/her finger or thumb, and other possible habits. Sometimes a patient may be unaware of the habit or unaware of its significance until questioned about it.

The clinical and radiographic signs should also be recorded. The important clinical signs are mobility; wear patterns; changes in tooth position; poorly contoured restorations; plunger cusps; excessive overbite or overjet; overdevelopment of the muscles of mastication; clicking, pain, or improper movement of the TMJ; and tooth sensitivity (Carranza, 1979; Goldman and Cohen, 1980; Ramfjord and Ash, 1971). It is important to remember that the presence of one or more of these signs does not mean that occlusal traumatism is present. These are indicators of potentially destructive forces, but the intensity, duration, and frequency of these forces and the resistance of the host to these forces are important factors in the development of occlusal traumatism. A force that causes destruction of the supporting structures of one person may not affect the supporting structures of another person. The key to occlusal traumatism is whether or not the force is causing damage to the supporting structures at the present time or is likely to cause destruction in the future. The destruction is best seen radiographically or histologically (Carranza, 1979; Goldman and Cohen, 1980; Zander and Polson, 1977).

Ramfjord and Ash (1981) have emphasized the role of plaque as an etiologic factor in periodontal disease associated with occlusal trauma. Destruction of the supporting structure due to plaque must be differentiated from occlusal traumatism.

The destruction of the supporting structures that can occur from occlusal trauma includes widening of the periodontal ligament space, necrosis of the periodontal ligament, cemental tears, loss of the lamina dura, bone resorption, and root resorption (Carranza, 1979; Goldman and Cohen, 1980; Zander and Polson, 1977). Widening of the periodontal ligament spaces, loss of the lamina dura, and bone or root resorption can be detected radiographically and should be recorded.

These signs and symptoms are important and, if detected, should be brought to the attention of the supervising dentist. A suggested format for an occlusal screening is shown below. Note the suggested questions for gathering the subjective data from the patient. Once an occlusal screening has been performed, the dentist may decide that an occlusal evaluation that examines the tooth-to-tooth relationships, the TMJ relationship, and the movements of the mandible needs to be performed.

SAMPLE
Occlusal screening form

PATIENT'S SUBJECTIVE FINDINGS
1. Are you pleased with the way your teeth look?
2. Have you noticed if any of your teeth have moved?
3. Do you have any problems speaking or eating because of your teeth?
4. Are any of your teeth bothering you? Are any of your teeth sore?
5. Do you clench or grind your teeth?
6. Do you bite or chew your lips, cheeks, or fingers?
7. Do you bite or chew any objects such as pencils or pipes?

CLINICAL FINDINGS: Record the tooth number of any tooth that exhibits
1. Mobility
2. Wear patterns
3. Malposition
4. Faulty restoration
5. Pain or clicking in TMJ
6. Excessive overjet or overbite
7. Malocclusion

RADIOGRAPHIC FINDINGS: Record the tooth number of any tooth that exhibits
1. Widened periodontal ligament space
2. Loss of continuity of lamina dura
3. Bone or root resorption

OCCLUSAL ANALYSIS

Several formats for performing an occlusal analysis are available (Nasedkin, 1978; Ramfjord and Ash, 1971; Rieder, 1975; Shore, 1980). An occlusal analysis involves palpation of the TMJ, auditory examination of the TMJ, and palpation of the lateral pterygoid muscles at least, in addition to examination of the tooth-to-tooth relationships. The occlusal analysis is presented here in a step-by-step format. It is recommended that a form to record findings be used such as the one shown below. The patient's subjective and radiographic findings discussed in the section on occlusal screening are also included in the occlusal analysis but do not need further discussion.

Extraoral findings

The patient's TMJ should be examined by placing the clinician's fingers over the TMJ and having the patient open and close his/her mouth. The clinician should record any clicking or excessive lateral movement of the TMJ. The TMJ can also be palpated by placing the little fingers into the patient's ears and having the patient open and close his/her mouth. This will allow the clinician to feel the posterior portion of the TMJ as the patient opens and closes his/her mouth (Nasedkin, 1978).

The lateral pterygoid muscle is palpated in two steps. If a patient is experiencing TMJ dysfunction (i.e., the TMJ is overly stressed), the lateral pterygoid muscle will be extremely sensitive. First, the patient opens his/her mouth, and the soft tissue posterior to the maxillary tuberosity is palpated. Then the palpation buccal to the maxillary tuberosity is performed. The patient may have to close the mouth part way. If the muscle is in spasm, the patient will experience pain during the palpation. Pain or tenderness should be recorded. Other mus-

---

SAMPLE

Occlusal analysis form

EXTRAORAL FINDINGS
1. TMJ
   a. Pain
   b. Clicking
   c. Lateral movement
2. Lateral pterygoid muscle
3. Other muscles
   a. Masseter
   b. Buccinator
   c. Temporalis
   d. Mentalis
4. Swallowing pattern

INTRAORAL FINDINGS
1. Angle's classification
2. Overbite
3. Overjet
4. Maximum opening
5. Pathway of closure
6. Amount of movement from centric relation to centric occlusion
7. Direction of movement from centric relation to centric occlusion

INITIAL CONTACT(S) IN CENTRIC RELATION

1	2	3	4	5	6	7	8		9	10	11	12	13	14	15	16
32	31	30	29	28	27	26	25	24	23	22	21	20	19	18	17

RIGHT LATERAL EXCURSION

1	2	3	4	5	6	7	8		9	10	11	12	13	14	15	16
32	31	30	29	28	27	26	25	24	23	22	21	20	19	18	17

LEFT LATERAL EXCURSION

1	2	3	4	5	6	7	8		9	10	11	12	13	14	15	16
32	31	30	29	28	27	26	25	24	23	22	21	20	19	18	17

PROTRUSIVE EXCURSION

1	2	3	4	5	6	7	8		9	10	11	12	13	14	15	16
32	31	30	29	28	27	26	25	24	23	22	21	20	19	18	17

cles of mastication—the temporalis, masseter, and buccinator—can also be palpated. Tenderness, swelling, or spasm should be recorded. At the minimum, the lateral pterygoid muscle should be palpated.

The patient should be asked to swallow, and the clinician should note if the swallowing pattern is normal. It should also be noted if the mentalis muscle is used during swallowing. If so, the patient may have an abnormal swallowing pattern that is affecting the occlusion.

Intraoral findings

The patient's Angle's classification, overbite, and overjet should be determined and recorded. The patient's *maximum opening* must also be recorded. The patient is asked to open his/her mouth as wide as possible, and then the opening from incisal edge to incisal edge is measured (Fig. 28-6). The usual maximum opening is about 40 mm (Nasedkin, 1978). As the patient closes the mouth, the *path of the mandible* should be observed, and it should be noted if the mandible deflects to the right or left. An unusually small maximum opening or a large deflection may indicate a problem in the TMJ.

Centric relation must be established next. If a patient is having occlusal problems, the muscles and ligaments guiding the mandible into centric relation may be in spasm, and centric relation may

be difficult to establish. It is easiest to do if the patient can relax the lower jaw and allow the clinician to guide it into centric relation. The first step is to stabilize the patient's head by holding the maxillary arch and grasping the chin to guide the mandible (Fig. 28-7). Then the clinician should try to move the mandible gently up and down until it feels relaxed. Once the mandible is relaxed, the clinician can guide the mandible upward and backward into centric relation (Fig. 28-7). Once centric relation has been established, the patient should be guided into centric relation; then the clinician can

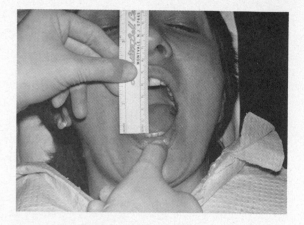

Fig. 28-6. Patient's maximum opening of mandible is measured.

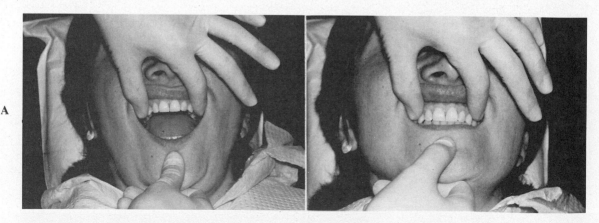

Fig. 28-7. Establishing centric relation. **A,** Patient's head is stabilized. **B,** Mandible is guided into centric relation.

watch the mandible and direct the patient to bite together into centric occlusion. While the patient is biting from centric relation into centric occlusion, the clinician should note the approximate distance from centric relation to centric occlusion and the direction the mandible deflects. This information should be recorded.

Again, the patient is guided into centric relation and asked to indicate which teeth/tooth contact first during centric relation. Once the patient has indicated the area, it is dried with a stream of air (Fig. 28-8) and articulating paper placed in the area. The patient is guided into centric relation with the paper in place; the patient then opens his/her mouth, and the initial contacts are recorded on the form. The initial contact or contacts are the teeth marked by the articulating paper (Fig. 28-8).

The lateral excursions are examined next. The patient should start from centric occlusion, and the clinician should guide the patient into a left lateral excursion (Fig. 28-9), observing the excursion to see if any teeth are contacting on the working or nonworking sides. The interferences should be identified with the use of articulating paper or dental floss and recorded (Figs. 28-10 and 28-11). The same procedure is repeated for the right lateral excursion and the protrusive excursion (Fig. 28-12).

Once the teeth have been examined, the occlusal analysis is complete and can be analyzed. All of the findings must be considered as a whole. An interference may or may not be significant. If the interference is accompanied by other findings, such as bone loss, widened periodontal ligament space, and tenderness of the lateral pterygoid muscle, the interference is probably significant.

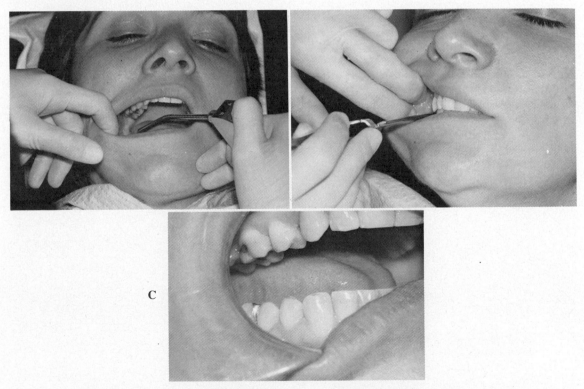

Fig. 28-8. Identifying initial contacts in centric relation. **A,** Drying teeth. **B,** Placement of articulating paper. **C,** Initial contact identified by markings.

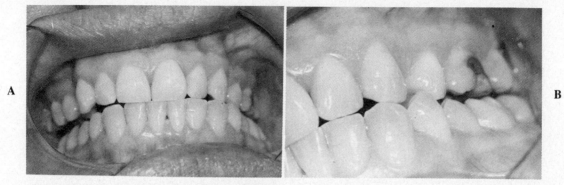

Fig. 28-9. Left lateral excursion. Mandible is shifted to left **A,** until cuspids are edge to edge, **B.**

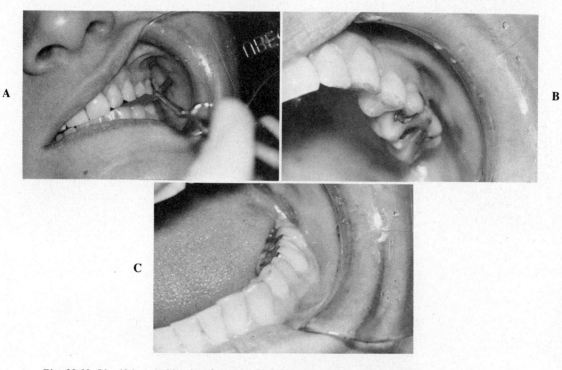

Fig. 28-10. Identifying working interferences of left lateral excursion. **A,** Articulating paper placed on dry teeth; left lateral excursion. Markings indicate interferences on maxilla **B,** and mandible, **C.**

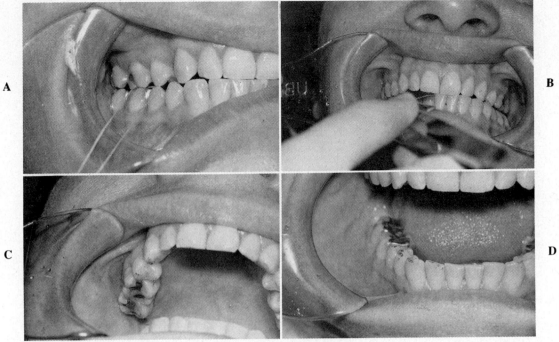

Fig. 28-11. Identifying nonworking interferences for left lateral excursion. **A,** Loop of floss is pulled from posterior to indicate interference. **B,** Articulating paper placed. **C** and **D,** Interferences are shown by markings.

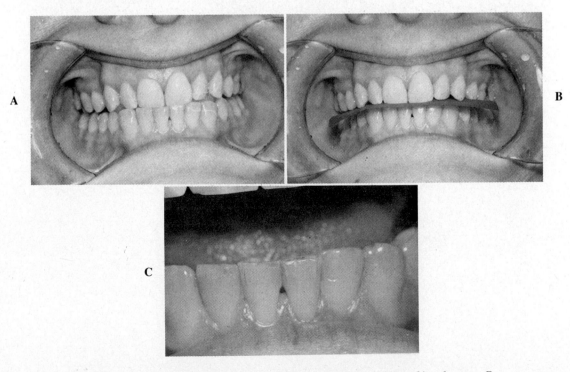

Fig. 28-12. **A,** Protrusive excursion. Articulating paper, **B,** shows markings of interferences, **C.**

SUMMARY

Occlusion is a complex human system that must be examined and considered as a whole. This chapter has presented information about the development of normal occlusion as well as occlusal trauma and occlusal analysis.

ACTIVITIES

1. Perform an occlusal screening for a partner.
2. Perform an occlusal screening as part of the baseline data collection for a patient.
3. Complete an independent study project on any of the following topics:
   a. Posselt envelope of mandible movement
   b. Centric relation versus centric occlusion
   c. Relationship of TMJ anatomy and occlusion
   d. Interrelationships among the TMJ, muscles of mastication, nerve supply, and teeth
4. Perform an occlusal analysis for a partner.

REVIEW QUESTIONS

1. Define the following terms:
   a. Overbite
   b. Occlusal trauma
   c. Occlusal traumatism
2. List five etiologic factors of occlusal traumatism.
3. List the subjective, clinical, and radiographic signs and symptoms of occlusal traumatism.
4. True or false. Correct each false statement.
   a. A patient may suffer from occlusal traumatism even though there is no damage to the supporting structure.
   b. Occlusal traumatism is serious because it causes the formation of periodontal pockets.
   c. If the force causing occlusal traumatism can be removed from the tooth, the supporting structures will in many instances repair themselves.

REFERENCES

Ash, M.M., and Ramfjord, S.P. 1982. An introduction to functional occlusion. Philadelphia: W.B. Saunders Co.

Borell, G. 1980. The development of normal occlusion. Alpha Omegan **73:**15.

Carranza, F.A. 1979. Glickman's clinical periodontology. Philadelphia: W.B. Saunders Co.

Ericsson, I., and Lindhe, J. 1982. Effect of longstanding jiggling on experimental marginal periodontitis in the beagle dog. J. Clin. Periodontol. **9:**497.

Glaros, A.G., and Rao, S.M. 1977. Effects of bruxism: a review of the literature. J. Prosthet. Dent. **38:**149.

Glossary of terms. 1977. J. Periodontol. (Suppl.)**48:**19.

Goldman, H.C., and Cohen, D.W. 1980. Periodontal therapy, ed. 6. St. Louis: The C.V. Mosby Co.

Hoople, S. 1976. Occlusal evaluation module. Seattle: University of Washington.

Jago, J.D. 1974. The epidemiology of dental occlusion: a critical appraisal. J. Public Health Dent. **34:**80.

Krauss, B.S., et al. 1969. Dental anatomy and occlusion. Baltimore: Williams & Wilkins.

Levine, N., and Pulver, F. 1979. Guiding the developing occlusion in children. Alpha Omegan **72:**49.

McDonald, R.E., and Avery, D.R. 1983. Dentistry for the child and adolescent. St. Louis: The C.V. Mosby Co.

Mosteller, J.H. 1980. Occlusion of the natural dentition. J. Ala. Dent. Assoc. **64:**36.

Nasedkin, J.N. 1978. Occlusal dysfunction: screening procedures and initial treatment planning. Gen. Dent. **26:**52.

Perry, H.T. 1976. Temporomandibular joint and occlusion. Angle Orthod. **46:**284.

Ramfjord, S.P., and Ash, M.M. 1971. Occlusion. Philadelphia: W.B. Saunders Co.

Ramfjord, S.P., and Ash, M.M. 1981. Significance of occlusion in the etiology and treatment of early, moderate, and advanced periodontitis. J. Periodontol. **52:**511.

Rieder, C.E. 1975. A simplified occlusal and temporomandibular examination procedure. CDA J. **3:**56.

Robinson, et al. 1969. Nocturnal teeth-grinding: a reassessment for dentistry. J. Am. Dent. Assoc. **78:**1308.

Schifter, C.C. 1979. Occlusal analysis module. Philadelphia: University of Pennsylvania.

Shore, N.A. 1980. Temporomandibular joint dysfunction: a review of successful diagnostic and therapeutic techniques. Alpha Omegan **73:**67.

Stallard, R.E. 1968. Periodontal disease and its relationship to pulpal pathology. Periodontol. Acad. Rev. **2:**80.

Thurow, R.C. 1977. Atlas of orthodontic principles, ed. 2. St. Louis: The C.V. Mosby Co.

Waerhaug, J. 1979. The angular bone defect and its relationship to trauma from occlusion and downgrowth of subgingival plaque. J. Clin. Periodontol. **6:**61.

Weinberg, L.A. 1982. The role of stress, occlusion, and condyle position in TMJ dysfunction—pain. J. Prosthet. Dent. **49:**532.

Weisgold, A.S. 1975. Occlusion: review of various concepts. Probe **16:**373.

Wirth, C.G. 1977. Occlusion. In Boundy, S.S., and Reynolds, N.J., editors. Current concepts in dental hygiene, vol. 1. St. Louis: The C.V. Mosby Co.

Woerth, J.H. 1979. Detecting occlusal dysfunction. Dent. Hyg. **53:**456.

Zander, H.A., and Polson, A.M. 1977. Present status of occlusion and occlusal therapy in periodontics. J. Periodontol. **48:**540.

29 FLUORIDE THERAPY

OBJECTIVES: *The reader will be able to*

1. Discuss the discovery of fluoride as an anticariogenic agent.
2. Explain the value of laboratory and animal experiments in testing fluorides.
3. Discuss the different fluoride compounds used with dentrifice or professional products.
4. Describe the problems in planning a successful clinical caries study.
5. Identify products currently accepted by the American Dental Association.
6. Justify water fluoridation and fluoride products.
7. List three types of topical fluoride preparations and compare their characteristics.
8. Describe factors involved in preparing the patient for a topical fluoride treatment.
9. Identify indications for application of fluoride solutions or gels.
10. Describe materials and techniques used for application of topical fluoride solutions.
11. Describe materials and techniques used for application of topical fluoride gels.
12. Discuss precautions and dangers in the misuse of high-concentration fluoride preparations.

In contrast to the practice of dentistry, which focuses on restorative aspects of care, dental hygiene has always emphasized preventive care (A.M. Horowitz, 1983). In the area of caries, fluorides are the primary preventive agent used and recommended by all dental professionals. Since the establishment of the National Institute of Dental Research over 25 years ago, the use of fluoride has been one of the primary methods studied for preventing caries. Although many other approaches have been attempted, fluoride remains the best available anticariogenic agent (H.S. Horowitz, 1973a). No other approach has been studied as extensively in the laboratory, in animals, or in humans (H.S. Horowitz, 1974).

In evaluating several national surveys on dental opinions, A.M. Horowitz (1983) reported the following: In 1972 about 70% of the respondents indicated that they had heard or read about fluoridation, but only about half of these respondents knew that fluoridation prevented tooth decay. A 1978 Gallup poll reported similar findings. Responses to a 1980 telephone survey asking for "the best way for people to keep from getting tooth decay" were:

> Oral hygiene measures 61%
> Going to the dentist 15%
> Not eating sweets 12%
> Using fluoride 1.5%

It is evident that while dental professionals are well aware of the benefits of fluoride therapy, many consumers are not.

DISCOVERY OF THE ANTICARIOGENIC ACTIVITY OF FLUORIDE

A thorough history of the notable research and epidemiologic studies that documented the anticariogenic properties of fluoride has been published in *Water Fluoridation: the Search and the Victory* (McClure, 1970) and in many reviews and other books (H.S. Horowitz, 1973a, 1973c, 1974, 1982; Imfeld et al., 1983; Katz, McDonald, and Stookey, 1979; Mellberg and Ripa, 1983; Stallard, 1982). Only highlights are presented here. The discovery of fluoride as a caries inhibitor occurred in the early 1900s. In the Rocky Mountain area of the United States, Dr. S.S. McKay noted brown discolored or stained teeth in many of his patients. He later found that patients with stain had less dental decay than those without stain. In the 1930s investigations directed by Dr. H. Trendly Dean determined a common factor that linked staining and reduced decay: all of these individuals lived in regions where the water contained a high amount of fluoride. The next step was to compare towns with varying degrees of natural fluoride in the water with towns having minimal fluoride levels to determine the

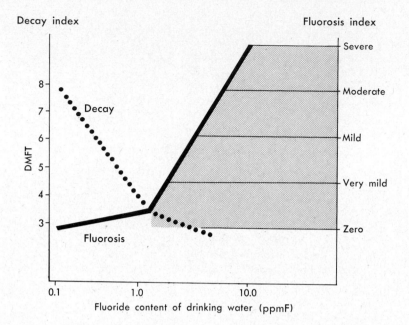

Fig. 29-1. With high fluoride content in drinking water, fluorosis increases and there are diminishing returns with regard to fluoride's caries-prevention effectiveness. Minimum fluorosis and maximum caries prevention occurs with 1 ppmF (parts per million fluoride). (Adapted for Horowitz, H.S. 1976. In Wei, S.H.Y., editor. Fluorides: an update for dental practice. New York: Medcom, Inc.)

optimum concentration for inhibiting decay without staining (Fig. 29-1). From these results it was determined that the optimum dosage level of fluoride in water was approximately 1 part per million (1 ppm). The next step in this research activity began in 1945 when cities such as Grand Rapids, Michigan, and Newburgh, New York, began adding fluoride to their water supplies at a level of 1 ppm. Before fluoridation was initiated, the resident population was examined for caries and bone structure and major organ systems. In addition, records of death rates from specific causes, disease incidence, birth statistics, infant mortality, and many other factors were maintained. Data were also collected from nearby "control" cities (i.e., Muskegon, Michigan, and Kingston, New York) where minimal fluoride was present and none was added to the drinking water. The results of these and subsequent studies showed significant reduction in caries as well as unequivocal safety (ADA Council, 1982; H.S. Horowitz, 1973a; McClure, 1970; Stallard, 1983; Wei, 1974). With fluoride established as being both safe and effective in reducing dental

caries, researchers turned their attention to determining the mechanism of action of fluoride as an anticariogenic agent.

Mechanism(s) of action of fluoride

As with the history of water fluoridation, many articles and books have been written on the potential mechanisms of action of fluoride as an anticariogenic agent (Brown and König, 1977; H.S. Horowitz, 1983; Katz, McDonald, and Stookey, 1979; Muhlemann, 1976; Myers, 1972; Newbrun, 1978; Stiles, Loesche, and O'Brien, 1976). Three of the areas most often researched to explain how fluorides work include (1) increasing enamel resistance, (2) remineralizing initial or precaries "white spot" lesions, and (3) antimicrobial effects. Again, only highlights are presented here to promote an initial understanding of this subject. The chemical name of the principal component of enamel is *hydroxyapatite,* and its chemical formulation is $Ca_{10}(PO_4)_6(OH)_2$. Fluoride converts the hydroxyapatite to a material termed *fluoroapatite*. Fluoride is substituted for the OH, and the chemical

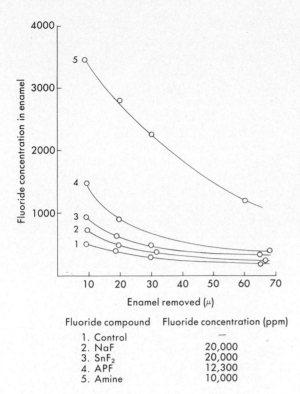

Fluoride concentration in enamel

Enamel removed (μ)

Fluoride compound	Fluoride concentration (ppm)
1. Control	—
2. NaF	20,000
3. SnF$_2$	20,000
4. APF	12,300
5. Amine	10,000

Fig. *29-2.* Fluoride in enamel. (Modified from Muhlemann, H.R. 1967. Die Quintessenz **18,** ref 3192, issues 5-8.)

formulation is $Ca_{10}(PO_4)_6F_2$. When fluoride is incorporated, two factors occur: the apatite structure is more stable, and it is less susceptible to being dissolved in acids. Knowledge of the ability of fluoride to promote remineralization, or rehardening, of the enamel is based primarily on laboratory studies. Clinically high fluoride levels can occur in plaque; fluoride may then be capable of killing organisms in plaque. Other antibacterial effects may include reducing the ability of plaque bacteria to adhere to enamel or, by decreasing the viability of the organisms themselves, inhibiting the ability of plaque organisms to produce acid.

Laboratory tests

The anticariogenic effects of topically applied fluorides were first determined in laboratory experiments (Brown and König, 1977). Three primary methods have been used. The first method determines the levels of fluoride taken up by enamel. This has been done with extracted human or animal teeth or with powdered hydroxyapatite.

As can be seen in Fig. 29-2, high fluoride levels occur even in the untreated, outer levels of enamel. With topical fluoride treatments, all levels can be significantly increased. The organic fluoride tested is taken up at higher levels at all depths of enamel, as compared with sodium or stannous fluoride (Muhlemann, 1967). The second method of testing determines the ability of fluoride to reduce enamel solubility in the presence of acid or acid buffer solutions. With increased uptake of fluoride in the enamel, acid dissolves less of the material. This correlates to the clinical situation wherein plaque organisms metabolize sugars to produce acids that can dissolve enamel. The third method of testing determines fluoride incorporation to or binding by enamel. In these studies, the amount of uptake of fluoride into the enamel or hydroxyapatite is measured as a function of time. It is highly desirable to have large amounts of fluoride taken up as rapidly as possible. Although laboratory tests are excellent as preliminary evaluations, they are not entirely satisfactory, primarily because exposure time to fluoride must be 15 minutes to 8 hours to obtain sufficient fluoride uptake to be quantitatively analyzed or to show protection against the effects of acid etching. Recently, several manufacturers have used remineralizing claims, such as "reverse the decay process before it starts," etc. (as advertised in the *Journal of the American Dental Association*). These statements are based on laboratory results wherein enamel has been exposed to fluoride for much longer time periods than during clinical use.

Animal tests

Many animal species have been used to study caries etiology and pathogenesis (Navia, 1977; Yankell, 1984). Sodium fluoride was demonstrated in the 1930s and 1940s to prevent caries in albino rats and hamsters. In general, fluoride in the water is more effective than when provided in the diet. To more closely simulate toothpaste use, brushing techniques have been used. Artists' camel's hair brushes, cotton-tipped applicators, and electric toothbrushes have been used (Savdir and König, 1964). Rats are the animals used most in testing fluoride products. The pathogenesis of caries in rats is similar to that in humans but is much more rapid (20 to 56 days). The three factors necessary to produce caries in animals (and in humans) have been defined as diet, bacteria, and host (susceptible teeth) (Keyes, 1962) (Fig. 29-3). A fourth factor, time, has been added as another perspective to be considered in caries development (Newbrun, 1978) (Fig. 29-4).

Clinical trials

Testing the clinical effectiveness of a new fluoride or other therapeutic agent is a difficult, expensive (Yankell and Emling, 1978), and long-term procedure (ADA Council, 1982; Horowitz and Heifetz, 1975; Stallard, 1983). Clinical trials must be conducted over 2, or preferably, 3 years. The studies must involve many subjects (i.e., 200 to 250 in each group at the end of the study). The conditions of use must be well defined. Each study must contain a test group that receives the active material and a control group that receives a placebo or material without a known active agent. With a fluoride agent, two studies must be conducted—the first in a nonfluoridated area and the second in a water-fluoridated area—to determine if an additive effect exists. Clinical studies can be influenced by many factors. These include:

1. Using products under supervised (observed) or unsupervised conditions.
2. The subjects' age, which determines the number of permanent teeth available at the beginning and/or end of the study.
3. Caries incidence in the subjects.
4. Caries evaluation methods (tactile and/or radiographic).
5. Reproducibility between or among investigators during scoring. A minimum of two investigators is required for each clinical study. Investigators must correlate diagnostic procedures; if one investigator is missing at any subsequent scoring time, the other(s)

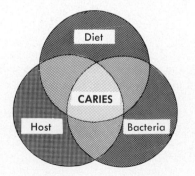

Fig. 29-3. Interrelationship of diet, bacteria, and host in development of caries. (Adapted from Keyes, P.H. 1962. Int. Dent. J. **12**:443.)

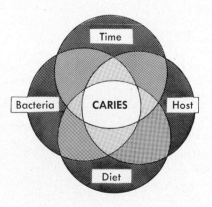

Fig. 29-4. Time is additional factor interrelating with diet, bacteria, and host in development of caries. (Adapted from Newbrun, E. 1978. Cariology. Baltimore: Williams & Wilkins.

will be available to monitor the entire populations.

6. Population stability. The stability of the population must be estimated in a school system. The turnover or dropout rate must be known to ensure an adequate number of subjects remaining at the end of the study.

7. Cooperation of the school and of community, local, and state professional individuals and organizations. This cooperation must be obtained to maximize participation throughout the study.

8. Statistics. Statistical assessments of the data. These must be critically defined before beginning the study.

Scoring clinical caries

Clinical caries examinations should be conducted with a mirror and a sharp sickle-shaped explorer. Radiography may or may not be recommended for the particular clinical situation (FDA Bureau, 1978; ''Oral Health Surveys,'' 1977).

The most common method for evaluating caries is to assess the *decayed (D), missing (M),* and *filled (F)* aspects of the permanent teeth in the mouth. This is done on *all surfaces (S)* and *all teeth (T)* in the mouth. The indices are therefore referred to as the *DMFS index* when the surfaces are analyzed or as the *DMFT index* when the teeth are the primary factors analyzed. Some investigators score all of the teeth in the mouth, whereas others select those categorized as more likely to demonstrate carious lesions (Marthaler, 1966). Several investigators use only the DFS or DFT aspects of the scoring. This may be more sensitive, since missing teeth could have been extracted for reasons other than caries (Muhlemann, 1976).

An extensive review of caries criteria evaluations has been published (Bibby and Shern, 1978).

SYSTEMIC FLUORIDE

Fluoride has been classified as an essential trace element and must be supplied in the diet or drinking water for optimum development of teeth and bones. As with other essential elements, systemic fluorides are ingested, absorbed through the digestive tract, and then circulated in the blood throughout the body. Systemic fluoride effects are topical as well as through the bloodstream and saliva (Brown and König, 1977; Harris, 1970). Thus benefits to teeth

can occur before and after eruption into the oral cavity. Fluoride can be deposited in enamel in three different stages: (1) during the period the enamel is forming and before the tooth erupts into the mouth; (2) after mineralization of the enamel is complete but before the tooth has erupted; and (3) at eruption and throughout the tooth's life span.

Community water fluoridation

The process of adjusting a community's water to the optimum level of 1 ppm fluoride (1 ppmF) for preventing dental caries is defined as community water fluoridation. Since fluoride is such a widely distributed element in the earth's crust, all water contains some fluoride. *Adjusting* is a key word in this definition (H.S. Horowitz, 1982).

Water fluoridation is the least expensive and most effective way to provide fluoride to large groups of people. Optimum benefit can be derived from water fluoridation when the individual resides in the community throughout his/her life. Water fluoridation also provides protection for caries-prone older children and adults after the enamel has calcified and the tooth has erupted (Driscoll et al., 1983, H.S. Horowitz, 1973a, 1973c; Katz, McDonald, and Stookey, 1979).

The safety of communal fluoridation has been extensively reviewed (Hodge, 1972; H.S. Horowitz, 1982; McClure, 1970; Silverstein, Wycoff, and Newbrun, 1972). Misconceptions about fluoridation related to cancer, kidney dysfunction, heart disease, allergies, blood anomalies, and fluoridation equipment have been indexed with pertinent references (Barrett and Rovin, 1980; Rapp, 1976).

School water fluoridation

Another systemic approach is being used in communities that lack a central water supply. In these areas levels 2.3 to 5 times the optimum recommended for community fluoridation have been tested in school water systems with the expectation that benefits would occur in erupted teeth and there would be minimal fluorosis. Decreases in DMFS have ranged between 30% and 50% in these studies, and no fluorosis has resulted from these test procedures (H.S. Horowitz, 1973).

Tablets/drops

Fluoride supplements are no longer approved in vitamin/mineral preparations administered to preg-

Table 29-1. Recommended doses of daily fluoride tablets or drops

| | *Fluoride concentration of drinking water (ppm)* | | | |
| | *Less than 0.3* | *0.3 to 0.7* | *More than 0.7* | |
Patient's age	*Recommended mg. of fluoride per day*			*Suggested product*
Birth to 2 years	0.25	0	0	Drops
2 to 3 years	0.50	0.25	0	Tablets or drops
3 to 13 years	1.00	0.50	0	Tablets

Modified from ADA Council on Dental Therapeutics. 1982.
Accepted dental therapeutics, ed. 39. Chicago: American Dental Association.

nant women. Research with prenatal administration of fluoride has indicated that fluoride could only be incorporated into primary incisors. Since other primary teeth are in formative stages until birth and completed crown calcification occurs after this time, the administration of fluoride supplements to pregnant women is considered to be of minimal value (H.S. Horowitz, 1973c; Katz, McDonald, and Stookey, 1979). Research on a limited number of subjects has indicated that fluoride tablets taken from the third to the ninth month of pregnancy resulted in consistent fluoride uptake in all teeth in the infant (Glenn, 1977).

Fluorides are supplemented as liquid solutions, tablets, or in combination with vitamin preparations (Parkins, 1976). All modes of administration have been documented as providing protection both systemically and topically against caries.

The most important factor to consider when giving fluoride supplements is the concentration of fluoride in the drinking water where the patient lives. A patient's age and tooth development are other primary factors considered when determining which supplement to prescribe (Table 29-1). While the teeth are developing in young children, benefits are both systemic and topical. After this, it is most beneficial for fluorides to be present in the oral cavity for longer periods of time, and topical administration is recommended.

TOPICAL ADMINISTRATION OF FLUORIDE

Sodium fluoride is the primary systemic fluoride source. Various fluoride compounds have been incorporated into commercial products for topical administration.

Sodium fluoride (NaF). Based on laboratory and animal studies, sodium fluoride was the first fluoride incorporated into dentifrice products. In several clinical studies no anticariogenic benefit was found. It is now known that the fluoride reacted with the calcium and/or phosphate of the abrasive and was no longer available to interact with the teeth in the mouth. Recently a sodium fluoride dentrifrice with a silica abrasive was clinically demonstrated to be effective and this product has been accepted by the American Dental Association (ADA Council, 1982) (Table 29-2).

Stannous fluoride (SnF_2). This compound was demonstrated to be significantly more effective than sodium fluoride in both laboratory studies and in caries studies in rats and hamsters. The stannous ion itself was shown to contribute to the efficacy of the fluoride compound. Since the optimum activity of stannous fluoride was in the acid pH range, toothpaste formulations were prepared with abrasives that were stable in the pH range and compatible with the active agent. This led to the development of the first clinically effective anticariogenic dentifrice product. There are several problems with stannous fluoride: it is not stable in water, and the stannous ion can cause staining. Perhaps because of these properties, there are no longer any major dentifrice products that contain this agent.

Acidulated phosphate fluoride (APF). Acidulated phosphate fluoride (APF) or sodium fluoride adjusted to an acid pH with phosphoric acid was developed as the result of laboratory studies that indicated enhanced fluoride uptake could be developed as a result of decreasing (i.e., making more acid) the pH of a neutral sodium fluoride solution

Table 29-2. ADA-accepted fluoride dentifrices

Product (trade name)	ADA acceptance date	% fluoride compound*	Abrasive(s)
Aquafresh	1978	0.76% MFP	Calcium carbonate Silica
Aim	1979 1980	0.4% SnF₂ 0.8% MFP	Silica Silica
Colgate	1969	0.76% MFP	Insoluble sodium metaphosphate Dicalcium phosphate
	1980	0.76% MFP	Dicalcium phosphate
Crest	1964 1980	0.4% SnF₂ 0.243% NaF	Calcium pyrophosphate Silica
Macleans	1976	0.76% MFP	Calcium carbonate

*MFP, Sodium monofluorophosphate; *NaF,* sodium fluoride; *SnF₂,* stannous fluoride.

(Brudevold et al., 1963). In initial clinical studies with APF, enhanced fluoride levels were observed in the teeth of subjects treated with APF as compared with those treated with neutral sodium fluoride. In more recent studies, however, the clinical efficacy of acidulated versus neutral sodium fluoride solutions was not related to the enamel fluoride levels (Aasenden, DePaola, and Brudevold, 1972).

Monofluorophosphate (MFP). This compound, which in actuality is sodium monofluorophosphate, is compatible with a wide range of calcium abrasive systems and other dentifrice ingredients and is unique in this regard (DePaola, 1983). Laboratory and animal studies have failed to document enhanced activity of this compound as compared with that of sodium fluoride. Clinical caries reductions, however, have been consistent with many MFP formulations (ADA Council, 1982). A combination of MFP and NaF has been shown to be more effective clinically than an MFP dentifrice, but the total fluoride level was higher in the combination product (Hodge et al., 1980). Extensive reviews of MFP have recently been published, since it is now the most commonly used anticaries compound in dentifrices (Gron and Ericksson, 1983), and the one most widely tested in the world (Mellberg and Ripa, 1983).

Fluoride mouth rinses

In the mouth rinse vehicle, a neutral sodium fluoride appears to be the agent of choice as compared with solutions of stannous fluoride or APF (Hagarty and Shannon, 1979; H.S. Horowitz, 1973b). Two concentrations have received the most attention in research (i.e., a 0.05% solution used daily and a 0.2% solution used once a week or once every other week). Rinses containing 0.05% solution of neutral sodium fluoride are available commercially as an over-the-counter product, and several products containing 0.2% sodium fluoride are available with a prescription. Many of these have been reviewed and accepted by the American Dental Association (ADA Council, 1982).

Dentifrices with fluoride

Our comments have been confined to those products that have been reviewed and accepted according to the criteria of the ADA Council on Dental Therapeutics (1982). The first dentifrice accepted by the American Dental Association was Crest, with stannous fluoride, in 1964 (Table 29-2). In 1969 Colgate, with MFP and an abrasive system with two components, was accepted. In the late 1970s three other products—Aim, with stannous fluoride, and Aquafresh and Macleans, both with MFP—were also accepted by the American Dental Association. In 1980 three of the ADA-accepted products made significant changes. Both Aim and Crest dropped stannous fluoride as the active ingredient. Aim developed an MFP product, and new Crest contained sodium fluoride. Colgate maintained its same fluoride, MFP, but changed the abrasive system to a single component. (A summary of this information is contained in Table 29-2). The maximum level of fluoride contained in dentifrices in the United States is 1000 ppmF (FDA Bureau, 1978).

Several stannous fluoride solutions in an anhydrous vehicle (to maintain stability) and a stannous fluoride tablet that can be prepared as a rinse just prior to use are also available. The tablet product, when prepared according to directions, contains 250 ppmF, as do nonprescription mouth rinses. The solutions contain 0.4% stannous fluoride, or 1000 ppmF (the same concentration as allowed in dentifrices or prescription mouth rinses). Several of these solution products are being promoted to dental professionals to replace professional topical products and with other major claims. The studies cited to support some of these claims (Yankell et al., 1982) have not used the same vehicles, modes of application, etc., to enable substantiation of these claims. The American Dental Association has only allowed anticaries claims for these products (1982).

Fluoride mouth rinses have several advantages over other methods of delivering topical fluorides. As a solution, mouth rinses are more accessible to interproximal areas that are not reached during tablet use or toothbrushing with a fluoride dentifrice. Depending on the volume of mouth rinse used, higher fluoride levels as compared with toothpastes will be available in the mouth (Yankell, 1978) (Table 29-3). Toothbrushing is usually followed by water rinsing; after mouth rinse use, it is recommended not to rinse the mouth with water to maintain the fluoride levels for a longer time period.

Table 29-3. Fluoride levels after product use

Product	Fluoride concentration (ppmF)	Amount of product used	Fluoride in oral cavity (mg)
Dentifrice	1000	1 g	1.0
Mouth rinse	250	5 ml	1.25
		10 ml	2.5
		15 ml	3.75
Prophylaxis pastes	12,500	1 g	12.5
Professional gels	10,000 to 25,000	10 to 15 g	125 to 375

Modified from Yankell, S. 1978. Interaction of anticaries agents with saliva. In Kleinberg, I., Ellison, S.A., and Mandel, I.D., editors. Saliva and dental caries. Microbiology Abstracts, Special Supplement. New York: Information Retrieval, Inc.

Table 29-4. Comparison of professionally applied topical fluoride agents

Characteristic	Sodium fluoride	Acidulated phosphate fluoride	Stannous fluoride
Form	Solution	Solution or gel	Prepared by dental professional
Frequency of application	Four consecutive 4-minute applications are given 1 week apart; repeated at ages 3, 7, 11, and 13	Semiannual; 4-minute applications	Semiannual; 4-minute applications
Fluoride concentration (ppmF)	10,000	12,300 to 12,500	20,000 to 25,000
Labeled concentration	2% (total compound)	1.23% to 1.25% (F)	8% to 10% (total compound)
Advantages	Can be stored in solution / No adverse effects on gingiva, teeth, or restorations	Can be stored / No adverse effects on gingiva, teeth, or restorations / Ease of application / Acceptable taste	Proved effective in children residing in fluoridated areas / Demonstrated effectiveness in arresting incipient lesions
Disadvantages	Requires four visits / No known effect on children in fluoridated areas or on adults	Relatively expensive	Stains hypocalcified tooth surfaces / Stains silicate restorations / Unpleasant taste and astringency / Must be mixed immediately before using, cannot be stored / May cause gingival irritation / Stains radiographs

Finally, it may be easier for the patient to use a mouth rinse on a routine basis than to take fluoride tablets or to brush with a fluoride-containing toothpaste. Mouth rinses provide a refreshing mouth sensation that is not experienced with tablet use and an ease or convenience that is not inherent in toothpaste use.

Professional gels or solutions

Products that are administered in the dental office have been formulated in either solution or gel vehicles and usually contain 10,000 to 12,500 ppmF. The fluoride materials contained in these gels or solutions include neutral sodium fluoride or APF. Stannous fluoride powder preparations are available that are 8% to 10% stannous fluoride (20,000 to 25,000 ppmF) when made into solution form. Many of these preparations have been accepted by the American Dental Association (ADA Council, 1982). Modes of application and treatment therapy advantages and disadvantages are different for each of the active agents in this category (Table 29-4).

When an agent is introduced into the mouth and in the various vehicles of a dentifrice, mouth rinse, or professionally applied product, several meaningful differences become apparent with regard to the level of fluoride available (Yankell, 1978). Approximately 1 g of dentifrice is applied with a toothbrush. This results in total fluoride of approximately 1 mg available in the oral cavity. Although adults use approximately 12 to 14 ml of a commercially available mouth rinse, children use much less, probably in the range of 7 to 10 ml. At these volume levels, with a 250 ppmF mouth rinse, much higher fluoride levels are available as compared with toothbrushing. It is interesting to note that with either of these products the amount of fluoride available in the oral cavity is significantly less than that administered during a professional treatment with materials containing 10,000 ppmF.

TOPICAL FLUORIDE THERAPY

It is important for the dental professional to be knowledgeable about all forms of fluoride and their effectiveness in reducing dental decay. Patients will turn to dental professionals for information and advice concerning the safety and effectiveness of community fluoridation, fluoride dentifrices, dietary fluoride supplements, and topical fluoride applications. The ability of dental professionals to provide accurate and up-to-date information is a critical component of educating dental consumers so that they can make well-informed decisions concerning the preventive options that are available to them. Dental professionals are also directly responsible for the application of professional-strength fluorides in the dental office. In this section the fluoride agents available for topical application in the dental office and the technique for their use are described.

There are two major categories of topically applied fluoride agents. First, there are those that are applied professionally in the dental office; these include fluoride solutions, gels, and prophylactic pastes. The second category comprises those agents that are self-applied by the patient. In most situations fluoride agents available for self-application by the patient have lower fluoride concentrations than professionally applied solutions or gels so that they can be used safely without the direct supervision of a dental professional. Examples of these products include fluoride dentifrices, fluoride mouth rinses, solutions or gels applied during toothbrushing, prophylactic pastes applied during toothbrushing, and tray application of gels. Self-application of topical fluorides may occur under direct supervision, such as in the dental office or in a classroom situation, or they may be performed by the individual in the home. After minimal instruction from the dental professional, most patients can safely and effectively apply the topical agent without professional assistance. These methods are more cost-effective in situations requiring frequent application of fluoride on a weekly or daily basis, such as patients with rampant dental decay or those undergoing irradiation for treatment of head and neck cancer. Self-application methods are also more cost-effective and efficient ways of delivering topical fluoride to large numbers of children in community or school-based dental programs. In these programs parents, teachers, school nurses, or other supervisory personnel can be instructed to monitor the use of topical fluorides by children so that cost factors and the need for professional dental supervision are minimized.

Professionally applied topical fluorides

There are three major types of fluoride solutions or gels that are used in professional applications.

They are acidulated phosphate fluoride (APF), sodium fluoride (NaF), and stannous fluoride (SnF_2). Table 29-4 provides information comparing these three topical agents and includes advantages and disadvantages of each type to aid dental professionals in their determination of which agent best suits their patients' needs. There is little proven difference in the effectiveness of the three types of fluorides. A large number of commercial brands of fluoride are available for professional use. Dental professionals should rely on recommendations and evaluations of the effectiveness of specific brands when choosing which ones to purchase. Yearly updates of this information are available in *Accepted Dental Therapeutics*. Within the list of accepted topical fluoride preparations, clinicians should also consider factors such as cost, taste, stability, and shelf life.

The patient's assessment data should be evaluated to determine the value of including topical fluoride therapy in the preventive treatment plan. Topical fluorides have consistently demonstrated effectiveness in reducing the incidence of dental decay among children in both fluoridated and non-fluoridated communities. As a preventive measure, fluorides should be incorporated into the treatment plans of children in the years when they are especially prone to dental caries. This includes the years from age 2 (after eruption of the primary dentition) until age 15 or 16 (at least 2 years after the eruption of the second permanent molars). Professional applications after this time should depend on the rate of caries in the individual. If this has not been brought under control, topical treatments may continue into the adult years. The demonstrated benefits for adults have not been as dramatic, since mature enamel does not appear to absorb the fluoride as readily as newly formed enamel and because the incidence of decay is not as high in adult population groups. Nonetheless, adults, especially those in high–caries risk groups, can benefit from topical fluoride applications.

The frequency of professionally applied fluoride applications has been associated traditionally with the 6-month recall interval. This approach does not take individual patient needs into consideration. A more cost-effective approach for determining the frequency of fluoride applications is to consider both the caries susceptibility of the patient and the total exposure to fluorides when determining the potential benefits of topical fluoride applications. It is difficult, for example, to justify the routine application of fluorides for a child with no history of dental decay, who demonstrates acceptable plaque control habits, and who has daily exposure to fluoridated water and a fluoridated dentifrice. The same conclusion may apply to an adult with no active decay and good oral hygiene. Individual patient needs should be considered in every aspect of treatment planning, including recommendations for topical fluoride therapy.

Certain patients fall into high-risk categories because of a high incidence of dental decay or increased susceptibility to dental decay. Fluoride therapy should be a high priority in the preventive treatment plan for these patients. Children and adults who are undergoing corrective orthodontics are more susceptible to decay because of the increased difficulty of performing effective home care procedures around the orthodontic appliances. It is particularly difficult for these patients to implement plaque control; interproximal and other smooth surfaces in the teeth of these patients are afforded increased protection by the topical fluoride agents. Patients with rampant or active caries rates are prime candidates for topical fluoride applications, as are patients who are experiencing recurrent or secondary decay. Although additional clinical research is needed to establish the effect of fluoride on root or cervical caries, fluoride therapy is still considered to be beneficial in these cases. Patients receiving therapeutic doses of radiation in the treatment of head and neck cancer and patients who are experiencing xerostomia (lack of salivary gland function) either because of medications or gland dysfunction are also considered at high risk for dental caries and require regular fluoride therapy.

After identifying the need for fluoride therapy in a patient, this conclusion and the assessment data on which it was based should be presented to the patient as part of the recommended treatment plan. It is important to explain to the patient in lay terms how the fluoride affects the teeth and what the benefits will be. The application procedure should be briefly described and questions should be solicited from the patient. After consent has been obtained, the procedure may be made part of the approved treatment plan.

Patient preparation

Before topical fluoride is applied to the patient's teeth, all deposits that might hinder the uptake of fluoride by the tooth surfaces should be removed. This means that all calculus deposits and extrinsic stains must be removed by scaling, root planing, or polishing with abrasives.

Necessity of a professional prophylaxis. There is some controversy as to whether or not all tooth surfaces must be polished free of plaque before a topical fluoride application will be effective. Those who favor this practice state that the prophylaxis is necessary to ensure that all surface deposits have been removed and to enable removal of the un-reactive enamel surface to expose enamel that will react more favorably with the fluoride (Katz, McDonald, and Stookey, 1975). Opponents of the practice of polishing believe that the procedure does more harm than good by removing the outer layers of enamel, which are the richest in fluoro-apatite concentration. If the goal is to increase the fluoride protection of the tooth, then this loss of outer enamel due to polishing will hinder rather than contribute to the desired effect. It is true that fluoride is able to penetrate through plaque and the acquired pellicle of the tooth to reach the enamel surface (Wei, 1974).

Steele et al. (1982) studied the effect of different methods of tooth cleaning on the uptake of fluoride in enamel. They compared the following methods of tooth cleaning: (1) toothbrushing without a dentifrice, followed by flossing with unwaxed floss; (2) polishing with a rubber cup and a fluoride-containing prophylaxis paste; (3) polishing with a rubber cup and a nonfluoride prophylaxis paste; and (4) no prior tooth cleaning at all. Topical fluoride was applied to all four groups of teeth. The results indicated that the teeth that had been cleaned with a toothbrush and floss showed the highest fluoride uptake, followed by polishing with a fluoridated paste, and then polishing with a nonfluoride paste. They concluded that the routine use of abrasive prophylaxis pastes prior to topical application of fluoride should not be recommended as the most effective method of preparing the enamel to enhance fluoride uptake. Thorough tooth cleaning with a toothbrush and floss appears to be better for that purpose. In addition, they found that the presence of prophylaxis paste in interproximal areas seemed to inhibit fluoride uptake on those surfaces.

This report confirmed similar findings by others (Mellberg and Nicholson, 1968; Vrbic and Brudevold, 1970; Vrbic et al., 1967) that certain components of prophylaxis pastes such as flavorings and humectants appear to interfere with fluoride uptake in enamel. This information should alert the clinicians who use these abrasive pastes prior to fluoride treatments that thorough rinsing and flossing of interproximal areas are imperative prior to the fluoride application procedure.

Tinanoff et al. (1974) found that there was no difference in fluoride uptake on the incisor teeth of school-age children following either cleaning with a toothbrush and water or a pumice prophylaxis. Bruun and Stoltze (1976) reported that not only was fluoride absorbed by both cleaned and plaque-covered teeth, but that the presence of plaque may even enhance the uptake of sodium fluoride . Ripa et al. (1983) also studied the need for professional prophylaxis prior to application of APF gel in school-age children. In this clinical study, one group received a complete prophylaxis performed by a hygienist, which was followed by the application of APF gel in trays for 4 minutes. The second group brushed their teeth using a non-fluoride dentifrice and flossed for 8 minutes. Brushing and flossing were supervised and evaluated with the aid of a disclosant by a hygienist/assistant team. Following tooth cleaning by this method, the same fluoride gel application technique was performed. The third group of children received no tooth cleaning prior to the fluoride gel treatment. Caries increments were measured by comparing baseline caries data with examinations performed after 2 years, with most groups receiving four fluoride treatments and a prescribed cleaning procedure. The differences between caries increments in all three groups were not statistically significant, indicating that the professionally applied prophylaxis did not improve the clinical effectiveness of the fluoride treatments. The results of this study were similar to those reported by Houpt et al. (1981, 1982). These laboratory and clinical studies suggest that there is a strong possibility that our previous assumptions regarding the need for a complete prophylaxis prior to the application of fluoride solutions or gels should be carefully reevaluated.

An additional word of caution should also be included about the relative effectiveness of fluoride-containing prophylaxis pastes. Although many have been shown to result in enamel fluoride uptake, the benefit is only a short-term one and should not be compared with the more significant caries reduction benefit following the application of fluoride gels or solutions. The use of these pastes alone is not a substitute for the 4-minute application procedure as a means for producing long-term preventive benefits (Barenie et al., 1976; Mellberg et al., 1976, Ripa, 1982).

In light of this current evidence regarding the necessity of a complete prophylaxis prior to topical fluoride treatments, dental professionals should begin to investigate other options for patient preparation. Within the dental practice, tooth cleaning is one of the priorities of treatment. The patient should be instructed and reinforced regarding the necessity of effective supramarginal plaque control. In addition, the professional bears the responsibility of removing those soft and hard deposits both supramarginally and submarginally that the patient cannot remove. During a preventive appointment, then, tooth cleaning (i.e., scaling, root planing, and prophylaxis) are important. There are a number of ways that the clinician can accomplish coronal cleaning other than with a rubber cup prophylaxis. One alternative might be to have the patient perform supervised brushing and flossing either with a fluoride paste or without one. In this way the professional could instruct and reinforce effective behaviors in the patient while accomplishing the tooth cleaning simultaneously. If a fluoride paste or gel is used during the brushing, the fluoride treatment or application is also accomplished in the same step. If no paste or gel is used, the brushing and flossing can be followed by a topical fluoride treatment if needed.

Another alternative to the traditional prophylaxis is selective polishing of only those teeth with stain that the patient cannot remove. The patient can then brush and floss to remove remaining plaque under professional supervision, and the topical fluoride can be applied. Both of these approaches open up new treatment alternatives that allow the clinician to spend more time with patients, instructing them on home care methods, and less time polishing plaque from the coronal surfaces. They also demonstrate to patients that the primary responsibility for supragingival plaque removal lies with them rather than with the professional.

Topical fluoride treatments become more cost-effective in community-based programs if the time and cost involved in providing a preparatory prophylaxis are not necessary. Fewer personnel are required to treat large numbers of children with topical fluorides, and the money saved on this procedure could be applied more effectively to meeting the treatment needs of targeted population groups. Dental professionals should continue to be aware of scientific advances and research findings that allow more cost-effective and efficacious treatment of their patients and the public in general.

Fluoride gel application

There are two different methods by which professional fluoride applications can be delivered. The first method of fluoride application to be discussed, the tray technique, is used to apply fluoride gels to the teeth. The second involves the application of fluoride solution. Since fluoride solution cannot be applied in trays because it would spill out into the mouth, it must be "painted" onto the individual tooth surfaces, using cotton-tipped applicators. This technique for applying fluoride solution is described later in the chapter.

The widespread use of fluoride gels for professional fluoride applications has significantly increased the ease and simplicity of applying topical fluorides. The gels are inserted into a tray, which is designed to fit over all the teeth of one arch at once, thereby eliminating the need to apply fluoride to individual teeth. The gel is more viscous or thick than the fluoride solutions and is transferred easily into the mouth, where it adheres to the tray and teeth with minimal or no leakage.

Tray selection. A wide variety of fluoride trays are commercially available for use in professional fluoride applications (Fig. 29-5). Although most trays are made of disposable materials, some use disposable liners in a reusable, arch-fitting base (Fig. 29-5, *top left, bottom middle left*). The clinician should consider several factors carefully to determine which type of tray design to purchase. The tray should be available in a variety of sizes to fit primary, mixed, and adult dentitions (Fig. 29-6). The length of the tray should provide complete coverage of all erupted teeth without extending beyond the most distal tooth's surfaces. The width and depth should provide both effective isolation of teeth and intimate contact of the fluoride gel and the tooth surfaces once it is in place. The

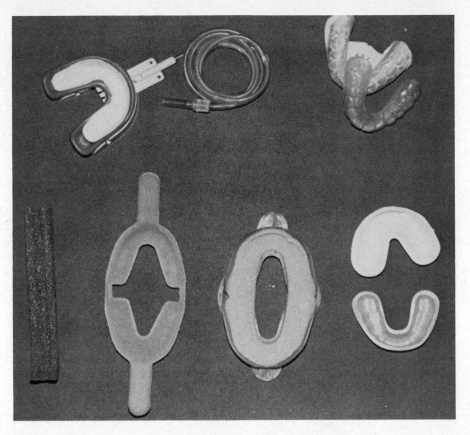

Fig. 29-5. A variety of fluoride trays are available for application of fluoride gels. *Clockwise from upper left:* Reusable tray with hard plastic base, rubber membrane liner, and paper inserts (note also saliva ejector attachment on tray); pliable plastic tray made by forming plastic material directly from patient's arch impressions; styrofoam trays; plastic disposable tray with foam insert; tray in which plastic and foam are fused; foam tray that can be cut and adapted to arch length at time of treatment.

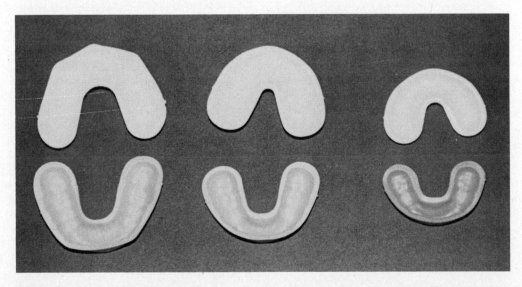

Fig. 29-6. Many disposable fluoride trays come in a selection of arch sizes to ensure optimal fit for each patient.

ends of the tray should be closed so that fluoride gel is not spilled into the mouth during the procedure. Trays that are custom fitted to the patient's mouth will provide the best fit, since they conform exactly to the teeth and arch (Fig. 29-5, *top right*). A custom-made fit improves the amount of contact between the teeth and the fluoride gel and promotes compression of the gel against the teeth and into interproximal areas. Another advantage of custom-fitted trays is that they require less gel to cover all surfaces of the teeth. Larger amounts of gel may be needed in mass-produced trays to ensure that all tooth surfaces are thoroughly coated during the treatment procedure. A technique that minimizes the amount of gel that will be needed is preferred because it reduces the chances that excess gel will be swallowed by the patient and retained as a result of the treatment. In addition to vacuum-molded custom-fitted trays, those with foam or air-filled liners may also enhance the adaptation of the fluoride to the teeth.

The trays should be made of a material that is comfortable for the patient and will not interfere with the contact of fluoride with the tooth. Use of custom-made wax trays is not recommended, because the waxy material can adhere to tooth surfaces and interfere with fluoride uptake. Trays should be easy to handle and to insert into the mouth when filled. Flexible sponge trays and trays that use paper inserts require slightly more handling than do other types of trays, increasing the procedure time (Fig. 29-5, *top left, bottom far left*). The use of disposable trays reduces the chances of cross-contamination and eliminates additional time and handling required to sterilize reusable trays. Since most reusable fluoride trays are made of heat-sensitive materials, chemical sterilization must be used to decontaminate them.

Le Compte and Doyle (1982) compared different types of fluoride trays and cotton swab fluoride application by measuring the amounts of fluoride that were retained in children's mouths following the use of each of the different application vehicles. They found that in all cases significant amounts of the 1.23% APF gel were retained orally following a topical fluoride treatment (e.g., 9.9 to 25.4 mg was retained before expectorating and 3.1 to 6.9 mg fluoride was retained after expectorating). Their results confirmed those of other studies (Ekstrand and Koch, 1980; Ekstrand et al., 1981; Owen et

al., 1979) and raises concern that the high levels of systemic fluoride resulting from the amount of fluoride retained after a professional fluoride treatment may contribute to the incidence of fluorosis in developing enamel. Their study emphasizes the necessity of minimizing the amount of retained fluoride through the use of well-fitting trays, conservative use of gel within the trays, and allowing patients to empty their mouths thoroughly after the trays have been removed. It was also noted that tray systems with some type of absorbent liner resulted in statistically less orally retained fluoride than occurred with other types of non-custom-made trays. The use of excessive amounts of gel within the tray encourages overflow and spillage of the excess gel into the mouth. McCall et al. (1983) also studied the amount of fluoride loss resulting from the use of commercially built and custom-made trays. Their results showed that excessive loss of fluoride may occur during APF application using most commercially designed trays, with minimal loss resulting from the use of closely fitting vacuum-formed custom-made trays. These studies emphasize the need for clinicians to exercise clinical judgment and care in all aspects of the application technique, especially when treating children, to minimize the amount of fluoride that is ingested by the patient.

Application procedure. The same major steps are followed for the application of fluoride solution or gel. Tray setups for solution application and gel application are shown in Figs. 29-7 and 29-8, respectively. The patient should be positioned in an upright position to facilitate evacuation of saliva and fluoride and also to reduce the possibility of gagging. All necessary supplies and materials for the procedure should be assembled, and the procedure should be explained to the patient. Patient consent should have already been obtained during the treatment-planning stage. It is important to reinforce the patient's knowledge regarding the benefits of the topical fluoride application at this time and to solicit any questions that the patient may have. After the best tray size has been selected for the patient's mouth (Fig. 29-9), both trays should be filled by placing a narrow strip of fluoride gel among the bottom of the tray. There must be enough gel to wet thoroughly all tooth surfaces when the tray is in place but not so much that it overflows the tray boundaries onto soft tissues and into the mouth.

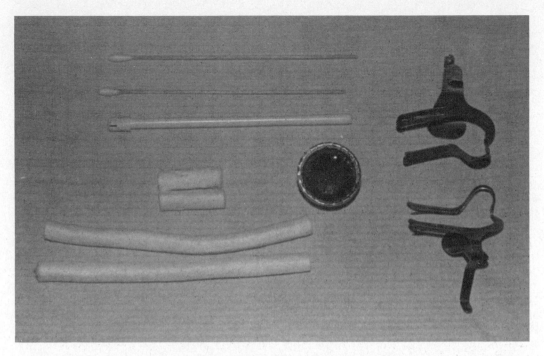

Fig. 29-7. Suggested tray setup for application of fluoride solutions includes cotton roll holders, cotton rolls in two lengths, saliva ejector tip, disposable applicators, and fluoride solution.

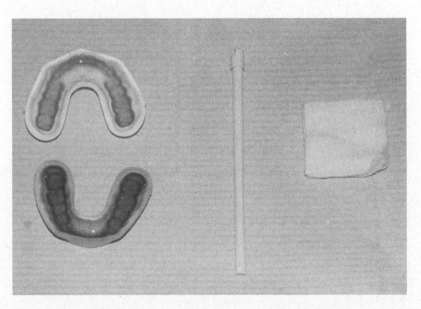

Fig. 29-8. Suggested tray setup for application of fluoride gels.

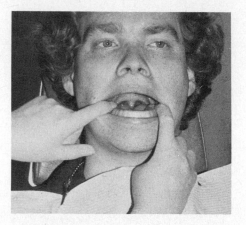

Fig. 29-9. Tray size is selected and tried in patient's mouth to make sure that all teeth will be contacted by fluoride gel.

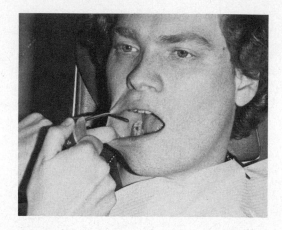

Fig. 29-10. Teeth should be carefully dried and kept as dry as possible until trays are placed. Each arch is dried separately immediately before tray is placed.

After all materials have been assembled and the patient has been adequately prepared, the first step is to dry all the teeth that will be treated. This should be done slowly and thoroughly to ensure that all tooth surfaces are free of saliva, which might dilute the fluoride concentration and reduce fluoride uptake. The patient should be informed that cooperation is needed to maintain the dry field until the trays are in place. Best results are obtained if the areas least likely to become rewetted are dried first, such as palatal surfaces. Areas near saliva ducts, such as maxillary buccal and mandibular lingual surfaces should be dried immediately before the fluoride is applied. Dry the teeth with an air syringe using the following pattern:

Mandibular arch. Dry buccal surfaces; then occlusal surfaces; finish on lingual surfaces.
Maxillary arch. Dry palatal surfaces; then occlusal surfaces; finish on buccal surfaces.

Retract the buccal mucosa and labial mucosa away from the dried teeth with either plastic retractors or the fingers of one hand until the tray is placed into position on the teeth with the other hand.

If both arches are to be treated simultaneously, position the mandibular tray first, then the saliva ejector over the tray, and finally insert the maxillary tray. Ask the patient to close the mouth and to bite gently on the trays. The slight pressure from biting will help force the fluoride gel around and between

all the teeth that are being treated. Begin timing the procedure after the trays are in position and all the teeth to be treated are thoroughly wetted with the fluoride. Supervise or monitor the patient for the entire 4-minute period. All patients, and especially children, should be discouraged from swallowing excess fluoride during the treatment and should be encouraged to rely on the saliva ejector. Patients usually appreciate having disposable tissues on hand to assist in the removal of excess saliva around their mouths during and after the procedure. These steps are shown in Figs. 29-10 to 29-14.

With some trays, such as the ion-fluoridation tray shown in Fig. 29-5, *top left,* only one tray is put in place at a time. This is because the saliva ejector is attached directly to the tray and because simultaneous use of both trays would be too bulky and uncomfortable for the patient. When using only one tray at a time, dry the arch to be treated. Then place the tray, add the saliva ejector, and ask the patient to close the teeth together gently.

At the end of 4 minutes, remove the trays from the mouth and remove excess fluoride and saliva by means of the saliva ejector or high-speed evacuation. Encourage the patient to expectorate any remaining fluids from the mouth. To ensure maximum fluoride uptake, do not permit the patient to rinse immediately after the fluoride trays are removed and give the patient instructions not to rinse,

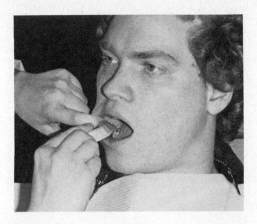

Fig. 29-11. One end of filled mandibular tray is inserted from side of patient's mouth rather than directly from front. This is similar to technique described for insertion of impression trays.

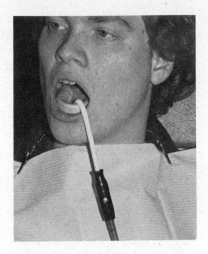

Fig. 29-12. Saliva ejector is inserted *before* maxillary tray is placed.

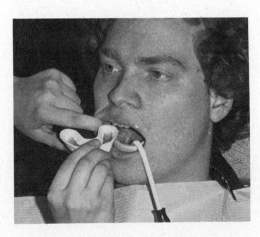

Fig. 29-13. Insertion of maxillary tray.

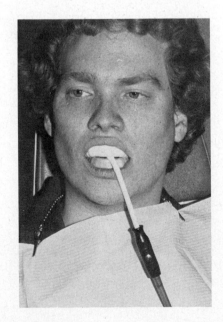

Fig. 29-14. With maxillary tray in place, patient is told to close his mouth gently, and 4-minute timing for fluoride application can begin.

drink, eat, or smoke for at least 30 minutes. A recent in vivo study confirms the need for these instructions by showing that rinsing immediately after tray removal reduced the amount of fluoride deposited in incipient enamel lesions by nearly one half compared to not rinsing for 30 minutes (Stookey et al., 1986).

The advantages of the tray application methods are:

1. Ease of application.
2. The whole mouth can be treated during a single 4-minute time period.
3. Trays are used only once, eliminating sterilization procedures.
4. Improved patient comfort.

The disadvantages of the tray application methods are:

1. Poorly designed or fitted trays may hinder fluoride uptake or allow leakage of gel into the mouth.
2. Cost of disposable supplies.

Fluoride solution application

Use of cotton roll holders. Fluoride in solution form requires the painting technique of application because it must be applied in small quantities and would flow easily out of trays and be swallowed. When solutions are used, the teeth are isolated and kept dry by means of cotton rolls, which are held in place adjacent to the teeth that will be treated so that the tongue, cheeks, and saliva do not touch them during the procedure. Cotton roll holders (i.e., Garmer clamps) are used to stabilize the cotton rolls in the mouth. Garmer clamps can be obtained in two sizes for adults and children. The cotton rolls are inserted onto metal prongs with a short roll on the lingual side of the clamp and a 6-inch roll on the buccal side (Fig. 29-15). The cotton roll holder is placed gently in the mouth so that the lingual cotton roll isolates the lingual surface of the teeth from the tongue and the lowest half of the buccal roll is lying in the mandibular buccal and labial vestibule with the rest extending out of the mouth. The holder should then be stabilized in the mouth by anchoring the clamp snugly under the patient's chin. The rest of the buccal cotton roll should then be securely positioned so that the free end curves up along the maxillary vestibule and returns labially to the central incisors.

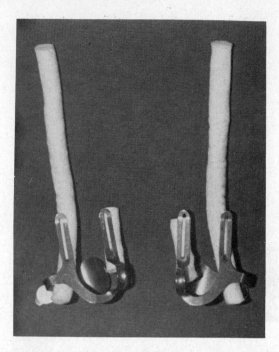

Fig. 29-15. Set of cotton roll holders known as Garmer clamps. Each holder secures two cotton rolls to isolate one half of mouth at a time. Short roll lies against lingual surfaces of mandibular arch, and longer roll isolates buccal surfaces of maxillary and mandibular teeth from mucosa.

A slight twist on the end of the cotton roll before placing the lip over it will hold the anterior end in place. A final check should be made to ensure that the cotton rolls are effectively isolating the teeth from the cheeks, lips, and tongue but are not touching the tooth surfaces to be treated.

The lingual roll should not extend beyond the distal surface of the last molar, where it might elicit gagging from the patient. Once the cotton roll holder is in place, the saliva ejector should be positioned and the teeth on the side to be treated should be dried thoroughly following the same pattern suggested earlier in the chapter.

Application procedure. Ask the patient to hold the fluoride solution close to his/her mouth, or place it on the bracket table near the mouth. Apply the solution first to the mandibular lingual surfaces using an application pattern that moves systematically around the quadrant as follows: posterior on the lingual surfaces, anterior on the occlusal surfaces, and posterior on the buccal surfaces. Apply solution to the surfaces of the maxillary arch by starting on the buccal aspect of the molars and moving forward; then wet the occlusal surfaces and finally the lingual or palatal surfaces. Apply the solution to each tooth liberally with a cotton-tipped applicator, taking care that all accessible tooth surfaces are thoroughly wetted. After all isolated teeth are covered with solution, begin timing the application. During the application period continue to apply solution to the teeth using the same pattern as before to ensure that they are continously bathed in fluoride. At the end of the recommended application time, remove the saliva ejector, then the cotton rolls and clamps. Suction all remaining fluoride solution and excess saliva from the mouth, and allow the patient to empty his/her mouth into a cuspidor or funnelsuction device (depending on the equipment available).

The entire procedure (isolation, drying, application) is then repeated on the opposite side of the mouth.

The advantages of this method of isolation are:
1. It provides effective isolation when fluoride solutions are used.
2. Garmer clamps can be autoclaved and are reusable, thereby reducing the cost of supplies.

The disadvantages of this method of isolation are:
1. The procedure is more time consuming and complicated than tray techniques.
2. Only half the mouth can be treated at one time.
3. Bulkiness of clamps and cotton rolls may be uncomfortable for the patient.

Special considerations

Dental professionals must exercise care in the application of fluoride solutions or gels to ensure that all necessary steps are taken to maximize fluoride uptake by the enamel and to minimize the amount of fluoride that is ingested systemically. With the increasing use of fluoride dentifrices and community water fluoridation, the unnecessary ingestion of high-dosage fluorides from professional applications could increase the likelihood of dental fluorosis in children. Although this does not pose a major health threat, it is a minor side effect that can be effectively controlled through proper application technique. A number of ways to control fluoride ingestion have been suggested in this chap-

ter. They include (1) using well-fitting trays that are designed for maximal coverage and minimal leakage, (2) applying only enough gel or solution to wet all treated tooth surfaces, (3) using the saliva ejector and the high-speed suction during and after the application, (4) encouraging the patient to avoid swallowing during the application, and (5) allowing the patient to expectorate thoroughly after the removal of trays or cotton rolls and to rinse with water at the end of the application procedure.

It is also important for the clinician to realize that although fluoride applied in recommended dosages and with recommended techniques is a safe and effective means of preventing dental caries, its misuse can result in illness and even death. The oral dose of sodium fluoride that may be lethal for adults is 5 to 10 g. Lesser amounts have been known to cause accidental poisoning or even death in children (ADA Council, 1982). Only fractions of this amount, perhaps 125 to 375 mg, are used during the professional fluoride applications unless negligent practices occur. (see Table 29-3).

Symptoms of fluoride poisoning include vomiting, severe abdominal pains, diarrhea, convulsions, and spasms. Antidotes for accidental fluoride poisoning include ingestion of milk or lime juice. Frozen lime juice can be stored in the freezer, or if refrigeration is not possible, powdered milk can be kept on hand and mixed if the need arises. Both of these substances can combine with fluoride in the stomach to form nontoxic and insoluble calcium fluoride. Preparations containing large amounts of aluminum or magnesium are also recommended (Duxbury et al., 1982). If for any reason a parent or clinician suspects that a child has ingested unknown or potentially dangerous amounts of fluoride, an antidote should be administered and immediate emergency medical treatment sought. Treatment for fluoride toxicity consists of intravenous glucose and calcium gluconate, gastric lavage, and conventional treatment for shock (ADA Council, 1982). Because of this potential danger, dental professionals should use concentrated topical fluoride solutions only in recommended amounts and should incorporate all precautions to ensure that only minimal amounts of fluoride are actually ingested. Young children should be closely supervised and monitored during fluoride application procedures and watched for signs of adverse reactions to the fluoride. In most cases if the flu-

---

Fluoride application procedure

Suggested check-off sheet

Mark **S** for satisfactory completion or **U** for unsatisfactory completion of each criterion in the appropriate space.

PERFORMANCE CRITERIA: Does the student   FACULTY | STUDENT

1. Assess the need for topical fluoride therapy
2. Explain the benefits of fluoride, describe the application procedure, and obtain the consent of the patient
3. Evaluate the teeth for removal of calculus, stain, and plaque
4. Assemble all necessary supplies
5. Seat the patient in an upright position

Tray technique

6. Select the appropriate-size tray and check the fit in the patient's mouth
7. Dispense the proper amount of gel into each tray
8. Dry the mandibular teeth and isolate them
9. Insert the mandibular tray
10. Insert the saliva ejector
11. Dry the maxillary teeth and isolate them
12. Insert the maxillary tray
13. Ask the patient to close his/her mouth and bite the teeth together gently
14. Begin timing the procedure
15. Monitor patient comfort
16. Remove the trays after the full 4-minutes have elapsed
17. Remove excess fluoride with a saliva ejector or high-speed evacuation
18. Allow the patient to expectorate.

Solution technique

6. Attach cotton rolls to holders properly for maximum effectiveness and patient comfort
7. Insert cotton roll holders and stabilize them in the mouth
8. Check the placement of the cotton rolls in relation to the soft and hard tissues
9. Dry the teeth using the prescribed pattern
10. Insert a saliva ejector
11. Apply the solution, using the prescribed pattern, to all tooth surfaces on the isolated side of the mouth
12. Begin timing the procedure after all surfaces have been covered
13. Repeat the application pattern throughout the 4-minute period to keep surfaces continuously wet with fluoride
14. Remove the cotton rolls and holder after the full 4-minute period has elapsed
15. Evacuate excess saliva and fluoride from the mouth, and allow the patient to expectorate
16. Repeat steps 6 through 15 for the other side of the mouth

oride procedure is performed competently and efficiently, few if any problems will ever be encountered.

MULTIPLE BENEFITS OF FLUORIDE

Maximum fluoride benefits are afforded the individual who optimizes his/her exposure to fluoride therapy. This includes a program combining community water fluoridation, professional fluoride applications, and daily brushing with an approved fluoride dentifrice. Although these benefits are not purely additive, they have been shown to be greater on a combined basis than any of the single components (Katz, McDonald, and Stookey, 1979). Fluoride is the most effective treatment available to prevent dental decay at this time. It is up to the dental professional to inform the public of its value and to recommend and implement its safe and effective use.

ACTIVITIES

1. Determine which students come from areas where the water supplies were fluoridated (optimum level), and relate this to the number of caries for each student. Can any trends be determined?
2. Divide the class into two groups, pro– and anti–water fluoridation. Discuss both viewpoints in relation to cancer, arthritis, death rates, etc.
3. Plan and discuss setting up a clinical study to investigate a new anticariogenic agent in your (or a hypothetical) town. Would you participate, or would you let your child, brother, sister, etc., participate if you knew you might receive the placebo product?
4. Do a DMFS and DFS on each member of the class. Compare the results. Which do you think is more accurate for this class? Why?
5. Invite representatives of dental manufacturing companies to discuss their fluoride products and supplies. Collect a wide variety of fluoride trays, and discuss advantages and disadvantages of each tray design.
6. Perform a topical fluoride treatment for a partner in your class.
7. Construct scenarios in which the clinician made errors during the topical fluoride procedure, and then have the class critique the procedures and discuss the possible results of the errors.
8. Demonstrate fluoride effectiveness by soaking an egg in a high-concentration fluoride solution overnight. Then take the test egg and a control egg and soak them in household vinegar. Compare the results.

9. Select several members of the class and have them each dispense fluoride gel into similar or different tray designs. Weigh each set of trays to determine how much gel was dispensed. Compare results and compute the total fluoride dosage that would be delivered to each patient. Are there differences? How much variation is there? Discuss ways to determine how much fluoride gel is actually needed for the topical procedure.
10. Check the most current edition of *Accepted Dental Therapeutics* for a list of fluoride products that have proven effectiveness. Identify products available to the public that are not on the list. Perform a literature search on these items to determine what claims have been made regarding their effectiveness or lack of effectiveness.

REVIEW QUESTIONS

1. Identify the following:
   a. ppm
   b. $Ca_{10}(PO_4)_6(OH)_2$
   c. $Ca_{10}(PO_4)_6F_2$
   d. DMFS
   e. DFT
   f. MFP
2. What are the approved or optimum fluoride levels in the United States in:
   a. Water
   b. Toothpastes
   c. Prophylaxis pastes
3. What are some of the proposed mechanisms of action of fluoride on enamel?
4. What products and method of fluoride application or adminstration are optimal for:
   a. In utero
   b. Children up to age 6
   c. Children ages 6 to 12
   d. Children age 12 and over
   e. Adults
5. Name three types of topical fluoride preparations and state their form and suggested frequency of application
6. What are the advantages and disadvantages of performing a complete prophylaxis prior to a topical fluoride treatment?
7. Describe, in order, the steps involved in performing:
   a. A tray application of fluoride gel
   b. The application of fluoride solution
8. When should the 4-minute timing of the fluoride application begin?
   a. After the teeth are dried
   b. As soon as the first tray is in place, or solution has been applied to the first treated teeth
   c. When all teeth to be treated have been thoroughly wetted with the fluoride gel or solution

9. State the lethal dose of fluoride for adults; for children. Compare these amounts with the amounts that are normally dispensed in a topical fluoride treatment.
10. Which of the following are effective antidotes for accidental fluoride poisoning?
    a. Milk
    b. Lime juice or lime water
    c. Preparations containing large amounts of magnesium or aluminum
    d. All of the above

REFERENCES

Aasenden, R., DePaola, P.F., and Brudevold, F. 1972. Effects of daily rinsing and ingestion of fluoride solutions upon dental caries and enamel fluoride. Arch. Oral Biol. **17**:1705.

ADA Council on Dental Therapeutics. 1982. Accepted dental therapeutics, ed. 39. Chicago: American Dental Association.

Barenie, J.T., et al. 1976. Effect of professionally applied biannual applications of phosphate-fluoride prophylaxis paste on dental caries and fluoride uptake: results after two years. J. Dent. Child. **43**:340.

Barrett, S., and Rovin, S. 1980. The tooth robbers. Philadelphia: George F. Stickley Co.

Bibby, B.G., and Shern, R.J., editors 1978. Methods of caries prediction. Microbiology Abstracts, Special supplement. Arlington, Va.: Information Retrievel, Inc.

Brown, W.E., and König, K.G., editors. 1977. Cariostatic mechanisms of fluorides. Caries Res. **11**:1.

Brudevold, F., et al. 1963. A study of acidulated fluoride solutions. I. In vitro effects on enamel. Arch. Oral Biol. **8**:167.

Bruun, C., and Stoltze, K. 1976. In vivo uptake of fluoride by surface enamel of cleaned and plaque-covered teeth. Scand. J. Dent. Res. **84**:268.

Cooley, R.L., and Barkmeier, W.W. 1983. Staining of composite and microfilled resin with stannous fluoride. J. Prosthet. Dent. **49**:346.

DePaola, P.F. 1983. Clinical studies of monofluorophosphate dentifrices. Caries Res. (Suppl. 1)**17**:119.

Driscoll, W.S., et al. 1983. Prevalence of dental caries and dental fluorosis in areas with optimal and above-optimal water fluoride concentrations. J. Am. Dent. Assoc. **107**:42.

Duxbury, A.J., et al. 1982. Acute fluoride toxicity. Br. Dent. J. **153**:64.

Ekstrand, J., and Koch, G. 1980. Systemic fluoride absorption following fluoride gel application. J. Dent. Res. **59**:1067.

Ekstrand, J., et al. 1981. Pharmacokinetics of fluoride gels in children and adults. Caries Res. **15**:213.

FDA 79-3075. Washington, D.C.: U.S. Government Printing Office.

FDA Bureau of Drugs Clinical Guidelines. 1978. Guidelines for the clinical evaluation of drugs to prevent dental caries.

Glenn, F.B. 1977. Immunity conveyed by a fluoride supplement during pregnancy. J. Dent. Child. **44**:391.

Gron, P., and Ericsson, Y. 1983. Caries Res. (Suppl. 1) **17**:1.

Hagarty, T.J., and Shannon, I.L. 1979. Enamel solubility reduction by commercial mouthrinses containing 0.05% NaF. Gen. Dent. **27**:46.

Harris, R.S., editor. 1970. Dietary chemicals vs. dental caries. Washington, D.C.: American Chemical Society.

Hodge, H.C. 1972. Evaluation of some objections to water fluoridation. In Newbrun, E., editor. Fluorides and dental caries. Springfield, Ill.: Charles C Thomas, Publisher.

Hodge, H.C., et al. 1980. Caries prevention by dentifrices containing a combination of sodium monofluorophospate and sodium fluoride. Br. Dent. J. **149**:201.

Horowitz, A.M. 1983. Health education and promotion to prevent dental caries: the opportunity and responsibility of dental hygienists. Dent. Hyg. **57**:(5)8.

Horowitz, H.S. 1973. Fluoride: research on clinical and public health applications. J. Am. Dent. Assoc. **87**:1013.

Horowitz, H.S. 1973. The prevention of dental caries by mouthrinsing with solutions of neutral sodium fluoride. Int. Dent. J. **23**:585.

Horowitz, H.S. 1973. A review of systemic and topical fluorides for the prevention of dental caries. Community Dent. Oral Epidemiol. **1**:104. (c)

Horowitz, H.S. 1974. Increasing the resistance of teeth. Adv. Caries Res. **2**:5.

Horowitz, H.S. 1976. In Wei, S.H.Y., editor. Fluorides: an update for dental practice. New York: Medcom, Inc.

Horowitz, H.S. 1982. Water fluoridation and other methods for delivering systemic fluorides: In Stallard, R.E., editor. A textbook of preventive dentistry, ed 2. Philadelphia: W.B. Saunders Co.

Horowitz, H.S., and Heifetz, S.B. 1975. Clinical tests of dentifrices. Pharmacol. Ther. Dent. **2**:235.

Houpt, M., et al. 1981. The effect of prior tooth cleaning upon the efficacy of semi-annual topical fluoride treatment. J. Dent. Res. **60**:504.

Houpt, M., et al. July-Aug. 1983. The effect of prior tooth-cleaning on the efficacy of topical fluoride treatment: two-year results. Clin. Prevent. Dent. **5**:8.

Imfeld, T., et al. 1983. Cariology, Zurich 1953-1983: some aspects of one man's stand: dedicated to Prof. H.R. Muhlemann. Swiss. Dent. **4**:7.

Katz, S., McDonald, J.L., and Stookey, G.K. 1979. Preventive dentistry in action, ed. 3. Upper Montclair, N.J.: D.C.P. Publishing.

Keyes, P.H. 1962. Recent advances in dental caries research: bacteriology: bacteriological findings and biological implications. Int. Dent. J. **12**:443.

Le Compte, E.J., and Doyle, T.E. 1982. Oral fluoride retention following various topical application techniques in children. J. Dent. Res. **61**:1397.

Marthaler, T.M. 1966. A standardized system of recording dental conditions. Helv. Odontol. Acta **10**:1.

McCall, D.R., et al. 1983. Fluoride ingestion following APF gel application. Br. Dent. J. **155**:333.

McClure, F.J. 1970. Water fluoridation: the search and victory. Bethesda, Md.: National Institutes of Health.

Mellberg, J.R., and Nicholson, C.R. 1968. In vitro evaluation of an acidulated phosphate fluoride prophylaxis paste. Arch. Oral Biol. **13**:1223.

Mellberg, J.R., and Ripa, L.W. 1983. Fluoride in preventive dentistry: theory and clinical applications. Chicago: Quintessence Publishing Co., Inc.

Muhlemann, H.R. 1967. The cariostatic effects of amine fluorides—10 year review: Die Quintessenz **18,** ref. 3192, issues 5-8.

Muhlemann, H.R. 1976. Introduction to oral preventive medicine. Berne, Switzerland: Hans Huber Publishers.

Myers, H.M. 1972. The mechanism of the anticaries action of fluoride ion. In Newbrun, E., editor. Fluorides and dental caries. Springfield, Ill., Charles C Thomas, Publisher.

Navia, J.M. 1977. Animal models in dental research. Birmingham: The University of Alabama Press.

Newbrun, E. 1978. Cariology. Baltimore: Williams & Wilkins.

Oral health surveys, basic methods. ed. 2. 1977. Geneva: World Health Organization.

Owen, D., et al. 1979. Monitoring ingestion and urinary excretion of topical fluoride. IADR Program and Abstracts **57**(1256):405.

Parkins, F.M. 1976. Prescribing fluoride supplements for home use. In Moss, S.J., editor. Fluorides: an update for dental practice. New York: Medcom, Inc.

Rapp, R. 1976. Popular misconceptions about fluoridation. In Moss, S.J., editor. Fluorides: an update for dental practice. New York: Medcom, Inc.

Recommended Dietary Allowances, revised 1980. Washington, D.C.: Food and Nutrition Board. National Academy of Sciences–National Research Council.

Ripa, L.W. 1982. Professionally (operator) applied topical fluoride therapy: a critique. Clin. Prevent. Dent. **4**(3):3.

Ripa, L.W., et al. 1983. Effect of prior toothcleaning on biannual professional APF topical fluoride gel-tray treatments: results after two years. Clin. Prevent. Dent. **5**(4):3.

Savdir, S., and König, K.G. 1964. An electrical toothbrush for use in caries experiments on rodents. Helv. Odontol. Acta **8**:24.

Shannon, I.L. 1982. Fluoride treatment programs for high-caries-risk-patients. Clin. Prevent. Dent. **4**(2):11.

Silverstein, S.J., Wycoff, S.J., and Newbrun, E. 1972. Sociological, economical and legal aspects of fluoridation. In Newman, E., editor. Fluorides and dental caries. Springfield, Ill.: Charles C Thomas, Publisher.

Silverstone, L.M. 1978. Preventive dentistry. London: Update books, Ltd.

Stallard, R.E., editor 1982. A textbook of preventive dentistry, ed. 2. Philadelphia: W.B. Saunders Co.

Stallard, R.E., editor. 1983. Proceedings, international conference on fluorides and dental health, Nairobi, Kenya. New Brunswick, N.J.: S & S Printing Services, Inc.

Steele, R.C., et al. 1982. The effect of tooth cleaning procedures on fluoride uptake in enamel. Pediatr. Dent. **4**:228.

Stiles, H.M., Loesche, W.J., and O'Brien, T.C., editors. 1976. Microbial aspects of dental caries. vols. 1-3. Microbiology Abstracts, Special Supplement. Arlington, Va.: Information Retrieval, Inc.

Stookey, G.K., et al. 1986. Post-application rinsing versus fluoride uptake with APF gel (abstract no. 589). J. Dent Res. **65** (Special Issue):235.

Swango, P.A. 1983. The use of topical fluorides to prevent dental caries in adults: a review of the literature. J. Am. Dent. Assoc. **107**:447.

Tinanoff, N., et al. 1974. Effect of a pumice prophylaxis on fluoride uptake in tooth enamel. J. Am. Dent. Assoc. **88**:384.

Vrbic, V., and Brudevold, F. 1970. Fluoride uptake from treatment with different fluoride prophylaxis pastes and from the use of pastes containing a soluble aluminum salt followed by topical application. Caries Res. **4**:158.

Vrbic, V., et al. 1967. Acquisition of fluoride by enamel from fluoride pumice pastes. Helv. Odontol. Acta **11**:21.

Wei, S.H.Y. 1974. The potential benefits to be derived from topical fluorides in fluoridated communities. In Forester, D.J., and Schulz, E.M., editors. International workshop on fluorides and dental caries reductions. Baltimore: University of Maryland School of Dentistry.

Yaffe, A., and Zalkind, M. 1981. The effect of topical application of fluoride on composite resin restorations. J. Prosthet. Dent. **45**:59.

Yankell, S.L. 1978. Interaction of anti-caries agents with saliva. In Kleinberg, I., Ellison, S.A., and Mandel, I.D., editors. Saliva and dental caries. Microbiology Abstracts, Special Supplement. New York: Information Retrieval, Inc.

Yankell, S.L. 1984. Oral disease in laboratory animals: rats and other laboratory animals. In Harvey, C.E., editor. Veterinary dentistry. Philadelphia: W.B. Saunders Co.

Yankell, S.L., and Emling, R.C. 1978. Understanding dental products: what you should know and what your patient should know. Continuing Dental Education, University of Pennsylvania School of Dental Medicine **1:** No. 7.

Yankell, S.L., et al. 1982. Clinical effects of stannous fluoride mouthrinses in a five day no oral hygiene study. J. Periodont. Res. **17**:374.

30 PIT AND FISSURE SEALANTS

OBJECTIVES: *The reader will be able to*

1. List three methods that have been used to prevent pit and fissure caries.
2. Discuss the role of sealants in a total preventive program.
3. Discuss research findings regarding sealant retention and caries reduction.
4. Describe the mechanism by which the sealant attaches to the tooth.
5. Discuss the effect that the shape of a pit or fissure has on the penetration of a sealant.
6. Discuss the factors to be considered when selecting teeth for the sealant application.
7. Describe two types of sealant material.
8. List the sequence of steps most commonly used when applying pit and fissure sealants.

One of the most recent advances in the prevention of caries has been the development of occlusal sealants. These materials effectively protect the pits and fissures from bacterial activity that creates carious lesions. It is interesting to note that although the occlusal surfaces account for only about 12.5% of the total surfaces at risk to caries, occlusal decay makes up almost 50% of the decay in children's teeth (Ripa, 1973).

Methods other than sealants have been attempted for lowering the rate of pit and fissure caries. These have included eradication of the occlusal anatomy by reshaping the occlusal grooves or by placing conservative occlusal restorations before decay actually occurs (Craig, O'Brien and Powers, 1979). Since both of these methods eliminate sound tooth structure, it seems unclear as to what is actually being prevented. An analogy is that of removing everyone's appendix at birth to prevent appendicitis. Obviously, the procedure is unnecessary for a number of people; thus the cost, time and inherent risks outweigh the benefits.

Obturation or closing the occlusal anatomy with materials such as silver nitrate, zinc chloride, potassium ferrocyanide, or red copper cement has been tried. Such procedures have been unsuccessful primarily because of the material's physical or chemical properties.

Fluoride seemed an obvious answer to the problem of occlusal decay, since it would have a systemic effect on the actual quality of the enamel. Indeed, fluorides do reduce the absolute number of caries, but studies indicate that the proximal and smooth surfaces, not the occlusal surfaces, enjoy the most benefit from systemic or topical fluoride therapy (Ripa, 1973).

Reducing the retentive nature of the occlusal anatomy is the key to a significant reduction in pit and fissure caries. A fissure that is less likely to harbor debris and/or bacteria is less likely to decay. The sealants used today are adhesive materials that coat the occlusal surface. In this way the sealant acts as a physical barrier to prevent oral bacteria and nutrients from developing the acidic conditions necessary to destroy tooth structure. The factor that has made today's sealants more successful than other coverage techniques is an acid-conditioning process that alters or enlarges the naturally occurring enamel pores. With the resultant increase in surface area due to this technique, the sealant is able to better penetrate the enamel and achieve a reliable mechanical bond (Gwinnett, 1973).

It is not surprising that sealants met with some controversy, considering the unsuccessful records of previous methods to curb occlusal caries. The following studies indicate the significance of currently used materials in the patient's total prevention program.

In a 2-year study of a single adhesive application, of 113 surfaces of permanent teeth covered, 87% had retained full coverage after 2 years. In the untreated control teeth, 60% became carious during the 2 years. Ninety-nine percent protection was obtained in the experimental surfaces of the permanent teeth (Buonocore, 1971).

In a 4-year clinical evaluation of pit and fissure sealants, 50% of the teeth had fully retained their single application of sealant. When sealant remained intact, the effectiveness in caries reduction was 84% (Going, 1977).

Retention and effectiveness of a single application of adhesive sealant after 5 years showed that 42% of the initially sealed sites retained their covering. When sealant was only partially lost, 93% of the sites remained caries-free. When sealant was fully retained, less than 1% became carious as compared with 18% of the untreated paired controls. When sealant was partially lost, 7% became decayed, missing, or filled as compared with 41% of the untreated pairs. Regardless of retention status, after 5 years of a single application of sealant a 39% effectiveness in preventing decay was attained (Horowitz, Heifetz, and Poulsen, 1977).

In a comparative study between a chemically polymerized fissure sealant resin and a light-cured resin, Rock et al. (1983) found almost identical retention figures at 6-month and 1-year intervals.

Mertz-Fairhurst et al. (1982) have reported a comparative clinical study of two pit and fissure sealants in which even 6 years after a single application, 49% of the teeth remained sealed with one product and 78% remained intact with the other product. Sealants are effective in prevention of caries and can be expected to be even more effective in a practice situation where reapplication of any lost material is a routine procedure.

THE BONDING MECHANISM

Buonocore (1975) has suggested that the occlusal surface of a tooth is similar to an iceberg: much of what exists cannot be seen. In fact, with conventional explorer examination much cannot be determined with tactile sense. The explorer may "catch" in the tooth because of anatomy alone. Three principal types of pit and fissure configurations have been described: V types, U types, and I types (Figs. 30-1 to 30-3). In addition, miscellaneous shapes exist as small round openings, fissures that have pits associated with their bases or walls, or continuous grooves that separate cusps (Fig. 30-4). To protect these anatomic defects from the inevitably high percentage of carious lesions, acid-etch resin sealants are useful. Success is dependent on a highly effective bonding technique and a leakage resistant material.

Mechanical bonding refers to a physical entrapment of material within pores or cavities occurring naturally or artificially created (Gwinnett, 1973). Etching or conditioning the occlusal or pitted surface with a 30% to 70% solution of acid, usually 30% unbuffered phosphoric acid, removes organic material and exposes a more reactive, porous surface. Microscopically, the conditioned enamel surface shows enamel rods that have lost material from rod cores (Fig. 30-5). The increased surface area created by the conditioning technique is the key to providing a competent mechanical bond. The studies mentioned previously indicate the degree of retention that is possible even after several years with only one application of sealant. In practice, sealants are examined regularly at recall intervals (3 to 6 months) and reapplied when necessary.

Since conditioning does remove enamel structure, does it harm the tooth? Generally, conditioning is confined to the cuspal planes of the occlusal surfaces that are to be covered with the sealant material. If conditioned enamel is left exposed, minerals in the saliva replenish the surface. This is similar to the remineralization that occurs after enamel constituents have been removed through routine prophylaxis procedures or during ingestion of acid-containing foods (fruits) (Buonocore, 1973).

The margins of sealed surfaces have been shown to resist leakage of dye and radioisotopes even after being boiled in water. Several researchers have reported that decay inadvertently sealed in a tooth does not appear to progress when the sealant is firmly bonded to the tooth. When sealant was removed and pits and fissures studied for caries activity, findings showed that the teeth remained caries-free. The nature of the sealant margin compares favorably with other current restorative material margins that, despite microscopic leakage, arrest the decay process and resist recurrence of caries to a high degree.

Dennison et al. (1980) compared the margins of amalgam restorations with sealants retained after 18 months. Margin deterioration occurred in 50% of the amalgam restorations. Sealant margins remained undetectable in 55% of the cases.

In clinical situations the sealants appear to be retained by the individual teeth in the following

Text continued on p. 528.

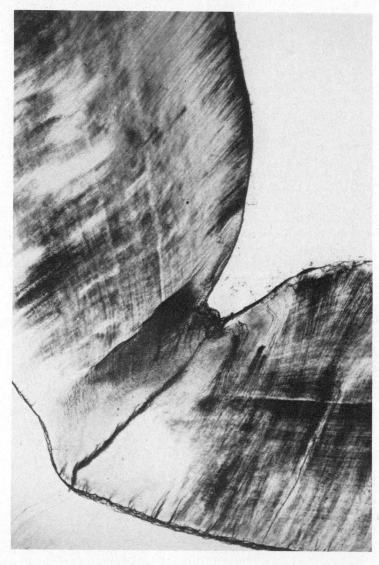

Fig. 30-1. Photomicrograph showing wide V-type fissure. (From Gwinnett, A.J. 1973. J. Am. Soc. Prevent. Dent. **3:**21.

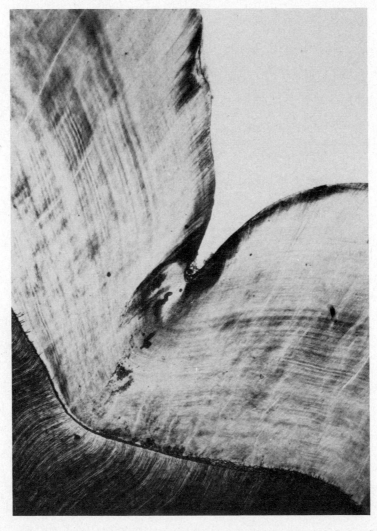

Fig. 30-2. Photomicrograph showing narrow V-type fissure. (From Gwinnet, A.J. 1973. J. Am. Soc. Prevent. Dent. **3**:21.

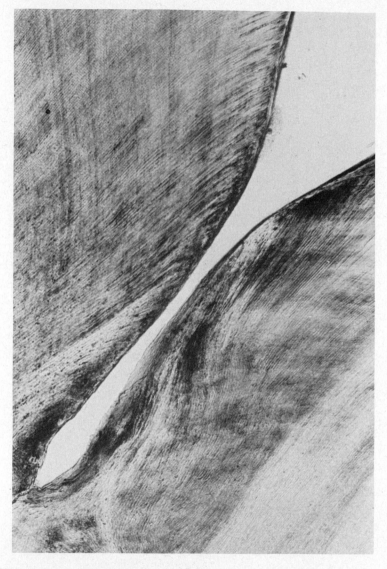

Fig. 30-3. Photomicrograph showing I-type fissure, a narrow constrictive configuration that is somewhat bulbous toward its base. (From Gwinnett, A.J. 1973. J. Am. Soc. Prevent. Dent. **3**:21.

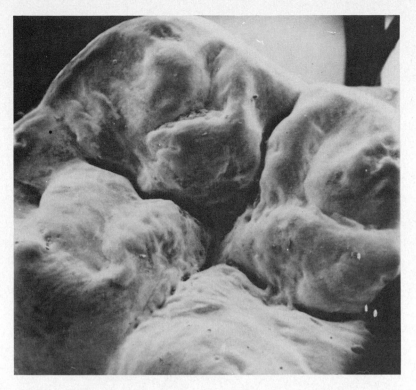

Fig. 30-4. Scanning electron micrograph showing random distribution of pits and fissures on occlusal surface. (From Gwinnett, A.J. 1973. J. Am. Soc. Prevent. Dent. **3**:21.

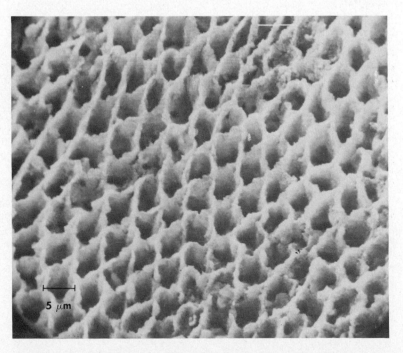

5 μm

Fig. 30-5. Scanning electron micrograph of enamel surface that has been etched (conditioned) with phosphoric acid for 60 seconds. Note loss of enamel prism core, which will encourage sealant retention. (From Silverstone, L.M. 1978. Preventive dentistry. Fort Lee, N.J.: Update Publishing International, Inc.)

way: Pit and fissure sealants have been shown to be better retained in the premolars than in the molars. First molars stay sealed more often than second molars. The distolingual groove of the maxillary molars is the most difficult site for retaining the sealant. In general, mandibular molars retain sealant material more frequently than maxillary molars (Messer et al. 1980). These findings may be influenced by tooth anatomy combined with the degree of isolation that can be achieved during the sealant application.

INDICATIONS FOR SEALANT APPLICATION

In selecting teeth to be protected by sealant, the patient's caries susceptibility is important. This is reflected by the number of restorations and/or caries present and the patient's preventive attitude. Occlusal sealants are not likely to be successful for reducing caries when adequate home care and dietary measures are lacking. Sealant protection is intended to be used as part of a total preventive program. Regular professional care, fluoride application (systemic and topical), and individual home care are the components of the preventive plan.

The patient's tooth anatomy is also a consideration. Deep, narrow pits and fissures tend to be more retentive of oral bacteria than teeth with shallow grooves, which retain less plaque and are more accessible to cleaning methods. In the permanent dentition, molars are more susceptible to caries than premolars. In the primary dentition, the second molars are more susceptible than the first molars (Ripa, 1973). If a tooth has been maintained caries-free for several years, surviving the period of childhood and adolescence, the sealing procedure will probably be insignificant. Of course, considering whether the patient's general caries susceptibility is being currently altered by systemic or local factors is necessary. In general, when a patient is identified as being caries susceptible, despite other preventive measures, the teeth should be protected as soon after eruption as possible.

A thorough radiographic examination should be performed. Occlusal sealing is contraindicated when proximal surfaces are carious, since the necessary restorative procedure will include a portion of the occlusal table. At the clinical evaluation and in conjunction with radiographic diagnosis, a careful examination of all teeth with compressed air and an explorer is important.

Table 30-1 provides a summary of indications and contraindications for sealants.

SEALANT MATERIALS

Most sealants are bisphenol A-glycidyl methacrylate (BIS-GMA) materials, which are polymerized by an organic amine or ultraviolet light (Craig, O'Brien, and Powers, 1983). Amine-accelerated materials are supplied as two-component systems and require mixing. Ultraviolet light–polymerized materials require no mixing.

To ensure success with either type of material, careful handling is necessary. It is especially important that the sealant material not be exposed to air during storage. This may cause evaporation, which would make the material less fluid and reduce penetration into the pits and fissures. Fresh sealant material should be used, and other sealant procedure equipment such as brushes and an ultraviolet light source should be well maintained.

Table 30-1. Indications and contraindications for occlusal sealing

Clinical condition	Do not seal	Seal*
Occlusal morphology	Well-coalesced pits and fissures; absence of pits and fissures	Deep, narrow pits and fissures that "catch" the probe
General caries activity	Many proximal lesions present	Occlusal lesions present (indicating occlusal susceptibility); few proximal lesions
Tooth age	Teeth that have remained caries-free for 4 or more years	Recently erupted teeth
Preventive program	If other caries preventive measures are not available	If patient cooperates in total caries preventive program

From Ripa, L.W. 1973. J. Am. Soc. Prevent. Dent. **3:**32.
*Only teeth with caries-free occlusal and proximal surfaces are indicated for sealing.

Ultraviolet light–accelerated BIS-GMA materials include Lee Seal (Lee Pharmaceuticals), and Nuva-Cote P.A. and Nuva-Seal P.A. (L.D. Caulk Co., Division of Dentsply International, Inc).

Amine-accelerated BIS-GMA materials include Concise White Sealant System and Concise Enamel Bond (3M Co.), Delton (Johnson & Johnson), Epoxylite 9075 (Lee Pharmaceuticals), and Kerr Pit and Fissure Sealant (Kerr Manufacturing Co., Division of Sybron Corp.).

SEALANT APPLICATION

Although manufacturers' products differ, the basic steps in sealant application are similar. It is essential to note that the quality of the end product is determined to a great extent by the clinician's attention to (1) strict clinical dryness, (2) accurate timing for conditioning, (3) fresh sealant material, and (4) adherence to recommended setting (polymerization) procedures.

Application technique

1. Prepare the tooth surface, cleaning it of hard and soft deposits. Polishing with a pumice and water is recommended. A polishing paste with fluoride or a fluoride treatment prior to the sealant application is contraindicated. The fluoride will interfere with the etching/conditioning technique (Silverstone, 1978). Rinse the teeth thoroughly with water.
2. Isolate the teeth with a rubber dam or a Garmer clamp with cotton rolls (Figs. 30-6 and 30-7). It is extremely important to keep the working area dry. The rubber dam procedure is recommended when the sealant is to be applied to several teeth in the quadrant. Satisfactory results can be obtained with frequent changing of cotton rolls. Once the teeth are isolated, dry the area with clean, dry compressed air (Fig. 30-8).
3. Apply the conditioner for the enamel-etching process. Follow the manufacturer's directions for acid concentration and conditioning time. A brush for painting the conditioner on the occlusal surface is recommended, although a cotton pellet can be used (Fig. 30-9). A fine brush is more accurate in placing the acid than a cotton pellet, which may absorb too much of the solution or cause air to be trapped in the fissure (Silverstone, 1983).
4. After the appropriate conditioning time (usually

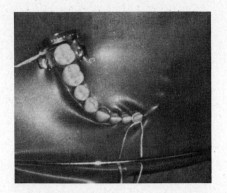

Fig. 30-6. One technique to maintain a dry working field during sealant procedure is to isolate teeth with a rubber dam.

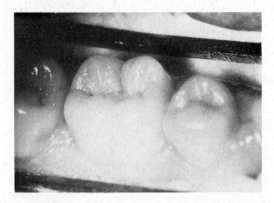

Fig. 30-7. Teeth are isolated with Garmer clamp and cotton rolls. (Courtesy L.D. Caulk Co., Milford, Del.)

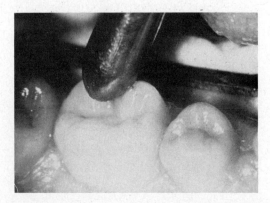

Fig. 30-8. Teeth are dried with compressed air. (Courtesy L.D. Caulk Co., Milford, Del.)

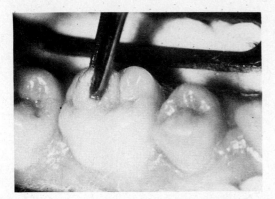

Fig. 30-9. Conditioner is applied according to manufacturer's directions. (Courtesy L.D. Caulk Co., Milford, Del.)

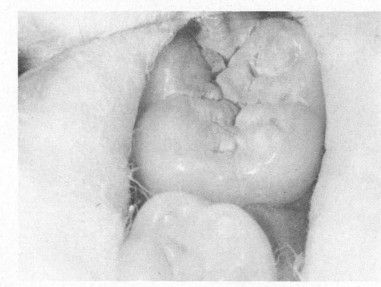

Fig. 30-10. Conditioner is rinsed off, and teeth are dried. Note dull, chalky appearance. (From Spohn, E.C., and Berry, T.G. 1979. Pit and fissure sealants. In Boundy, S.S., and Reynolds, N.J., editors. Current concepts in dental hygiene, vol. 2. St. Louis: The C.V. Mosby Co.)

60 seconds), rinse the area with water to thoroughly remove the conditioning solution. Immediately dry the teeth and replace the cotton rolls if necessary. Take care not to let saliva contact the conditioned surface, since this will interfere with the bonding of the sealant. This is the most critical period in the sealant application. Inspect the teeth for a dull, chalky surface (Spohn and Berry, 1979) (Fig. 30-10). If

the entire surface to be sealed does not appear chalky or if the teeth have been contaminated with saliva, repeat the conditioning procedure.
5. Apply the sealant by brushing the liquid on the conditioned tooth surface (Fig. 30-11). Concentrate the sealant in the central pits and fissures (Fig. 30-12). Apply the sealant to the cuspal planes to complete the coverage (Fig. 30-13). Take care not to apply an excess of

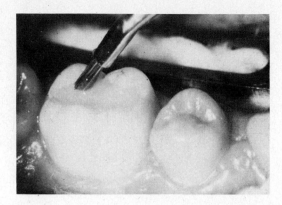

Fig. 30-11. Sealant is brushed on conditioned surface. (Courtesy L.D. Caulk Co., Milford, Del.)

Fig. 30-12. Sealant is concentrated in central pits and fissures. (Courtesy L.D. Caulk Co., Milford Del.)

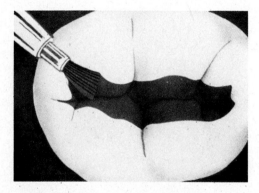

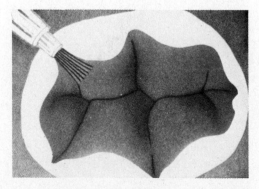

Fig. 30-13. Inclined planes of cusps are covered to complete coverage of occlusal surface. (Courtesy L.D. Caulk Co., Milford, Del.)

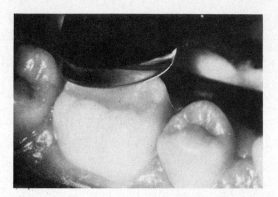

Fig. 30-14. Liquid sealant is polymerized with ultraviolet light according to manufacturer's directions. (Courtesy L.D. Caulk Co., Milford, Del.)

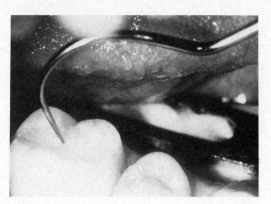

Fig. 30-15. Surface is evaluated with an explorer or probe to check total coverage. (Courtesy L.D. Caulk Co., Milford, Del.)

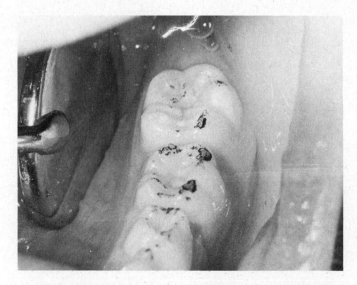

Fig. 30-16. Occlusal relationship is checked. In this case minimal occlusal contact occurs on sealant. (From Spohn, E.C., and Berry, T.G. 1979, In Boundy, S.S., and Reynolds, N.J., editors. Current concepts in dental hygiene, vol. 2. St. Louis: The C.V. Mosby Co.)

sealant or to let the sealant flow into the contact area.

6. If polymerization is to occur chemically, follow the manufacturer's directions for the appropriate period of time (usually 1 minute). If ultraviolet light is needed for polymerization, follow directions for placement of the light wand and for correct exposure time. Not only do current ultraviolet machines vary in their output, but they also become less effective in time as a result of deposits occurring on the ultraviolet lamp (Silverstone, 1983). Maintain the light source according to the manufacturer's specifications (Fig. 30-14).

7. After polymerization occurs, rinse and wipe the occlusal surface. This removes any excess sealant from the tooth surface. Evaluate the surface with a probe or carefully with an explorer to ensure that a smooth, hard surface has been achieved (Fig. 30-15).

8. Check the occlusal relationship with articulating paper (Fig. 30-16). Check the contact between the teeth with floss.

CONCLUSION

Research continues to verify the role of sealants in the practice of preventive dentistry. Because of the time and expertise involved in successfully applying this material, the procedure seems especially suited to the expanded-function dental auxiliary. Reexamination and reapplication of sealants at recall intervals help improve the success rate of this procedure and increase the clinician's involvement in providing a total preventive program for his/her patients.

In summary, these well-documented conclusions can be stated about pit and fissure sealants (Pullman, 1983):

1. Pit and fissure sealants are effectively retained on occlusal surfaces of posterior teeth.

2. Pit and fissure sealants are effective in reducing the incidence of occlusal caries.

3. Sealant failures do not increase the susceptibility of the occlusal surface to caries. Partially retained sealants still provide significant protection against caries.

4. Pit and fissure sealants are retained more effectively in premolars than in molars. Also, mandibular teeth show better sealant retention than maxillary teeth.

5. Caries sealed under sealants does not progress but tends to regress.

6. When auxiliaries are trained properly, the cost-benefit ratio and the effectiveness of the sealant can be favorable.

7. Generally, teeth are most susceptible to caries during the first year after eruption. Therefore for the maximum preventive effect, pit and fissure sealants should be placed as early as possible after eruption.

ACTIVITIES

1. Practice sealant technique on a typodont or on extracted teeth using various manufacturer's products.

2. Practice techniques for isolation with rubber dam application or a clamp and cotton roll.

3. Practice a four-handed technique for sealant application.

4. Identify an appropriate patient, and apply a pit and fissure sealant.

REVIEW QUESTIONS

1. Compare the significance of pit and fissure sealants in preventing occlusal caries with two methods of caries prevention attempted previously.

2. How might the following list of factors be considered in determining whether the sealant application is appropriate for this particular patient?

   Patient age: 12 years old
   New resident; moved from nonfluoride area
   Teeth No. 3, No. 14, No. 19, and No. 30 restored
   Teeth No. 18 and No. 31 erupted recently
   No current interproximal caries radiographically
   Home care and plaque control: good
   Parents concerned about diet and regular dental care

3. List the steps to be followed in the sealant application procedure.

REFERENCES

Buonocore, M.G. 1971. Caries prevention in pits and fissures sealed with an adhesive resin polymerized by ultra violet light: a two year study of a single adhesive application. J. Am. Dent. Assoc. **82:**1090.

Buonocore, M.G. 1973. Sealants: questions and answers. J. Am. Soc. Prevent. Dent. **3:**44.

Buonocore, M.G. 1975. The use of adhesives in dentistry. Springfield, Ill.: Charles C Thomas, Publisher.

Craig, R.G., O'Brien, W.J., and Powers, J.M. 1983. Dental materials: properties and manipulation, ed. 3. St. Louis: The C.V. Mosby Co.

Dennison, J.B., et al. 1980. A clinical comparison of sealant and amalgam in the treatment of pit and fissures. I. Clinical performance after 18 months. Pediatr. Dent. **2:**167.

Dennison, J.B., et al. 1980. A clinical comparison of sealant and amalgam in the treatment of pit and fissures. II. Clinical application and maintenance during an 18 month period. Pediatr. Dent. **2:**176.

Going, R.E., et al. 1977. Four year clinical evaluation of a pit and fissure sealant. J. Am. Dent. Assoc. **95:**972.

Going, R.E., et al. 1978. The viability of microorganisms in carious lesions five years after covering with a fissure sealant. J. Am. Dent. Assoc. **97:**455.

Gwinnett, A.J. 1973. The bonding of sealants to enamel. J. Am. Soc. Prevent. Dent. **3:**21.

Handelman, S.L. 1983. Effect of sealant placement on occlusal caries progression. Clin. Prevent. Dent. **4**(5):11.

Handelman, S.L., et al. 1972. A preliminary report on the effect of a fissure sealant on bacteria in dental caries. J. Prosthet. Dent. **27:**390.

Handelman, S.L. 1981. Use of adhesive sealants over occlusal carious lesions: radiographic evaluation. Community Dent. Oral Epidemiol. **9:**256.

Horowitz, H.S., Heifetz, S.B., and Poulsen, S. 1977. Retention and effectiveness of a single application of an adhesive sealant in preventing occlusal caries: final report after five years of study in Kalispell, Montana. J. Am. Dent. Assoc. **95:**1133.

Katz, S., McDonald, J., and Stookey, G. 1979. Preventive dentistry in action. Upper Montclair, N.J.: D.C.P. Publishing.

Mertz-Fairhurst, E.J., et al. 1979. Clinical progress of sealed and unsealed caries. I. Depth changes and bacterial counts. J. Prosthet. Dent. **42:**633. (a)

Mertz-Fairhurst, E.J., et al. 1979. Clinical progress of sealed and unsealed caries. II. Standardized radiographs and clinical observation. J. Prosthet. Dent. **42:**633. (b)

Mertz-Fairhurst, E.J., et al. 1982. A comparative study of two pit and fissure sealants: six year results in Augusta, Ga. J. Am. Dent. Assoc. **105:**237.

Messer, L.B., and Cline, J.T. 1980. Relative caries experience of sealed versus unsealed permanent posterior teeth: a three year study. ASDC J. Dent. Child. **61:**405.

Pullman, T.M. 1983. The effectiveness of pit and fissure sealants. J. Mich. Dent. Assoc. **65**(2):91.

Ripa, L.W. 1973. Occlusal sealing: rationale of the technique and historical review. J. Am. Soc. Prevent. Dent. **3:**32.

Ripa, L.W. 1982. Occlusal sealants: rationale and review of clinical trials. Clin. Prevent. Dent. **4**(5):3.

Rock, W.P., et al. 1982. A comparative study between a chemically polymerised fissure sealant resin and a light cured resin. Br. Dent. J. **152**(7):232.

Silverstone, L.M. 1978. Preventive dentistry. Fort Lee, N.J.: Update Publishing International, Inc.

Silverstone, L.M. 1983. The current status of adhesive sealants. Dent. Hyg. **57**(5):44.

Simonsen, R.J. 1980. The clinical effectiveness of a colored pit and fissure sealant at 24 months. Pediatr. Dent. **2:**10.

Simonsen, R.J. 1982. Potential uses of pit and fissure sealants in innovative ways: a review. J. Pub. Health Dent. **42:**305.

Spohn, E., and Berry, T. 1979. Pit and fissure sealants. In Boundy, S.S., and Reynolds, N.J., editors: Current concepts in dental hygiene. vol. 2. St. Louis: The C.V. Mosby Co.

Takahashi, Y., et al. 1980. The effect of sodium fluoride in acid etching solution on sealant bond and fluoride uptake. J. Dent. Res. **59:**625.

31 CONTROL OF TOOTH HYPERSENSITIVITY

OBJECTIVES: *The reader will be able to*

1. Discuss the interrelationships of dentin, cementum, enamel, the dentoenamel junction, and Tome's fibers as they relate to hypersensitivity.
2. Describe the three general categories of stimuli that elicit pain response and give examples of each.
3. Discuss the importance of plaque in the prognosis of treating hypersensitivity.
4. Describe antihypersensitive products available for home care.
5. Select and justify in-office procedures for treating sensitivity.
6. Comment on the current American Dental Association and Food and Drug Administration positions for desensitizing products.

Dentinal sensitivity has been defined as a painful response to an irritation when the root of the tooth is exposed (Gedalia et al., 1978). Pain in the area of the cementoenamel junction is one of the more difficult and challenging management problems to both the patient and the dental professional. Usually the pain is directly related to the stimulating agent (i.e., pain begins immediately when the stimulus is applied and ceases soon after the stimulus is removed).

It has been estimated that approximately 40 million adults in the United States have dentinal hypersensitivity at one time or another and more than 10 million have long-term or chronic hypersensitivity (Kanapka, 1982). While the development of better periodontal procedures has enabled treatment and maintenance of many teeth, this can be accompanied by gingival recession or exposed root surfaces, which are prone to developing sensitivity (Goldman, 1982; Green, Green, and McFall, 1977).

There is little concrete evidence regarding the etiology or cause of tooth sensitivity, the process by which pain sensation is transferred from the exterior of the tooth to the pulp (Tronstad, 1982), the ultimate prognosis of the problem, or the treatment regimens that are beneficial for the majority of patients (Yankell, 1982; Wycoff, 1982). The areas of concern, however, are easily identified;

examination of the sensitive area often reveals that either the enamel and cementum or both have eroded or been planed away, thus leaving exposed dentin (Goldman, 1982; Wycoff, 1982).

ETIOLOGY OF HYPERSENSITIVITY

Tooth sensitivity is a problem that patients often recognize. Often when an individual reports to the dental office with this problem, it is due (1) to caries that have penetrated through the enamel into the dentinal area to leaking margins of restorations, (2) to gingival recession resulting from periodontal disease, or (3) to exposure or abrasion of the enamel and/or cemental tooth layers covering the dentin.

Dental procedures can contribute to or initiate the onset or progression of hypersensitivity. Periodontal therapy techniques may create or increase exposure of root surfaces, and it is recommended that concepts of hypersensitivity be explained to the patient when such procedures as root planing and other scaling procedures in the gingival margin area are to be performed. The root surface is covered with cementum, which is softer than calculus and often is removed by hand scaling or with ultrasonic cavitation to expose the dentinal surface.

Caries or crown preparations by the dentist may also elicit sensitivity. For example, if temporary filling materials are in contact with the dentin for an excessive length of time after a cavity preparation has been performed, sensitivity may result. Temporary or permanent crowns on prepared teeth may create sensitivity problems during placement or, if leakage results, around the exposed root surface.

Stimuli that may elicit hypersensitivity have been classified in three primary areas (Grant, Stern, and Everett, 1979). A direct *mechanical* stimulation can occur during dental instrumentation (e.g., during exploratory procedures or scaling). Direct trauma can result during brushing, especially when toothbrushes with firm-textured bristles are being used, or during eating when a metal utensil may inadvertently hit a sensitive tooth area. The second type of stimuli that causes tooth sensation is *thermal*. Responses can occur when hot or cold foods or liquids are consumed or when cold air reaches the exposed dentinal areas. *Chemical* stimuli can also cause pain, especially with sweet, sour, or highly acidic foods. Plaque is also associated with chemically induced pain. For example, after the consumption of sweets or carbohydrates plaque microorganisms can metabolize these materials to produce acid pH levels.

MECHANISMS OF PAIN SENSITIVITY

The rationale for using specific desensitizing materials has not been fully defined (Everett, Hall, and Phatak, 1966; Grant, Stern, and Everett, 1979; Peden, 1977). The techniques used focus on four primary mechanisms of action. One procedure is designed to *deposit or precipitate an insoluble material* at the ends of the nerves or fibrous areas to act as a barrier to painful stimuli. Fluorides are thought to work in this manner. Another approach has attempted to *denature the superficial ends of the nerve endings or Tomes' fibers* in dentin with agents such as silver nitrate or calcium phosphate. A third procedure attempts to *stimulate secondary dentin formation* with calcium hydroxide, thus forming an insulating barrier to protect the pulp from external stimuli. The fourth method has been to *reduce hyperemia in the pulp* through the use of antiinflammatory compounds such as corticosteroids.

The mechanism of action of agents used to treat hypersensitivity has not been related to dental morphology (Avery, 1974; Stanley, 1974; Susi, 1978). Nerve fibers have not been demonstrated to extend from the pulp through the dentin to the dentoenamel junction (DEJ) (Tronstad, 1982). It also has not been established why the area closest to the DEJ appears to be the most sensitive. The most common explanation is based on the extensive branching and anastomosing of dentinal tubules as they approach the DEJ. Thus it appears that a stimulus affecting a few tubules can be transmitted to many other tubules and eventually result in an increased number of nerve fibers being stimulated. The unique feature of pulp in dentin is that, regardless of the stimuli (mechanism, thermal, or chemical), only one sensation is elicited—that of pain. This is based on the theory that pulp contains only free pain receptor nerve endings.

TREATMENT OF HYPERSENSITIVITY

Although there are many products available for use either by the patient or in a professional office, there is no one accepted modality that gives maximum or consistent benefit (Chasens, 1974; Everett, Hall, and Phatak, 1960; Goldman, 1982; Grant, Stern, and Everett, 1979; Peden, 1977; Yankell, 1982; Wycoff, 1982).

Since early in dental research, many agents have been tested for treating hypersensitive teeth. The essential criteria used to select agents to be tested have not changed since they were developed by Grossmann (1935). They are as follows:

1. Easy to use and apply
2. Nonirritating
3. Minimum number of dental appointments required (applications)
4. Painless
5. Minimum application time
6. Will not discolor teeth
7. No danger to teeth or soft tissues
8. Minimum of expense

These criteria apply to both professional and over-the-counter (OTC) products.

Clinical studies to determine the effectiveness of agents or products for desensitization are difficult to conduct because of the following factors:

1. Sole use of subjective evaluations
2. Lack of proper controls
3. Lack of objective measurements
4. High control response

Many evaluations have been based on subjective reactions. In these studies, the person's reaction to the products being tested has been based on his/her impressions of whether there was poor, fair, good, or excellent improvement. In addition, several studies have been based on the patient's evaluation under unsupervised use and without using a placebo or control product (i.e., a product containing no known effective agent). Methods used to quantitate pain also have been poor. One common method for eliciting a sensitive reaction has been to use a sharp probe at the sensitive tooth site. Responses are based on the subject's subjective indication of the amount of pain induced by this mechanical stimulation. This method has drawbacks, including the reliability of the amount of pressure applied and the need for ensuring that the probe is placed in the same critical, sensitive area. Other approaches to monitoring product effectiveness have included thermal stimuli (e.g., cold stimuli such as ice or ethyl chloride or the use of solutions at defined temperatures).

Two types of instrumentation have been developed that can be applied to the tooth surface to produce specified temperatures at the probe site (Kanapka, 1982, Smith and Ash, 1964a, 1964b; Tarbet et al., 1982). This equipment has been used to critically evaluate agents with desensitizing potential and has recently resulted in acceptance of two products by the American Dental Association (Chasens, 1974; Kanapka, 1982).

A major problem with testing desensitizing agents or products can be the high degree of reduction in sensitivity that occurs in groups treated with control products. This may be due to a general decline over a period of time (often observed with sensitivity problems) or to improved cleaning by patients who become aware of being seen routinely by the dental professional.

Home care procedures should be emphasized as a primary factor when initiating treatment of sensitivity. It is important to have adequate plaque control procedures well developed by the patient before professional treatments are started (Chasens, 1974; Grant, Stern, and Everett, 1979; Green, Green, and McFall, 1977; Peden 1977) and for long-term benefits (Wycoff, 1982). In addition to proper brushing and flossing procedures, the use of other topical and interdental aids to achieve cleaning and/or burnishing should be initiated. It is also important to discuss diet with the patient and, if necessary, to eliminate foods that are acidic or sour, as well as those that are fermentable carbohydrates, which can produce acids in plaque. It is also important to evaluate the patient's toothbrush and dentifrice product. It is suggested that soft or ultrasoft toothbrushes be used as well as dentifrices with minimum abrasive properties. There is no uniformity among toothbrush manufacturers as to the texture of the toothbrush bristles, and one manufacturer's soft bristles may be firmer than another manufacturer's medium bristles (Yankell and Emling, 1978). As discussed in Chapter 26, toothpaste abrasiveness is difficult to monitor clinically, and it is up to the dental professional to individualize the dentifrice used by each patient. Regardless of treatment, it has been indicated that tooth sensitivity can improve with a change in oral hygiene procedures (Gedalia et al., 1978; Hiatt and Johansen, 1972).

Commercially available products

Desensitizing toothpastes are widely promoted to both the dental profession and the public. Recently the ADA Council on Dental Therapeutics has classified two toothpastes containing potassium nitrate as the active agent (Hodosh 1974) as effective in relieving dental hypersensitivity. One of these, Denquel (Richardson-Vicks, Inc.) has been classified as "accepted," allowing the product to use the statement "an effective densensitizing dentifrice that with regular brushing can be of significant value in relieving sensitivity to hot and cold in otherwise normal teeth" on their packaging and in their advertising (ADA Council, 1982). The product Promise (Block Drug Co., Inc.) has received "provisional acceptance," indicating that initial studies have shown reasonable evidence of usefulness but that additional studies are still needed.

Three other products are specifically marketed as densensitizing dentifrices. Two of these, Sensodyne (Block Drug Co., Inc.) and Thermodent (Chas. Pfizer & Co.), contain strontium chloride as the claimed active ingredient. The third product, Protect (J.O. Butler), contains dibasic sodium citrate in a pluronic gel as the claimed active ingredient. These products have not been classified by the ADA Council on Dental Therapeutics. While fluoride toothpastes are often recommended by dental professionals for use in treating hypersensitivity, and indeed theoretically should provide some benefit, none of the currently marketed fluoride products have been tested or classified for this claim.

Another proposed method of treating dental hypersensitivity is *iontophoresis*. The purpose of this procedure is to enhance movement of ions by electric currents. With this system, a negative ion such as fluoride would be pushed away from the toothbrush surface and encouraged to penetrate dental enamel. Another mechanism of action attributed to iontophoresis is the formation of secondary dentin. Several clinical studies have been reported on the use of iontophoresis alone or coupled with the use of fluoride material or a strontium chloride preparation. In general, iontophoresis alone has been claimed to be effective against hypersensitivity; when this procedure has been coupled with an active agent, an enhanced benefit has been reported. The American Dental Association has reviewed these studies but has not concluded that efficacy has been proved (ADA Council, 1982).

Professional products

The products used by dental professionals have not changed significantly in content or method(s) of application since they were comprehensively reviewed by Everett, Hall, and Phatak in 1966, and as described in many textbooks and review articles since then (Chasens, 1974; Grant, Stern, and Everett, 1979; Peden 1977). None of these products has been classified as effective by the ADA Council on Dental Therapeutics (ADA Council, 1982) or the Food and Drug Administration.

Initial preparation of the teeth must be done before any desensitizing agent is professionally applied. Teeth must be free of all hard and soft deposits as assured by scaling, root planing, and polishing with a porte polisher if the teeth are very sensitive. In addition, 3% hydrogen peroxide can be applied to the teeth with a cotton pellet for further cleansing. Teeth are rinsed with warm water, dried, and isolated prior to treatment. Care should be taken to use air lightly or to dry the sensitive areas with cotton rolls. Rather than refer to specific products, only the active claimed ingredient(s) of products are indicated here.

Formalin in a concentration of 40% is claimed to precipitate albumin or denature Tomes' fibers. A small amount of the solution is placed on a cotton pellet and rubbed into the sensitive area. A porte polisher is used to continue rubbing for a defined time period. This agent should not contact the mucosa, since a reaction (precipitation of protein) with the tissues will occur, resulting in soft tissue irritation.

A solution of basic or ammoniated *silver nitrate* is stated to precipitate albumin and denature Tomes' fibers. This solution is applied directly to the sensitive area and then is precipitated with a reducing agent such as eugenol. This preparation may be irritating to soft dental tissue and cause tooth discoloration.

Solutions of 40% *zinc chloride* and 20% *potassium ferrocyanide* are used in a two-step process. The clinical result of this combination is protein precipitation and denaturization of Tomes' fibers. The solution of zinc chloride is applied with a moist cotton pellet or porte polisher. With the use of unwaxed floss or tape, the zinc chloride is rubbed vigorously on the interproximal surfaces and allowed to remain on the tooth for 1 minute. Excess solution is removed from the gingival margin. While the teeth are still moist, the second solution of potassium ferrocyanide is applied. This solution is rubbed vigorously until a white precipitate forms. Again, dental floss is worked interproximally. One minute is allowed for the reaction to occur, and then the excess is removed from the gingival margin.

Professional *fluoride gels and solutions* for caries treatment are used to treat hypersensitivity. As with caries prophylaxis, the teeth should be scaled and stain removed prior to fluoride treatment. With generalized sensitivity or many areas of gingival recession, tray or painting procedures are used. If specific teeth are sensitive, fluoride can be burnished into the area with a porte polisher. There are also fluoride products with claimed desensitization properties available. The first contains equal amounts of sodium fluoride, kaolin, and glycerin. This product is rubbed into the dried isolated sensitive area with a porte polisher for 1 to 5 minutes. The mechanism of action is attributed to the deposition of insoluble salts. Two products are available that contain *sodium silicofluoride*. The first of these is a saturated solution containing 0.7% in cold water or 0.9% in hot water. This preparation is rubbed into sensitive areas for 5 minutes. A calcium gel forms, which is stated to be an improved insulating barrier. Sodium silicofluoride is also combined with calcium hydroxide in a two-step procedure. Initially, the sodium silicofluoride is applied and allowed to react for 1 to 2 minutes. Then the area is painted with 5% calcium hydroxide and allowed to stand for 1 minute. This combination treatment is claimed to aid in a more rapid and complete precipitation and a more effective desensitization.

A *stannous fluoride* paste containing 8.9% stannous ion is being promoted for use in the treatment of sensitivity. During prophylaxis this paste should be rubbed into sensitive areas, preferably with a porte polisher.

In all of the aforementioned fluoride treatments, the suggested regimen is to apply the material at weekly intervals at least three times to obtain optimum results.

Corticosteroid products also are available for dentin hypersensitivity. These products are used primarily for sensitivity due to cavity preparations but are also used for dentin hypersensitivity. Usually the agent is administered by being rubbed into the sensitive site. The mode of action is considered to be that of decreasing pulp hyperemia.

There are several professional iontophoresis units available. Two are discussed here. The first of these is the Chayes-Siemon apparatus. This contains a 9-volt battery and an ammeter that must register 20, or about 0.4 milliampere, to ensure ion transfer. The patient holds the grip, or positive charge, of the equipment. The dental professional then applies the negatively charged end of the equipment, a sable brush dipped into a 1% sodium fluoride solution, in contact with the sensitive area for 1 minute. Because of a fairly high current, the patient may experience slight pain on initial contact with this equipment.

The second apparatus is the barrel-shaped Lemonstron apparatus with a sable brush at one end. The clinician moistens the brush with a 2% sodium fluoride solution and applies this to the sensitive tooth area. The circuit is completed by the clinician touching the patient. The brush is allowed to contact the sensitive area for 1 minute. Since this unit operates with two penlite batteries and there is no ammeter, the clinician is unsure of the quantity of current being dispensed.

Although only products or agents commercially available to the public or to the professional have been reviewed here, many compounds have been tested. Following is a list of agents or combinations (Chasens, 1974; Everett, Hall, and Phatak, 1966; Goldman, 1982; Grant, Stern, and Everett, 1979; Peden, 1977; Yankell, 1982; Wycoff, 1982):

Calcium hydroxide (Leven, Yearwood, and Carpenter, 1973)
Calcium phosphate (Hiatt and Johansen, 1972)
Corticosteroids
Formalin
Fluorides (APF, MFP, sodium, sodium silicofluoride, stannous)
Glycerin
Magnesium hydroxide (Levin, Yearwood, and Carpenter, 1973)
Phenol
Potassium nitrate (Hodosh, 1974)
Potassium hydroxide
Silver nitrate
Strontium chloride plus sodium fluoride (Gedalia et al., 1978)
Zinc chloride plus potassium ferrocyanide

ACTIVITIES

1. Determine if members of the class have areas of gingival recession and/or tooth sensitivity. Test both areas with the following: ice, a blast of air, cold water, hot water, and a sharp probe. What is the most severe reaction in terms of speed of reaction and pain? Do areas of recession and sensitivity differ? Why? What parameters do you think would be best for testing a new antihypersensitive agent?
2. Review two publications on desensitizing products, pre- and post-1970. Comment on the use of placebo reaction and on the measurements used.

REVIEW QUESTIONS

1. What are the primary areas where tooth sensitivity occurs?
2. What professional procedures contribute to tooth sensitivity?
3. What are the three stimuli that elicit hypersensitivity?
4. Classify the mechanisms of action of desensitizing agents.
5. True or false
   a. Several sensitivity products are classified as effective by the ADA Council on Dental Therapeutics and the Food and Drug Administration.
   b. The tooth area closest to the DEJ is the most sensitive.
   c. The placebo effect often occurs in treating sensitivity.
   d. Regardless of treatment, improved oral hygiene can reduce sensitivity.
6. Describe how the fluoride treatment for caries is:
   a. Different from the fluoride treatment for sensitivity
   b. Similar to the fluoride treatment for sensitivity

REFERENCES

ADA Council on Dental Therapeutics. 1982. Dental therapeutics, ed. 39. Chicago: American Dental Association.

Avery, J.K. 1974. Anatomic considerations in the mechanisms of pain and sensitivity in the teeth and supporting tissues. In Chasens, A.I., and Kaslick, R.S., editors. Mechanisms of pain and sensitivity in the teeth and supporting tissues. Rutherford, N.J.: Fairleigh Dickinson University.

Chasens, A.I. 1974. The management of tooth pain and sensitivity. In Chasens, A.I., and Kaslick, R.S., editors. Mechanisms of pain and sensitivity in the teeth and supporting tissues. Rutherford, N.J.: Fairleigh Dickinson University.

Everett, F.G., Hall, W.B., and Phatak, N.M. 1966. Treatment of hypersensitive dentin. J. Oral Ther. Pharmacol. **2:**300.

Gedalia, I., et al. 1978. The effect of fluoride and strontium application on dentin: *in vivo* and *in vitro* studies. J. Periodontol. **49:**269.

Goldman, H.M. 1982. Dental sensitivity: a periodontist's perspective. Comp. Contin. Educ. Dent. (Suppl.)**3:**S110.

Grant, D.A., Stern, I.B., and Everett, F.G. 1979. Periodontics: in the tradition of Orban and Gottlieb, ed. 5. St. Louis: The C.V. Mosby Co.

Green, B.L., Green, M.L., and McFall, W.T., Jr. 1977. Calcium hydroxide and potassium nitrate as desensitizing agents for hypersensitive root surfaces. J. Periodontol. **48:**667.

Grossman, L.I. 1935. A systematic method for the treatment of hypersensitive dentin. J. Am. Dent. Assoc. **22:**592.

Hiatt, W.H., and Johansen, E. 1972. Root preparation. I. Obturation of dentinal tubules in treatment of root hypersensitivity. J. Periodontol. **43:**373.

Hodosh, M. 1974. A superior desensitizer—potassium nitrate. J. Am. Dent. Assoc. **88:**831.

Kanapka, J.A. 1982. A new agent. Comp. Contin. Educ. Dent. (Suppl.)**3:**S118.

Levin, M.P., Yearwood, L.L., and Carpenter, W.N. 1973. The desensitizing effect of calcium hydroxide and magnesium hydroxide on hypersensitive dentin. Oral Surg. **35:**741.

Peden, J.W. 1977. Dental hypersensitivity. J. West. Soc. Periodontol. **25:**75.

Smith, B.A., and Ash, M.M., Jr. 1964. Evaluation of a desensitizing dentifrice. J. Am. Dent. Assoc. **68:**639. (a)

Smith, B.A., and Ash, M.M., Jr. 1964. A study of a desensitizing dentifrice and cervical hypersensitivity. J. Periodontol. **35:**222. (b)

Stanley, H.R. 1974. Dentin permeability and sensitivity. In Chasens, A.I., and Kaslick, R.S., editors. Mechanisms of pain and sensitivity in the teeth and supporting tissues. Rutherford, N.J.: Fairleigh Dickinson University.

Susi, F.R. 1978. Sensory receptor morphology in the teeth and their supporting tissues. Dent. Clin. North Am. **22**(1):3.

Tarbet, W.J., et al. 1982. Home treatment for dentinal hypersensitivity: a comparative study. J. Am. Dent. Assoc. **105:**227.

Tronstad, L. 1982. The anatomic and physiologic basis for dentinal sensitivity. Comp. Contin. Educ. Dent. (Suppl.)**3:**S99.

Yankell, S.L. 1982. At home treatment. Comp. Contin. Educ. Dent. (Suppl.)**3:**S115.

Yankell, S., and Emling, R.C. 1978. Understanding dental products: what you should know and what your patient should know. Continuing Dental Education, University of Pennsylvania School of Dental Medicine **1:** No. 7.

Wycoff, S.J. 1982. Current treatment for dentinal hypersensitivity: in-office treatment. Comp. Contin. Educ. Dent. (Suppl.)**3:**S113.

PAIN AND PAIN CONTROL: TOPICAL AND LOCAL ANESTHESIA

OBJECTIVES: *The reader will be able to*

1. Explain the relevance of psychosomatic, topical, and local anesthesia to dental hygiene practice.
2. Define pain, pain perception, and pain reaction; discuss the influences on pain reaction.
3. Develop an approach to be used to assist patients in coping with the pain that may be associated with dental treatment.
4. Explain why a thorough knowledge of the pharmacology, chemistry, and modes of action of anesthetic agents and vasoconstrictors and the possible medical complications is necessary for any dental personnel applying topical anesthestic or administering local anesthesia.
5. Draw and label the nerve anatomy supplying the maxilla and the mandible.
6. Identify the tissues innervated by each of the nerves associated with dental local anesthesia.
7. Identify the tissues anesthetized by topical and local anesthesia.
8. Given several dental procedures, select the appropriate injections to be administered to achieve the desired anesthesia and identify the injection site.
9. Describe preliminary procedures to be performed prior to the administration of an injection.
10. When indicated, properly apply a topical anesthetic.

Pain and dental care go hand in hand for many people as is shown by the many cartoons and comedy routines centered around dental pain. This fear of being hurt or feeling pain prevents some people from seeking routine dental care. Dental personnel have used various methods to alleviate patients' pain, such as verbal reassurance, topical anesthetics, local anesthetics, conscious sedation, acupuncture, sedative premedication, general anesthesia, and hypnosis. As hygienists' responsibilities have increased to include the various expanded duties, pain control procedures such as application of topical anesthesia, administration of local anesthetics, and nitrous oxide and oxygen conscious sedation have been viewed as necessary procedures to be added to the hygienists' responsibilities. Some states' laws have been modified to permit dental hygienists to perform these procedures.

PAIN

Pain is a universal condition that everyone has experienced at some time. There is a dual aspect to pain, namely pain perception and pain reaction. *Pain perception* is the physical aspect, the process by which the pain is received and transmitted via the nervous system (Bennett, 1984). The nerve end organs, pain perceptors, sense the painful stimulus, and it is transmitted through the peripheral nervous system to the central nervous system. Pain perception is the same for most healthy persons, unless the nervous system has been damaged by injury or disease (Bennett, 1984). *Pain reaction*, the other aspect of pain, is a person's expression of or reaction to the perceived pain. Pain reaction varies from person to person, being influenced by conscious and unconscious thinking as well as emotional, cultural, and ethnic factors (Burstein et al., 1979; Christensen, 1980; Foreman, 1979; Spear, 1977). Persons having minimal reactions to pain are said to have low pain reaction and high *pain reaction thresholds;* the pain reaction threshold is inversely related to pain reaction (Bennett, 1984). Pain reaction is discussed in greater detail on pp. 542 and 543.

PAIN CONTROL

Within dentistry, various methods are used to alleviate the patient's pain—both perception and reaction. These methods are referred to as *pain control;* some of the methods are listed at the beginning of the chapter. As described by Bennett (1984), there are essentially five methods of pain control. The first is *removal of the cause,* which is not always possible. If the cause of gingival pain during a scaling procedure is the clinician's use of a curette at too open an angle, the cause of the pain can be removed by closing the angulation. If, however, the cause of the pain is edematous tender tissue, the use of a topical or local anesthetic may be needed, since the cause (swollen gingiva) cannot be removed. A second method of pain control is the use of *psychosomatic methods,* such as verbal instruction or suggestion, hypnosis, relaxation techniques, and distraction methods. Psychosomatic methods alleviate the patient's pain by lessening his/her pain reaction. A third method of pain control is the use of a drug to *block the pathway of the painful impulse.* Topical and local anesthestic agents are used in this method to block the impulse before it is carried to the central nervous system. Blocking the impulse interferes with pain perception, thus lessening or eliminating pain. Both Bennett (1984) and Malamed (1980) present discussions of how the painful impulse is blocked and should be consulted by the reader. A fourth method of pain control is to *raise the pain reaction threshold* with drugs that have analgesic properties; this method is referred to as *conscious sedation* (Bennett, 1984). One method of conscious sedation—nitrous oxide and oxygen analgesia—is discussed in Chapter 33. Many drugs have analgesic properties. Narcotics such as codeine or meperidine hydrochloride (Demerol), as well as other types of drugs including barbiturates and psychosedatives, have analgesic properties and are used in dentistry. These drugs can be used alone or in combination to achieve conscious sedation (Bennett, 1984). The fifth method of pain control is achieved through *depression of the central nervous system* with general anesthetic agents. The general anesthesia prevents the patient's reaction to pain (Bennett, 1984).

An introduction to psychosomatic methods and the use of topical and local anesthetic agents are presented in this chapter. After reading this chapter, the reader should be able to use some of the psychosomatic methods and topical anesthestic agents for pain control. Although the educational background of dental hygienists provides the prerequisite knowledge (i.e., chemistry, pharmacology, medical evaluation, anatomy, and emergency detection and procedures) as well as other knowledge necessary for a thorough local anesthesia course, before administering local anesthetics, any dental personnel—dentist or dental hygienist—should participate in an in-depth local anesthesia course, which provides information about anesthetic agents, including the effects, contraindications, complications, reactions, patient evaluation and management, and technique. The administration of local anesthetics must be taken seriously by the practitioner; a foreign substance is being placed into a person's body, and a drug is being administered that will probably produce the desired effect but that may also produce undesired effects. The practitioner must be able to differentiate among the desired and undesired effects of local anesthetics and initiate the appropriate care. A properly educated dental hygienist is capable of assuming the added responsibilities associated with the administration of local anesthetics, but *proper formal education is essential* (American Association of Dental Schools, 1980). This chapter provides only a general overview of local anesthesia and emphasizes determining when a local anesthetic is needed and which injections will provide the desired anesthesia. The skill of administering an injection is not presented. The ability to determine which injection is needed, even if the hygienist does not perform the injection, allows the hygienist to request the proper injection; prepare the necessary armamentarium; and prepare the patient, including the application of the topical anesthetic. In addition, an understanding of the uses and limitations of topical anesthesia and local anesthesia will provide the dental hygienist with a realistic understanding of the capabilities of each agent for pain control.

INFLUENCES ON PAIN REACTION

As previously mentioned, pain reaction varies from person to person and may even vary for the same person depending on his/her mental and physical condition. Factors that influence a person's interpretation of an event as being painful can be divided into three catagories: cognitive, emotional, and symbolic (Wepman, 1978).

Cognitive factors are those that influence how

persons think about pain or when they interpret a sensation as being painful. There is evidence that what the clinician says can modify how patients think and react to painful stimuli. For example, Steblay and Beaman (1982) showed that telling patients that some of their physiologic sensations, such as temporarily increased heart rates, were due to the local anesthetic allowed the patients to properly associate the feelings with the anesthetic. This in turn seemed to allow the patients to be less fearful and experience less pain.

Wepman (1978) has reported an experiment in which patients were told that they would experience less pain if they listened to music through earphones during treatment (Melzack, 1973). The patients seemed to develop ways to cope with the pain, or to distract themselves from it, by tapping a foot, fingers, or humming. The patients reported less pain.

The above example helps illustrate the concept that people are less susceptible to pain, fear, or anxiety when they feel they have some control over a situation. Developing a way to cope with pain, as above, indicates having some control. When patients feel helpless or not in control, they are likely to experience greater pain. Thus it is important to allow the patient to have some control in managing the pain whenever possible (Wepman, 1978).

Emotional factors such as anxiety greatly influence patients' tolerence for pain. In general, increased anxiety is associated with decreased tolerance for pain, a high pain reaction, and a low pain reaction threshold (Bennett, 1984). For example, a patient, nervous about a scaling procedure, who jumps when the clinician establishes a fulcrum has a high pain reaction and a low pain reaction threshold. Increased anxiety is many times exacerbated by patients' feelings of helplessness or of not being in control of the situation. Certainly, dental treatment is a situation in which patients have a limited amount of control. In order to decrease anxiety and thus increase patients' pain reaction thresholds, it is important to allow patients to have a sense of control and assist them in relieving their anxiety. The verbal instructions given by Steblay and Beaman (1982) gave patients information that allowed them to have a sense of control and thus decreased their anxiety.

Events in patients' lives such as marriage, the birth of a child, change in a job, loss of a job, divorce, or the death of a loved one may also affect their ability to cope with pain. Since such events create stress and its associated anxiety, it is likely that patients may have a decreased pain reaction threshold. Careful listening, as described in Chapter 7, will help the clinician discern if life events are affecting a particular patient and perhaps her/his pain reaction.

The *symbolic factors* affecting pain are unique to each person, but universally pain symbolizes an attack, damage, or a threat. All persons have unconscious symbolizations and feelings of which they are unaware and usually unable to explain. These unconscious feelings and symbolizations regarding pain affect patients' pain reactions (Wepman, 1978). The dental health professional can recognize that all persons react to pain and are affected by their unconscious feelings. It is not the role of the dental health professional to analyze why a patient reacts to pain in a certain manner. Rather, the role of the professional is to listen and observe to discern when patients are in pain and to take steps to alleviate the pain associated with dental treatment.

A variety of other factors such as fatigue, sex, race, and ethnicity may affect persons' pain reactions. When persons are tired or fatigued, their pain reaction thresholds are decreased (Bennett, 1984). Various authors have indicated that pain reaction may be influenced by one's sex (Bennett, 1984), and race or ethnicity (Bennett, 1984; Christensen, 1980; Spear, 1977; Wepman, 1978). For example, men have a higher pain reaction threshold than women; Latin Americans and Southern Europeans have a lower pain reaction threshold than North Americans or Northern Europeans. Since different groups have different cultures that regard expression of emotions and pain in a variety of ways, it is not surprising that pain reactions may vary. Yet, these are generalizations that may be true for the majority of persons from a particular ethnic group; certainly, there are many exceptions. Thus these generalizations may be helpful to the clinician, but every patient must be treated as an individual with particular reactions to pain (Wepman, 1978).

PSYCHOSOMATIC METHODS OF PAIN CONTROL

In order to provide as painless dental treatment as possible, the health care provider must incorporate knowledge about pain reaction and psychosomatic methods into a general approach to pain control. Some suggestions for a general approach to pain control, including psychosomatic methods, are presented in this section. Perhaps the most important element of an approach is to develop helping relationships with patients (see Chapter 7) in which they can trust the health care provider. This is more than establishing rapport, such as asking the obligatory "How are you" (Wepman, 1978). Rather, it is offering a relationship in which the provider genuinely cares about patients' well-being, especially their dental health. The health care provider must be truthful and honest with patients about procedures that are painful. It is highly inappropriate for the health care provider to tell patients that procedures will not hurt or will only hurt a second if the health care provider knows otherwise. The health care provider should take seriously patients' reports of pain and use methods to alleviate the pain. Patients' complaints of pain may sometimes be verbal, but many times they are nonverbal communications such as knitted eyebrows, rolling eyes, or white knuckles clinging to the chair's arms. The astute clinician will be attuned to such communications and question the patient to determine the source of the pain.

In addition to developing a helping relationship and being honest with the patient regarding pain associated with treatment, the health care provider must develop skills to alleviate pain. Some psychosomatic approaches include telling the patient about sensations associated with medication or treatment. Use of a soothing, not singsong, voice can help to relax or soothe the patient. The patient can be instructed to take a few deep breaths to help relax and ease tension. If the clinician is familiar with relaxation techniques such as tensing and relaxing muscle groups, these may be helpful for some patients (Atterbury, 1978; Foreman, 1979). Use of these techniques within a trusting, helping relationship may help the patient feel at ease with the clinician and more in control, thus increasing the patient's pain reaction threshold. Other methods that require further training, such as hypnosis, biofeedback, or progressive relaxation, can be used. The use of psychosomatic methods within a trusting, helping relationship has been presented because these pain control methods are many times overlooked, as is the importance of the quality of the relationship between patients and the health care provider. These methods can potentiate other pain control measures such as topical or local anesthesia, nitrous oxide and oxygen conscious sedation, and general anesthesia. Psychosomatic methods alone are rarely successful in controlling the pain associated with dental treatment. The health care provider should use other pain control measures as necessary to alleviate the patient's pain. The remainder of this chapter presents the use of local and topical anesthetic agents.

LOCAL ANESTHESIA

An overview of local anesthetic agents, their use, and sites of injection are presented prior to the use of topical anesthetics. An understanding of local anesthetics will enable the reader to better understand topical anesthetic agents and their use.

Local anesthetic agents

Local anesthetics are water-soluble hydrochloride salt solutions that have three components: the intermediate linkage, the hydrophilic group, and the lipophilic group (ADA Council on Dental Therapeutics [ADA-CDT], 1982; Bennett, 1984; Giovannitti and Bennett, 1979). Local anesthetics are classified as either *esters* or *amides,* depending on the type of intermediate linkage; the linkage is either an ester or an amide and determines many of the properties of the local anesthetic agent. The hydrophilic group functions to carry the solution through the interstitial tissues to the nerve; the lipophilic group promotes penetration of the anesthetic agent into the lipid-rich nerve. The lipophilic group also contains the charged portion of the agent, which interacts with the nerve fibers to block the nervous impulse and, hence, prevent the patient from experiencing pain (ADA-CDT, 1982; Bennett, 1984).

The ester type of local anesthetic was the first type of anesthetic agent used successfully in dentistry. The best known ester is procaine (Novocain). Other types of esters are tetracaine (Pontocaine) and propoxycaine (Ravocaine) (ADA-CDT, 1982; Bennett, 1984). Additional types of anesthetic agents (nonesters) were developed because the esters produce allergic reactions in some patients. The esters are broken down primarily in the plasma and in the liver; it is thought that the allergic reactions may be due to the esters being partially broken down in the plasma (Bennett, 1984; Giovannitti and Bennett, 1979; Larson, 1977).

The amides were developed after the esters had been used for a period of time. The most commonly used amides include lidocaine (Xylocaine), mepivacaine (Carbocaine), and prilocaine (Citanest). The amides are broken down in the liver, and there have not been any documented cases of allergic reactions to any of the *pure* amides (Bennett, 1984; Giovannitti and Bennett, 1979; Larson, 1977). Some allergic reactions have been reported as a result of amides that contain the preservative methylparaben (Bennett, 1984; Larson, 1977). Methylparaben is chemically similar to an ester, and it is thought that some patients have allergic reactions to this agent rather than to the amide anesthetic. Some amides are available without methylparaben.

Vasoconstrictors are added to some local anesthetics to increase their effectiveness and duration and to permit administration of smaller amounts. The vasoconstrictor constricts the blood vessels in the area, so that the anesthetic is carried away from the nerve at a slower rate. Commonly used vasoconstrictors include epinephrine, norepinephrine, levonordefrin, and others (ADA-CDT, 1982; Bennett, 1984) (Table 32-1).

Potency, toxicity, concentration, and maximum safe dose. The *potency* of a local anesthetic

Table 32-1. Sample of local anesthetic agents and vasoconstrictors

Anesthetic agent	Vasoconstrictor
Esters	
Procaine 2%	Epinephrine 1:50,000
Procaine 2%, tetracaine 0.15%	Neo-Cobefrin 1:20,000
Procaine 2%, propoxycaine 0.4%	Levophed 1:30,000
Amides	
Lidocaine HCl 2%	None
Lidocaine HCl 2%	Epinephrine 1:50,000
Lidocaine HCl 2%	Epinephrine 1:100,000
Mepivacaine HCl 3%	None
Mepivacaine 2%	Neo-Cobefrin 1:20,000
Prilocaine HCl 4%	None
Prilocaine Forte HCl 4%	Epinephrine 1:200,000

*Modified from Bennett, R.C. 1979. Monheim's local anesthesia and pain control in dental practice, ed. 6. St. Louis: The C.V. Mosby Co.; and ADA Council on Dental Therapeutics. 1982. Accepted dental therapeutics, ed. 39. Chicago: American Dental Association.

agent is the amount necessary to produce the desired effect. *Toxicity* refers to the amount of local anesthetic or vasoconstrictor necessary to produce a toxic overdose. Usually, the greater the potency of an agent, the greater the chance of a toxic overdose (Bennett, 1984). A toxic overdose occurs when the level of drug present in the blood or plasma is too high (Malamed, 1979). The signs, symptoms, and treatment of a local anesthetic or vasoconstrictor toxic overdose are discussed in Chapter 10. The blood plasma level of a local anesthetic or vasoconstrictive agent can become too high if (1) too much is given, (2) it is injected intravascularly, (3) it is rapidly absorbed, (4) it is metabolized slowly, or (5) it is unable to be excreted. Thus a toxic overdose can occur if the clinician's technique is faulty (1 and 2) or if the patient is medically compromised (3, 4, and 5). In either case it is essential that the clinician use proper injection techniques, such as aspirating and injecting slowly, and that the patient's medical history be reviewed carefully.

Local anesthetic and vasoconstrictive agents are available in various *concentrations* (Table 32-1) according to their potency. A weakly potent agent would be produced in a higher concentration in order to achieve the desired anesthetic or vasoconstrictive effect.

Each local anesthetic and vasoconstrictive agent has a *maximum safe dose (MSD);* the estimated greatest amount that can safely be given to a healthy 150-pound person (Bennett, 1984; Dafoe, 1982; Malamed, 1979; Rogo, 1982). Table 32-2 lists the MSDs for some local anesthetic and vasoconstrictive agents.

It should be noted that the MSDs are expressed in milligrams and that the anesthetic and vasoconstrictive agents are expressed in milligrams per milliliters. Whenever local anesthetic or vasoconstrictive agents are administered, the clinician should calculate the amount of each agent given to ensure that the MSD is not exceeded and record the amount in the patient's record (Fig. 4-1). A standard cartridge contains 1.8 ml. A 1.0% solution contains 10 mg/ml, so a cartridge of 1% solution is equivalent to 18 mg of anesthetic agent. One cartridge of 2.0% solution is equivalent to 36 mg of anesthetic agent. Thus if a patient were given two cartridges of a 1.0% local anesthetic agent, the patient would have received 36 mg of the agent

Table 32-2. Maximum safe doses for a healthy 150-pound person

	Amount	
Local anesthetic agents		
Procaine (Novocain)	400 mg	
Tetracaine (Pontocaine)	30 mg	
Lidocaine (Xylocaine)	300 mg	
Mepivacaine (Carbocaine)	300 mg	
Prilocaine (Citanest)	400 mg	
	Amounts for	
	Healthy persons	Medically compromised persons
Vasoconstrictive agents		
Epinephrine	0.2 mg	0.004 mg
Levophed (Norepinephrine)	0.34 mg	0.14 mg
Nordefrin (Cobefrin)	1.0 mg	0.4 mg
Levonordefrin (Neo-Cobefrin)	1.0 mg	0.4 mg

Modified from Bennett, R.C. 1979. Monheim's local anesthesia and pain control in dental practice, ed. 6. St. Louis: The C.V. Mosby Co.

(Bennett, 1984; Dafoe, 1982) (see box, p. 547).

The amount of vasoconstrictor administered should also be calculated and the MSDs observed. Epinephrine, the most commonly used vasoconstrictor, has an MSD of 0.2 mg for a healthy person and 0.004 mg for a person with a cardiac condition (Bennett, 1984). Again, the concentration of the agent must be considered in order to calculate the amount of drug administered. If one cartridge of solution containing epinephrine 1:100,000 is given, the patient will receive 0.018 mg of epinephrine. The box on p. 547 presents the formulas and information necessary to calculate the amounts of local anesthetic and vasoconstrictive agents administered.

When local anesthetic and vasoconstrictive agents are used in conjunction, one of the two agents will determine the MSD. For example, the MSD for epinephrine may be reached before the MSD for the local anesthetic, and no more can be given.

The health care provider must adjust the MSD for patients with compromised medical histories. Patients with heart conditions, such as cardiac arrhythmias or hypertension, should have reduced amounts, or no vasoconstrictors (Bennett, 1984; Malamed, 1979) (see Table 32-2). The MSD should also be adjusted downward for persons

weighing less than 150 pounds (Bennett, 1984; Malamed, 1979). By weight, the MSD for Citanest is 3.6 mg per pound up to a maximum of 600 mg (Malamed, 1979). Therefore a healthy person weighing 60 pounds can be given 216 mg, or three cartridges of prilocaine (Malamed, 1979). Calculating the MSD according to patients' weights appears to be becoming the preferred method, particularly for children (Bennett, 1984; Malamed, 1979; Rood, 1981). The MSDs given in Table 32-2 are helpful guidelines when working with healthy patients, but the practitioner must keep in mind that the amounts are to be adjusted for medically compromised and lighter persons. Many times, the package insert accompanying the local anesthetic agent will assist the practitioner in determining the appropriate dosages and the MSD.

Medical considerations

A complete and thorough review of the patient's medical history and vital signs is essential prior to the administration of a local anesthetic. Some patient's conditions may contraindicate a local anesthetic agent and/or vasoconstrictor. For example, patients with liver dysfunction should not be given an amide, since the liver's ability to break down the amide is compromised. Patients with heart conditions such as arrhythmias or hypertension should

---

Computation of amounts of agents administered

Local anesthetic agents

FORMULA:

1.8 ml per cartridge × Number of cartridges × Concentration of solution = mg administered

$$1\% = 10 \text{ ml}$$
$$2\% = 20 \text{ ml}$$
$$3\% = 30 \text{ ml}$$
$$4\% = 40 \text{ ml}$$

EXAMPLE: 2 cartridges of lidocaine 2%

$$1.8 \times 2 \times 20 = 72 \text{ mg}$$

Vasoconstrictive agents

FORMULA:

1.8 ml per cartridge × Number of cartridges × Concentration of agent = mg administered

Epinephrine
$$1:50,000 \ \ = 0.02 \text{ mg}$$
$$1:100,000 = 0.01 \text{ mg}$$
$$1:200,000 = 0.005 \text{ mg}$$

Norepinephrine
$$1:30,000 \ \ = 0.03 \text{ mg}$$

Nordefrin
$$1:10,000 \ \ = 0.1 \text{ mg}$$

Levonordefrin
$$1:20,000 \ \ = 0.05 \text{ mg}$$

EXAMPLE: 2 cartridges containing epinephrine 1:100,000

$$1.8 \times 2 \times 0.01 = 0.036 \text{ mg}$$

---

be given reduced amounts of vasoconstrictors or none at all. Patients with hyperthyroidism, unable to tolerate vasoconstrictors, should not receive them at all (Bennett, 1984). These examples of medical complications emphasize the importance of reviewing patients' medical histories prior to the administration of local anesthetics and vasoconstrictors. If the clinician is unsure of the impact of these agents on a particular medical condition, the dentist or the patient's physician should be consulted. It is also important to be aware of other medications the patient may be taking. For ex-

ample, if a patient were taking a sulfonamide, procaine would be contraindicated because it interferes with the action of the sulfonamide (Bennett, 1984).

Allergic reactions to local anesthetics are mentioned earlier in the chapter and in Chapter 10. Once the agent has been administered, the patient should be observed for at least 3 to 5 minutes, since most reactions occur within that amount of time. If any untoward reaction occurs, the dentist should be informed, proper treatment provided, and the incident recorded in the patient's chart.

Administration

A knowledge and understanding of the anatomy of the nervous, vascular, osseous, and muscular structures of the head and oral area are necessary to determine which injections should be given and the technique for administration. Fig. 32-1 illustrates the innervation of the teeth and associated structures that are of interest to local anesthesia. The nerves supplying the oral structures pictured in Fig 32-1 are branches of the fifth cranial nerve, the trigeminal nerve. Specific injections and injection techniques have been developed to anesthetize the nerve trunks and nerve branches. A nerve can be anesthetized along the nerve trunk before it branches; this is called *block anesthesia* (Haglund and Evers, 1972; Sicher and DeBrul, 1975). A branch of a nerve trunk can be anesthetized by depositing solution in the area of the nerve branch so that the solution filters through the underlying bone to reach the nerve; this is called *infiltration* or *field anesthesia* (Haglund and Evers, 1972; Sicher and DeBrul, 1975). Infiltration anesthesia depends on the solution filtering through the tissues and bone to reach the nerve; its effectiveness is dependent, in large part, on the thickness of the bone.

Table 32-3 lists the various injections along with the nerves and tissues anesthetized by each injection. Figs. 32-2 to 32-11 illustrate the injection sites. This can help the clinician determine which injections could be given to achieve anesthesia in a given area. It is important to determine if soft or hard tissue anesthesia is necessary, since all of the injections do not provide both. For example, the long buccal injection only anesthetizes the soft tissues over the mandibular molars; if the molars must be anesthetized, an inferior alveolar block must also be given. In some instances more than one combination of injections may be administered to achieve the desired anesthesia. In those instances the clinician decides which injections to give based on such factors as which combination requires the fewest penetrations, which requires the least amount of solution, the desired duration, the patient's medical condition, and other factors as well.

A local anesthetic may be required when the patient is experiencing pain in the gingiva and/or in the teeth. If verbal reassurance does not alleviate the pain, the clinician can consider nitrous oxide and oxygen conscious sedation and/or local anesthesia. Local anesthesia will provide complete an-

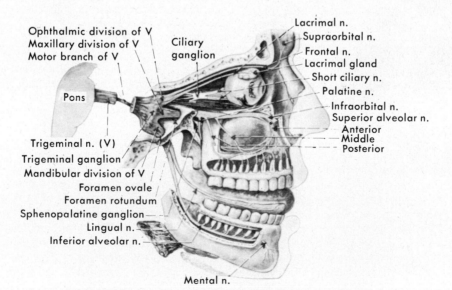

Fig. 32-1. Innervation of dental structures by trigeminal nerve. (From Bennett, C.R. 1978. Monheim's local anesthesia and pain control in dental practice, ed. 6. St. Louis: The C.V. Mosby Co.)

Table 32-3. Branches of the trigeminal nerve related to dental local anesthesia

Nerve	Tissues innervated/anesthetized	Injection
Maxillary division		
Greater palatine	Hard tissue: none Soft tissue: palatal tissue from teeth to midline from distal of third molar to cuspid	Greater palatine
Nasopalatine	Hard tissue: none Soft tissue: palatal tissues from left cuspid to right cuspid	Nasopalatine
Posterior superior alveolar (PSA)	Hard tissue: second and third molars; first molar excluding mesiobuccal root; associated supporting structures Soft tissue: overlying buccal tissues	Posterior superior alveolar (PSA)
Middle superior alveolar (MSA) branch of infraorbital	Hard tissue: first and second premolars, mesiobuccal root of first molar, and associated supporting structures Soft tissue: overlying buccal tissues and cheek or lip	Middle superior alveolar (MSA)
Anterior superior alveolar (ASA) branch of infraorbital	Hard tissue: cuspid and incisors and associated supporting structures Soft tissue: overlying facial tissues and lip	Anterior superior alveolar (ASA)
Infraorbital (includes both MSA and ASA)	Hard tissue: premolars, cuspid, incisors, and associated supporting structures Soft tissue: overlying facial tissue, cheek, and lip	Infraorbital
Individual terminal branches of MSA or ASA	Hard tissue: individual premolars, cuspid, incisors, and associated supporting structures Soft tissue: facial tissue and lip overlying individual teeth	Maxillary infiltration
Free nerve endings	Hard tissue: none Soft tissue: individual papillae	Interpapillary
Mandibular division		
Buccal (long buccal)	Hard tissue: none Soft tissue: buccal tissue of molars	Long buccal
Lingual	Hard tissue: none Soft tissue: lingual tissue from molar to midline, including anterior two thirds of tongue	Lingual
Inferior alveolar (includes dental, mental, and incisive branches)	Hard tissue: molars, premolars, cuspid, and incisors to midline, as well as associated supporting structures Soft tissue: facial tissue anterior to mental foramen, including lip	Inferior alveolar or mandibular block
Mental branch of inferior alveolar	Hard tissue: none Soft tissue: facial tissue and lip anterior to mental foramen	Mental
Incisive and mental branches of inferior alveolar	Hard tissue: premolars, cuspid, incisors, and associated supporting structures Soft tissue: facial tissue and lip anterior to mental foramen	Incisive and mental
Individual terminal branches of mental and incisive	Hard tissue: individual cuspids, incisors, and sometimes premolars Soft tissue: facial tissue and lip overlying individual teeth	Mandibular facial infiltration
Anterior portion of lingual nerve	Hard tissue: none Soft tissue: lingual tissue in area of injection	Mandibular lingual infiltration
Free nerve endings	Hard tissue: none Soft tissue: individual papillae	Interpapillary

Data from Bennett, 1984; Reed and Sheppard, 1976; and Sicher and DeBrul, 1975.

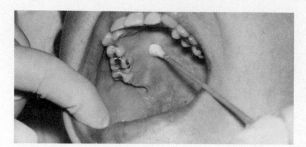

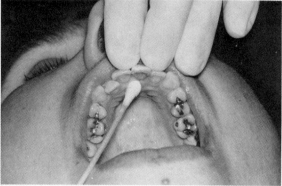

Fig. 32-2. Placement for greater palatine injection is at height of hard palate between first and second molars.

Fig. 32-3. Placement for nasopalatine injection is incisive papilla.

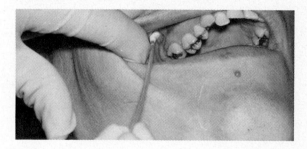

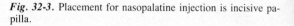

Fig. 32-4. Placement for posterior superior alveolar injection is at height of mucobuccal fold, distal to second molar.

Fig. 32-5. Placement for anterior superior alveolar injection is at height of mucobuccal fold between premolars.

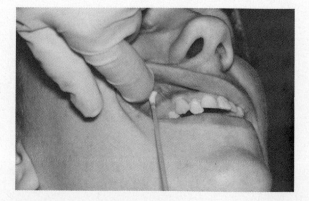

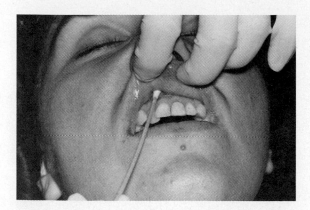

Fig. 32-6. Placement for maxillary infiltration is at height of mucobuccal fold over tooth.

Fig. 32-7. Placement for inferior alveolar and lingual injection is distal to retromolar pad.

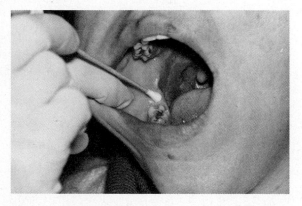

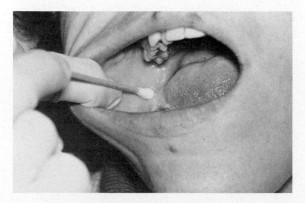

Fig. 32-8. Placement for long buccal injection is buccal to ramus and at height of molar.

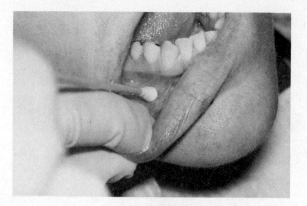

Fig. 32-9. Placement for mental infiltration in mucobuccal fold, between premolars, approximating mental foramen.

Fig. 32-10. Placement for mandibular facial infiltration is at depth of mucobuccal fold at tooth.

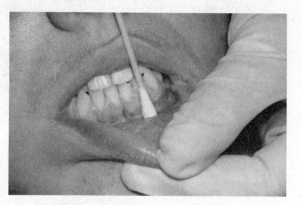

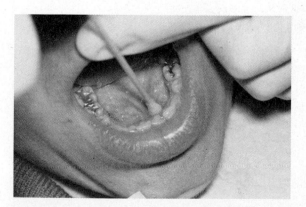

Fig. 32-11. Placement for mandibular lingual infiltration is at depth of floor of mouth adjacent to tooth.

esthesia for a localized area from a single tooth to a quadrant of half of the mouth. It is rare that a patient is subjected to local anesthesia in all four quadrants at the same time; the maximum safe dose would be approached, and the patient may not appreciate a completely numb mouth. Most clinicians anesthetize a sextant or a quadrant to perform dental hygiene or periodontal procedures.

The clinician is concerned with the osseous, vascular, and muscular anatomy during the administration of an injection. (Bennett, 1984; Haglund and Evers, 1972; Reed and Sheppard, 1976) The osseous structures are the most reliable landmarks, since they are constant in shape and location. The musculature is important because penetration and trauma to the muscles must be kept to a minimum to avoid muscle trismus or soreness after the injection. A knowledge of the probable location of the blood vessels is important, since depositing solution intravascularly or rupturing a vessel can cause internal bleeding and the formation of a hematoma. The clinician must *always aspirate*—pull back the plunger—to create a negative pressure in the cartridge, which will draw blood into the cartridge if the tip of the needle is in a vessel. There are blood vessels associated with each of the nerves. Aspiration will help the clinician avoid injecting into the major blood vessels and decrease the chances of a hematoma or toxic overdose.

Armamentarium

The armamentarium necessary for an injection is illustrated in Fig. 32-12. The syringe is an aspirating syringe; the clinician can pull back the plunger by pulling back the ring. The tray also includes a topical anesthetic, an antiseptic, cotton-tipped applicators, gauze to retract, dry, and hold movable tissues, and the assembled syringe. Fig. 32-13 shows the proper assembly of the syringe, cartridge, and needle. Needles are available in short or long lengths and a variety of gauges. The short needle is used for infiltration anesthesia, and the long needle is used for block anesthesia, including the posterior superior alveolar, mental, and inferior alveolar blocks. The gauge of a needle refers to the diameter of the opening; the most common gauges used in dentistry are 25, 27, and 30. The 25-gauge needle is recommended because

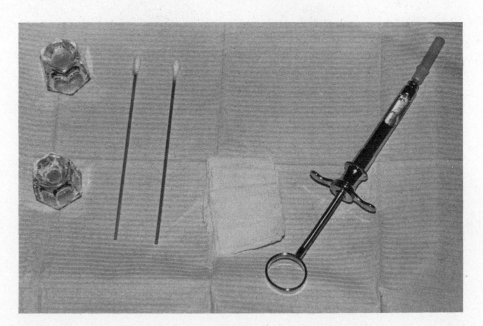

Fig. 32-12. Tray setup for administration of local anesthesia: topical anesthesia, antiseptic, cotton-tipped pad applicators, gauze, and assembled syringe.

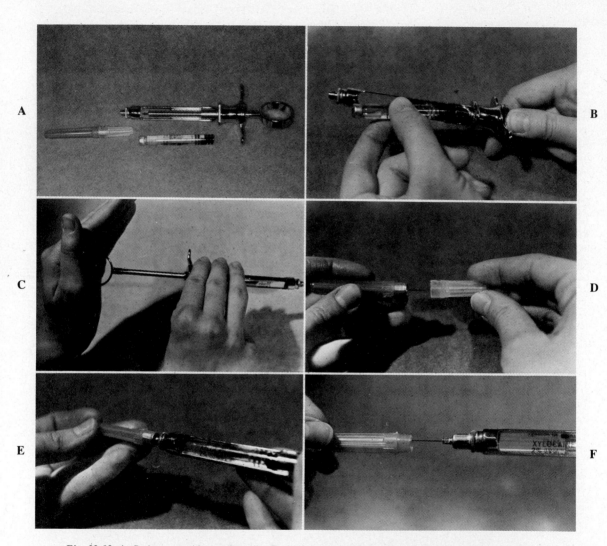

Fig. 32-13. **A,** Syringe, cartridge, and needle. **B,** Aspirator assembly is drawn back, and cartridge is inserted. **C,** Aspirating tip is engaged into plunger with several firm taps against ring. **D,** End of needle to be inserted into cartridge is uncovered. **E,** Needle penetrates diaphragm of cartridge and is screwed into syringe. **F,** Needle is exposed.

it is believed to be the smallest gauge through which blood can be successfully aspirated (Bennett, 1984).

Aseptic technique must be observed to protect the patient from a bacteremia or an infection. The needle should not touch anything except the patient's tissues; therefore the cap should remain on the needle unless the setup is being tested or the syringe is being used. Bennett (1984) has advocated the use of an antiseptic solution on the penetration site to lessen the chances of carrying bacteria and debris from the oral cavity into the tissue. The antiseptic solution is applied to the site just before the needle penetrates the tissue. In addition, some practitioners recommend using topical anesthetics on the penetration site to lessen the pain of the needle penetrating the tissue (Bennett, 1984; Haglund and Evers, 1972).

Once the clinician has identified the injection to be given, he/she should palpate the landmarks to locate the penetration site. The penetration site is

dried, and the topical anesthetic is applied to the area for the appropriate amount of time (Fig. 32-14). The topical anesthetic is rinsed and suctioned away, and the movable tissue is retracted so the clinician can see the penetration site (Fig. 32-15). If possible, the clinician should establish a fulcrum against which to rest the syringe so it can be held steady during the penetration, aspiration, and administration of the solution (Fig. 32-16). Just prior to the penetration, the antiseptic should be applied. Prior to and during the injection the clinician should talk to and reassure the patient. After appropriate penetration and aspiration techniques are performed, the solution should be injected slowly to increase the patient's comfort and to reduce the chance of a toxic reaction. When the desired amount of solution has been administered, the needle and syringe are removed and the needle should be recapped. The clinician may massage the area to distribute the anesthetic solution. The clinician or another properly trained person should

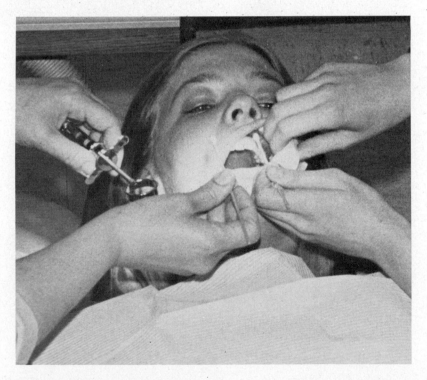

Fig. 32-14. Topical anesthetic being applied. Assistant is ready to pass cotton-tipped applicator with antiseptic to clinician. Antiseptic will be applied after topical anesthetic is rinsed and suctioned away.

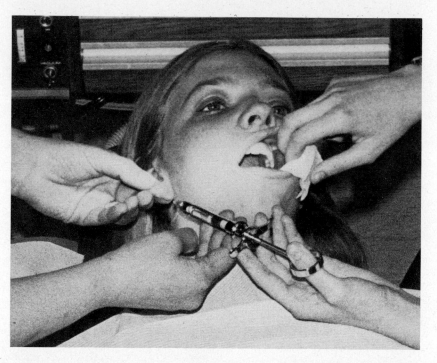

Fig. 32-15. Clinician grasps movable tissue with sterile gauze square and retracts tissue to achieve accessibility and visibility. Clinician is receiving syringe from assistant.

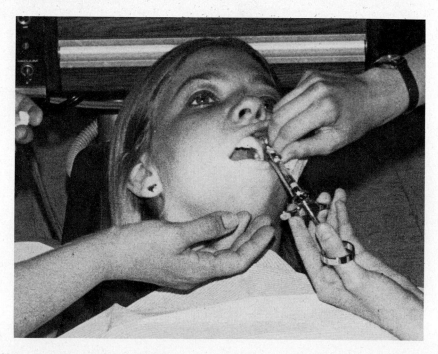

Fig. 32-16. Clinician establishes fulcrum for syringe against thumb to help steady syringe and needle during penetration, advancement, aspiration, deposition, and removal.

remain with the patient for several minutes after the injection has been given, since an immediate reaction such as syncope, a toxic reaction, or an allergic reaction could occur (see Chapter 10). After several minutes, the clinician may tap the tissue and teeth to determine if anesthesia has been achieved. At the end of the appointment the patient should be reminded not to chew or bite the soft tissues that are numb. The patient should be instructed to call the office if any unusual sensations or rashes are experienced.

Some modifications in technique are necessary during the administration of local anesthesia to children. Malamed (1979) and Rood (1981) should be consulted if anesthesia is being given to children.

TOPICAL ANESTHESIA

Topical anesthesia is achieved by direct application of an anesthetic agent onto the mucous membrane surface (Bennett, 1984). Once placed on the mucous membrane, the agent is absorbed by the free nerve endings in the area, creating an anesthetic effect. Only the free nerve endings are affected; since the topical anesthetic is not injected into the tissue, neither the nerve trunk nor its branches are affected. The topical anesthetic is absorbed by the blood vessels in the affected area, making a toxic reaction possible (Bennett, 1984; Rogo, 1982). In fact, a toxic reaction is even more likely to occur with a topical anesthetic than with a local anesthetic because topical anesthetics are supplied in much higher concentrations.

Topical anesthetic agents

Chemically, topical anesthetics are similar to local anesthetics. There are two groups of topical anesthetics: amides and esters. The amide used as a topical anesthetic is lidocaine (Xylocaine), and the main two esters used as topical anesthetics are tetracaine (Pontocaine) and ethyl aminobenzoate (benzocaine). Benzyl alcohol is also used as a topical anesthetic. In order for these agents to be effective, they are produced in greater concentrations than local anesthetics; for example, lidocaine is used in a 5% concentration; tetracaine is used in a 2% concentration; and benzocaine is available in 10%, 15%, and 20% concentrations (Bennett, 1984; Rogo, 1982). Since such high concentrations are placed in areas of the mouth where they are

rapidly absorbed into the bloodstream, there is a danger of a toxic reaction. Many practitioners regard topical anesthetics as relatively harmless agents. Nothing could be further from the truth; thus this emphasis on the chance of toxic overdose.

Topical anesthetics are available in three forms: gel, liquid, and spray. The gels and liquids are recommended for use prior to local anesthesia or during scaling procedures for superficial soft tissue anesthesia. Some practitioners also use topical anesthetics during radiographic series or impression taking to lessen patients' gag reflexes. Use of a topical anesthetic in these last two instances must be done judiciously to ensure that the patient maintains some of the necessary protective gag reflex. The use of topical anesthetic sprays is highly discouraged because their application is difficult to control and the patient and clinician can inhale the agent, which is not recommended.

The precautions observed when selecting a local anesthetic, such as patient sensitivity to esters or methylparaben and compromised medical histories, also apply when selecting a topical anesthetic. If a patient has a history of allergy to ester anesthetics, then lidocaine topical anesthetic should be used. Methylparaben is used with some amide topical anesthetics so if a patient has a history of allergic reaction, the clinician should check the package insert accompanying the product to see if methylparaben is used. Patients with liver disease or dysfunction should not be given amide topical anesthetics, since they are broken down in the liver; rather, an ester should be used (Bennett, 1984; Rogo, 1982). Topical anesthetics do not contain vasoconstrictors, so the medical conditions affected by vasoconstrictors do not apply to topical anesthetics.

A complication of topical anesthetics, unlike local anesthetics, is tissue irritation. Since a topical anesthetic is applied directly to the mucous membrane, it has the potential to irritate or damage the tissue. This is of particular concern with benzocaine topical anesthetics because they are produced in very high concentrations. Benzocaine topical anesthetics can cause tissue sloughing if left in contact with the tissue too long.

Application

The use of a topical anesthetic prior to the injection of a local anesthetic and during a scaling procedure are presented in this section. Topical anesthetics are only effective on the soft tissue and are most effective on unkeratinized soft tissue, since they are more readily absorbed.

Prior to an injection, a topical anesthetic can be applied to the injection site. Figs. 32-14 to 32-16 illustrate the application of a topical anesthetic to some of the injection sites listed in Table 32-3. Prior to applying the topical anesthetic, the area should be dried with either a gauze square or a stream of air (Fig. 32-17). Drying the tissue helps keep the agent in the desired area, and it also ensures that the desired amount is being applied. If there is saliva in the area, the topical anesthetic will be carried away, lessening the amount applied and producing undesired anesthesia in other areas of the mouth. The topical anesthetic should be applied with a cotton-tipped applicator that has been dipped into the agent. In order to maintain asepsis, the topical anesthetic should be removed from the container and placed into a dappen dish so that the container is not contaminated. The topical anesthetic on the cotton-tipped applicator (Fig. 32-18) is held in place for the appropriate amount of time. The length of application depends on the agent used and is determined by reading the manufacturer's directions accompanying the product. The highly concentrated benzocaine agents usually have very short application times of about 15 seconds; the less concentrated agents, such as lidocaine and tetracaine, may have longer application times of 30 to 60 seconds. The manufacturer's directions should be observed in order to obtain the desired effect and avoid tissue irritation.

Once the length of application is complete, the cotton-tipped applicator should be removed and the area should be thoroughly rinsed to remove the agent. Ideally, the area should be suctioned as it is rinsed. In no situation should the patient swallow the rinse water. If a suction is not available, the patient should expectorate the rinse water and topical anesthetic. After the area is rinsed, an antiseptic, if one is used, is applied to the injection site and the injection is begun (Fig. 32-19).

The *application of a topical anesthetic during a scaling procedure* requires some modifications to the previous technique. It is still important to dry the area with either a stream of air or a gauze square, but the topical anesthetic can be applied in one of two ways. It can be applied with a cotton-tipped applicator or with a curette. Application

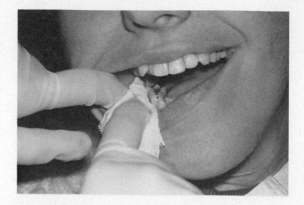

Fig. 32-17. Drying area with gauze prior to application of topical anesthetic.

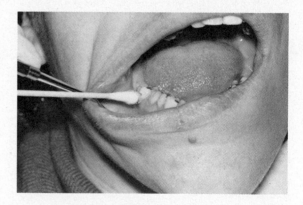

Fig. 32-18. Applying topical anesthetic for interpapillary injection with cotton-tipped applicator.

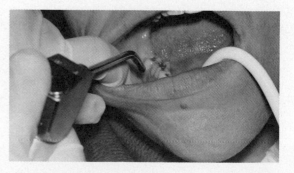

Fig. 32-19. Rinsing area at end of application time.

with a cotton-tipped applicator will allow the topical anesthetic to reach the outer surface of the papilla and marginal gingiva but will not reach into the sulcus. Since the most sensitive tissue is likely to be the lining of the sulcus, it is recommended that one dip the curette into the topical anesthetic and carry it into the sulcus in this manner. Liquid topical anesthetic is most easily carried into the sulcus on a curette. The application time must still be observed and the area thoroughly rinsed.

During a scaling procedure the topical anesthetic of choice would provide a relatively long anesthetic effect and have a low toxicity. The MSDs of the agents (see Table 32-2) must be observed. Benzocaine has a longer anesthetic effect and a lower toxicity than lidocaine or tetracaine. Benzocaine's longer effect and lower toxicity is due to its low water solubility; thus it is slowly absorbed. But also keep in mind that benzocaine is an ester and that tissue sloughing is more likely. If the patient is not allergic to ester drugs and the clinician observes the application time, benzocaine can provide adequate topical anesthesia. Lidocaine and tetracaine also provide adequate anesthesia and are less likely to produce an allergic reaction and tissue sloughing. As with many agents, the clinician should use several and develop his/her own preference, to be modified by the patient's medical history.

In general, the least amount possible of topical anesthetic necessary to produce the desired effect should be used. Also, the use of a topical anesthetic in highly vascular areas such as the floor of the mouth should be done with care. Observation of the application times and thorough rinsing are essential.

SUMMARY

Some psychosomatic, topical anesthetic, and local anesthetic approaches to pain control have been presented in this chapter. If the practitioner develops helping relations with patients and uses the appropriate methods of pain control, his/her patients should have very little or no pain associated with dental treatment.

ACTIVITIES

1. Make up a sample of dental hygiene procedures that may require local anesthesia and decide which injections could be given. Refer to Table 31-3.

2. The innervation of the maxilla and mandible described in Table 31-3 is for the permanent dentition. Look up the innervation of the primary and mixed dentitions, and compare and contrast the innervations.

3. Obtain a copy of the laws that govern the practice of dental hygiene in the state. Is administration of local anesthesia permitted? If not, does the class think it should or should not be permitted? What can or cannot be done about the practice act in the state?

4. Participate in a formal local anesthesia course that is open to dental hygienists to learn how to administer local anesthetics.

5. Root plane or scale a patient's teeth with local anesthesia. How does the benefit of local anesthesia affect the clinician's process during the scaling and/or root planing, and how does it affect the results of the procedure?

REVIEW QUESTIONS

1. A dental hygienist graduated from a dental hygiene program that did not teach local anesthesia. The hygienist is now living in a state where he/she can administer local anesthesia. What additional education, if any, does the hygienist need? Why?

2. Draw and label the following nerves:
   a. Posterior, superior, middle superior, and anterior superior
   b. Lingual, buccal, and inferior alveolar

3. Name the tissues innervated by each of the following nerves:
   a. Posterior superior alveolar
   b. Greater palatine
   c. Buccal (long buccal)
   d. Infraorbital

4. Name the injections that should be given for each of the following procedures:
   a. Soft tissue curettage on the facial and lingual aspects of the mandibular right quadrant
   b. Class II mesioocclusal amalgam preparation on the maxillary left first molar. A rubber dam clamp will be placed on the second molar
   c. Root planing on the mandibular central incisor without soft tissue curettage

REFERENCES

ADA Council on Dental Materials, Instruments, and Equipment 1983. Status report: the periodontal ligament injection. J. Am. Dent. Assoc, **106:**222.

ADA Council on Dental Therapeutics. 1982. Accepted dental therapeutics, ed. 39. Chicago: American Dental Association.

Adriani, J., and Campbell, D. 1956. Fatalities following topical application of local anesthetics to mucous membranes. JAMA **162:**1527.

Aldrete, T.A., and O'Higgins, T.W. 1971. Evaluation of patients with a history of allergy to local anesthetics. South Med. J. **64:**115.

American Association of Dental Schools. 1980. Special report: curricular guidelines for comprehensive control of pain and anxiety in dentistry. J. Dent. Educ. **44:**279.

Atterbury, R. 1978. Relaxation by vocal pre-sedation in dentistry. CAL **43:**18.

Bateman, P.M. 1974. Multiple allergy to local anesthetic including prilocaine. Med. J. Aust. **2:**449.

Bennett, R.C. 1984. Monheim's local anesthesia and pain control in dental practice, ed. 7. St. Louis: The C.V. Mosby Co.

Burstein, A., et al. 1979. Injection pain: memory, expectation, and experienced pain. N.Y. J. Dent. **49:**183.

Christensen, L.V. 1980. Cultural, clinical, and physiological aspects of pain: a review. J. Oral Rehabil. **7:**413.

Dafoe, B.R. 1982. Providing pain control: local anesthesia. RDH **2**(3):46.

Foreman, P.A. 1979. Behavioral considerations in patient management. Anesth. Prog. **26:**161.

Fry, B.W., et al. 1980. Concentration of vasoconstrictors in local anesthesia change during storage in cartridge heaters. J. Dent. Res. **59:**1163.

Gangarosa, L.P., Sr. 1981. Newer local anesthetics and techniques for administration. J. Dent. Res. **60:**1471.

Gill, G.J., and Orr, D.H. 1979. A double-blind crossover comparison of topical anesthetics. J. Am. Dent. Assoc. **98:**213.

Giovannitti, J.A., and Bennett, R.C. 1979. Assessment of allergy to local anesthetics. J. Am. Dent. Assoc. **98:**701.

Haglund, J., and Evers, H. 1972. Local anaesthesia in dentistry. London: Astra Läkemedel.

Johnson, W.T., et al. 1983. Hypersensitivity to procaine, tetracaine, mepivacaine and methylparaben: a report of a case. J. Am. Dent. Assoc. **106:**53.

Larson, C.E. 1977. Methylparaben—an overlooked cause of local anesthesia hypersensitivity. Anesth. Prog. **24:**72.

Malamed, S.F. 1979. An update on pain and anxiety control in pediatric dentistry. II. Inhalation sedation and local anesthesia. Alpha Omegan **72:**29.

Malamed, S.F. 1980. Handbook of local anesthesia. St. Louis: The C.V. Mosby Co.

Malamed, S.F. 1982. The periodontal ligament (PDL) injection: an alternative to inferior alveolar nerve block. Oral Surg. **53:**117.

Melzack, R. 1973. The puzzle of pain. New York: Basic Books, Inc. Publishers.

Mollen, A.J., et al. 1981. Needles—25 gauge vs 27 gauge—can patients really tell? Gen. Dent. **29:**417.

Mumma, R.D., Jr., et al. 1977. Survey of administration of infiltration anesthesia. Dent. Hyg. **51:**159.

Peterson, D.S., et al. 1981. Pain sensation related to local anesthetics injected at varying temperatures. Anesth. Prog. **25:**164.

Prensky, H.D. 1981. Current concepts in pain control. Clin. Prevent. Dent. **3**(1):8.

Reed, G.M., and Sheppard, V.F. 1976. Basic structures of the head and neck. Philadelphia. W.B. Saunders Co.

Rogo, E.S. 1982. Providing safe comfortable pain control. RDH **1:**12.

Rood, J.P. 1981. Notes on local anesthesia for the child patient. Dent. Update, **8:**377.

Reed, G.M., and Sheppard , V.F. 1976. Basic structures of the head and neck. Philadelphia: W.B. Saunders Co.

Sharp, J. Nov. 1979. Should dental hygiene students be taught to administer local anesthesia? N.M. Dent. J. **30:**8.

Sicher, H., and DeBrul, E.L. 1975. Oral anatomy, ed. 6. St. Louis: The C.V. Mosby Co.

Siskin, L. 1978. Anaphylaxis due to local anesthesia hypersensitivity: report of case. J. Am. Dent. Assoc. **96:**841.

Spear, F.C. 1977. Cultural factors in clinical pain assessment. Int. Dent. J. **27:**284.

Steblay, N.M., and Beaman, A.L. 1982. Reduction of fear during dental treatment through reattribution technique. J. Am. Dent. Assoc. **105:**1006.

Wepman, B.J. 1978. Psychological components of pain perception. Dent. Clin. North Am. **22:**101.

Yaacob, H.B., et al. 1981. The pharmacological effect of Xylocaine topical anesthetics—a comparison with a placebo. Singapore Dent. J. **6:**55.

Yoeman, C.M. 1982. Hypersensitivity to prilocaine. Br. Dent. J. **153:**69.

33 NITROUS OXIDE AND OXYGEN CONSCIOUS SEDATION

OBJECTIVES: *The reader will be able to*

1. State the indications for nitrous oxide and oxygen conscious sedation in dental hygiene practice.
2. Define the term *conscious* as used in the philosophy of conscious sedation.
3. State several methods of monitoring the patient's conscious state.
4. Describe the chemical nature of nitrous oxide.
5. Describe the pharmacologic mechanism that renders nitrous oxide effective.
6. Provide a list of representational examples of patient responses as the concentration of nitrous oxide is increased from 10% to 50%.
7. Complete a preoperative evaluation of a patient.
8. State the contraindications to nitrous oxide and oxygen conscious sedation.
9. Describe the safety features that a nitrous oxide and oxygen conscious sedation system should include.
10. Calculate the percentage of nitrous oxide delivered to a patient.
11. Prepare a patient for receiving nitrous oxide and oxygen conscious sedation.
12. Describe and demonstrate the technique for administering and monitoring nitrous oxide and oxygen conscious sedation.

For many patients, visiting the dental office is an anxiety-producing situation. Because of past experiences or current discomfort the patient worries that further discomfort is inevitable. Modern dentistry offers excellent pain control techniques. Local anesthetics are effective in blocking pain perception. Such techniques are necessary for most periodontal procedures and restorative dentistry. Before some patients are receptive to local anesthetic techniques, sedation techniques are helpful. Nitrous oxide and oxygen conscious sedation is a conscious inhalation sedation method that is used in many dental offices and clinics.

The hygienist performs procedures that may cause the patient discomfort. Patients who rely on nitrous oxide and oxygen conscious sedation for other restorative dental procedures may require it for deep subgingival scaling, root planing, soft tissue curettage, and placement of temporary restorations or crowns. In such cases the hygienist may be called on to monitor a patient undergoing inhalation sedation or administer conscious sedation if the state law permits trained hygienists to perform this function.

Nitrous oxide has been used in dentistry for over 100 years. Horace Wells, a dentist, first demonstrated its effectiveness during a surgical procedure in 1844 (Langa, 1976). Since that time, the properties and effects of nitrous oxide used with oxygen have been studied and documented.

Nitrous oxide and oxygen conscious sedation is most beneficial to dentistry because it comforts and relaxes the patient. Nitrous oxide alters pain reaction, which is a very individualized interpretation of actual pain perception. By raising the patient's pain reaction threshold, the patient is able to relax and cooperate better during dental procedures. As an additional effect, nitrous oxide and oxygen conscious sedation alters the patient's perception of time, so dental appointments seem to pass more quickly. With a relaxed, conscious, and cooperative patient the appointment can be handled efficiently. Less stress results for both the patient and the clinician.

The basis of an understanding of nitrous oxide and oxygen conscious sedation is an appreciation of the conscious state. At no time during the administration of this form of inhalation sedation should the patient lose consciousness. The American Dental Society of Anesthesiology, Inc., defines *conscious* in this way: "A patient is said to be conscious if he/she is capable of rational response to command and has all protective reflexes intact, including the ability to clear and maintain his/her airway in a patent state" (Bennett, 1978). All parts of this definition must be observed. Rational response to command will be especially important in monitoring the patient's conscious state. Retaining the ability to breathe automatically and cough so that aspiration is avoided enables inhalation sedation to be administered without sophisticated technical support personnel and equipment. With nitrous oxide and oxygen inhalation sedation, vital signs and the function of cardiovascular and respiratory systems will remain within normal limits (Bennett, 1978; Roberts et al., 1982).

The patient will experience an alteration of his/her mood, and the pain reaction threshold will increase. Nitrous oxide depresses the cerebral cortex, thalamus, hypothalamus, and reticular activating system. This results in nerve impulses either not being relayed to the cortex or being interpreted differently (Swepston, 1976).

Conscious sedation with nitrous oxide and oxygen does not significantly reduce pain or the reflex reaction to pain stimulus. Nitrous oxide is mildly potent and a weak anesthetic when compared with the standard anesthetic morphine. *Potency* refers to the amount of medication necessary to achieve a desired effect. A clinical measure of relative potency has been experimentally determined. This is called the *mean alveolar concentration (MAC).* MAC is defined as the concentration of anesthetic agent required to prevent movement (reflex reaction to pain) at the time of surgical incision in 50% of patients (DeMartina and Garber, 1979). A very potent medication such as halothane, a general anesthetic, has a MAC of 0.77%. Nitrous oxide has a MAC of 101% (Fordham, 1974). Since it is impossible to deliver a 101% concentration of pure nitrous oxide gas because of atmospheric conditions, relieving response to frank pain perception cannot be relied on. In a dental procedure where hard or soft tissue pain will be significant for the patient, nitrous oxide and oxygen conscious sedation must be accompanied by local anesthesia. Increasing the concentration of nitrous oxide will not significantly reduce true pain perception. A patient responding to pain while under nitrous ox-

ide and oxygen conscious sedation will not be comfortable or cooperative for long.

Nitrous oxide is a colorless, nonexplosive, and sweet-smelling inorganic agent. It is prepared by heating ammonium nitrate crystals in an iron retort at 240° C (Bennett, 1978). This produces nitrous oxide and water. Commercially, nitrous oxide is supplied in pressurized cylinders as a liquid and a gas.

Nitrous oxide is nonallergenic and does not react with body tissues. It diffuses across tissue membranes much more rapidly than oxygen. When inhaled, nitrous oxide diffuses across the alveolar membrane in the alveoli of the lungs, entering the bloodstream. With a very low blood gas solubility (0.47) the nitrous oxide molecule travels unchanged in the blood. Nitrogen molecules are usually displaced in the bloodstream by the nitrous oxide. As long as the patient continues to breathe the flow of nitrous oxide and oxygen, a concentration of nitrous oxide that will affect the central nervous system will be maintained in the bloodstream. By controlling the external concentration of nitrous oxide and oxygen as it comes from the sedation equipment, the patient's alveolar concentration is controlled (DeMartina and Garber, 1979).

To calculate nitrous oxide concentration, a percentage is determined. The flow of nitrous oxide, expressed in liters per minute, is placed over the total flow of nitrous oxide and oxygen, creating a fraction which can then be converted to a percentage (Bennett, 1978):

Example 1: $\dfrac{2 \text{ liters of } N_2O}{2 \text{ liters of } N_2O + 8 \text{ liters of } O_2} = \dfrac{2}{10} = 20\%$

Example 2: $\dfrac{3 \text{ liters of } N_2O}{3 \text{ liters of } N_2O + 6 \text{ liters of } O_2} = \dfrac{3}{9} = 33\tfrac{1}{3}\%$

The alveolar concentration, or percentage of nitrous oxide delivered, determines the sedative effect on the central nervous system that the patient will experience. Table 33-1 summarizes the range of responses possible at given concentrations (Bennett, 1978).

The sedation (depression) of the central nervous system resembles the state one experiences just prior to falling asleep. At concentrations higher than necessary for dental procedures sleep indeed occurs. To maintain the definition of consciousness, the patient must remain awake and responsive to verbal commands at all times. If the patient is unable to keep his/her mouth open or is falling

Table 33-1. Signs and symptoms in response to nitrous oxide and oxygen conscious sedation

Concentration N₂O	Response
10% to 20%	Body warmth
	Tingling of hands and feet
20% to 30%	Circumoral numbness
	Numbness of thighs
20% to 40%	Numbness of tongue
	Numbness of hands and feet
	Droning sounds present
	Hearing distinct but distant
	Dissociation begins and reaches peak
	Mild sleepiness
	Analgesia (maximum at 30%)
	Euphoria
	Feeling of heaviness or lightness of body
30% to 50%	Sweating
	Nausea
	Amnesia
	Increased sleepiness
40% to 60%	Dreaming, laughing, giddiness
	Further increased sleepiness, tending toward unconsciousness
	Increased nausea and vomiting
50% and over	Unconsciousness and light general anesthesia

From Bennett, C.R. 1978. Conscious sedation in dental practice, ed. 2. St. Louis: The C.V. Mosby Co.

asleep, the amount of nitrous oxide being delivered must be reduced.

In addition to being relaxed and having time perception altered, the patient may experience dissociation (DeMartina, 1979; Minnis, 1979). This refers to an effect on the patient's ability to maintain his/her spatial orientation. The patient may describe floating or sinking into the chair. The clinician's voice and sounds in the operatory may seem distant. Most people enjoy a slight bit of "escape" from the dentistry at hand. Other patients may interpret dissociation as a feeling of losing control of themselves or the situation. This in itself may be alarming to the patient, thereby reducing the comfort that the patient expects to feel.

Patient reactions vary a great deal at any given concentration of nitrous oxide. The clinician must be sensitive to the physiologic and psychologic personality of the patient. Observing the patient's responses constantly ensures that a comfortable level of sedation is maintained at all times.

A few parameters are noteworthy. When nitrous oxide is administered above a 40% concentration, the patient generally becomes increasingly sleepy and responds sluggishly to commands (Bennett, 1978; Hamburg, 1980). The patient may begin to perspire, look uncomfortable, move in an uncoordinated manner, and complain of nausea. Any of these signs indicate that the inhaled concentration is too high for the patient. Although vomiting is rare at recommended levels, it is potentially dangerous and unpleasant for everyone concerned.

A concentration of 30% to 35% is accepted as a range for maximum nitrous oxide and oxygen conscious sedation (Bennett, 1978). Many patients are comfortable at lower concentrations. An administration technique in which the concentration is preset is unacceptable. The patient is induced with small amounts of nitrous oxide and a constant flow of at least 6 liters of oxygen per minute. After a few minutes at each increment of nitrous oxide, the concentration is increased until a comfortable state is achieved.

From one appointment to another the same patient may achieve desired sedation at different concentrations. The time of day, level of fatigue, general mood of the patient, and a variety of other factors influence this. In any case, delivering an excess of medication is, at worst, capable of producing a bad experience for the patient and, at best, unnecessary and wasteful.

PATIENT SELECTION

Before a patient experiences nitrous oxide and oxygen conscious sedation, a review of the medical status is necessary. Conditions that contraindicate this type of sedation include (DeMartina and Garber, 1979):

1. Recent myocardial infarction (within 6 months)
2. Chronic obstructive pulmonary disease (e.g., emphysema)
3. The first trimester of pregnancy
4. An active asthmatic condition
5. Nasal obstruction resulting from current upper respiratory tract infection
6. Inability to communicate (very young children, severely retarded patients)

Patients with a history of recent myocardial infarction may be more likely to have a recurrent episode. Elective dental treatment is generally postponed until the patient is again medically stable.

Patients with emphysema, chronic bronchitis, or

bronchial asthma in which the pulmonary system is chronically compromised may be prone to hypoxia. This refers to a lack of necessary oxygen in the bloodstream to adequately supply the patient's functional demand. If lack of oxygen is a problem for some, too much oxygen can also create a problem. Some patients, especially patients with emphysema, may rely on a lower level of oxygen circulating in the blood to stimulate the oxygen drive "reflex," which actually induces breathing. When abundant oxygen is delivered along with nitrous oxide, the drive to breathe is suppressed. Room air contains approximately 20% oxygen as compared with 70% to 80% delivered with inhalation sedation.

In the early stages of pregnancy, the use of all medications is best avoided. Although studies do not confirm serious fetal effects, an unnecessary risk at this critical time in development is to be avoided.

The patient with active asthma is prone to breathing difficulty and may pose a serious problem should bronchospasm occur.

Since nitrous oxide and oxygen conscious sedation relies on inhalation for its effectiveness, an upper respiratory tract infection and associated "stuffed" nose make the procedure useless. Because of the chance of cross-infection, elective dental care at this time is generally not advised.

The ability to communicate is essential, since this is a primary sign of the patient's consciousness. In patients with compromised ability, monitoring the patient is difficult.

The effects of nitrous oxide and oxygen conscious sedation are especially beneficial to the mild to moderately anxious and tense patient. Patients with more severe anxiety or less control of their emotions may not be helped with inhalation sedation of this type.

For patients with hypertension, the sedative effect of nitrous oxide is very beneficial because it keeps the blood pressure within the patient's normal limits.

Older patients who have Addison's disease or who have been taking corticosteroids should be carefully screened. If steroid therapy has been discontinued recently, the reaction to stress may be poor. The physician should be consulted about the possible need for steroids being reinstituted prior to treatment (Riklin, 1978).

For some medically compromised patients, the analgesia produced by nitrous oxide and oxygen may prove superior to other anesthetic/analgesic measures. Kaufman et al. (1982) have reported the success of nitrous oxide and oxygen conscious sedation for the treatment of a hemophiliac, a patient with severe cerebral palsy, and a patient with severe disabilities caused by familial dysautonomia.

The clinician's discretion and the physician's consultation may be necessary for patients with epilepsy, multiple sclerosis, questionable emotional status, central nervous system disorders, and other medically compromised conditions. In general, no procedure should be performed for a patient unless the office personnel are able to support the patient should an emergency or life-threatening situation occur (DeMartina and Garber, 1979).

EQUIPMENT FOR NITROUS OXIDE AND OXYGEN CONSCIOUS SEDATION

Nitrous oxide and oxygen conscious sedation equipment is available as a portable or central system.

A portable unit is shown in Fig. 33-1. The small tanks of oxygen and nitrous oxide permit mobility of the unit throughout the office or clinic. If inhalation sedation is used frequently, changing the empty tanks may create a problem. The "E" size oxygen tank contains 165 gallons of oxygen. At a

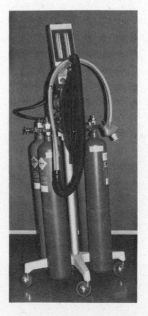

Fig. 33-1. Portable nitrous oxide and oxygen conscious sedation equipment.

permittable flow of 6 liters per minute, the tank is emptied in 104 minutes. The "E" size nitrous oxide tank contains 420 gallons (Bennett, 1978). Fig. 33-2 illustrates the regulators that attach to the portable unit tanks. These gauges indicate the pressure of the gas in the cylinder. Oxygen is supplied at a pressure of 2100 pounds per square inch (psi). As the oxygen is used, the pressure of the gas falls in direct proportion to this amount. Therefore if one half of the tank has been used, the regulator gauge will read 1050 psi.

Nitrous oxide is present as both a liquid and a gas and is supplied in cylinders at a pressure of 750 psi. The pressure remains the same in the tank until all the liquid is converted into gas. A nitrous oxide tank that is half empty will still read 750 psi; once all the liquid is converted, the pressure will drop until the tank is empty. A tag should be placed on the tank to keep track of the nitrous oxide used, with the date a full tank was opened and the dates and lengths of subsequent appointments when nitrous oxide was administered.

Central systems run from a bank of several large nitrous oxide and oxygen cylinders. These are called "H" and "G" tanks, respectively. With a central system, lines run to several wall hookups where the flow meter and mask unit are attached (Fig. 33-3). In addition to showing the pressure in

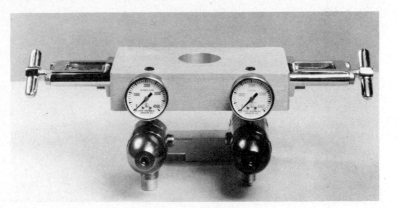

Fig. 33-2. Nitrous oxide and oxygen regulators that affix to portable analgesia machine. Pressure gauges indicate pressure of gas contained in cylinders. (Courtesy Fraser Sweatman, Inc. From Bennett, C.R. 1978. Conscious sedation in dental practice, ed. 2. St. Louis: The C.V. Mosby Co.)

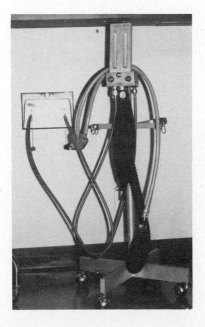

Fig. 33-3. Wall hookup for centralized nitrous oxide and oxygen conscious sedation system.

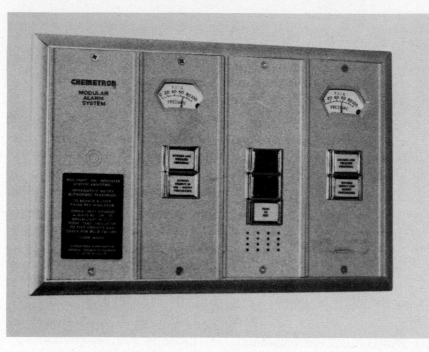

Fig. 33-4. Wall alarm system for centralized system.

the tanks, central systems usually include a wall- or desk-mounted alarm system that lights up or sounds if supplies are low (Fig. 33-4).

Several safety systems and devices have been developed to ensure proper use of inhalation sedation equipment (Bennett, 1978; DeMartina and Garber, 1979):

Universal color coding. The tanks and associated parts of the equipment (tubing, regulator gauge mount, flow controls) are colored *green* for oxygen and *blue* for nitrous oxide.

Pin index or diametric index system. The connection for the tanks and hoses for nitrous oxide will not adapt to the oxygen hookups. This prevents a person from mistakenly interchanging the gas systems.

Minimum oxygen flow. A preset flow of oxygen is provided at all times when the unit is on. This prevents the administration of pure nitrous oxide.

Fail-safe system. If for some reason the oxygen supply runs below the minimum level, the nitrous oxide automatically shuts off and begins to whistle.

Flow meter. This is a visual indication of liters per minute flow of both nitrous oxide and oxygen. The flow control valve (dial or lever) is color coded and labeled for each gas (Fig. 33-5). Automatic flow meters are available in which the concentration of nitrous oxide is dialed in. The machine adjusts to higher or lower concentrations automatically when the dial is changed.

Nonrebreathing system. Expired gases are not recirculated.

Analgesia machine circuit. The analgesia machine circuit is a set of two tubes connected to the machine and to the nasal mask. The nasal mask has two valves—air dilution and exhalation. The air dilution valve would allow the patient to dilute the flow of nitrous oxide by inhaling room air. This is not desirable, because the clinician no longer can accurately estimate the alveolar concentration of nitrous oxide and oxygen being delivered by the equipment. This valve, if present on the mask, is always in a closed position (Fig. 33-6). The exhalation valve allows the patient to exhale the previously circulated gases. This valve is always in the open position (Fig. 33-7). This is a nonscavenging system.

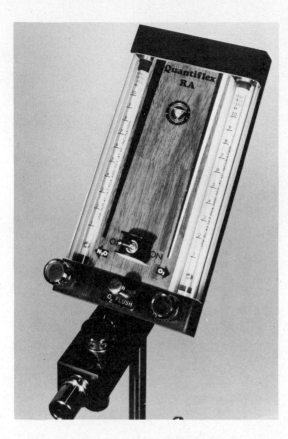

Fig. 33-5. Fraser Sweatman analgesia machine with dials to regulate gas flow. (Courtesy Fraser Sweatman, Inc. From Bennett, C.R. 1978. Conscious sedation in dental practice, ed. 2. St. Louis: The C.V. Mosby Co.)

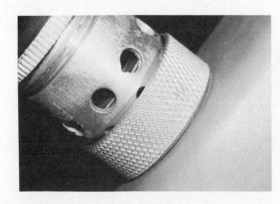

Fig. 33-6. Nasal mask with air dilution valve in *incorrect* position. Small holes indicate that air dilution valve is open.

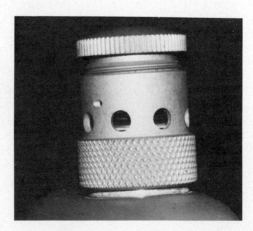

Fig. 33-7. Nasal mask with valves in *correct* position. Exhalation valve (large holes) open; air dilution valve (small holes) closed.

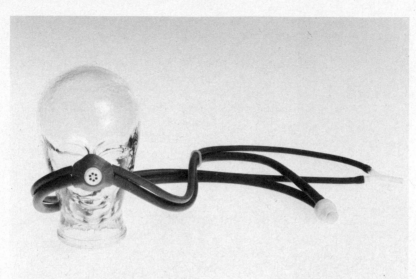

Fig. 33-8. Scavenging nasal mask. (Courtesy Narco McKesson. From Bennett, C.R. 1978. Conscious sedation in dental practice, ed. 2. St. Louis: The C.V. Mosby Co.)

Scavenging system. This includes a mask or other device to remove expired gases from the operatory (Fig. 33-8). Studies on the effects of long-term exposure to small amounts of nitrous oxide and other anesthetic gases indicate that use of such a system is a prudent safety precaution.

Reservoir bag. The reservoir bag is filled by fresh gas and is large enough to accommodate the volume of the patient's greatest inspiration.

Flush valve. By activating this valve, the clinician is able to deliver 100% oxygen at a high flow rate. This also enables the machine to be used in manual resuscitation.

Attention to nitrous oxide and oxygen conscious sedation equipment is essential. The installation of such equipment should be completed by qualified professionals. After installation, the equipment must be maintained and checked regularly to ensure proper functioning. The equipment must not be altered in any way, and guidelines from the manufacturer for safe handling must be followed.

CONCERN ABOUT ENVIRONMENTAL CONTAMINATION

In the last several years interest has been shown in the possible effects of chronic exposure to anesthetic gases. Although few studies have looked at nitrous oxide as a single agent, evidence does suggest that trace contamination of anesthetic gases may be a health hazard (Cohen et al., 1980; Jastak and Greenfield, 1977).

Major topics of study have included miscarriage, congenital malformation, cancer, and psychologic disorders. Knill-Jones et al. (1972) found that working female anesthesiologists reported an abortion rate of 18.2% as compared with 14.7% in nonanesthesiologists.

In a study sponsored by the American Society of Anesthesiologists, female respondents reported a 1.25 rate of congenital abnormality per 100 live births as compared with a 0.21 rate reported by women responding from the American Academy of Pediatrics. The rates of the wives of men responding in the two associations were 1.56 and 0.9, respectively (Cohen et al., 1974).

In a 20-year study of the cause of death among anesthesiologists, Bruce et al. (1968) found that the rate of lymphoid malignancy was significantly higher than normally expected.

In studies of psychologic effects, it has been found that traces of anesthetic gases may affect memory, reaction time, or temperament. Swepston (1976) has outlined a case presentation in which after 3 months of daily misuse of nitrous oxide, a clinician experienced and was hospitalized for paranoid delusions.

When comparing individuals not exposed to inhalation anesthetics with those who were, Cohen et al. (1980) found that male dentists had a 1.7-fold increase in liver disease, a 1.2-fold increase in kidney disease, and a 1.9-fold increase in neurologic disease.

Although an exact cause-and-effect relationship has not been determined, it seems that available safety precautions are indicated.

Swenson (1976) studied the mean concentration of halothane and nitrous oxide, measured 15 inches in front of the nasal mask. In a nonrebreathing system in which partial recirculation of exhaust occurs, 1955 parts per million (ppm) of nitrous oxide were found. In a system in which no recirculation of exhaust occurs, 172 ppm of nitrous oxide were found. Scavenging devices and well-ventilated operatories are helpful in reducing the amount of exposure to nitrous oxide for dental personnel.

The National Institute for Occupational Safety and Health has recommended 50 ppm exposure to nitrous oxide waste gas. In a study with pediatric patients, Badger et al. (1982) has noted that levels above the recommended persist in operatories in spite of scavenging equipment. This suggests that better methods for delivering analgesia, eliminating waste gases, and monitoring trace gases in the dental environment must be developed.

In the years to come, investigators will continue to define the dangers and to determine safety standards for this facet of dental practice.

Guidelines for nitrous oxide scavenging and waste gas monitoring equipment are published by the ADA Council on Dental Materials and Devices (1977).

ADMINISTRATION

Once the patient is identified as a candidate for nitrous oxide and oxygen conscious sedation, preparation for the experience is in order.

Often an initial experience is helpful for the patient. This is done at a time when no dentistry is to be performed. The patient is familiarized with the sedation equipment and experiences the relaxation effects. In that way the patient looks forward to a comfortable dental appointment. This step may

in itself create an important change in the patient's attitude.

Occasionally the patient may have heard about nitrous oxide, or "laughing gas," and may be afraid he/she will do something embarrassing. The clinician should explain to the patient that this will not occur. The level of sedation will produce pleasant relaxation, but the patient will be aware of and in control of all actions. The patient is able to control the level of sedation by breathing deeply through the nose (increase effect) or by breathing through the mouth (decrease effect). These maneuvers affect the external concentration, thereby increasing or reducing alveolar concentration.

The clinician maintains a professional attitude. The patient's comments are listened to, and positive reassurance is offered. This encourages confidence in the clinician. During sedation, it will be important that the patient trust the clinician's suggestions.

Other suggestions prior to the dental appointment include attention to diet and dress. Before nitrous oxide and oxygen conscious sedation, the patient does not need to restrict diet altogether. A light meal 1 hour or so before the appointment is recommended. For patient comfort neither an empty stomach nor a full stomach is suggested.

Comfortable, loose clothing is ideal. If desired, clothing at the neck can be loosened.

Technique

Following are the steps for administering nitrous oxide and oxygen conscious sedation.

1. Review the patient's medical history. Take vital signs.

2. Discuss the procedure with the patient.

3. Prepare the sedation equipment by cleaning the nasal mask with disinfectant. Check to make sure that the supply of oxygen and nitrous oxide is sufficient to complete the procedure. Once the patient is seated in the operatory, the sedation equipment can be shown to the patient. Never force sedation on a patient. He/she should agree to trying the experience. Reaffirm the comfortable feelings the patient will experience.

4. Turn the oxygen on to a flow of 6 to 8 liters per minute. This flow will be maintained throughout the procedure. The patient can hold the mask and feel the flow of oxygen. If the system does not include a scavenging mask, check the exhalation

valve to be sure it is set at *open* and check the air dilution valve to be sure it is set at *closed*.

5. Fill the reservoir bag by activating the flush valve. The patient seats the nasal mask himself/herself and adjusts it to a comfortable position. A gauze square may be helpful if placed under the edges of the mask on sensitive areas of the face. This pads the mask against the face and closes any leaks around the mask if a perfect fit is not possible. It is especially important to have the oxygen flowing and the reservoir bag filled so that the patient may take a comfortable first breath of pure oxygen.

6. Allow the patient a few minutes to breathe the oxygen. Have the patient practice breathing through the mouth to show the patient how he/she has control of the inhalation technique.

7. Inform the patient that he/she may smell a sweet odor as the nitrous oxide is started at 0.5 to 1 liter per minute. Reassure the patient that the procedure is going well. Ask the patient to take a few deep breaths while relaxing arms, hands, and legs. Suggest that the patient rest back in the dental chair for a comfortable and enjoyable dental appointment. The patient may begin to show signs of less tension: relaxed facial expression, relaxed hands, and less movement of the eyes around the room. If the patient feels uncomfortable, he/she will usually say so or look distressed.

If the patient comments that nothing has changed, increase the nitrous oxide level another ½ or 1 liter per minute. Suggest the reactions that the patient will generally feel at that particular nitrous oxide concentration, such as, "You may be feeling warm or notice tingling in your hands and feet. Everyone responds a bit differently, but a feeling of floating comfortably or relaxing into the chair is common. These feelings are part of the relaxation technique."

Once a patient is started on a sedation procedure, he/she should never be left alone. The operatory and supplies should be fully arranged before the sedation procedure is begun. Constant monitoring must be maintained (Fig. 33-9). One can arrange instruments, write notes, or begin examination procedures while observing the patient. Hanging on the patient's every feeling may be anxiety producing if the patient senses he/she is not feeling what has been suggested.

Careful observation of the patient will determine whether the nitrous oxide should be increased to

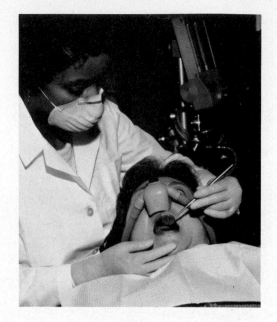

Fig. 33-9. Monitor patient at all times for consciousness, comfort, and cooperation.

the next step. When the patient is comfortable, he/she may sigh, readjust the body to a more relaxed position, become quiet, and smile slightly. Voices and other operatory noises may be exaggerated or muffled. Speak in a quiet voice, at a slower rate, and in a calming manner.

Minnis (1979) has noted that a person under nitrous oxide and oxygen conscious sedation is in a very suggestible state. The effect of the clinician's verbal and nonverbal communication is crucial. How things are said is often more important than what is said. The softness and sincerity of the clinician's voice may be one of the best instruments for relaxing and reassuring the patient.

The comfort range for each patient is individualized. The optimum concentration of nitrous oxide should never exceed 35%. Use the formula mentioned earlier to compute the percentage.

8. Once a comfortable level of sedation has been achieved, a local anesthetic can be administered.

9. Proceed with the appointment plan.

10. Monitor the patient constantly for consciousness, comfort, and cooperation. If the patient

is becoming very lethargic, closing his/her mouth often and tending toward sleep, reduce the percentage of nitrous oxide ½ to 1 liter per minute to lighten the level of sedation.

11. Nearing the end of the appointment, reduce the nitrous oxide concentration. The patient will usually maintain satisfactory relaxation if simple procedures are performed, such as polishing, flossing, carving amalgam, or checking occlusion. Place sensible limits on the duration of sedation in the individual case.

About 5 minutes before the end of the appointment, turn the nitrous oxide off completely.

12. Allow the patient to breathe 6 to 8 liters of pure oxygen per minute for at least 5 minutes. This step is necessary to avoid diffusion hypoxia, which may precipitate syncope.

Since nitrous oxide diffuses more rapidly than oxygen, the concentration of nitrous oxide in the bloodstream begins to diffuse into the alveolar spaces rapidly when the nitrous oxide is shut off. A temporary state of hypoxia (lack of oxygen) may occur if adequate oxygen is unable to diffuse from the lungs into the bloodstream during the phase of exhaling the nitrous oxide concentration. A lack of adequate oxygen or an increase in carbon dioxide levels in the bloodstream may produce syncope or other adverse cardiac and respiratory effects. By oxygenating the patient for several minutes following termination of the nitrous oxide flow, diffusion occurs gradually and a hypoxic state is avoided.

Generally, under short-term conditions such as are used in conjunction with outpatient dental treatment, the patient should be largely recovered after a 5-minute exposure to 100% oxygen at the conclusion of the appointment. However, further benefit is apparently gained from a somewhat longer recuperation before the patient engages in any activity requiring exacting psychomotor skills (McKercher et al., 1980).

13. Remove the nasal mask.

14. Slowly seat the patient in a semisupine position. Following the 5 minutes of breathing 100% oxygen, breathing room air for 10 to 15 minutes is appropriate. In most cases this much time is necessary to complete appointment procedures prior to dismissal. The patient remains in the chair until all sedation effects are gone. The patient should feel normal and be pleased with the dental appointment.

15. Disinfect the mask and equipment. Shut the entire system off after each administration if sedation is used infrequently or at the end of the day if the system is used frequently.

Because of the rapid euphoric effects nitrous oxide is capable of creating, there is potential for abuse of this medication. In fact, one or two deaths occur each year because of misuse of nitrous oxide (Swepston, 1976). Lock portable equipment and secure the central system to discourage any unfortunate occurrences.

16. Record the experience in the patient's chart. Note vital signs before nitrous oxide administration, concentrations of nitrous oxide and oxygen administered, length of time, and effects on the patient or reactions that may be helpful for future reference.

Conditions during sedation

If a patient becomes uncomfortable or anxious and tries to remove the nasal mask, gently prevent this from occurring, since it predisposes the patient to diffusion hypoxia. Immediately flush the system with 100% oxygen while at the same time verbally reassuring the patient that you understand what is occurring and realize the patient feels uncomfortable (DeMartina and Garber, 1979). Ask the patient to breathe deeply as the pure oxygen is delivered. Within a few moments the patient will begin to feel better. Reassure the patient that everything is fine. He/she is safe and will be feeling better as each breath of oxygen is taken.

When a relaxed state is again achieved, complete the dental procedure. Do not let the patient have a bad experience with sedation. At the end of the appointment compliment the patient on his/her cooperation and the successful dental appointment.

An occasional patient may become nauseated and vomit. This usually does not happen when sedation is maintained with nitrous oxide and oxygen below a 35% concentration. If the patient felt well before the appointment and ate lightly prior to the dental appointment, this situation probably will not occur.

If vomiting does occur, help the patient to a position that will prevent aspiration from occurring. Hold the head over the cuspidor and use suction to assist evacuation (Swepston, 1976). Again, maintain the mask and flush the system so that the patient is breathing 100% oxygen. Supply the patient with a cool, wet towel to clean up. Refresh the operatory as quickly as possible. The patient will no doubt be embarrassed. Handle the situation promptly, comfort the patient, and finish the dental procedure. Prevention is possible by maintaining comfort at a lower level of nitrous oxide and observing the early signs of patient distress.

Conditions following sedation

In general, an episode of nitrous oxide sedation has no residual effects. The medication is inhaled, it influences the central nervous system while it circulates in the bloodstream, and it is exhaled unchanged. Depending on the nature of the patient and the length of sedation, the patient may retain a relaxed feeling. Often the dental procedure is itself tiring, and the patient may feel a bit fatigued.

Normal functioning or driving is not contraindicated specifically because of nitrous oxide and oxygen conscious sedation, but the dentist or hygienist may recommend precautions according to the procedures performed or the patient's health status.

Patients returning to professions that require operating heavy machinery, using highly skilled motor coordination, or making critical decisions may need to use discretion in returning to these functions. In general, recovery occurs within 10 to 15 minutes, with the patient feeling fine and able to perform as normal.

CONCLUSION

Nitrous oxide and oxygen conscious sedation permits a safe and effective means for providing comfortable dentistry to an important group of patients. It is a justifiable means to a successful end. As the anxious patient gains confidence in the clinician and experiences several successful appointments, the patient may be ready to be weaned from nitrous oxide. One may find that increasing positive suggestion and decreasing nitrous oxide concentration produce the desired sedation. The patient is usually pleased with the realization of this new behavior. Seeing such a patient approach and accept dental care without fear is possibly the greatest benefit of nitrous oxide and oxygen conscious sedation.

ACTIVITIES

1. Given patient profiles, discuss the indication for nitrous oxide and oxygen conscious sedation.
2. Watch a demonstration of administration technique. Observe the experience of a clinic patient with nitrous oxide and oxygen conscious sedation.
3. Simulate administration of or actually administer nitrous oxide and oxygen conscious sedation to a lab partner. If actually administering sedation, share the variety of responses that were noted in the group.
4. Administer nitrous oxide and oxygen conscious sedation to an appropriate clinic patient.*

REVIEW QUESTIONS

1. Nitrous oxide and oxygen sedation is a form of conscious sedation. What does this mean (include a definition of conscious in your answer)?
2. Consider each of the following pairs. Check the characteristic that best describes nitrous oxide.
   a. Organic inhalation agent, odorless, and flammable
   a′. Inorganic inhalation agent, sweet smelling, and nonflammable
   b. Has a high blood gas solubility as compared with oxygen
   b′. Has a low blood gas solubility as compared with oxygen
   c. Eliminated unchanged by the lungs
   c′. Eliminated by the lungs as nitrogen
   d. An extremely potent anesthetic when administered with oxygen
   d′. A mildly potent anesthetic when administered with oxygen
   e. Affects the body's physiologic reaction to pain perception
   e′. Affects the person's psychologic reaction to pain perception
3. State the reason nitrous oxide and oxygen conscious sedation is contraindicated for persons with the following conditions:
   a. Patient with emphysema
   b. Patient with an upper respiratory tract infection
4. Calculate the percentage of nitrous oxide being delivered to a patient at the flow of 4 liters per minute of nitrous oxide and 6 liters per minute of oxygen. How does this percentage relate to the level recommended for optimal sedation? If this patient were having a tooth extracted, would local anesthesia be indicated?
5. Identify three signs that indicate that the inhaled concentration of nitrous oxide is too great.

---

*An instructor qualified to administer nitrous oxide and oxygen conscious sedation must supervise a student providing sedation to a clinic patient. Direct supervision during the induction phase and continued priority attention to this student and patient throughout the appointment are necessary.

REFERENCES

ADA Council on Dental Materials and Devices. 1977. Expansion of the acceptable program, nitrous oxide scavenging equipment and nitrous oxide trace gas monitoring equipment. J. Am. Dent. Assoc. **95:**791.

ADA Council on Dental Therapeutics. 1982. Accepted dental therapeutics, ed. 39. Chicago, Ill.: American Dental Association.

Badger, G., et al. 1982. Nitrous oxide waste gas in the pediatric operatory. J. Am. Dent. Assoc. **104:**480.

Bennett, C.R. 1978 Conscious sedation in dental practice, ed. 2. St. Louis: The C.V. Mosby Co.

Bruce, D.L., et al. 1968. Causes of death among anesthesiologists: a 20 year survey. Anesthesiology **29:**565.

Bruce, D.L., et al. 1974. Trace anesthetic effects on perceptual, cognitive and motor skills. Anesthesiology **40:**453.

Cohen, E.N., et al. 1974. Occupational disease among operating room personnel: a national study. Anesthesiology **41:**321.

Cohen, E.N., et al. 1975. A survey of anesthetic health hazards among dentists. J. Am. Dent. Assoc. **90:**1291.

Cohen, E.N., et al. 1980. Occupational disease in dentistry and chronic exposure to trace anesthetic gases. J. Am. Dent. Assoc. **101:**21.

Control of occupational exposure to N₂O in the dental operatory. 1977. HEW Pub. No. (NIOSH) 77-171. Cincinnati: US Dept. of Health, Education and Welfare, Public Health Service Center for Disease Control, National Institute for Occupational Safety and Health.

DeMartina, B.K., and Garber, J.G. 1979. Analgesia in dental practice. Continuing Dental Education, University of Pennsylvania School of Dental Medicine **2:** No. 5.

Dionne, R.A. 1981. The pharmacological basis of pain control in dental practice: N₂O₂. Compend. Contin. Educ. Dent. **2:**271.

Fordham, K.C. 1974. Analgesia (medicated air). Booklet accepted for course credit by the Academy of General Dentistry, 304 King of Prussia Road, Radnor, Penn. 19087.

Getter, L. 1977. Review and current status of scavenging and monitoring devices: report of ad hoc committee on trace anesthetics as a potential health hazard in dentistry. J. Am. Dent. Assoc. **95:**788.

Hamburg, H.L. 1980. Establishing a standard technique for nitrous oxide/oxygen sedation. Dent. Surv. **56(**3):28.

Jastak, J.T., and Greenfield, W. 1977. Trace contamination of anesthetic gases: a brief review. J. Am. Dent. Assoc. **95:**758.

Kaufman, E., et al. 1982. Nitrous oxide analgesia in selected dental patients. Anesth. Prog. **29:**78.

Knill-Jones, R.P., et al. 1972. Controlled survey of women anesthetists in the United Kingdom. Lancet **1:**1326.

Langa, H. 1976. Relative analgesia in dental practice, inhalation analgesia and sedation with nitrous oxide, ed. 2. Philadelphia: W.B. Saunders Co.

Littner, M.M., et al. 1983. Occupational hazards in the dental office and their control. IV. Measures for controlling contamination of anesthetic gas, nitrous oxide. Quintessence Int. **14:**461.

McKercher, T.C., et al. 1980. Recovery and enhancement of reflex reaction time after nitrous oxide analgesia. J. Am. Dent. Assoc. **101:**785.

Minnis, R. 1979. Psychological effects of conscious sedation. Anesth. Prog. **26:**150.

Riklin, B.M. 1978. Nitrous oxide–oxygen sedation for the geriatric patient. J. Am. Soc. Geriatr. Dent. **13(**2):8.

Roberts, G.J., et al. 1982. Physiological changes during relative analgesia—a clinical study. J. Dent. **10:**55.

Swenson, R.D. 1976. Scavenging of dental anesthetic gases. J. Oral Surg. **34:**207.

Swepston, B.A. 1976. The practical use of oxygen–nitrous oxide conscious sedation in dental practice. Plano, Tex.: Happiness Seminars.

Swepston, B. 1980. Dental phobia becomes euphoria: advances of nitrous oxide, parts 1 and 2. Dent. Pract. **1(**5):60; **1(**6):42.

Wald, C. 1983. Nitrous oxide—are there any real contraindications? Quintessence Int. **14:**213.

34 MODIFICATION OF DENTAL HYGIENE CARE FOR PATIENTS WITH SPECIAL NEEDS

OBJECTIVES: *The reader will be able to*

1. Identify patients with special needs for whom dental hygiene care should be modified.
2. Modify dental hygiene care for patients with special needs in the areas of:
   a. Communication
   b. Appointment planning
   c. Environmental considerations such as equipment positioning and patient positioning
   d. Instruction for individualized home care
   e. Safety precautions in treatment
3. Identify the reasons for seeking specific resources to gain additional information regarding patients with sensory and physical limitations.

Every patient needs to be treated as an individual with a unique personality, set of senses, and physical self. In fact, modifications in dental care are made regularly for patients with special needs. These patients include those who are very tall, very short, pregnant, or very young, as well as overweight and extremely fearful patients, patients with busy schedules, older patients, and patients who live far from the office.

In general, the professional team deals with these patients by modifying communication, appointment planning, chair and equipment considerations, and individualized instruction for home care. This same attention applies to patients who are handicapped in a mental, physical, or sensory way.

COMMUNICATION

Communication differs with each person. For patients who can see, looking at pictures, reading information, looking at and handling equipment, and observing other patients during dental procedures does much to acquaint them with care. Patients without sight can use hearing, touch, smell, and taste to explore dentistry. Depending on the sensory limitation, communication by way of the remaining senses helps the patient experience dentistry without fear. The clinician who takes time to reach out to these patients and to create a good dental experience will no doubt make friends as well as ensure the patients' cooperation.

Careful introductory procedures are useful for patients who are deaf or blind. These patients lack essential sensory cues for determining what procedures are about to occur. A deaf person may be able to lip-read. If so, the dental professional should speak to the patient only when the patient can see the professional's lips. It is usually annoying and embarrassing for the lipreading patient if the dental professional accentuates mouth movements in speaking or shouts. Speaking slowly but normally is usually most acceptable. A helpful tool for communication is to know sign language for the deaf or to write out a series of descriptions and questions for the patient.

For the blind patient, it is possible to describe procedures and allow the patient to feel the components of the dental operatory. Sharp instruments for obvious reasons should be felt only with caution and careful direction or not at all. Disinfection should follow the guided tour of equipment, and sterile instruments should replace those handled by the patient. This process should be explained to the patient to avoid arousing concern over why changes are being made.

Patients who may not understand the visual or verbal introduction to dentistry will need to take one step at a time. Every patient does better when surprises are minimized in a new and potentially frightening situation. Human qualities of friendliness, a calm manner, light touch, and gentle tone indicate in a universal language that the professional cares.

ALTERING THE APPOINTMENT PLAN

For most patients with a disability, the appointment plan is dependent on their individual tolerance of the procedure. Perhaps only one half of the mouth or one tooth at a time can be completed. Unless access to care is an extreme problem, creating a good experience without overdoing the length of the appointment is the main consideration. As much as possible, the patient should be introduced to an appointment routine that will be followed each time. For example:

1. Check the mouth with a mirror.
2. Check with an explorer.
3. Clean the teeth with a toothbrush.
4. Clean the teeth with an instrument.
5. Clean the teeth with a rubber cup.
6. The patient looks in a mirror or feels the teeth.
7. Apply fluoride.

Such a routine creates a comfortable familiarity. (Nowak, 1976) Attention to the appointment schedule as far as the time of day or length of time may be significant for the patient. A rested and nourished patient is usually most receptive. A midmorning appointment might be the best time to treat a patient needing a moderate amount of modification in care.

MODIFYING THE ENVIRONMENT FOR CARE

The dental clinic or office should be equipped to handle a patient in a wheelchair. This includes access ramps, a suitable rest room, and an operatory area where patient transfer is possible.

Several wheelchair transfer techniques are described in the following section.

Transfer techniques from a wheelchair to a dental chair*

General considerations for all transfers

1. When lifting, always use the knees and hips—not the back.
2. Consult with the patient or attendant on the transfer method he/she prefers.
3. Be sure that the patient's toilet needs are met before transferring.
4. Be cognizant of the following: catheters and cushion padding (to prevent decubiti).
5. Brakes must be engaged.
6. Front wheels should be set forward and the lock engaged, if present.
7. Footrests and legrests on the wheelchair that would interfere with the transfer should be removed.
8. According to transfer technique, the wheelchair armrest adjacent to the dental chair may require removal.
9. The dental chair armrest adjacent to the side of transfer is moved into an appropriate position to permit access.

Transfer technique for hemiplegics

1. Position the wheelchair facing the dental chair at about a 45-degree angle with the patient's unaffected side adjacent to the dental chair.
2. Stand in front of the patient and slightly to the affected side.
3. The patient moves forward in the wheelchair and leans forward.
4. Be sure the patient's feet are flat on the floor with a fairly wide base for support.
5. Using the unaffected arm, the patient pushes off from the wheelchair armrest to a standing position (Fig. 34-1).
6. If assistance is needed in standing, lock the affected knee with your knees and place your hand(s) under the patient's axilla.
7. Once standing and balanced, have the patient grip the furthermost armrest (if the left extremity is the normal one) or the closest armrest (if the right extremity is the normal one), positioning the thumb on the inside of the armrest, and pivot on the unaffected leg.

---

*By permission of C. Staman Kleiman, C.D.A., R.D.H., B.S. 1978. Philadelphia: Moss Rehabilitation Hospital.

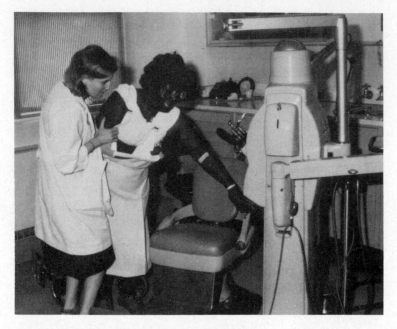

Fig. 34-1. Transfer technique for hemiplegics. Using unaffected side, patient pushes off from wheelchair armrest. (Courtesy Moss Rehabilitation Hospital, Philadelphia.)

8. Have the patient lower himself/herself slowly into the dental chair, using the unaffected arm and leg for support (Fig. 34-2).
9. Adjust the dental chair armrest.

One-person transfer technique for quadriplegics and paraplegics (Stiefel et al., 1978)

1. Position the wheelchair parallel to the dental chair.
2. Grasp the patient under the thighs and lifting slightly, pull forward until the buttocks rest just ahead of the rear wheel.
3. Place the patient's feet so that the outside of the balls of the feet are firmly within your instep.
4. While bending at the knees, place your knees around the patient's knees (Fig. 34-3).
5. Lean the patient forward until the head rests on your left shoulder.
6. Lock your chin on the patient's shoulder.
7. Help the patient place his/her arms around your neck.
8. Place your arms around the patient's back below the rib cage and use one hand to grasp your opposite wrist.
9. Rock forward slightly on the balls of your feet, then rock back, initiating the lift.
10. Pull the patient forward using your leg muscles to provide strength for the lift.
11. Pivot toward the dental chair and seat the patient (Fig. 34-4).
12. With your right hand, lift both legs and swing them onto the dental chair.

Two-person transfer technique for quadriplegics and paraplegics (Stiefel et al., 1978)

1. Position wheelchair parallel to the dental chair.
2. First person: stand behind the patient and reach under the patient's arms, clasping your right hand over patient's left hand and your left hand over his/her right.
3. Pull the arms toward you and just under the patient's rib cage.
4. Second person: stand on the patient's right and place one arm just above the knees and one arm under the patient's feet (Fig. 34-5).

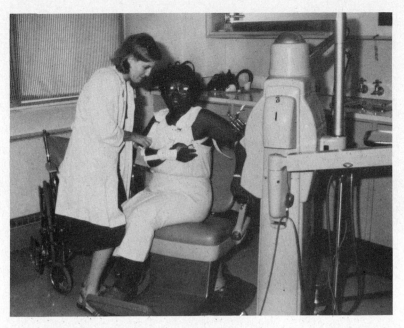

Fig. 34-2. Patient grasps dental chair armrest, and clinician pivots patient on unaffected side for lowering into dental chair. (Courtesy Moss Rehabilitation Hospital, Philadelphia.)

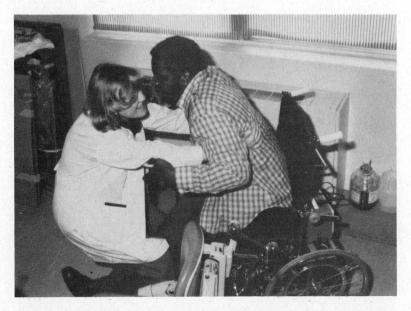

Fig. 34-3. One-person transfer technique for quadriplegics and paraplegics. After patient is positioned forward in wheelchair, clinician bends at knees and places his/her knees around patient's knees. (Courtesy Moss Rehabilitation Hospital, Philadelphia.)

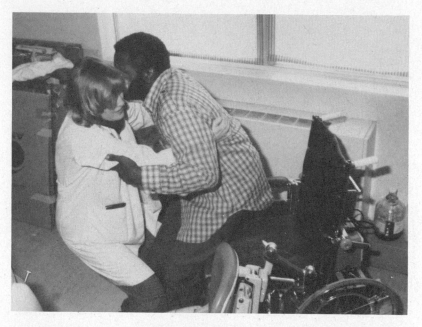

Fig. 34-4. Clinician rocks forward and back to initiate lift, then pivots patient and lowers patient into dental chair. (Courtesy Moss Rehabilitation Hospital, Philadelphia.)

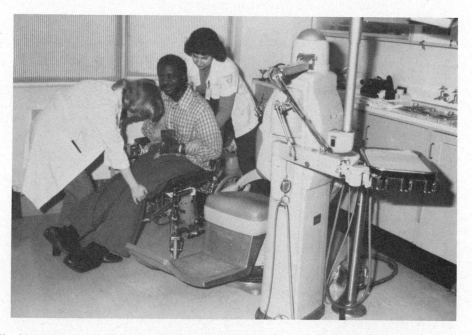

Fig. 34-5. Two-person transfer technique for quadriplegics and paraplegics. Wheelchair is positioned next to dental chair. One person grasps patient under arms benath rib cage. Second person supports patient's legs under knees. (Courtesy Moss Rehabilitation hospital, Philadelphia.)

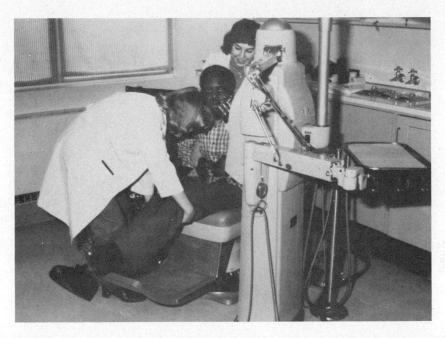

Fig. 34-6. In unison, both persons lift patient into dental chair. (Courtesy Moss Rehabilitation Hospital, Philadelphia.)

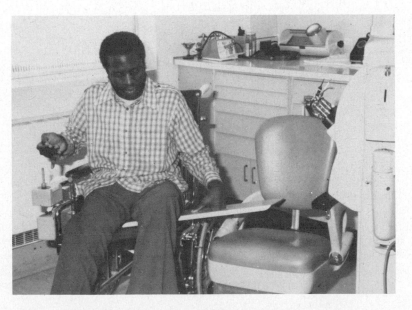

Fig. 34-7. Sliding board transfer. Board is placed under patient and across dental chair. (Courtesy Moss Rehabilitation Hospital, Philadelphia.)

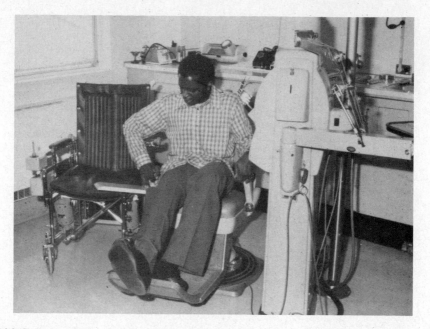

Fig. 34-8. Patient eases himself along board until position in dental chair is achieved. Assistance with legs may be necessary. After transfer, board is removed. (Courtesy Moss Rehabilitation Hospital, Philadelphia.)

5. In unison, lift the patient to the other chair (Fig. 34-6).

Transfer technique with a sliding board (Stiefel et al., 1978)

1. Place wheelchair parallel and as close as possible to the dental chair.
2. First person: stand behind the patient and grasp the patient's arms as described in step 2 of the two-person transfer technique.
3. Tilt the patient away from the dental chair and slightly forward.
4. Second person: slide the board under the buttocks and across the dental chair.
5. Second person: move to the patient's right.
6. Together: simultaneously lift the patient's legs and torso with the weight being supported on the sliding board.
7. First person: elevate the patient slightly forward and to the left as the second person removes the board (Figs. 34-7 and 34-8).

Other equipment modifications

If transfer is not possible, portable equipment such as a headrest attachment, a mobile unit with handpieces, and access to a suitable light and central suction system are adequate.

For patient and clinician safety, implements have been designed to prevent excess body movement, to keep the jaw in working position, and to prevent laceration or aspiration.

The use of restraints is necessary to treat some highly mobile or spastic patients. The human touch is advised if the condition can be adequately controlled by placing a hand or arm on the limb to restrict motion. If this cannot be accomplished, special wraps (Pedi-wrap, Papoose Board), seat belts, and harnesses are available to ensure that the patient cannot harm himself/herself or the clinician (Luke, 1977; Nowak, 1976).

Similarly, working in the oral cavity with hands and sharp or motorized instruments is potentially dangerous if patient cooperation cannot be relied on. Mouth props and bite blocks can be made or purchased in various sizes to suit the patient's mouth (Fig. 34-9). Unbreakable steel mirrors are advised in place of glass mirrors. A thimble can be altered to make a protective finger covering.

To avoid laceration or aspiration, a rubber dam

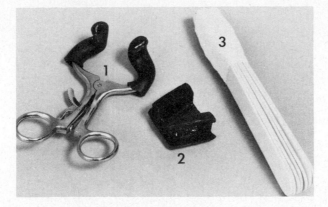

Fig. 34-9. Mouth props. *1.* Molt mouth gag; *2,* McKesson mouth prop; *3,* multiple tongue blades taped together to form mouth prop. (From Nowak, A.J. 1976. Dentistry for the handicapped patient. St. Louis: The C.V. Mosby Co.)

is recommended whenever possible. Other supplies placed in the mouth such as clamps, gauze, bite blocks, or cotton rolls should be secured by tying a strand of floss to the object so that it may be readily retrieved.

INSTRUCTION FOR INDIVIDUALIZED HOME CARE

One of the most important aspects of care for patients with disabilities is helping the patient establish a preventive home care routine. Many studies report the universal prevalence of periodontal disease, as well as significantly poorer oral hygiene in the handicapped population when compared with control groups (Nowak, 1976). The daily care for some handicapped patients is so overwhelming that oral care may seem trivial. Explaining the high degree of sensitivity of this area of the body in relation to expression and nourishment may help the patient focus on oral care. If the patient is able to comprehend the value of prevention, extensive time must be devoted to illustrating prevention and dealing with the patient's physical limitations. The objectives for removing plaque are the same as described in Chapter 17. With the individual patient, the hygienist will be able to determine how to clean the crowns and oral soft tissues.

Modifying the tools for oral hygiene is a special help for the patient with a disability. Perhaps an appointment or part of one can be used for experimenting with a variety of cleaning aids. The time spent to study the patient's abilities will help the clinician create a workable tool. Price (1980) has suggested that patients with limited arm movement can often use a toothbrush with an elongated handle. Taping the brush handle to a wooden dowel or a plastic item such as a ruler may create a brushing tool the patient can work independently. Patients unable to flex their fingers are helped by tools with oversized handles. A rubber ball or sponge may be useful for mounting the brush in. Other patients with limited finger movement but good arm movement can use a brush strapped to the finger or hand. An interlocking tape can be useful for making a modification such as this. In a study to evaluate the efficacy of a digital brush (a brush that is attached to the patient's finger), Goho (1980) found that plaque levels were reduced by as much as 20% in the patient's home care routine. The digital brush is a good idea for a patient who has arm and wrist movement but cannot grasp a regular brush.

For patients with no arm movement, an electric toothbrush can be mounted on the wall. Patients who have head and trunk movement can position themselves to use this type of apparatus (Price, 1980).

By carefully heating the plastic handle of a regular brush in a Bunsen burner, the plastic becomes flexible so that almost any shape or turn of the brush head can be made. A patient may need several brushes modified to reach all areas of the mouth.

With all modifications, it is important to consider the cost and safety of each item. To keep the tools as sanitary as possible, items should be selected that can be washed and dried or disposed of and replaced. It is important for the clinician to see the tool in use by the patient to check for the safety of the design. These tools will need to be replaced frequently. The clinician can make several and keep a copy of the "original" so that more can be made as needed. The time taken to create a tool that is special will help the patient realize the value the clinician places on home care for the patient's well-being. It is individualized care and instruction at its best.

If the patient is unable to handle a modified brush, automatic brush, or help in cleaning the teeth, another person must assume responsibility for oral care. Appreciating the importance of daily plaque control may be an attitude that develops slowly on the part of the patient, parent, or other person providing care.

Many handicapped patients have anomalies of the dentition, receive special or soft-textured diets, or take medications that alter oral conditions. The hygienist can stress the role of healthy teeth and oral tissues in limiting infection, improving mastication, enhancing the patient's sociability, and preventing the need for restorative procedures. In-struction with the patient and helper must be supportive if a successful preventive routine is to be established.

Disclosing solution is excellent for making the plaque a visible target for removal. Instructions for brushing in a systematic routine should be given. After brushing, flossing bimanually or with a floss holder is recommended. If this can be done only once daily, the routine is advised before the patient is put to bed at the end of the day. Rinsing the mouth after meals and snacks, and wiping the teeth with a soft cloth are helpful cleaning measures to be used throughout the day. Taking the time to teach patient positioning and the use of the mouth prop may facilitate the entire process. At a follow-up visit the home care steps should be reviewed and any problems that may be occurring can be discussed.

SUGGESTIONS FOR PATIENT POSITIONING

1. Oral hygiene can be accomplished with the patient seated. The clinician stands behind the patient and uses one arm to support the patient's head. The other arm and hand are used to manipulate the brush and floss (Fig. 34-10).
2. With the patient lying down, the clinician sits next to the patient. Restraining one arm with

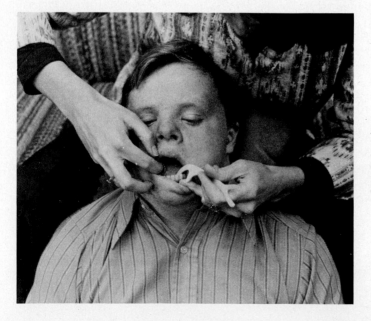

Fig. 34-10. Clinician stands or sits behind patient and supports head. Note thimble on clinician's finger for protection and to prop mouth open. Other hand is free to clean teeth. (From Nowak, A.J. 1976. Dentistry for the handicapped patient. St. Louis: The C.V. Mosby Co.)

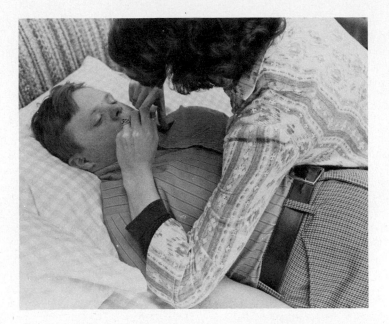

Fig. 34-11. Position of one person to clean teeth of patient with uncontrollable movements. Note position across chest of patient, as well as use of arm to control patient's arm. (From Nowak, A.J. Dentistry for the handicapped patient. St. Louis: The C.V. Mosby Co.)

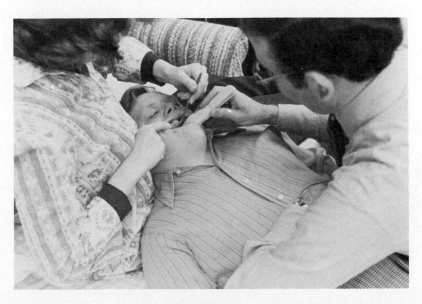

Fig. 34-12. Positioning of two people to clean teeth of patient with uncontrollable movements. (From Nowak, A.J. 1976. Dentistry for the handicapped patient. St. Louis: The C.V. Mosby Co.)

the body, the clinician leans across the patient and holds the other arm. The free hand is used to clean the teeth (Fig. 34-11).

3. If two people are available, a patient who needs considerable restraint can be held by one person. The other person can then support the head and complete the cleaning procedures (Fig. 34-12).

DENTAL CARE FOR PREGNANT PATIENTS

A few modifications in care are necessary for pregnant patients. Women of childbearing age should be questioned about pregnancy through the medical history or recall history update prior to treatment. During the first trimester of pregnancy, the fetus is undergoing critical development of all organs and tissues. At this stage, called organogenesis, the unborn child is most susceptible to substances or events that could disturb normal growth. Exposure to certain medications and radiation could adversely affect the well-being of the mother and developing fetus. If there is a possibility that the patient may be pregnant, the taking of diagnostic radiographs should be delayed. Routine prophylaxis and examination can be performed if the patient is feeling well. Otherwise, all elective dental work can be postponed until the second trimester of pregnancy or until after the child is delivered.

It is best to provide treatment for the pregnant patient in the last half of the second trimester (fifth or sixth month). At this point, organogenesis is completed. The patient may be feeling quite well, and the weight and size of the fetus will generally not cause the patient discomfort when she is in the supine position. In later stages of pregnancy, the enlarged fetus puts pressure on major abdominal veins, causing blockage of venous return from the legs when the patient is supine. Hypotension and syncope can result if the patient is reclined for too long.

In general, all medications should be avoided throughout pregnancy. However, routine restorative dentistry can be provided with local anesthesia during the second and third trimesters. Additional vasoconstrictors are not necessary in anesthetic solutions. Nitrous oxide analgesia and general anesthesia are contraindicated. In emergency situations, many medications can be administered safely during pregnancy. The clinician should have the full support of the patient's obstetrician before prescribing or administering any type of analgesic, sedative, or antibiotic.

If radiographic diagnosis is essential, radiographs may be taken late in the second trimester or in the early part of the third trimester. To limit radiation to the patient, only a single film of the area in question should be exposed. The x-ray unit should have proper collimation and shielding. High-speed film and a long-cone/high-voltage technique are recommended. The patient is also protected by the lead shield drape as usual (Gier and Janes, 1983).

Patient education is important for the pregnant patient. This is an ideal time for the clinician to lay to rest the myths about decalcification of the mother's teeth and loss of teeth due to pregnancy. It is an especially good time to review the need for good home care habits and plaque control. In 1965 Loe studied 121 prenatal and postnatal women for signs of clinical inflammation. Gingival changes occurred in 100% of the subjects. Changes were noted as early as 8 weeks' gestation and were most severe by 8 months' gestation. The accumulation of plaque paralleled the gingival changes. When complete removal of plaque was accomplished, resolution of gingivitis usually occurred. Other factors contribute to gingivitis and oral problems during pregnancy. For example, preexisting periodontal conditions may be aggravated by hormonal changes. Home care habits may change as a result of general fatigue. Nausea and vomiting associated with "morning sickness" may make oral hygiene difficult. If the gag reflex is easily stimulated, the patient may avoid brushing and flossing. Vomiting will produce a temporary acidic state in the oral cavity, leaving the teeth more susceptible to attack. Providing understanding and support for the pregnant patient is as important as encouraging good oral hygiene habits and a noncariogenic diet.

The clinician should ask whether the patient is receiving nutritional information in conjunction with prenatal classes at the medical clinic or hospital. If not, this is something the dental staff should provide. The pregnant patient has increased demands for protein, calories, calcium, iron, and vitamins A, B-complex, C, and D (Williams, 1982). The function of these nutrients during gestation and the types of food or supplements they may be found in is important information to cover. (See Chapter 20 for more nutritional information.) The teeth begin to develop in the fetus at 6 weeks. Substances consumed during pregnancy can affect the development of the teeth. Overconsumption of fluoride during gestation can cause fluorosis of the deciduous teeth. Some antibiotics taken during pregnancy may stain developing teeth (Cheney and DePaola, 1979). A discussion of the importance of supplemental fluoride after the birth of the child to prevent decay can be mentioned at this time also. Ideally, the mother and child can be seen at a future appointment to review fluorides, eruption dates, and the beginnings of home care for the infant.

While the patient is pregnant is a good time to review the role of plaque and the frequency of sugar consumption as related to tooth decay. This will be beneficial to the patient and will be useful information in feeding the child later. Baby bottle syndrome is a condition that fits in nicely with such a discussion of sugar and decay. The patient may not be aware of the danger to the teeth when a child is put to bed with a bottle of milk or juice to nurse through the night. Characteristic rampant decay on the facial surfaces of the teeth can result from such a practice.

Usually the pregnant patient is very receptive to any information concerning the well-being of the expected child in addition to being interested in having a safe and healthy pregnancy. The clinician should be ready to act as a resource for any questions the patient may have throughout this time. If gingival problems occur, an appointment to remove irritating calculus and review plaque control may be appreciated. A parent who is informed and motivated about dental health will be an excellent model for the child. Seemingly routine information provided to the pregnant patient may be more meaningful than ever before.

DENTAL CARE FOR PATIENTS RECEIVING CANCER THERAPY

It is more and more likely that the clinician today will have the opportunity to treat patients who have received or are undergoing cancer therapy. These would be patients who have either had (or will have) an intraoral tumor removed or patients who require the management of oral complications resulting from systemic chemotherapy or radiation therapy for a tumor in another part of the body.

When a patient is facing removal of an oral cancer, the surgeon, prosthodontist, general dentist, and dental hygienist can be involved in preparing the patient. Before surgery, every attempt is made to obtain a high degree of health in the oral cavity. Decisions will be made about teeth and bone that will be sacrificed during tumor removal. Teeth that can be preserved may be restored to act as abutments or support for a prosthesis that will be placed after surgery. If at all possible, a prosthesis that will provide as close to normal function and aesthetics as possible will be constructed. Impressions and study models of the patient's oral cavity will be made to work from. In some cases a maxillary prosthesis can be made prior to surgery. Most commonly, this is some type of obturator that will replace part or all of the palate to close the oral-nasal or pharyngeal defect. Such a prosthesis placed immediately after surgery can minimize scar contracture and disfiguration. It also may allow the patient to eat, breathe, and speak more reasonably during the initial healing phase. As healing occurs and the patient recovers function, adjustments are likely in all prostheses. It usually takes 4 to 6 months after surgery for the ideal prosthesis to be constructed.

Mandibular reconstructions are complicated by the unilateral removal of bone and muscle. The remaining healthy side pulls the mandible out of functional position. Reconstruction and successful rehabilitation will depend on (1) the extent of the remaining mandible, (2) the degree of deviation of the remaining mandible, (3) the quality of the remaining alveolar ridge, and (4) the number and state of remaining natural teeth (Carl, 1980). Manual exercises are generally started as soon as possible after surgery to help the remaining muscles realign the mandible in the direction of the original position. For a patient who wears a maxillary denture, another row of denture teeth may be added to the palatal side of the arch. This will provide a wider surface for the mandibular prosthesis to bite on when the mandible has been displaced to one side. If the patient has natural anterior and posterior teeth remaining in the maxilla and mandibular teeth in the anterior of the resected mandible, a flange prosthesis can be made. This consists of a maxillary and mandibular framework that holds the mandible in place for near-normal function. To support the forces of such a prosthesis, the remaining teeth have to be in excellent periodontal health.

Restorative and prosthetic dentistry is becoming more sophisticated to offer better alternatives to oral cancer patients. Maintaining a healthy periodontium will be extremely important. Routine professional care for teeth and tissues in addition to monitoring home care habits will continue. Modifications in tools used for oral hygiene, cleaning the teeth, and stimulating tissues may be necessary for each patient. Emotional support through the treatment and rehabilitation phase will be part of comprehensive care.

All adult patients should be examined at recall visits for tissue changes that may require biopsy. Teaching the oral self-assessment and oral cancer self-examination to detect early changes in the oral cavity may save a life. (See Chapter 19 for these examinations.)

Care for patients receiving chemotherapy

Chemotherapy is used for the treatment of many types of cancer. These include carcinomas, sarcomas, lymphomas, melanomas, and leukemia. Chemical agents that are selectively cytotoxic are used because they are more toxic to the tumor cells than to normal cells. Most chemotherapeutic agents cause bone marrow depression, decreasing platelets and white blood cells. This affects the immune system of the patient. The chemical agents also damage the basal cell layer. In the case of the oral cavity, where rapid cell turnover occurs, mucosa, which usually sloughs, is not readily replaced. The basal layers are inhibited in developing new cell structure. Approximately 5 to 7 days after the start of chemotherapy, mucosal inflammation and ulceration may appear and will continue for 4 to 10 days following the completion of therapy (Daeffler, 1980).

The chief oral complications related to these effects of chemotherapeutic agents include hemorrhagic disorders, spontaneous bleeding from periodontal sites, delayed healing after extraction, stomatitis (inflammation of the mucosa), mucositis (ulceration of the mucosa), and chemocaries.

The general health of the periodontium will contribute to the degree of difficulty the patient will have with chemotherapy. Acute and chronic periodontitis will be aggravated during therapy. Extractions, restorations, and periodontal treatment including prophylaxis, root planing, and soft tissue curettage prior to chemotherapy will reduce the potential pathways of infection.

Hemorrhagic conditions occur as a result of bone marrow depression. Areas of the periodontium that are not sound will spontaneously ooze during oral hygiene. Transfusions to replace platelets may be necessary to correct this complication. Sometimes a periodontal pack can be placed to control bleeding if an isolated area is identified (Carl, 1980).

Stomatitis may be caused by a toxic effect of the chemotherapeutic agent on the mucosa or by an infection of the mucosa (Fischman, 1983). Infections may be caused by common organisms: bacteria, viruses, or fungi. Greenberg et al. (1982) found that the patient's own oral cavity was a significant source of septicemia in patients with acute leukemia. Pericoronitis and periodontal disease are the oral diseases most frequently related to septicemia. Oral candidiasis and herpetic lesions are also seen. The ulcerations of the mucosa described as mucositis are large, often exceeding 1 cm in diameter. The ulcers may affect the lips, tongue, and esophagus. These are extremely painful. Eating or even talking can be uncomfortable. Treatment consists of decreasing the chance of secondary infection with appropriate antibacterial or antifungal preparations. Palliative treatment is advisable to make the patient as comfortable as possible.

The hypertrophic and sensitive conditions of the gingival and mucosal tissues demand that regular oral hygiene measures be altered. Rinsing the mouth with an antibiotic mouthwash or a cleansing agent such as saline and hydrogen peroxide may be all that can be done for a time. Wiping the teeth with a soft cloth, a foam stick, or cotton swab is helpful in removing food and plaque if the patient can tolerate this. Irrigation with a bulb syringe, Water Pic, power spray, or other device can be beneficial and refreshing to the patient. Brushing with a soft toothbrush and flossing can be instituted as soon as the patient's oral lesions have subsided.

Chemocaries may occur with long-term chemotherapy. This condition consists of small areas of decalcification that begin near the gingival margin and proceed laterally on the buccal and labial surfaces of the teeth. Daily topical fluoride treatments can be prescribed to prevent and control these caries. In some cases restorations may need to be placed.

In general, a consultation with the patient's physician is essential before all dental procedures in patients with a history of chemotherapy. Antibiotic coverage is recommended when a bacteremia is anticipated. Precautions should be taken against bleeding. Extractions may be necessary in the hospital setting if a transfusion of platelets is required (Fischman, 1983). The length and type of chemotherapy will vary with each condition. The patient's physical and emotional response will also be individualized. Close communication between the patient, hospital, and dental staff will determine what measures can be taken to help the patient through therapy and during recovery.

Care for patients receiving radiation therapy

Ionizing radiation is similar to chemotherapy in that normal tissues are affected when cytotoxic doses are administered to destroy the tumor cells. The amount of tissue damage will depend on the field of radiation and the dose. The tissues of the head and neck that are most susceptible to radiation include the salivary glands, the taste buds of the tongue, and the mucosa. The blood supply to the bone can be destroyed, causing pain and osteonecrosis. Dermatitis and trismus may result from irradiation of skin and muscles of mastication.

The salivary glands are very sensitive to radiation. The salivary flow will be decreased, and the nature of the saliva will change, becoming viscous and more acidic. The subsequent dry mouth condition is known as xerostomia. When the lubricating and cleansing functions of the saliva are lost, speech and swallowing are difficult. The patient is more prone to dental caries. For some patients salivary function may increase within 6 to 12 months after therapy, but for others the flow remains inadequate indefinitely (Fischman, 1983). Frequent rinsing with water or chewing sugarless gum has been helpful for some patients. New developments with artificial saliva products will have to be assessed to determine their place in easing the problems of xerostomia.

Because the patient is vulnerable to caries, topical fluoride treatments are important for the patient on a daily basis. As with chemocaries, the cervical area of the teeth is the most common site. Fluoride solutions for mouth rinsing or gels in a tray application technique can be used by the patient without difficulty. Patient motivation is critical in fostering compliance with the need for daily fluoride treatments.

Mucositis, as described in the section on chemotherapy, will also occur with radiation therapy. The inflammation and ulcers of the mucosa begin 5 to 7 days after treatment begins and will heal within 2 weeks of the completion of therapy. Attempts to keep the patient comfortable and free of infection during the outbreak of the lesions will be the goal. An opportunistic infection such as candidiasis may occur, necessitating treatment with an antifungal preparation.

Soft tissue other than the mucosa will be affected by radiation. The taste buds of the tongue are sensitive to radiation and may be obliterated, creating a partial or complete loss of taste during treatment. Usually the cells regenerate within 4 months' time after therapy, but permanent injury may result (Fischman, 1983).

All of the previously mentioned conditions—xerostomia, mucositis, loss of taste (ageusia), and caries—may cause major problems in the patient's ability and desire to eat. Encouragement is necessary to help the patient maintain proper nourishment despite discomfort. Inadequate nutrition and weight loss may only compound the patient's other problems and affect recovery time.

Oral hygiene measures will need to be altered as described in the chemotherapy section. Regular toothbrushing and flossing may be impossible during therapy. Frequent mouth rinsing and wiping the teeth may suffice for a number of days. Daeffler (1980) surveyed 69 cancer institutions for agents used in oral hygiene for cancer patients. She summarized the responses from 41 institutions. Many hospitals make up their own mouthwashes for patients. These include combinations of a variety of agents, such as an antibiotic and a pain reliever, a commercial mouthwash and hydrogen peroxide, mineral oil (lubricant) followed by a mouthwash, a normal saline and bicarbonate of soda mixture, and so forth. It is clear that no particular combination of agents has been proved to be better than others. The respondents stress that treatment must vary with the condition and what is most readily accepted by the patient. Some of the other points summarized from the survey are as follows:

A regular assessment of the oral cavity is done by tongue blade and flashlight.

Weekly cultures of oral flora are obtained.

Routine mouth care is provided before and after meals and throughout the day as the patient feels necessary.

A mouth-rinsing regimen is started at the same time therapy begins.

Nystatin (an antifungal preparation for candidiasis) is started as a preventive measure in mouth breathers.

Special mouth care is given every 2 to 4 hours to patients with leukemia, stomatitis, dehydration, and those receiving nothing by mouth.

Careful mouth care is necessary when platelets are decreased.

A hydrogen peroxide and water rinse is soothing to patients.

A bicarbonate of soda solution is effective and well accepted by patients.

Anesthetic throat lozenges relieve pain and dryness.

A viscous lidocaine (Xylocaine) solution offers short-term pain control prior to meals.

Mineral oil is best tolerated to loosen crusted mucus or saliva.

Gauze wrapped around a finger may be too abrasive for patients with mucositis.

A toothbrush is not used if stomatitis is present.

Self-irrigation with a bicarbonate solution has a salutary effect.

A good result was noted with a Water Pic and hydrogen peroxide.

A power spray is excellent for keeping the mouth and suture lines clean.

The approach to oral hygiene patient care is individualized and supportive. Time and continued data collection will hopefully identify oral hygiene measures that are most beneficial to the patients receiving cancer therapy.

Whenever possible, the dental staff and hospital staff should begin communication prior to the start of radiation therapy. Ensuring that the oral cavity is as healthy as possible will reduce and prevent problems for the patient later. Removing calculus, root planing, performing soft tissue curettage, and restoring periodontally sound teeth constitute appropriate care before radiation treatments begin. Teeth that are irreversibly damaged as a result of the periodontal condition or that are in need of extensive restoration should be identified for extraction. The patient's motivation to maintain oral hygiene will have a bearing on how aggressive pretherapy extractions need be. If the patient is not interested in following oral hygiene measures, daily fluoride treatments, or maintaining regular professional care, a conscientious assessment of each tooth is necessary.

The most serious oral complication of radiation treatment is osteoradionecrosis. The normal vasculature of the bone is decreased as a result of radiation exposure. If circulation is severely diminished, the bone will die. The mandible is most susceptible to this condition. The decreased blood supply may cause extreme pain, result in poor post-surgical healing, and precipitate a need for boney resection. Patients with periodontally involved teeth, because of the source of infection and possible need for extraction after radiation, have the highest risk of osteonecrosis. Patients who are edentulous at the time of therapy have a relatively low risk for this serious complication.

When extractions are performed prior to radiation therapy, 7 to 10 days of healing should be allowed before radiation begins. When extractions are necessary after radiation, antibiotic coverage is recommended. All boney edges should be trimmed and the site closed with sutures. The extractions should be limited to two or three at a time. Although healing may be delayed, osteonecrosis is not inevitable (Carl, 1980). Fischman (1983) has noted that the risk of osteonecrosis is related to the radiation dose, indicating that the risk to each individual may vary.

Summary

Regular dental care for patients with a history of cancer therapy is particularly important. The emphasis is on preventing future problems and helping the patient cope with existing ones, which may include the discomfort provided by abnormal saliva, loss of taste, increased susceptibility to infections, dental caries, and loss of function related to removal of part of the oral cavity or adjustment to an oral prosthesis. For these special patients, as with all people, the clinician should support a good preventive attitude, encourage excellent home care habits, and help the patient maintain a high level of oral health through frequent recall visits.

MANAGEMENT OF PATIENTS ENCOUNTERING DENTISTRY FOR THE FIRST TIME

Occasionally a dental professional sees an *adult who is encountering dentistry for the first time.* If fear of pain was the primary reason the patient avoided dental care, the "day of reckoning" when the patient does appear may be the zenith of anxiety for the patient. The very reason for the visit may be to alleviate the pain of a toothache or badly inflamed oral tissues. Thus the patient is in pain and is fearing further pain; a situation such as this requires careful handling. Even if the patient's long delay in seeking dental care is not directly related to fear, the messages about dentistry that people see on television, in cartoons, in comic routines, and in other media frequently connote pain and discomfort for the dental patient.

The key in working with a patient during his/her first dental visit is to briefly explain each procedure and each piece of equipment before picking it up to use and to be especially aware of the patient's verbal and nonverbal responses. The patient should be introduced to the basic parts of the dental unit. It may be wise to explain to the patient why the supine position is currently used before laying the patient out flat. The procedures for the guided self-assessment presented in Chapter 19 may be especially useful in helping the patient develop an understanding of his/her oral cavity and dentistry.

The patient in pain should be assisted promptly so that pain is relieved. Since this may require an injection, techniques to relax and distract the patient are critical to ensure a tolerable experience with anesthesia (see Chapter 32). The patient should be encouraged to share concerns about procedures and outcomes and to ask questions. The patient may be terrified of the anticipated evils that can be inflicted with an innocent tri-syringe; such terror can be avoided if the patient feels free to ask, "What is that?"

Working with a *child patient*, especially one making a first visit, is similar. In the case of the child, the introduction to dentistry may be more guided and experiential.

Infants who have a developmental disorder or whose parents have poor dental health should see the dentist not later than 6 months of age. Other children should be seen for their first appointment between the ages of 18 and 24 months (Wei and Nowak, 1982).

The infant or toddler should be escorted into the operatory with the parent. The parent should sit in the dental chair and hold the child. The child's head should be placed in the crook of the parent's arm, with the other arm holding the child's body. This will help control the movements of the child and prevent accidents (Wright, Starkey, and Gardner, 1983). The clinician should focus on examining the oral structures for normal eruption patterns and overall proper growth and development. Counseling regarding diet, the use of pacifiers, the effects of finger- or thumb-sucking, and what to expect in the coming months with regard to eruption of teeth can occur during these early-age appointments.

Once the child has a reasonable complement of primary teeth, dental appointments shift to deplaquing the teeth. The child and parent are shown the evidence of plaque with disclosing solution, and a toothbrush and fluoride paste are used to remove the plaque, instructing the parent and the child in the proper use of the brush. The parent should be shown how to support the child's head while brushing his/her teeth, but the child should be given the opportunity to use the brush to imitate the proper motions. The goal is to remove all the plaque during the appointment and for the parent to ensure that it is removed daily, with both brush and floss, in order to minimize caries and gingival inflammation (Wei and Nowak, 1982).

Dietary evaluation is an important part of early dental care. Patterns of snacking and foods typically eaten during mealtime should be examined for cariogenicity and for a good balance of essential nutrients. Fluoride supplements should be prescribed if the water supply is not fluoridated.

If a child of 2 or 3 years of age (or older) has never visited a dental office, time will need to be spent introducing the child to the dental equipment and procedures. The child may be encouraged to push the buttons once or twice or to make the "spaceship chair" rise and descend. The brave health care provider may even let the child operate the air and water "squirt gun" as long as the target is well-defined, such as a cup or sink (Figs. 34-13 and 34-14).

The mouth mirror and explorer may be the only two instruments needed for the first visit. The mirror is usually easily understood as a magic way to see the backs of the teeth and to shine light into the dark corners. The explorer is a magic wand that counts sparkles on the teeth and checks to see if the teeth are strong. The child can hold a hand mirror while the clinician checks for caries and

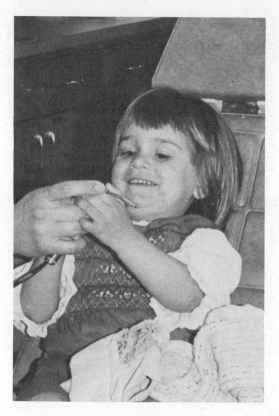

Fig. 34-13. Introducing a child to the dental environment should be experiential. Child may be given an opportunity to push buttons that cause the "spaceship chair" to rise and descend and to use the "squirt gun."

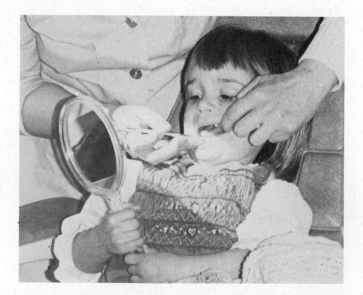

Fig. 34-14. Counting teeth with child observing in mirror involves child in beginning stages of care and familiarizes child with having a metal instrument and mouth mirror in her mouth.

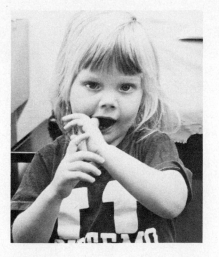

Fig. 34-15. Feeling teeth "way in the back" can help child be more aware of how far back the brush needs to reach.

counts sparkles. For a preliminary procedure, it can be used to count teeth. Most children are amazed to learn that they have 20 or more teeth. While counting molars, it is possible to point out the large teeth that are nestled way in the back that need extra brushing (Fig. 34-15). The clinician should always place a fingertip next to the sharp point of the explorer when moving in or out of the mouth of when moving from one tooth to another, in order to prevent sticking the child.

Occasionally, small pieces of calculus may be found on the lingual surfaces of the mandibular anterior teeth and on the facial surfaces of the maxillary molars; these can be removed with a scaler or curette. If the child is comfortable with the explorer feeling the teeth, the scaler should be easily accepted also. It may be necessary to gently caution the child to sit very still during the critical moments of adaptation. Asking the child to open wide, "like an alligator," helps keep a space available for getting hands and instruments inside the mouth. If the child has a tendency to inadvertently close slowly, the first and second fingers of the hand holding the mirror can be placed between the maxillary and mandibular arches to ensure at least a two-finger width space for access to the teeth. For the child whose jaws gently drift close, this technique is quite useful and is tolerated well by the child. This

technique becomes highly undesirable if the child closes forcibly. The resultant pain experienced by the clinician can be considerable. A rubber mouth prop is a better choice for this patient.

If stains are present on the teeth, it may be necessary to polish selected teeth with an abrasive. If a motor-driven handpiece is to be used, it can be described as an electric toothbrush. An unattached rubber cup can be handed to the child to squeeze to see how soft it is. The unattached cup can then be rubbed on the child's fingernail to prove its harmlessness and then on the front of a central incisor. Explaining that toothpaste goes in the rubber cup helps the child figure out why the electric toothbrush has no brush.

It helps to show how the cup attaches to the prophylaxis angle and then to the handpiece. With all the parts assembled, the cup should again be rubbed on the tooth to show that it feels the same. A critical point is when the handpiece is activated and begins to hum or whistle. To prepare for that, it can be explained that the cup could be rubbed by hand on the teeth but that it would take a long time to do it. Most children have plans for some pleasant activity following a dental appointment, which they do not wish to delay. The electric toothbrush helps make sure the child will not be late. The rotating cup should be applied with *light intermittent pressure* on the fingernail and then on an incisor. Then polishing paste ("toothpaste") is added, and stains are polished off.

The saliva ejector attachment (a "straw") for the high-volume suction should be used to evacuate saliva and the abrasive, since small children cannot easily control swallowing and expectoration.

In many cases neither calculus nor stain will be evident on the teeth. Both scaling and polishing are in these cases unnecessary. More appropriate is the use of a disclosant with the child locating the plaque and brushing (and flossing with assistance) to remove it.

After all plaque is removed, a topical fluoride treatment may be appropriate. (See Chapter 29 for a discussion of fluoride therapy.) Care must be taken that the child does not swallow the fluoride. Ingesting the fluoride gel can cause nausea, vomiting, and illness. Large quantities can cause death.

Dental hygiene care procedures do not cause great discomfort; in many instances, there is none at all. Therefore the dental hygiene appointment can be an important opportunity to build a trusting relationship, free from fear, which can focus on preventing maladies that could require less pleasant dental appointments.

A few general guidelines are helpful in preparing for a child patient (Bailey, 1979; Goose and Kurer, 1973; Huggins, 1973; McDonald and Avery, 1983; Roche, 1975; Wei and Nowak, 1982; and Wright, Starkey, and Gardner, 1983):

1. Do not keep the child waiting.

2. Call the child by name, touch him/her gently, and give the child a big smile. Project that you are happy to see the child.

3. Gently guiding the child to the operatory or to the sink and plaque-counting area while holding the child's hand helps the child feel confidence in the clinician. For first visits it may be wise to start with plaque counting and finish with exploring and any necessary scaling, polishing, and fluoride treatment.

4. If the child is crying, it may help to whisper in the child's ear, "I can't understand you when you cry," or "You can't hear me when you cry." The whispering may do the trick; it is a shocking contrast to most people's response to crying. Another phrase that may help is, "Why are you crying?" whispered in the ear. After hearing the child's answer (usually "I want to go home"), point out all the assets of the day: "How many teeth do you think you have? We were going to count them! And we were going to make sure that your teeth are bright and shiny! If you go home, we're going to miss all that. Besides, I've been waiting all day to meet you. I'd really like to spend a little time with you."

5. Be *truthful*.

6. A voice intonation that reflects calm, firm, gentle control and understanding is often more important than the content of what is said.

7. "Attention must be obtained for communication to take place, and communication *must* occur before behavior shaping commences" (Wright, Starkey, and Gardner, 1983).

8. *Do not use baby talk*. Use a gentle adult-to-adult tone with some simple words.

9. If the child will not open his/her mouth, it can be useful to teasingly say, "I bet you don't have any teeth in there. Do you have teeth in there? Give me just a peek." As soon as the teeth peek out, praise them and exclaim, "I guess you *do*

have teeth. How many?" The child will probably suggest a number such as 6, 7, or 58. Counting them answers the question and permits some preliminary inspection and caries detection.

10. Usually the parent of a child over 3 years of age remains in the reception area during treatment. However, if the parent must be in the room, it is wise to suggest that the conversation be limited to hygienist and child. A three-way discussion is confusing for the child, overly directive or distracting, and counterproductive. The parent should be fully involved during dental health education.

11. When working with a chairside assistant, be certain conversation is directed toward the child. The child should be the center of attention.

DENTAL CARE FOR THE ELDERLY AND FOR HOSPITALIZED PATIENTS

The changes that occur in the body from the aging process may affect the physical, mental, and environmental needs of the elderly patient. It is important for the clinician to realize that not all these changes may be present in all elderly patients. As pointed out in the assessment chapters of this text, each patient is an individual and must be assessed for individual treatment needs. The purpose of this section is to point out some significant findings that may help the dental professional in caring for the elderly patient. It has been organized according to segments of treatment during which modifications may be necessary. Although the same considerations should be afforded the elderly patient as were mentioned in the beginning of the chapter, there are some special considerations that may make the elderly person's treatment in the dental office more comprehensive and comfortable.

The *medical history* of the geriatric patient typically contains evidence of multiple health problems. Foremost among these are cardiovascular problems, including arteriosclerotic heart disease; problems involving bones, joints, and muscles, particularly arthritis; skin problems, including dry skin and neoplasms, both benign and malignant; urinary tract diseases; and emotional problems.

There are many pitfalls involved in taking the medical histories of elderly patients. They may supply information that is incorrect or incomplete as a result of confusion or loss of memory. Some patients may report a chief complaint that is relatively trivial in nature while ignoring or failing to mention major problems that exist. The descriptions of illnesses or symptoms may be vague. Many elderly patients take multiple drugs but may not remember what the names of the drugs are or why they were prescribed. To ensure that an accurate medical history is formulated, it may be necessary for the clinician to allow extra time to gather the information from the patient and to go over all questions carefully and in detail with the patient so that there is little doubt of understanding. It may also be necessary to consult with both the patient's family and the patient's physician if questions or concerns exist.

With regard to the *oral examination,* common problems of the geriatric patient include loss of teeth, caries, xerostomia (dry mouth), changes in the color and elasticity of tissues, an increased incidence of oral tumors and cancer, tissue changes resulting from nutritional deficiencies, and irritation related to dentures. Drug-induced conditions such as moniliasis and angular cheilosis are also common.

Frequent oral examinations are important for the elderly patient. The incidence of oral cancer increases with age, so it is critical that early tissue changes be detected and diagnosed to improve the prognosis of treatment and recovery. The patients themselves often are unaware of changes occurring in their own mouths. Since most malignant and benign lesions are asymptomatic, it is essential that the dental professional provide education and frequent examination.

Caries in the elderly person is a problem for several reasons. Drugs and the aging process both tend to affect the quantity and characteristics of saliva, limiting its self-cleansing effects on teeth. Elderly patients experience a loss of taste sensation, causing them to seek foods that may be sweeter to compensate for this loss. Home care may be diminished because of loss of hand and arm function or coordination. Loss of tactile sensations in the mouth prevents the patient from detecting the presence of food debris and plaque with the tongue. Patients may also simply forget to brush. All these factors tend to increase the incidence of dental caries and periodontal disease.

The loss of teeth and diminished chewing function, coupled with a loss of taste sensations, greatly affect the nutrition of elderly patients. Since they are no longer able to chew meats and firmer vegetables and fruits, they turn to a soft diet, which may be lacking in nutritional balance. These nutritional imbalances will show themselves in the overall health of the patient and may be reflected orally as a red, sore tongue, angular cheilosis, tissue inflammation, and poor healing response to injury or disease.

As it ages, the skin becomes dry, wrinkled, and less elastic. The skin may also display increased incidence of visible blemishes and localized thickening. The mucous membrane becomes drier and less elastic. Fordyce granules may increase in number and prominence. Conditions related to drug therapy, such as moniliasis, may be detected during the oral examination. It is especially important to examine all areas of the head, neck, and oral mucosa for signs of change. Salivary glands should be examined for function and texture.

In planning *dental health education,* the clinician should conduct assessments for vision and hearing impairment, difficulty in communication (stroke victims), decreased hand and arm function, loss of muscle coordination, and other problems that might affect treatment for the elderly patient. The clinician should discuss current home care methods with the patient to determine current practices, problems, and preferences. Planning for dental health education should include any special needs identified during the assessment stages.

When implementing education and instruction, it may be helpful for the patient if distinct, slow, and specific instructions are given. Many patients who have difficulty remembering instructions will benefit from repetition of simple instructions. Modification of oral hygiene aids as discussed earlier may be necessary to compensate for lack of motor ability. Visual aids for instruction are helpful, and their value may be enhanced for those with poorer vision by large lettering and adequate illumination. Patients who wear reading glasses should have them on during instructional sessions so that visual aids and demonstrations are of maximum benefit. If the patient is unable to perform personal home care, the person who will be responsible for this task should be present at the appointment for explanations and instructions.

Older patients who demonstrate problems with walking or who have poor balance will require assistance in and out of the dental chair. They require time to adjust between the supine and upright *positioning* of the chair, since their ability to adapt to sudden changes may be slower than normal. A supine position is recommended for most dental procedures, as with any other patient, unless medical complications prohibit the patient from being comfortable in that position.

The reaction of the young body's healthy tissues to injury or disease is one that can be characterized as acute, dramatic, self-limiting, and fast-repairing. In contrast, the tissues of the elderly patient may respond in ways that are chronic, insidious, asymptomatic, progressive, and slow-repairing. Because of these differences, the *tissue healing response* of the elderly patient may not be as dramatic and will occur more slowly after home care procedures or other treatment has been completed. The extent of tissue manipulation and tissue trauma must be minimized during treatment. One suggestion that may be helpful in treating patients whose lips are extremely dry is to moisten them before beginning any intraoral treatment. Petroleum jelly or a similar lubricant is satisfactory for this purpose.

Contrary to some beliefs, the pain threshold in elderly persons is not different from that in younger persons. They feel pain as acutely as anyone, although they may not wish to complain about it. *Pain control* is as necessary for the elderly patient as it is for anyone else, but its implementation may deserve some special considerations. Anyone with decreased kidney or liver function or with a history of other complicating medical problems may have an altered reaction to drugs. Precautions should be taken to reduce the possibility of adverse toxic effects from the anesthetic solution. Patients who are taking a variety of drugs are likely to suffer from undesirable drug interactions if care is not taken. The clinician should be acquainted with the actions and complications involved between anesthetic agents and other drugs that the patient may be taking (Baum, 1981; Reichel, 1978).

All too often, dental hygiene care for *patients who are hospitalized* or in *nursing homes* does not have the high priority that it deserves. When dental care is in the hands of nurses and nurse's aides, they should be instructed in the importance of frequent oral examinations and mouth cleansing. They also need to be instructed in the delivery of oral health instructions to patients who may be capable of performing some of these procedures themselves. For those individuals who cannot perform their own plaque control, daily mouth cleansing and inspection of dentures for damage and for cleaning should be performed. In long-term care facilities it is important that all dentures be identified with the patient's name or initials to prevent mix-ups and trading among patients.

When mouth care is performed at the bedside for a helpless patient, the following suggestions may be helpful:

1. Be sure that there are no contraindications or modifications to treatment suggested in the patient's medical record.
2. Assemble portable equipment and supplies at the bedside.
3. Move the patient to the edge of the bed, and elevate the head slightly to facilitate access and removal of liquids.
4. Drape the patient, and position an emesis basin under the chin.
5. Apply petroleum jelly or another lubricant to the lips.
6. A mouth prop may be useful if the patient cannot keep his/her mouth open.
7. Brush the teeth, and floss them. A dentifrice may be used but is not necessary and requires extra rinsing and suction.
8. Gently brush the tongue.
9. The mouth may be rinsed with a syringe, or the patient may be able to rinse with assistance. Care should be taken to ensure that fluids are not aspirated.
10. Apply a fluoride gel if indicated for long-term patients.
11. Swab the buccal mucosa with a glycerine swab to lubricate the mouth.
12. Remove equipment, and return the patient to his/her original position.

Whether the clinician is working with hospitalized, elderly, handicapped, very young, or other patients with special needs, it is extremely important to avoid biasing one's expectations of the limitations of the patient on the basis of stereotypes or one's own fears of the unusual needs and circumstances of others. It is especially important to draw on solid assessment data and on a personal approach to each patient that avoids categorizing patients according to malady, age, supposed interests and expectations, or other common stereotypes.

The clinician must become acquainted with the patient's background, medical status, and abilities. After a degree of rapport has been established, an individualized dental plan can be designed for each person. If the clinician is not willing to communicate with patients who have special needs or cannot take the time to provide specialized care, those patients belong with someone who can. In most cases modifications for care are quite reasonable. The clinician should reach out to the patient with a special need.

ACTIVITIES

1. Invite a panel of pedodontists and dental hygienists who work with children to discuss management of behavior problems associated with fear or resistance to care.
2. With a laboratory partner practice patient transfer techniques as described on pp. 575 to 580.
3. Invite a clinician who works with handicapped patients in private practice or in an institutional setting to discuss practical modifications in care.
4. Experience sensory deprivation during a clinic or classroom session by dimming the lights, wearing waxed paper over lenses of prescription or safety glasses, wearing gloves, and putting cotton in your ears. After being a patient or a student under these conditions, discuss what frustrations were experienced as a result of the sensory deprivations. Relate these frustrations to those that an elderly or disabled patient might experience during treatment or patient education.

REVIEW QUESTIONS

1. True or false. If a child patient is reluctant to cooperate in receiving care, it is best to send the child home and suggest that he/she return when older.
2. In working with a patient who is new to dentistry (whether an adult or a child), it is wise to _____.
3. Describe several modifications in communication that are appropriate when treating a patient who is visually handicapped.
4. State how the following modifications in care help make the patient with special needs more comfortable:
   a. Following an appointment routine
   b. Scheduling a midmorning appointment
5. List four (or more) implements that can be used to ensure safe delivery of care for a mobile patient.
6. Identify several different modifications of treatment that should be assessed before treating the elderly patient.
7. At what age should a child first see a dentist or hygienist?
8. Should a child's teeth be polished as part of a dental hygiene appointment?
9. What type of brushing tool modification would be appropriate for a patient with limited arm movement?
10. List three areas of patient education to cover with a pregnant patient.
11. State reasons why a dental consultation/treatment is advised before a patient begins cancer therapy.

REFERENCES

Bailey, B.E. 1979. Psychological management of the pedodontic patient. In Boundy, S.S., and Reynolds, N.J., editors. Current concepts in dental hygiene, vol. 2. St. Louis: The C.V. Mosby Co.

Baum, B.J. 1981. Current research of aging and oral health. Special Care Dentist. **1:**105.

Braham, R. 1977. The role of dentistry in the treatment of malignant disease. J. Prevent. Dent. **4**(1):28.

Carl, W. 1980. Dental management of head and neck cancer patients. J. Surg. Oncol. **15:**265.

Cheney, H.G., and DePaola, D.P. 1979. Preventive dentistry. Post-graduate dental handbook series. Littleton, Mass.: PSG/Wright, Inc. Publishing Co.

Daeffler, R.D. 1980. Oral hygiene measures in patients with cancer, parts I and II. Cancer Nurs., pp. 347; 427.

Fischman, S.L. 1983. The patient with cancer. Symposium on the patient with increased medical risks. Dent. Clin. North Am. **27:**235.

Gier, R.E., and Janes, D.R. 1983. Dental management of the pregnant patient. Symposium on the patient with increased medical risks. Dent. Clin. North Am. **27:**419.

Goho, C.D. July/Aug. 1980. Oral hygiene for the handicapped patient: digital brushing. Dent. Stud. **58:**35.

Goho, C.D. March-April 1983. A digital brushing technique for patients with perceptuomotor difficulties. Clin. Prevent. Dent. **5:**6.

Goose, D.H., and Kurer, J. 1973. A guide to children's dentistry. London: Henry Kimpton, Publishers.

Greenberg, M., et al. 1982. The oral flora as a source of septicemia in patients with acute leukemia. Oral Surg. **53:**322.

Hall, B.R. 1978. Oral hygiene for the hospitalized patient: an oral presentation and table clinic. Miami: Annual Meeting of the American Dental Hygienists' Association.

Huggins, B. 1973. Practical paedodontics. Edinburgh: Churchill Livingstone.

Loe, H. 1965. Periodontal changes in pregnancy. J. Periodontol. **36:**209.

Luke, D.J. 1977. People with physical and mental disabilities. In Boundy, S.S., and Reynolds, N.J., editors. Current concepts in dental hygiene, vol. 1. St. Louis: The C.V. Mosby Co.

McDonald, R.E., and Avery, B.S. 1983. Dentistry for the child and adolescent, ed. 4. St. Louis: The C.V. Mosby Co.

Morrish, R.B., et al. 1981. Osteonecrosis in patients irradiated for head and neck carcinoma. Cancer **47:**1980.

Nowak, A.J. 1976. Dentistry for the handicapped patient. St. Louis: The C.V. Mosby Co.

Price, V.E. 1980. Toothbrush modifications for the handicapped. Dent. Hyg. **54:**467.

Reichel, W. 1978. The geriatric patient. New York: H.P. Publishing Co.

Roche, J.R. 1975. Preventive pedodontics. In Vernier, J.L., and Muhler, J.C. Improving dental practice through preventive measures, ed. 3. St. Louis: The C.V. Mosby Co.

Sonis, S.T., et al. 1978. Oral complications in patients receiving treatment for malignancies other than that of the head and neck. J. Am. Dent. Assoc. **97:**468.

Stiefel, D.J., et al. 1978. Wheelchair transfers in the dental office. Project Dental Education for Care of the Disabled. Seattle: University of Washington School of Dentistry.

Swerdloff, M. March 1980. The problems and concerns of the handicapped. Dent. Educ. **44:**131.

Wei, S.H.Y., and Nowak, A.J. 1982. Implementing a preventive pedodontics practice. In Stewart, R.E., et al., editors. Pediatric dentistry: scientific foundations and clinical practice. St. Louis: The C.V. Mosby Co.

Williams, S.R. 1982. Essentials of nutrition and diet therapy, ed. 3. St. Louis: The C.V. Mosby Co.

Wright, G.Z., Starkey, P.E., and Gardner, D.E. 1983. Managing children's behavior in the dental office. St. Louis: The C.V. Mosby Co.

35 RESTORATIVE PROCEDURES

OBJECTIVES: *The reader will be able to*

1. Rubber dam
   a. List and explain the advantages and disadvantages of rubber dam isolation.
   b. Discuss the rationale for the use of a rubber dam.
   c. Identify the armamentarium needed to place and remove a rubber dam.
   d. Identify the clamps that can be used on each tooth.
   e. Explain the procedure to a partner or patient.
   f. Place a rubber dam on and remove it from a typodont.
   g. Evaluate a placed rubber dam and determine if the dam is clinically acceptable.
   h. If laboratory competency is achieved, place a rubber dam on a partner's teeth.
   i. Explain the importance of assuring that all fragments of the rubber dam are removed from the patient's mouth.
   j. Briefly describe alternative methods for placing the rubber dam.
2. Matrix band
   a. Explain the rationale for placing a Tofflemire matrix and wedge.
   b. Indicate the types of cavity preparations that require the use of a matrix for restoration.
   c. Identify the armamentarium necessary to place and remove a Tofflemire matrix system.
   d. Identify the parts of the matrix retainer.
   e. Indicate which portion of the matrix retainer and which portion of the matrix band are placed toward the occlusal surface.
   f. Explain the importance of burnishing a contact area into the band.
   g. List the criteria to be met for an acceptable matrix band placement.
   h. Place a matrix and wedge on a typodont.
   i. After laboratory competence has been achieved, place and remove a Tofflemire matrix and wedge for a partner.
3. Zinc oxide–eugenol Class II temporary restoration
   a. Discuss the rationale for a temporary restoration.
   b. List the criteria for a clinically acceptable temporary restoration.
   c. Differentiate between a clinically acceptable and a clinically unacceptable restoration.
   d. Identify the armamentarium necessary to place a temporary restoration.
   e. Place a zinc oxide–eugenol Class II restoration in a typodont.
   f. After laboratory competence has been achieved, place a zinc oxide–eugenol Class II restoration as dictated by the patient's needs.
4. Overhang removal (margination)
   a. Explain the rationale for performing margination procedures.
   b. List and discuss the indications and contraindications for amalgam overhang removal.
   c. Classify amalgam overhangs by size.
   d. Identify the armamentarium necessary for a margination procedure.
   e. Explain the function of the knife and various files used for the procedure.
   f. Define *excess, deficiency,* and *open margin.* Explain how each condition is detected.
   g. List the criteria for a clinically acceptable overhang removal—both the process and the product.
   h. Perform margination on a typodont tooth or on an extracted tooth.
   i. After laboratory competence has been achieved, perform an overhang removal procedure as dictated by the patient's needs.

5. Amalgam finishing and polishing
   a. State the rationale for finishing and polishing an amalgam restoration.
   b. List and describe the indications and contraindications for performing an amalgam finishing and polishing procedure.
   c. Identify the armamentarium necessary for an amalgam finishing and polishing procedure.
   d. List the criteria for a clinically acceptable polished amalgam restoration.
   e. Differentiate between a clinically acceptable and clinically unacceptable amalgam polishing procedure.
   f. List sequentially the order of instrumentation used for polishing an amalgam.
   g. Perform an amalgam finishing and polishing procedure on a typodont.
   h. After laboratory competence has been achieved, perform amalgam finishing and polishing procedures as dictated by patient's needs.

Restorative procedures are relatively new procedures for dental auxiliaries. In many states these procedures are called *expanded duties* and dental assistants and/or dental hygienists are allowed to perform none, some, or all of the restorative expanded duties. The most liberal states permit reversible restorative expanded duties: placement of a rubber dam; matrix band; temporary, tooth-colored, and amalgam restorations; stainless steel crowns; and temporary crowns; as well as overhang removal, amalgam polishing, and other reversible procedures. At the present time no state practice acts permits dental auxiliaries to cut hard or soft tissue or to take final impressions (i.e., an impression for a crown or a bridge). This chapter presents some of the expanded duties: placement and removal of a rubber dam and Tofflemire matrix band, placement of a zinc oxide–eugenol temporary restoration, overhang removal, and amalgam polishing. In this chapter a technique for each of these procedures is introduced; the reader will need background information in dental anatomy and dental materials to completely understand and integrate the material. Several excellent packets of teaching materials are available, including audiovisual tapes that can be used to augment the material presented here.

RUBBER DAM PLACEMENT AND REMOVAL

A rubber dam is a piece of rubber that is stretched over the teeth to expose only those teeth that are to be treated. The rubber dam is held in place by a rubber dam clamp and the rubber dam frame.

The dam isolates the area; keeps the area dry; protects the patient's lips, cheeks, and tongue; prevents the patient from aspirating or swallowing any of the materials; and improves the clinician's visibility and accessibility. All of these advantages allow the clinician to place and carve a high-quality restoration. The disadvantages of the rubber dam are that the clamp can be irritating to the gingiva, placement of the dam can be time-consuming for the beginning clinician, and some patients are sensitive to the rubber. Overall, the consensus is that the advantages of using a rubber dam outweigh the disadvantages, unless the patient is allergic to rubber.

Some dentists prefer to have the dam placed before the tooth is prepared so that visibility and accessibility are improved during the preparation; others believe the dam is an interference, especially if a tooth with a proximal lesion is being prepared.

The armamentarium needed for placement and removal of a dam is shown in Fig. 35-1. The dam material is available in several weights—light, medium, heavy, and extra heavy—and three colors—green (mint flavored), light, and dark. The dark material is usually used for restorative procedures because it provides a color contrast to the teeth and is more soothing to the clinician's eyes than light material. Heavy material is usually used because it provides adequate retraction of the lips and cheeks but does not tear easily during placement. Light-colored and lightweight material are used more often in endodontics, since only one tooth is isolated, tearing is less of a problem, and the lighter

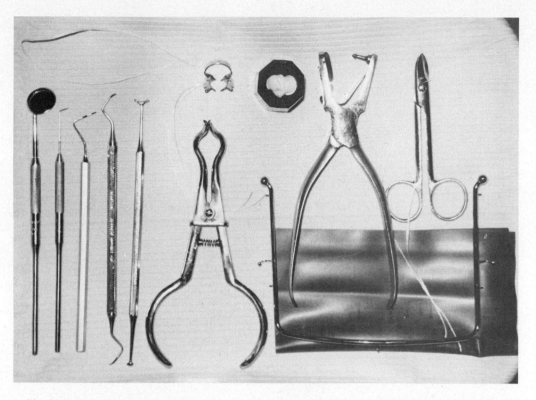

Fig. 35-1. Armamentarium for placement and removal of rubber dam: mirror, explorer, probe, curette, T-ball burnisher, clamp forceps, lubricant, punch, scissors, frame, floss, and rubber dam material.

material is easier to manipulate. Following are the steps for one method of placing a rubber dam; these steps are illustrated in Figs. 35-2 to 35-24.

Armamentarium

The necessary armamentarium includes the dam, which can be stamped with a pattern; a forceps to place the clamps; clamps; a rubber dam punch; a frame to hold the dam away from the patient's face; floss to floss the patient's teeth and to floss the dam through the contact areas; a blunt instrument such as a plastic instrument or a T-ball burnisher to turn the edge of the dam into the sulcus; lubricant for the patient's lips; lubricant for the dam to ease it over the teeth and through the contacts; a tri-syringe; and suction. When a rubber dam is being placed, the help of an assistant is invaluable.

There are a variety of rubber dam clamps to fit the variety of teeth in the mouth (Fig. 35-2). In Fig. 35-3 the clamps produced by two manufacturers are identified by number and location of use in the mouth. There are also several types of rubber dam holders (Fig. 35-4). One of the most commonly used holders is Young's frame. It is a metal U-shaped frame, which holds the dam away from the patient's face. The Woodbury holder is an elastic band that is wrapped around the back of the patient's head and attached to the sides of the dam with three clips on each side; this holder provides excellent lip and cheek retraction. A similar holder is the Wizard holder, which has two clips on each side. There are also some plastic rubber dam holders, which hold the dam away from the patient's face and allow the dam to be easily loosened. These plastic frames are useful for endodontic procedures because they allow radiographs to be taken without completely removing the dam and without the image of the metal frame appearing in the radiograph.

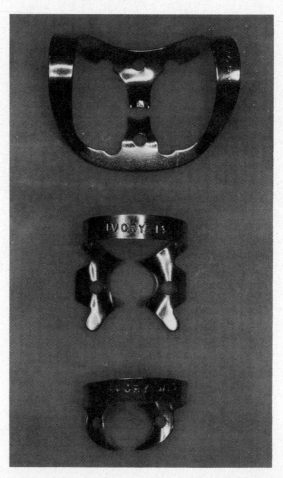

Fig. 35-2. Three types of rubber dam clamps. *From top to bottom:* Gingival retractor clamp, winged clamp, and wingless clamp.

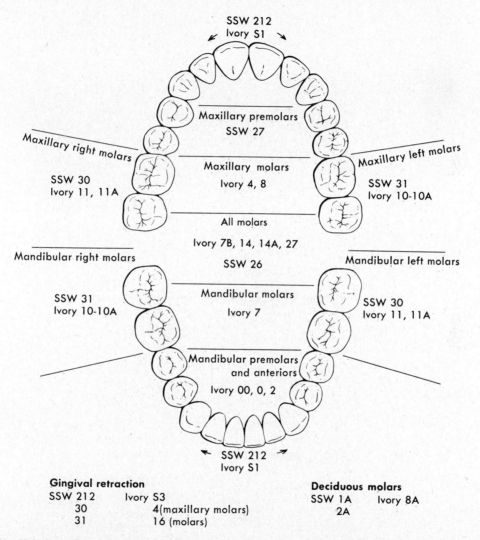

SSW 212
Ivory S1

Maxillary premolars
SSW 27

Maxillary right molars

SSW 30
Ivory 11, 11A

Maxillary molars
Ivory 4, 8

Maxillary left molars

SSW 31
Ivory 10-10A

All molars

Ivory 7B, 14, 14A, 27

SSW 26

Mandibular right molars

SSW 31
Ivory 10-10A

Mandibular molars
Ivory 7

Mandibular left molars

SSW 30
Ivory 11, 11A

Mandibular premolars
and anteriors

Ivory 00, 0, 2

SSW 212
Ivory S1

Gingival retraction		Deciduous molars	
SSW 212	Ivory S3	SSW 1A	Ivory 8A
30	4(maxillary molars)	2A	
31	16 (molars)		

Fig. 35-3. Chart of suggested clamps to be used in various areas of mouth. (From Howard, W.W., and Moller, R.C. 1981. Atlas of operative dentistry, ed. 3. St. Louis: The C.V. Mosby Co.)

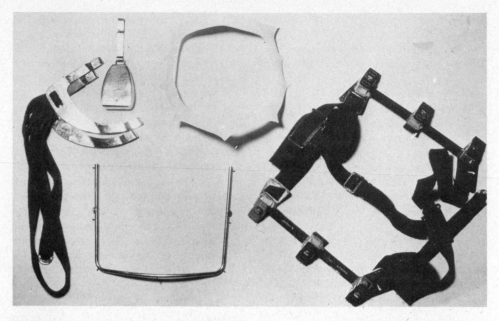

Fig. 35-4. Some examples of rubber dam holders. *Clockwise from upper left:* Wizard holder, weight, plastic frame, Woodbury holder, and Young's frame. (From Gilmore, W.H., et al. 1982. Operative dentistry, ed. 4. St. Louis: The C.V. Mosby Co.)

Patient preparation

The purpose of the rubber dam should be explained to the patient, especially if the patient has never experienced a rubber dam placement during previous dental treatment. The advantages to the patient, such as not having to taste or feel the materials in the mouth and receiving a better restoration, should be presented. The procedure should also be briefly explained to the patient so that the patient knows what to expect and what it will feel like. The patient will not be able to talk with the dam in place, so the clinician may want to suggest signals to the patient in case the patient needs to communicate with the clinician. The next part of preparing the patient is directly related to placing the dam. The patient's lips should be lubricated with petroleum jelly, since the lips will be stretched during the procedure. The clinician should floss the patient's teeth to determine if there will be difficulty in passing the dam between any of the teeth. If any of the contacts cannot be flossed the hygienist should determine the cause; if the cause is calculus

or an overhang, the clinician should remove the debris and/or overhang. If it is another problem, it should be brought to the supervising dentist's attention. The patient's occlusion is also checked before the dam is placed to determine if any unusual anatomy such as a plunger cusp may interfere with the restoration that is about to be placed. If a problem does exist, it should be brought to the attention of the supervising dentist.

Rubber dam preparation

The rubber dam must be punched before it can be placed. The clinician should look at the patient's mouth for missing teeth in the area to be isolated and for malaligned teeth in the area. The dam may be stamped with a guide for an ideal mouth, but the person punching the dam must modify the pattern according to the patient's unique conditions (Fig. 35-5). According to P. Cunningham et al. (1969), the isolation should extend from two teeth distal to the tooth being treated, if possible, to the central incisor on the opposite side of the mouth.

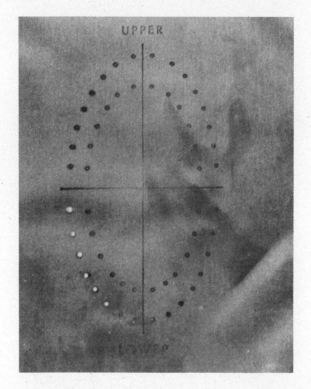

Fig. 35-5. Rubber dam punched according to ideal pattern stamped on dam.

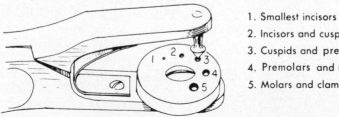

1. Smallest incisors
2. Incisors and cuspids
3. Cuspids and premolars
4. Premolars and molars
5. Molars and clamps

Fig. 35-6. Suggested sizes of holes to be punched in dam for various teeth. (Modified from Howard, W.W., and Moller, R.C. 1981. Atlas of operative dentistry, ed. 3. St. Louis: The C.V. Mosby Co.)

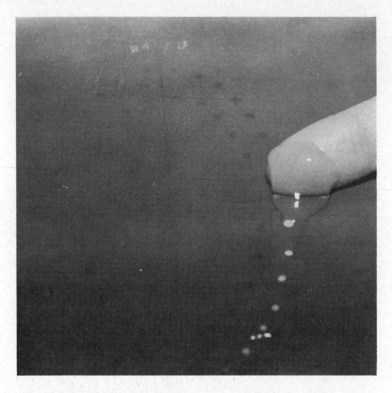

Fig. 35-7. Sterile lubricant being applied to dam to help ease it through contacts.

When an anterior tooth is being isolated, the area exposed is from cuspid to cuspid. Rubber dam punches have different-sized holes so that the dam can be punched to correspond to the sizes of the teeth. Usually five or six holes are punched; Fig. 35-6 illustrates the use of a five-hole punch. If a six-hole punch is used, the holes, from smallest to largest, are used for (1) mandibular incisors, (2) maxillary incisors, (3) cuspids, (4) premolars, (5) molars, and (6) an anchor tooth and clamp. After the dam is punched, the side of the dam that is to be against the teeth is lubricated lightly with liquid soap, shaving cream, or a sterile lubricant to help ease the dam over the teeth and through the contact areas (Fig. 35-7).

Clamp preparation

The rubber dam clamp is selected on the basis of the anatomy of the anchor tooth. *Anchor tooth* is the name given to the tooth that is being clamped.

The chart in Fig. 35-3 will be helpful in determining which clamps are most likely to fit particular teeth. When a clamp is selected to be tried onto the tooth, dental floss is attached to the clamp to permit retrieval of the clamp if it slips off the tooth. The floss may be looped around the bow of the clamp or tied through the buccal forceps hole (Figs. 35-8 and 35-9). The clamp is placed on the tooth by engaging the lingual prongs of the clamp against the lingual surface of the anchor tooth. After the clamp is placed on the lingual surface, the clamp is rotated onto the buccal surface so that the prongs are also contacting the buccal surface of the tooth. When the clamp is properly placed, all four prongs should be touching the tooth cervical to the height of contour (Fig. 35-10). The clamp should be stable; it should not rotate on the tooth; and the prongs of the clamp should not be impinging on the gingiva (Fig. 35-11). If any of these criteria are not met, the clamp should be adjusted to meet the criteria.

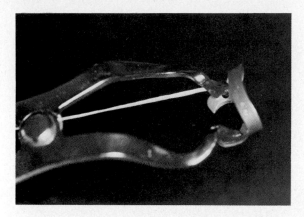

Fig. 35-8. Forceps tips engaged in clamp forceps holes.

Fig. 35-9. Clamp being placed on lingual surface and then on buccal surface.

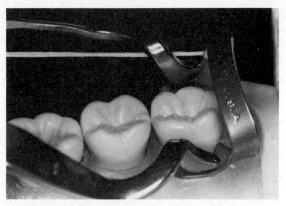

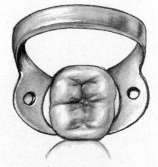

Fig. 35-10. All four prongs of clamp should be in contact with tooth. (From Howard, W.W., and Moller, R.C. 1981. Atlas of operative dentistry, ed. 3. St. Louis: The C.V. Mosby Co.)

Fig. 35-11. Stability of clamp is checked with light pressure.

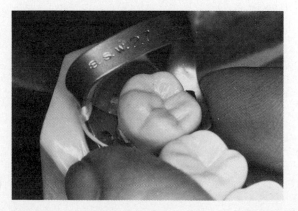

If the clamp rotates on the tooth, slides off the tooth, or rests on the papilla, it is probably too big; if the clamp does not fit over the heights of contour or seems to pop off the tooth, the clamp is probably too small. The clinician should always use care when placing a rubber dam clamp, since the prongs are pointed and can cut the gingiva or gouge the root surface. If the position of the clamp must be adjusted, forceps should be used to disengage the prongs from the tooth.

Rubber dam placement

P. Cunningham et al. (1969) have suggested that the powdered side of the dam be placed facing the clinician to reduce the glare that can be caused by the light reflecting off the dark dam material. The less powdered side of the dam will be placed toward the patient. A liquid soap, shaving cream or sterile lubricant is placed around the holes on the less powdered side; this lubricant allows the clinician and the assistant to ease the dam over the teeth and through the contact areas. The posterior portion of the dam material is rolled up and held by the clinician while he/she stretches open the hole to be placed over the anchor tooth. The dam is stretched over the bow of the clamp first, and then the tension is slightly loosened while the dam is eased over the lingual wings and then the buccal wings of the clamp (Figs. 35-12 to 35-15). This procedure places pressure on the clamp, but if the clamp is properly fitted and placed, it will not be dislodged. There are other methods for placing the clamp and dam, which are discussed at the end of this section.

After the dam is placed over the clamp, the terminal tooth, usually the central incisor on the opposite side of the mouth, is isolated. A piece of dental floss can be tied around the terminal tooth to hold the dam in place during the rest of the placement (Fig. 35-16). The frame is placed next to hold the dam away from the patient's throat and face; the frame also holds the dam away from the clinician's and assistant's work field (Fig. 35-17). The next step is to pass the rubber dam through the contact areas. While the clinician stretches the dam over each contact area, the assistant uses waxed dental tape or floss to carry the dam through each interproximal area (Fig. 35-18). If working alone, the clinician uses the tape or floss to carry the dam through the interproximal areas. It is preferable to use waxed tape rather than waxed floss

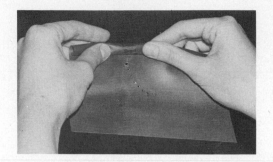

Fig. 35-12. Posterior portion of dam is rolled up to be placed in patient's mouth.

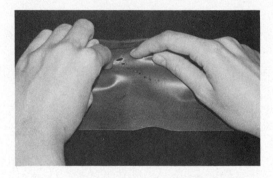

Fig. 35-13. Hole for anchor tooth is stretched open.

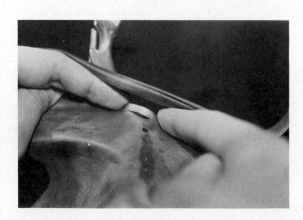

Fig. 35-14. Dam is being stretched over bow of clamp.

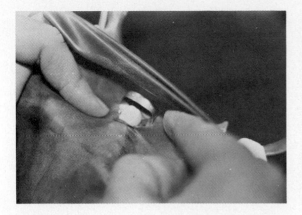

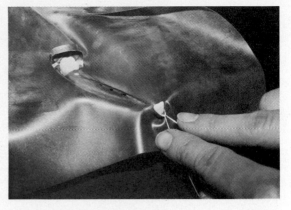

Fig. 35-15. Dam being stretched over lingual jaw of clamp. Pressure is released, and then dam is stretched over buccal jaw.

Fig. 35-16. Most anterior tooth is isolated and ligated.

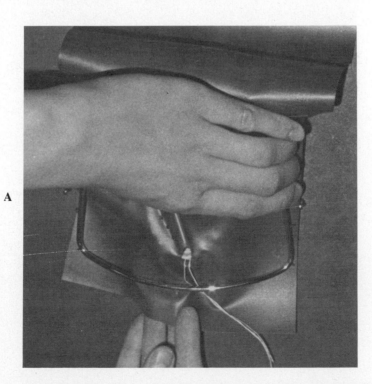

A

Fig. 35-17. Young's frame is placed by, **A**, pulling dam over lower portion of frame and then, **B**, pulling dam around side portions of frame. **C**, Frame after this initial placement.

Continued.

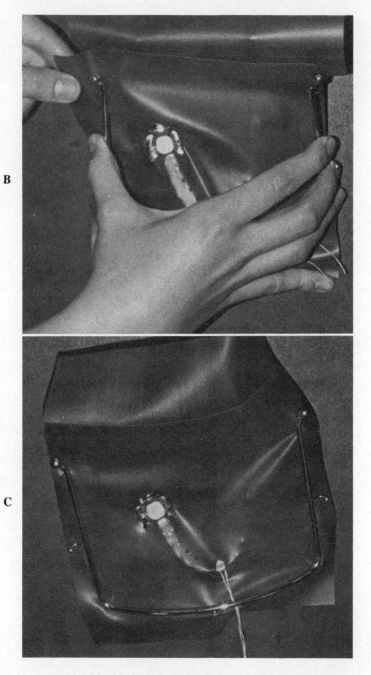

B

C

Fig. 35-17, cont'd. For legend see p. 607.

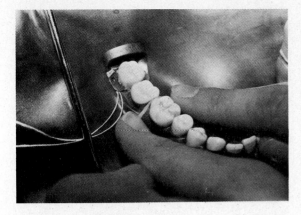

Fig. 35-18. Interdental portions of dam are carried through contacts.

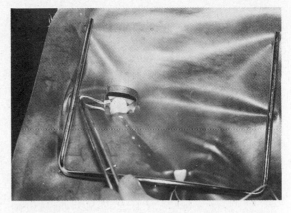

Fig. 35-19. Floss on clamp is pulled up to outer surface of dam.

or unwaxed floss, since the flosses are likely to tear the dam instead of carrying it through the contacts. If waxed tape is too thick for a particular patient's contact areas, waxed floss can be used. Carrying the dam through the contact areas at this stage will greatly ease the later step of tucking the dam into the sulci.

After the dam is through each of the contact areas, the frame is readjusted to hold the dam more tightly; the frame should also be as centered as possible and not endanger the patient (i.e., the ends of the frame should be away from the patient's eyes). The floss on the clamp should be pulled up to the outer surface of the dam (Fig. 35-19). The next step is to tuck, or invaginate, the dam into the sulcus around each tooth to prevent seepage of the sulcular fluid and saliva from the oral cavity onto the surface of the rubber dam (Fig. 35-20). The tucking can be accomplished in several ways. It is important that the flossing of the dam through the contact areas be done completely, since that procedure usually tucks the interproximal areas into the sulci. If the dam is not tucked in the interproximal areas, it will be difficult to tuck the dam into the facial and lingual sulci. The clinician may want to repeat the flossing in the resistant interproximal areas. A blunt instrument can be used to tuck the rest of the dam by placing the instrument against the cervical portion of the tooth at a 90-degree angle to the long axis of the tooth and then sliding the instrument from one line angle of the

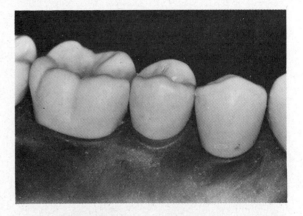

Fig. 35-20. Material around second premolar is not tucked, as compared with material around adjacent teeth, which is tucked.

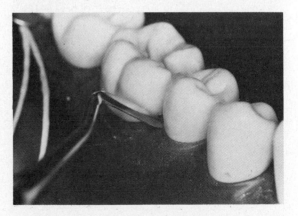

Fig. 35-21. Tucking dam with blunt instrument.

tooth to the next line angle in a continuous stroke (Fig. 35-21). For example, the instrument is placed at the distobuccal line angle of tooth No. 29 and slid to the mesiobuccal line angle of tooth No. 29. If the dam was tucked interproximally from the flossing, the blunt instrument will carry the facial and lingual portions of the dam into the sulcus. Another way to tuck the dam is to wrap dental tape around the tooth while the assistant places a blunt instrument on the lingual side of the tooth so that the floss is cervical to (under) the instrument, which is tipped into the sulcus (Fig. 35-22). When the instrument and floss are placed properly, the clinician crosses the floss once on the buccal surface and pulls the ends tight with a see-saw motion.

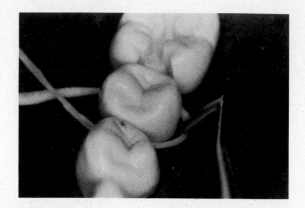

Fig. 35-22. Floss and blunt instrument being used to tuck dam.

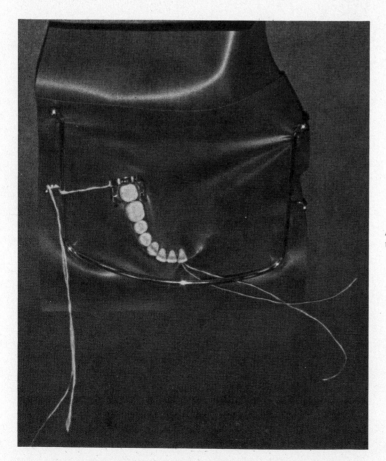

Fig. 35-23. Rubber dam properly placed on typodont.

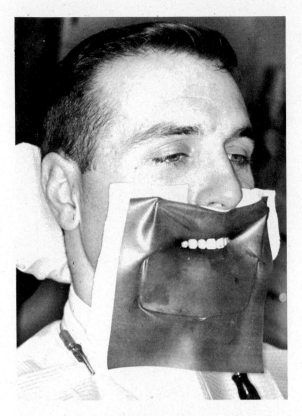

Fig. 35-24. Rubber dam properly placed on patient. Cotton rubber dam napkin has been placed between patient's face and rubber dam, and frame is on the underside of dam. (From Howard, W.W., and Moller, R.C. 1981. Atlas of operative dentistry, ed. 3. St. Louis: The C.V. Mosby Co.)

The floss will carry the dam into the sulcus, since the floss will conform to the cervical areas of the tooth. Another way to tuck the dam is to slide the blunt instrument from line angle to line angle while the assistant uses the tri-syringe to direct air on the instrument tip and toward the sulcus. If the instrument is slightly angled into the sulcus, the pressure of the air may force the dam into the sulcus. Once the dam is completely tucked, the final step is to cleanse the area with the tri-syringe and the suction. Properly placed rubber dams are illustrated in Figs. 35-23 and 35-24.

Rubber dam removal

At the completion of the placement of the restoration, the dam must be removed so that the cli-

nician can complete the carving of the restoration. The excess debris is removed from the dam with suction. A water rinse should not be used at this time, because it would interfere with the setting of the restorative material. It is important to remove the debris, especially small pieces of restorative material, to prevent it from catapulting off the dam into the patient's, assistant's, or clinician's eyes. After the dam is cleared of debris, the ligature on the most anterior tooth is cut, the buccal side of the dam is stretched away from the teeth, and the clinician or the assistant places one finger under the stretched dam to protect the patient's lips and cheeks while the interdental areas of the dam are cut (Figs. 35-25 and 35-26). The scissors should engage and cut an entire septa with one stroke (Fig. 35-26).

Pulling the dam up through the contacts or snipping the interproximal areas in stages may cause thin pieces of dam to tear or remain around the tooth. The rubber dam would be an irritant and could cause severe damage to the gingiva and supporting structures. For example, if a ring of the dam remained around the tooth, it would act like a rubber band and would progress toward the apex of the tooth, since the apex is the most constricted area of the tooth. As the rubber dam progressed apically, it could cause severe bone destruction and possibly cause loss of the tooth. H. Abrams et al. (1978) reported a case in which a gingival abscess developed because of a retained piece of rubber dam material. All of the interproximal areas are cut from the facial aspect, and the dam is then freed from the lingual surfaces (Fig. 35-27). The clamp ligature is held while the clamp is removed to prevent the clamps from slipping off the tooth unexpectedly. The clamp, dam, and frame are removed at the same time (Fig. 35-28). While the assistant rinses the patient's mouth with the tri-syringe and suction, the clinician lays the dam on a flat surface and checks the dam to make sure it matches and that there are no small pieces of dam missing that could remain in the patient's mouth (Fig. 35-29). The patient should be cautioned not to bite down on the newly placed restoration, because the restoration could be extended above the occlusal plane and could fracture with occlusal forces. The clinician will adjust the occlusion during the final carving.

There are other methods for placing a rubber

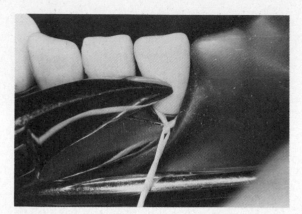

Fig. 35-25. Ligature is cut.

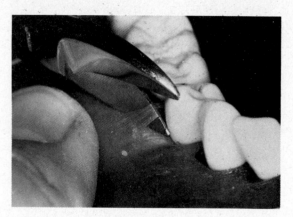

Fig. 35-26. Dam is stretched facially, blade of scissors is placed under entire interdental septa, and septa is cut.

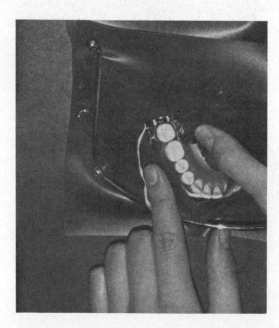

Fig. 35-27. Interdental areas of dam are freed from lingual surface.

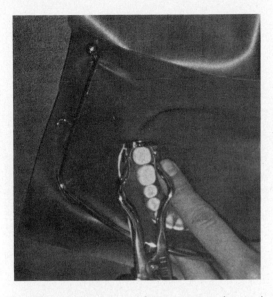

Fig. 35-28. Clamp, dam, and frame are removed as a unit.

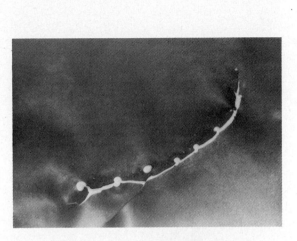

Fig. 35-29. Dam is inspected for missing pieces.

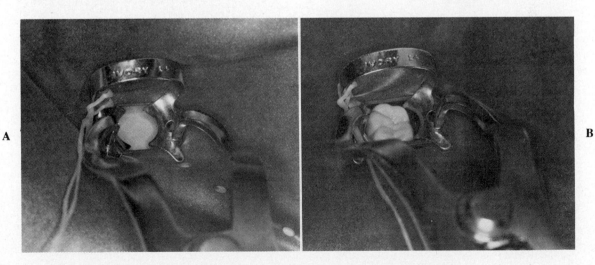

A

B

Fig. 35-30. Placing clamp and dam at same time. **A,** Dam is placed on winged clamp, and forceps are inserted. **B,** Clamp and dam are placed on tooth.

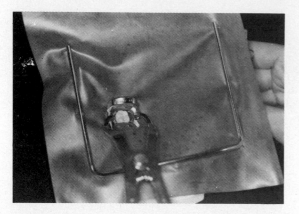

Fig. 35-31. Dam, with frame, is put onto winged clamp: all three are placed on tooth at once.

Fig. 35-32. Gingival retractor clamp being placed. Clamp will be stabilized with compound. (From Howard, W.W., and Moller, R.C. 1981. Atlas of operative dentistry, ed. 3. St. Louis: The C.V. Mosby Co.)

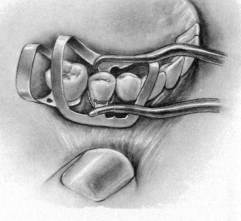

dam. The dam and clamp can be placed simultaneously, or the clamp, dam, and frame can all be placed in one step (Chasteen, 1978) (Figs. 35-30 and 35-31). In some instances (i.e., when a gingival retractor clamp is used) the dam is placed first (Fig. 35-32). Modifications in the placement technique are appropriate if the final dam is clinically acceptable.

TOFFLEMIRE MATRIX RETAINER AND BAND PLACEMENT AND REMOVAL

Matrix bands are used during the placement of a restoration that extends into the proximal area of a tooth. The matrices are used when amalgams or temporary cements are being placed into Class II and some Class III and V cavity preparations. The matrix is necessary for several reasons: (1) it provides contour for the proximal surface, which was removed during the preparation of the tooth; (2) it provides a surface against which the clinician can condense (pack) the restorative material into the preparation; (3) it helps to form a contact area with the adjacent tooth; and (4) it permits overfilling the proximal area of the tooth so that the marginal ridge can be carved to the proper height. There are several types of matrix systems; the placement and removal of the Tofflemire matrix system are described in this chapter. The armamentarium needed to place a matrix and wedge is illustrated in Fig. 35-33.

The Tofflemire matrix retainer (Fig. 35-34) holds the matrix band, which forms a loop around

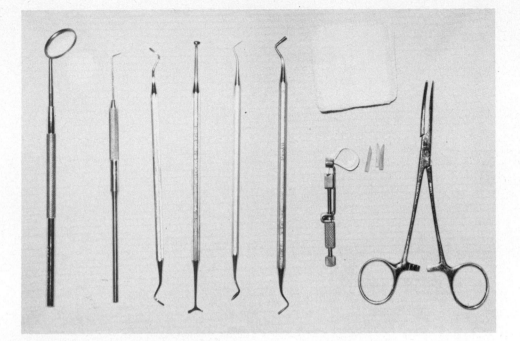

Fig. 35-33. Armamentarium for placement and removal of Tofflemire matrix band system: mirror, explorer, curette, T-ball/football burnisher, Hollenback carver, condenser, gauze, retainer, band, wedges, and hemostat.

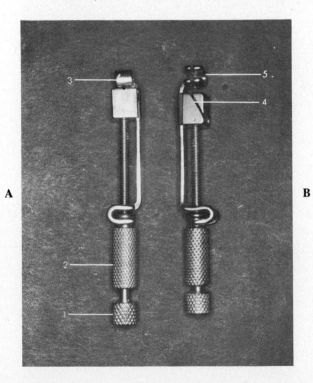

Fig. 35-34. **A,** Occlusal view of retainer: *1,* small locking knob; *2,* large adjustment knob; *3,* curved portion of prongs. **B,** Gingival view of retainer: *4,* groove for matrix band; *5* prongs.

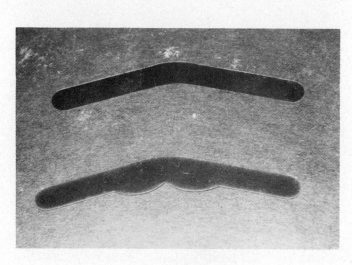

Fig. 35-35. Universal *(top)* and No. 2, gingival extension *(bottom)*, matrix bands.

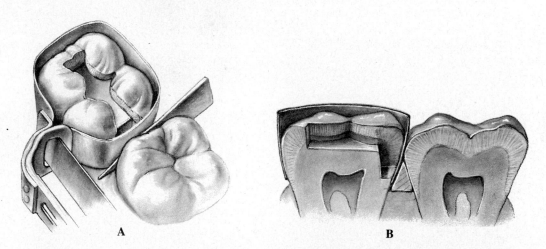

A   B

Fig. 35-36. A, Occlusal view of matrix band and wedge properly placed. **B,** Cross section. Note that band extends occlusally and cervically. (From Howard, W.W., and Moller, R.C. 1981. Atlas of operative dentistry, ed. 3. St. Louis: The C.V. Mosby Co.)

the tooth. The holder has two knobs that hold the band and increase or decrease the size of the loop. The small locking knob at the end of the holder holds the band in the holder, and the larger adjustment knob adjusts the size of the loop.

Several shapes of matrix bands are available to be used for various-sized cavity preparations. A universal matrix band is for cavity preparations with small to moderately deep proximal areas (Fig. 35-35). The No. 2 band is used for preparations with deep proximal areas because it has mesial and distal gingival extensions, which are placed cervically. The cervical extensions of the No. 2 band can be cut with scissors to the proper height. The matrix band must be wide enough to extend 1 to 2 mm gingivally to the cervical portion of the proximal area and 1 to 2 mm occlusally to the height of the marginal ridge (Fig. 35-36). This extension above the occlusal surface permits overfilling, and the extension cervical to the preparation reduces the chance of an overhang (with the use of a wooden wedge). There are also matrix bands with windows that can be used with Class V cavity preparations as well as plastic matrix bands that are used with anterior tooth-colored restorative materials.

In addition to the retainer and matrix band, wooden wedges are used to hold the matrix band against the constricted cervical area of the tooth. In cross section, the wedge is triangular in shape (like a Stim-U-Dent); the base of the wedge is placed toward the gingiva, and the apex of the wedge is placed toward the occlusal surface but apical to the contact area.

Placement of the band system and wooden wedge

The cavity preparation should be examined visually and with an explorer so that the clinician is familiar with the cavity preparation before the band is fitted and placed. The proper band should be selected according to the depth of the interproximal area of the preparation. Once the proper band is selected, it must be placed in the retainer properly. When the band is formed into a loop, the clinician will notice that there is a large and a small opening (Fig. 35-37). The smaller opening is placed toward the cervical area of the tooth to conform to the constricted anatomy, and the larger opening is placed toward the occlusal surface. The larger opening of the loop is placed in the matrix band so that it is directed toward the curved portion of the prongs that hold the band in place. The larger opening and the curve should face the occlusal surface. One way to remember this is that the larger loop allows for the ''large'' occlusal surface, and

A 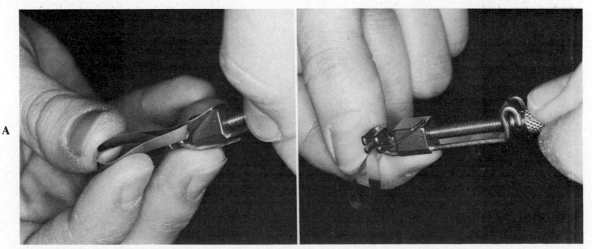 B

Fig. 35-37. **A,** Band is placed in groove of retainer and then, **B,** slid into prongs and bent through appropriate side.

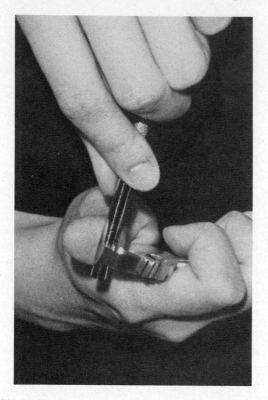

Fig. 35-38. Contouring band with rounded instrument to give band an even circumference.

the curve of the prongs is shaped like the cusp of a posterior tooth, which is on the occlusal surface. It is important to place the curved portion of the prongs facing the occlusal surface as an aid to removing the retainer. The loop of the matrix band should be placed in the prongs so that the retainer can be on the facial surface of the teeth and the knobs of the band can extend anteriorly out of the patient's mouth (Fig. 35-37). The band is then contoured as shown in Fig. 35-38.

The band is placed in the retainer and tightened with the small locking knob; then the size of the loop is adjusted with the larger adjustment knob to allow the band to be placed over the greatest circumference of the tooth. The opening of the prongs should be centered on the facial surface of the tooth and the band tightened until it is snug around the cervical area of the tooth. Sometimes pressure must be applied to the band with the pad of the thumb to push the band through the contact areas. If extreme pressure is needed to push the band through the contact area, the clinician should stop and assess the situation. Sometimes extremely close teeth may have to be slightly separated with a mechanical separator or a wooden wedge to permit passage of the band. The supervising dentist should be consulted in these instances. When the band is placed, the interproximal areas and some parts of the facial and lingual portion of the band will be slightly subgingival. At this time the band should be evaluated visually and with a mirror and explorer to see if the band extends cervically and occlusally 1 to 2 mm beyond the preparation.

One of the functions of the matrix band is to provide a contact area with the adjacent tooth. At the present stage the band is forming a flat surface from the occlusal to the cervical area, which is not the normal contour of an interproximal surface. The band must be burnished—an indentation is made in the band by rubbing an instrument along a portion of the band to form a contact area.

There are several ways to burnish a contact area into a band (Fig. 35-39). One way is to mark the area to be burnished by scratching the band with an explorer in the area of the contact while the band is on the tooth; the band is then loosened and removed from the tooth. Then the band, with or without the retainer attached, is placed on a pliable surface such as gauze or a paper mixing pad and is rubbed with a rounded instrument in the scratched area to mark the contact area. A football burnisher, beaver-tail burnisher, or the back of a large spoon excavator can be used to burnish the band. The band and the retainer are placed back on the tooth with the burnished contact area replaced in the proper position. Another way to burnish the band is to burnish a groove from the occlusal to the gingival margin of the band in the estimated area of the contact area, before the band is fitted onto the tooth. Then the band is slightly adjusted on the tooth to be sure the contact area is in the proper area. This procedure saves time, and with experience the clinician is able to estimate the location of the contact area fairly accurately. Another way to burnish the contact is to use a beavertail burnisher or the back of a large spoon excavator to rub the contact area when the band and retainer are in place on the tooth. This method also is time-

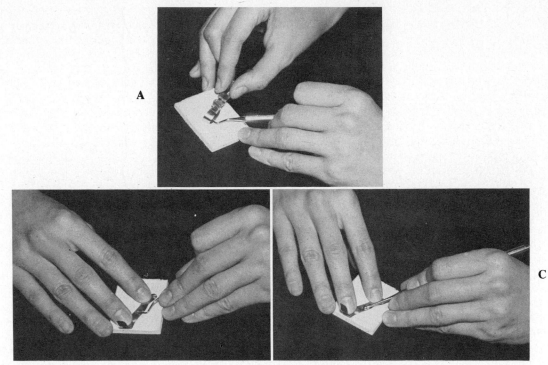

Fig. 35-39. Burnishing contact, **A,** with back of a spoon excavator while band is in the retainer; **B,** while band is removed; and **C,** with football burnisher.

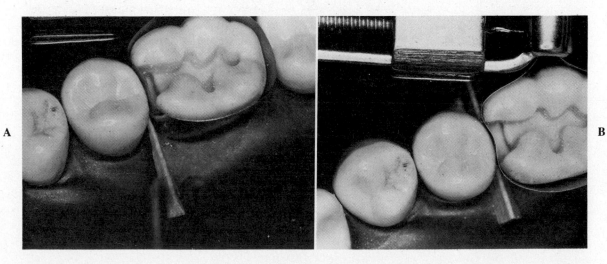

Fig. 35-40. **A,** Wedge being inserted from lingual aspect with cotton pliers. **B,** Wedge in place.

saving, but the contact area produced will not be as definite with this method as it would be with the other two approaches.

The wooden wedge is placed next with the base oriented gingivally, the apex placed occlusally, and the point placed toward the buccal aspect. Inserted from the lingual aspect (the lingual embrasure spaces are larger than the buccal embrasure spaces), the wedge is slid under the contact area and toward the buccal aspect; sometimes the point of the wedge is visible on the buccal surface (Fig. 35-40). The purposes of the wedge are (1) to hold the cervical area of the band tightly against the tooth to prevent any of the restorative material from extending beyond the preparation and eventually forming an overhang; (2) to separate the teeth slightly so that the contact area can be completely formed; and (3) to compensate for the thickness of the matrix band. The wedge must be checked carefully to be sure it is placed properly and is not impinging on the gingiva or extending into the preparation. The wedge is checked visually and with an explorer (Fig. 35-41). The explorer is moved along the gingival margin of the preparation to make sure the band is tight against the tooth. Then the explorer is moved from the gingival margin of the preparation toward the occlusal surface. If the clinician can clearly detect the occlusal portion of the wedge and if it feels like a ledge, then the wedge is impinging into the preparation and will cause a ditch in the restoration. The wedge should be removed and contoured with a sharp instrument so that it can slide under the contact without extending into the preparation (Fig.

35-42). If the explorer can be inserted between the band and the tooth, the wedge is too small and should be replaced with a larger one. Sometimes double wedging—inserting two wedges from the lingual aspect—is necessary.

After the evaluation the matrix placement is complete, and the tooth should be rinsed and dried gently. The band placement should be evaluated according to the criteria included on the check-off sheet at the end of the chapter.

Removal of the band system

At the completion of the condensation of the restorative material into the preparation and of the initial carving, the retainer, wedge, and matrix band must be removed to permit the final carving of the restoration (Fig. 35-43). The matrix retainer is removed from the band by the small knob being loosened and the retainer being lifted off the band. The retainer is pulled toward the occlusal surface while the band is stabilized by the pad of the thumb. The wedge is removed with cotton pliers or a hemostat. The band is first removed from the interproximal area that was not restored, and then the band is held straight with both hands. The band is eased out from the restored area by the lingual portion being removed first and the band being rotated out of the interproximal area from lingual to buccal aspect. If the restoration is an MOD, the band is removed from one interproximal area at a time. If the clinician is working with an assistant, the assistant can gently hold a large condenser on the marginal ridge of the newly placed restoration to help guide the band away from the ridge during

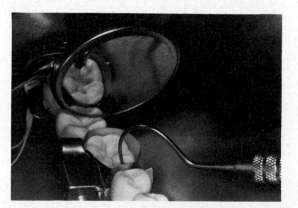

Fig. 35-41. Wedge placement being checked with mirror and explorer.

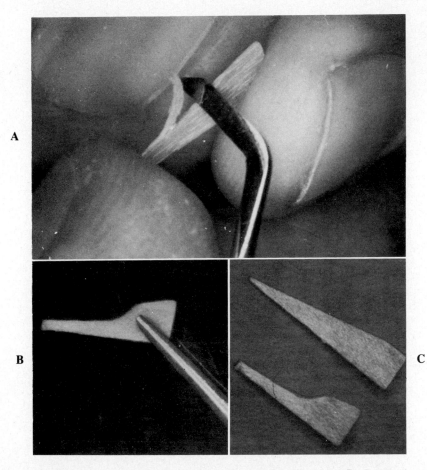

Fig. 35-42. A, Wedge is contoured with amalgam knife or Hollenback carver. **B,** Contoured wedge. **C,** Contoured and uncontoured wedges. (From Gilmore, W.H., et al. 1982. Operative dentistry, ed. 4. St. Louis: The C.V. Mosby Co.)

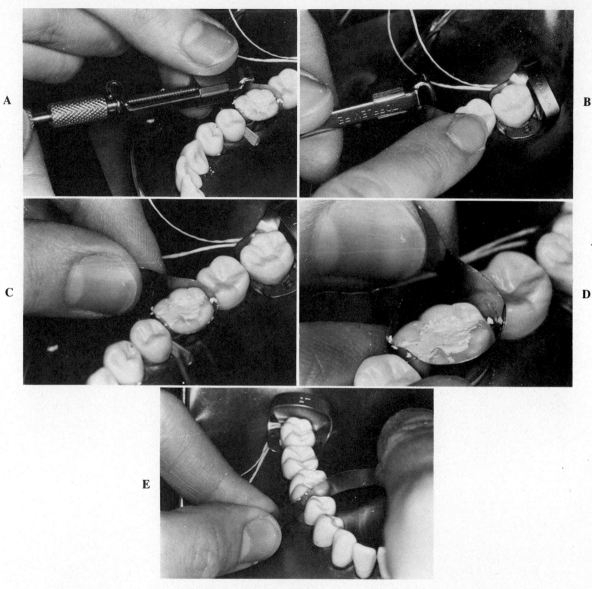

Fig. 35-43. Removal of matrix band and retainer. **A,** Retainer is loosened. **B,** Band is stabilized while retainer is removed. **C,** Wedge is removed. **D,** Distal portion of band is removed. **E,** Mesial portion of band is removed.

removal. It is possible to fracture the marginal ridge of the newly placed restoration while removing the band, so care must be taken.

PLACEMENT OF A ZINC OXIDE–EUGENOL TEMPORARY RESTORATION

Zinc oxide–eugenol temporary restorations are placed in cavity preparations in several instances: for caries control, to replace a permanent restoration that has fractured or fallen out, to restore a preparation that is not final, or to soothe the pulp of a tooth that has been slightly traumatized. The zinc oxide–eugenol restoration can remain in the tooth for up to 6 weeks, depending on the type of zinc oxide–eugenol restoration used. In all cases the zinc oxide–eugenol restoration is truly temporary and will be replaced by a permanent type of restoration such as an amalgam or a gold inlay. Zinc oxide–eugenol temporary restorations can be placed in Classes I to V cavity preparations; in this chapter a technique for placing zinc oxide–eugenol into a two-surface Class II preparation is described. The technique is similar for the other types of prep-

arations, but different matrix bands or no matrix bands are used, depending on the preparation. When placing a Class II zinc oxide–eugenol temporary restoration, the clinician should place a rubber dam and a Tofflemire matrix band in the appropriate area according to the procedures presented earlier in this chapter. Once the matrix band and wooden wedge are placed, the clinician should once again inspect the cavity preparation. The clinician should pay particular attention to the outline form of the preparation so that it can be reproduced during the carving of the temporary restoration.

The armamentarium necessary to place and carve a zinc oxide–eugenol temporary restoration is illustrated in Fig. 35-44. The spatula is used to mix the zinc oxide–eugenol according to the manufacturer's directions. One end of the plastic instrument is used to wipe the zinc oxide–eugenol into the preparation; the other end is a condenser, which is used to pack the zinc oxide–eugenol into the preparation. There are three carving instruments on the tray: a No. 1/2 Hollenback, a small

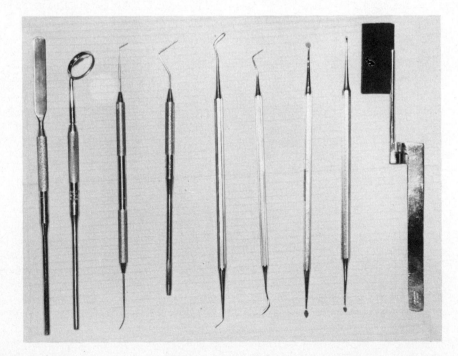

Fig. 35-44. Armamentarium for placement of zinc oxide–eugenol restoration: spatula, mirror, explorer, probe, placement instrument, No. 1/2 Hollenback and cleiod-discoid carvers, and articulating paper.

cleoid-discoid, and a large cleoid-discoid. The Hollenback carver is used to carve the interproximal and occlusal surfaces and the cleoid-discoid carvers are used to carve the occlusal surface. The articulating paper is used to check the occlusion at the end of the carving procedure. Carving technique is discussed later in this chapter.

Before the clinician or the assistant mixes the zinc oxide–eugenol, the clinician should be certain that the particular instruments can be used in the preparation; sometimes the instruments are too large to fit into the preparation and smaller instruments must be used. The beginning clinician can practice the entire procedure by adapting each instrument to the tooth in the order of use before the beginning of the procedure.

The zinc oxide–eugenol should be mixed to a thick puttylike consistency according to the manufacturer's recommendations. Once the zinc oxide–eugenol is mixed to the proper consistency, the clinician takes a small amount of the zinc oxide–eugenol on the placement instrument and wipes it into the proximal area of the tooth (Fig. 35-45). The condenser is used to pack the zinc oxide–eugenol into the proximal area (Fig. 35-46). A great deal of pressure is not needed, since the zinc oxide–eugenol has a puttylike consistency. When pressing the zinc oxide–eugenol into the preparation, the clinician should press the material against all areas of the proximal area (i.e., against the walls of the preparation, straight down, into the angles of the preparation, and against the matrix band). It is particularly important to press the zinc oxide–eugenol against the band in the contact area to make sure the temporary restoration will contact the adjacent tooth. Small increments are added and condensed into the proximal area and then into the rest of the preparation until the preparation is overfilled (Figs. 35-47 and 35-48). During the condensing, the instrument can be dipped in alcohol or extra powder to prevent the zinc oxide–eugenol from clinging to the instrument.

Next the clinician uses the explorer to clear the excess zinc oxide–eugenol away from the marginal ridge area of the matrix band (Fig. 35-49). The explorer tip is placed against the band with the side of the explorer angled against the restoration and is moved from buccal to lingual aspect to remove the excess. This frees the zinc oxide–eugenol from the matrix band, makes the removal of the band

easier, helps to shape the marginal ridge, and lessens the chance of fracturing the marginal ridge. The matrix band is then removed according to the procedure presented previously.

After the removal of the band, the first area to be carved is the proximal area: the buccal, lingual, and gingival margins of the proximal portion and the embrasures. It is important to remove all of the excess restorative material from the proximal area to promote gingival and supporting tissue health. The No. 1/2 Hollenback instrument is angled into the proximal area so that part of the blade is on the tooth and part of the blade is on the zinc oxide–eugenol (Fig. 35-50). All of the excess is not removed at once; trying to remove too much excess with one stroke could cause the restoration to fracture. Shaving strokes that preserve the contact area and do not reach all the way up to the marginal ridge are used. Oblique and upward-and-downward vertical strokes can be used to remove the excess and to carve and shape the interproximal area.

The discoid end (round end) of the large cleoid-discoid carver is used to establish the height of the marginal ridge to be even with the marginal ridge of the No. 1/2 Hollenback carver is rested in the ginal ridge height is established, the No. 1/2 Hollenback carver can be used to clear the excess zinc oxide–eugenol from the occlusal surface. The tip of the No. 1/2 Hollenbach carver is rested in the central groove area, and the side of the blade is rested on the tooth. Careful, shaving strokes, guided by the tooth's anatomy, are used to remove the excess. Either the No. 1/2 Hollenback or the cleoid (pointed) end of the smaller cleoid-discoid can be used to carve the final shape of the occlusal surface (Figs. 35-52 and 35-53). Whichever instrument is used, part of the blade should be resting on the tooth surface and part of the blade should be on the zinc oxide–eugenol. The portion of the instrument on the tooth should guide the carving of the restoration. The restoration should be carved until the material is even with the margins of the preparation and the original outline of the preparation has been reproduced. The restoration can be smoothed by using long strokes while finishing the anatomy.

When the clinician believes the carving is almost complete, the area is cleared of debris, the rubber dam is removed, and the occlusion is checked by placing the articulating paper in the patient's mouth

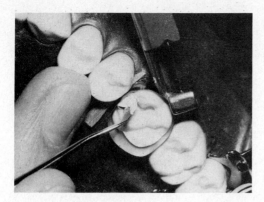

Fig. 35-45. Wiping zinc oxide–eugenol into preparation.

Fig. 35-46. Condensing zinc oxide–eugenol into proximal area.

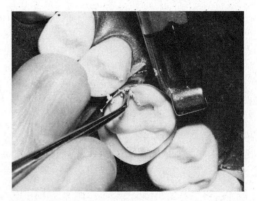

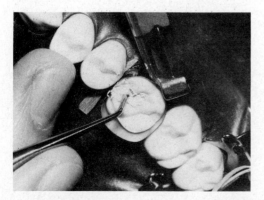

Fig. 35-47. Condensing zinc oxide–eugenol into rest of preparation.

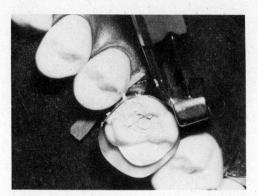

Fig. 35-48. Preparation overfilled with zinc oxide–eugenol.

Fig. 35-49. Zinc oxide–eugenol is cleared from matrix band. Note placement and angulation of instrument.

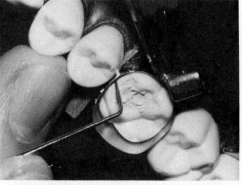

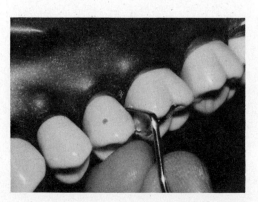

Fig. 35-50. Proximal area is carved with No. 1/2 Hollenback carver.

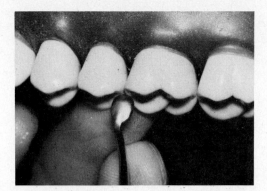

Fig. 35-51. Establishing height of marginal ridge with round end of large cleoid-discoid carver resting on adjacent marginal ridge.

Fig. 35-52. Occlusal surface is carved with No. 1/2 Hollenback carver.

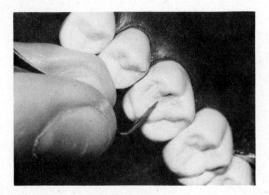

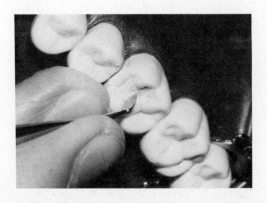

Fig. 35-53. Occlusal surface is carved with pointed end of small cleoid-discoid carver.

and having the patient *lightly* tap the teeth together and slide the mandible from side to side. The markings from the articulating paper should be light and evenly distributed over the contacts of the tooth. Zinc oxide–eugenol does not withstand the forces of mastication very well; therefore some practitioners recommend that the zinc oxide–eugenol restoration be slightly overcarved so that it does not occlude with the opposing tooth. If the restoration is too far out of occlusion, the opposing tooth will begin to extrude. Thus the opposing tooth (teeth) should *slightly* contact the tooth with the temporary restoration.

When the restoration is complete, the clinician should evaluate his/her work according to the criteria on the check-off sheet; then the supervising dentist should be asked to evaluate the restoration.

AMALGAM OVERHANG REMOVAL (MARGINATION)

An overhang is an extension of restorative material beyond the margin of the preparation and the surface of the tooth. Overhangs are usually at the gingival margin of a restoration, but sometimes the restorative material will be flush with the tooth in the gingival area and there will be a bulbous area just occlusal to the margin. The contour of the entire proximal surface (i.e., the shape of contact area, occlusal embrasure space, and buccal and lingual embrasure spaces) is evaluated and reshaped as necessary during the margination procedure. The presence of an overhang or of an improperly contoured proximal surface is of concern because both form plaque-retentive areas. Such plaque-retentive areas contribute to and exacerbate gingival inflammation and breakdown of the supporting structures.

Overhangs vary in size and shape (Fig. 35-54). The overhangs can be small, moderate, or large; margination is most successful with small to moderate overhangs. Many times, restorations with large overhangs must be replaced, but this decision depends on the opinion of the supervising dentist. Jeffcoat et al. (1980) have defined the size of an overhang according to the percentage of the interproximal space occupied by the overhang. An overhang is small if less than 20% of the interproximal space is occupied, medium if 20% to 50% is occupied, and large if greater than 50% is occupied.

Overhangs are usually caused during the placement of the restoration. Faulty placement of the matrix band and/or wedge can cause an overhang by permitting the amalgam to be condensed between the band and the tooth. Not using a matrix band and/or wedge at all during the placement of an amalgam restoration will certainly cause an overhang. Other factors such as rotated teeth, lack of patient cooperation, or other such difficulties can lead to an overhang. The clinician must use extreme care during the placement and carving procedures to avoid an overhang.

Rationale for margination

Coxhead et al. (1978) performed a radiographic survey of teeth restored with amalgam and determined that of 2108 proximal surfaces restored, 1094, or 52%, had overhangs. Thus the problem of amalgam overhangs seems to be rather common.

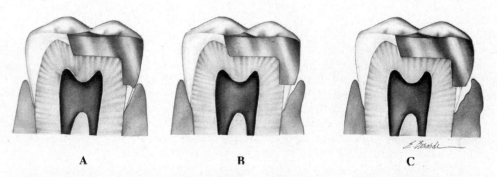

Fig. 35-54. A, Small overhang. **B,** Moderate overhang. **C,** Large overhang. Note effect that overhang has on adjacent tissues.

Amalgam overhangs have been associated with gingival inflammation and alveolar bone loss (Hakkarainen and Ainamo, 1980; Jeffcoat et al. 1980; Leon, 1977). The overhang impinges on the gingival tissue, but, more important, the overhang is a plaque-retentive object in an already susceptible and difficult-to-clean area. Thus the destructive effect of the overhang is due to the increased accumulation and entrapment of plaque, plaque byproducts, and other debris. Margination of overhangs, in conjunction with plaque removal procedures by the patient and by the professional, has been shown to improve the health of the gingiva and supporting structures (Axelsson, 1981; Gorzo et al., 1979; Highfield and Powell, 1978; Rodriguez-Ferrer et al., 1980). Clearly, the procedure of margination, along with professional and personal plaque removal, is essential to improve and maintain a patient's periodontal status.

Overhanging amalgam restorations and margination are the focus of this section of the chapter. It should be noted, however, that there are indications that even properly contoured restorations extending subgingivally contribute to gingival inflammation through plaque retention (Gullo and Powell, 1979; Leon, 1977). The surface of an amalgam restoration is rough, especially if it is not finished and polished, and plaque retentive. Thus it is of great importance that the interproximal surfaces of restorations be as smooth as possible. Marginating, finishing, and polishing amalgam restorations are procedures the dental health professional can perform to achieve smooth restored surfaces.

Detection

Overhangs can be detected visually, tactilely, and radiographically, as discussed in Chapter 11. Once the clinician has detected the overhang, he/she should determine the location, size, and shape of the overhang, just as one would do with a calculus deposit. An explorer and bitewing radiographs are valuable during this assessment of the overhang. The clinician should reach a decision about the size of the overhang—small, medium, or large—before the procedure is begun. If the overhang is small or medium and can be removed, the rest of the restoration should be evaluated for other involvements such as recurrent decay, a fracture, an open contact, or caries on another surface of the tooth, any of which would contraindicate

the overhang removal procedure. Many times, *very small overhangs* can be removed as part of the scaling procedure, but anything more involved should be approved by the supervising dentist.

Armamentarium

The armamentarium necessary for removing overhangs is pictured in Fig. 35-55. This section presents a margination technique in which hand instruments are used rather than burs or diamond stones. The amalgam knife is used to shave away some of the gross excess and to reach into the tight area around the contact area. The files are used to remove the amalgam, especially in the gingival area and on the buccal and lingual surfaces. Universal curettes are used to remove small amalgam extensions and to smooth the amalgam. Disks and strips are used to finish the contours, and floss with pumice is used to polish the area.

The first step is to use the knife with shaving strokes as shown in Fig. 35-56. Removing an overhang is different from removing calculus in that the amalgam is literally shaved away; the instrument is not placed under the entire overhang and activated to remove the overhang in one stroke. Calculus will break away from the tooth with such a stroke, but the amalgam may fracture, necessitating placement of a new restoration. The amalgam knife in cross section (Fig. 35-57) looks like an upside-down sickle scaler. The apex of the triangle is the cutting edge, which means that the instrument is angled differently than a scaler during the working stroke. The cutting edge of the amalgam knife is turned more toward the tooth than is the cutting edge of the sickle scaler. Care must be used with the amalgam knife because it is extremely sharp; the clinician should *never* run his/her finger along the cutting edge of the knife to remove debris because the edge will cut the soft tissue.

When the blade of the knife is activated, the posterior part of the blade should be against the surface of the tooth and the anterior portion of the blade against the amalgam. Vertical and oblique strokes can be used with the knife, but the clinician should not allow the instrument to proceed through the contact area between the teeth. If the instrument passes through the contract area, an open contact could be created.

The files are used after the knife. There are three sets of files that can be used: heavy, medium, and

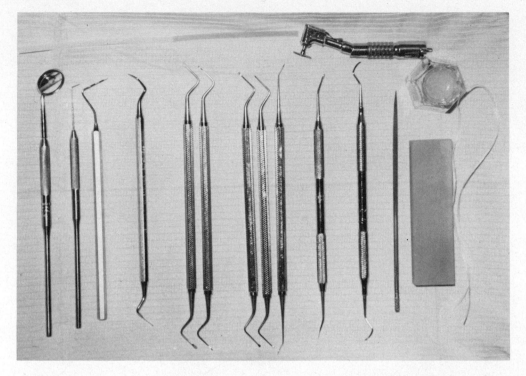

Fig. 35-55. Armamentarium for removal of overhang: mirror, explorer, probe, amalgam knife, Orban files, Hirshfeld files, Rhein file, curette, sharpening stones, floss, finishing strip, contra-angle, and disks.

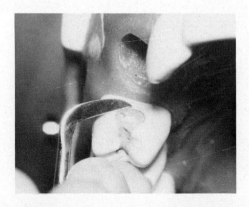

Fig. 35-56. Amalgam knife is placed against tooth and amalgam.

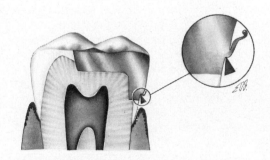

Fig. 35-57. Cross section of amalgam knife being used to shave away an overhang.

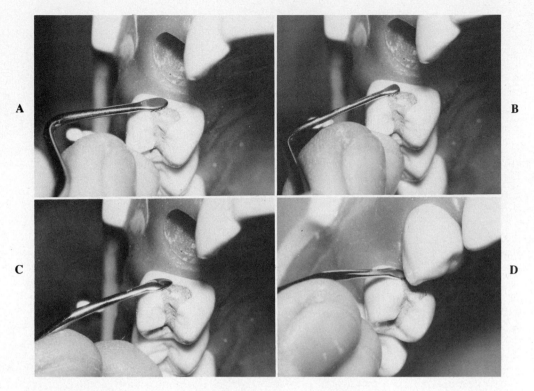

Fig. 35-58. Files being used to remove an overhang. **A,** Orban file. **B,** Hirshfeld file. **C,** Rhein No. 31/32 file. **D,** File adapted with adjacent tooth present.

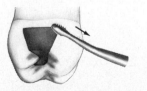

Fig. 35-59. File is placed on tooth and amalgam and is used with a pull stroke directed obliquely or horizontally.

finishing files (Figs. 35-58 and 35-59). Orban files are considered heavy files because they have only a few large serrations and remove large amounts of amalgam. Hirschfeld files are moderately heavy files because they have smaller-sized serrations and remove less amalgam. A file such as the Rhein file No. 31/32 is a very fine file, having about 20 serrations, and removes very little amalgam. The Rhein No. 31/32 file should be used after the other files because it produces the fewest striations on the surface of the amalgam. The file is placed on the tooth and amalgam surface and is pulled in either oblique or horizontal strokes. The files are used in order from heaviest to finest so that the deep striations are removed by each successively finer file. If an overhang is small, the Orban files may not be needed.

After the files are used, a universal curette can be used to smooth the interproximal surface further.

As the amalgam is being reduced, the clinician should check his/her progress with an explorer. After the knife, file, and curette have been used, the amalgam should be flush with the tooth. The explorer should be able to move smoothly from the amalgam to the tooth and back again. If *excess* remains, the explorer will pass from the amalgam to the tooth but will catch when passed from the tooth to the amalgam. If a *deficiency* has been created (too much amalgam removed) the explorer will catch when passed from the amalgam to the tooth. If an *open margin* has been exposed (an area where the amalgam does not meet the tooth), the explorer will catch when it is passed in both directions: from tooth to amalgam and from amalgam to tooth. If there is still some excess, the clinician should evaluate the location and the size of the overhang and use the instrument that seems most appropriate to remove the excess. If a deficient margin or an open margin is detected, the supervising dentist should be asked to evaluate the area, since hard tissue may have to be cut to remedy the situation or the restoration may have to be replaced. A clinician can produce a deficient or open margin by incorrectly using the instruments during the procedure; the instruments must be used with care.

Alternative methods

Alternative methods for removing the excess amalgam are available: surgical blades, ultrasonic scalers, and reciprocating motor-driven diamond tips. The use of surgical blades is similar to the use of an amalgam knife, but even greater care must be used. Ultrasonic scalers can be used, but there are two concerns. First, since the scaler removes the overhang rapidly, it is easy to remove too much and create a deficiency. Thus the clinician must proceed with caution and check progress with an explorer frequently. The second concern is one of safety. Mercury vapor is dangerous; inhalation and absorption of mercury can lead to mercury poisoning (ADA Councils, 1983). When an ultrasonic scaler is used, mercury is spewn throughout the perioral area and endangers the patient, clinician, and assistant. It is essential that a high-velocity suction be used when overhangs are removed with an ultrasonic scaler; in most instances this requires that a dental assistant work with the clinician.

Another method of removing overhangs is with a reciprocating motor-driven diamond tip such as the Eva Prophylaxis System (Unitex Manufacturing Co.). The tips are embedded with diamond particles on one side and can remove the overhang efficiently and effectively (Axelsson, 1981; Gelsky, 1982; Vale and Caffesse, 1979). The tips are triangular and designed to be adapted to the proximal surface of the teeth. Axelsson (1981) has recommended that the overhang removal be followed by finishing, polishing, complete plaque removal, and application of fluoridated paste with a plastic tip.

Disks and strips

Once the excess amalgam has been removed, the interproximal surface must be finished and polished so that it will be as plaque resistant and easily cleaned as possible. Finishing disks and strips are used to finish the area. This step is also performed during the amalgam and polishing procedure, which is discussed in the next section.

Disks are available in four sizes: 1/2, 5/8, 3/4, and 7/8 inches; the 1/2 and 5/8-inch sizes are most commonly used. The disks are attached to a mandrel that is inserted into a contra-angle. There are two types of mandrels: snap-on and screw-in; therefore disks are either snap-on or pinhole to fit the respective mandrels. Disks are made of plastic or paper; the paper ones are preferable because they are more flexible and pliable. Disks are available in a variety of grits (Craig, O'Brien, and Powers, 1983). The most commonly used grits for recontouring the interproximal surfaces of amalgam are garnet and cuttle. Garnet is a coarser abrasive and is used when a great deal of recontouring is to be done or if the surface of the amalgam is tarnished, corroded, or pitted. Cuttle disks are used for minor adjustments and after a garnet disk has been used. As discussed in Chapter 26, progressively finer abrasives must be used to achieve a smooth, plaque-resistant final product; therefore a cuttle disk is always used after a garnet disk. In most instances a fine garnet is the most abrasive disk used; it should be followed by a fine cuttle. The disks are used to recontour bulbous or broad contact areas with wiping strokes around the contact area. The disk should rotate from tooth to amalgam (from occlusal to gingival). The disk can also be used to reduce excess buccal and lingual margins to be flush with the tooth and to recontour the occlusal

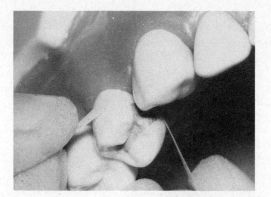

Fig. 35-60. Finishing strip placed on tooth and amalgam.

embrasure space. The disk must be used with intermittent strokes to prevent the creation of flattened areas.

A finishing strip can be used next to smooth the gingival margin of the restoration (Fig. 35-60). The portion of the finishing strip that is gritty should never be passed through the contact area because it can create an open contact. If gapped strips are used, the gapped portion of the strip can be passed through the contact. If ungapped strips are used, one end of the strip should be cut into a point and the strip should be threaded cervical to the contact area, the way a floss threader is carried under a contact. Once the finishing strip is cervical to the contact area, it is positioned so that half of the height of the strip is on the tooth and half is on amalgam; then a see-saw back-and-forth motion is used to remove the striations. If the strip is only on amalgam, the edge of the strip could rest at the gingival margin of the amalgam, and a deficient or open margin could be created.

Pumice and tin oxide

The next step is to floss the area with pumice and tape. The pumice and tape can be carried through the contact. The entire interproximal surface should be flossed to try to smooth the amalgam as much as possible; however, the contact area should be flossed with care. The final step is to rinse the area thoroughly and to floss the area without any pumice. It is important to provide thorough lavage of the area to remove all loose pieces of amalgam and other debris.

The finished product should be evaluated by the clinician and then by the supervising dentist. The product is considered acceptable if the following criteria are met: (1) the margins of the amalgam are flush with the tooth; (2) a contact with the adjacent tooth is present; (3) the contour of the interproximal area reproduces the contour of the original tooth; (4) no damage has been caused to the adjacent hard and/or soft tissues; (5) no debris is present; and (6) the interproximal area is smooth.

Many practitioners follow up the overhang removal procedure by finishing and polishing the rest of the amalgam. The technique for that procedure is presented in the following section.

FINISHING AND POLISHING AN AMALGAM RESTORATION

The majority of restorations placed by dental personnel are amalgam restorations. The life expectancy of an amalgam restoration is 8 to 15 years; this expectancy is increased by finishing and polishing the restoration. The finishing and polishing procedure removes *tarnish, corrosion products,* and *roughness* from the surface of the amalgam. The roughness weakens the amalgam and is plaque retentive. The corrosion products are due to a chemical reaction between the amalgam and sulfur and other components in the saliva, which produces a rough, pitted surface. Tarnish is merely a surface discoloration on the amalgam. Finishing and polishing an amalgam creates a smooth, shiny surface, which is resistant to tarnish and corrosion.

An amalgam restoration may be polished any time beyond 24 hours after the amalgam was placed in the mouth; the amalgam is not completely set and hardened until 24 hours after placement. This is true even for the high copper amalgam alloys. There has been discussion and experimentation with polishing high copper amalgams within 10 minutes of placement (Corpron et al., 1982; Creaven et al., 1980; Schemlitzer et al., 1982), and some practitioners recommend the practice (Nitkin, 1979). However, it is presently recommended that at least 24 hours pass before any amalgam restoration is polished (Creaven et al. 1980; Craig, 1980; Schemlitzer et al., 1982). Some practitioners have an appointment with a patient about 1 week after the amalgam was placed to polish the amalgam. Other practitioners polish the amalgam at the recall appointment. In either of these situations, the procedure could be delegated to the dental hygienist.

Sequence of abrasives

Several sequences of abrasive instruments can be used to finish and polish amalgam restorations (Charbeneau, 1965; Craig, 1980; J. Cunningham, 1977; Gilmore et al., 1982; Simon, 1978; Solow, 1981). The primary concept is that progressively finer abrasives are used to contour, shape, and smooth the amalgam restoration. Class II and III (such as a distolingual on a cuspid) amalgams are finished and polished in two stages. The interproximal surface, as discussed in the margination section, is done first with disks, strips, pumice and tin oxide. The occlusal (or lingual aspect of a Class III restoration) surface is done next. Many abrasives have been suggested for polishing and finishing these surfaces, such as green stones, white stones, rubber wheels, burs, pumice, silex,

tin oxide, and chemically impregnated cups and points. The use of rubber wheels is not recommended because of their excessive heat production and ensuing damage to the pulp (Cooley et al., 1978). Green and white stones also produce a great deal of heat, though less than rubber wheels, and must be used with great care. One acceptable sequence for polishing the occlusal surface includes green and/or white stones, various-shaped finishing burs, pumice or silex, and tin oxide. This sequence can also be used to finish and polish the lingual surface of a Class III amalgam. An acceptable sequence for polishing Class V amalgams includes the use of green and/or white stones, finishing burs, disks, pumice or silex, and tin oxide. It is acceptable to use chemically impregnated cups and points, in place of pumice or silex and tin oxide, in any of these sequences. The armamentarium for an amalgam polishing procedure is shown in Fig. 35-61.

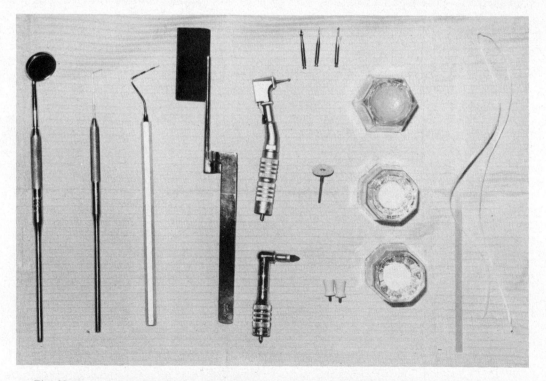

Fig. 35-61. Armamentarium for amalgam polishing procedure: mirror, explorer, probe, articulating paper, contra-angle, prophylaxis angle, burs, disk, cups, pumice, tin oxide, strips, and floss.

Assessing the restoration

The restoration is assessed visually and tactilely to determine if the margins are flush, excess, deficient, or open (see discussion of overhang removal) (Figs. 35-62 and 35-63). At the completion of the polishing, all of the margins should be flush; areas with excess or with slight deficiencies (0.5 mm) can be finished. Margins that are more than slightly deficient or that are open cannot be corrected during the polishing procedure; these conditions are considered contraindications to polishing. Other contraindications include open contacts, fractured restorations, marginal ridges below the plane of occlusion, large overhangs, restorations in teeth to be extracted or crowned, recurrent decay, and excessively deep occlusal anatomy. Some examples of contours that could be improved during the finishing polishing procedure are broad contact areas; high areas of the amalgam that contact first; marginal ridges that extend above the height of occlusion (if a marginal ridge is excessively high, it would be fractured by the forces of occlusion); and indistinct occlusal anatomy. If an amalgam has a slight to moderate overhang, it should be removed before the amalgam is polished; margination is done first.

Evaluating the occlusion

The occlusion should be evaluated with articulating paper for areas of the restoration that occlude prematurely; these areas will be identified by darker markings on the restoration. The markings should be of the same intensity at the points of contact. The high areas should be reduced with a bur and checked with articulating paper (see Chapter 28).

Isolating the teeth

The teeth should be isolated during the polishing procedure; ideally, a rubber dam should be placed. If only one amalgam (or single amalgams in one or more of the quadrants) is being polished, cotton roll isolation can be used. Rubber dam isolation is

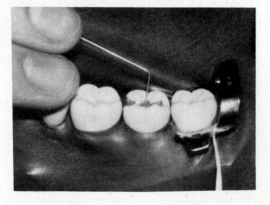

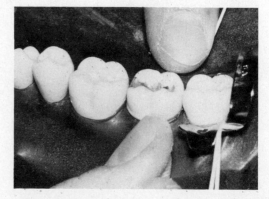

Fig. 35-62. Margins being evaluated with an explorer.

Fig. 35-63. Floss used to check for positive contact.

best because it permits thorough rinsing of the area between the steps and it prevents the abrasives from entering other areas of the patient's mouth. The rubber dam is especially good to use when a quadrant of restorations is being polished. The use of the rubber dam prevents the tooth from being bathed by saliva. When a dam is used, the tooth should be cooled with a stream of air periodically.

Finishing versus polishing

Finishing and polishing are two separate procedures performed with different abrasives. Finishing involves contouring, shaping, and defining the anatomy of the restoration and is done with stones, burs, disks, and strips. Polishing, done with pumice or silex and tin oxide or impregnated stone, removes the scratches and produces a smooth, shiny surface. Finishing is done before polishing, so when more than one surface is being done, all of the surfaces are finished and then all are polished. A procedure for finishing and polishing a two-surface Class II amalgam is described in the following sections. Similar procedures, as discussed later, are used for other classes of amalgam restorations.

Finishing the interproximal surface

The interproximal surface is finished with disks and strips as described in the margination section (see pp. 632 and 633) (Fig. 35-64). At the completion of these procedures, the margins should be checked with an explorer and the contours should be checked visually. The margins should be flush,

and the original contours of the tooth should be reproduced. If these criteria are not met, the disks and/or strip should be used again.

Finishing the occlusal surface

The first abrasive that can be used on the occlusal surface is the green stone. If the amalgam is tarnished or corroded and pitted, the green stone is used to remove the pitted surface. As is true when using any rotary instrument, short, light, intermittent strokes are used to reduce the heat produced by the instrument. This is especially true when using a stone, since a stone produces heat more quickly; if an assistant is available, he/she can direct a stream of air at the tooth for further cooling. A pointed green stone is most commonly used. It is rotated in a counterclockwise direction, placed on the amalgam with the point in the central groove and the side on the amalgam and tooth, and moved in a back-and-forth direction. As the stone is moved, it is guided by the tooth's anatomy, so it is raised to accommodate the ridges and lowered to conform to the grooves and fossae. The green stone will remove surface tarnish and corrosion; it will not create definitive anatomy.

A pointed white stone is used in the same manner after the green stone to further smooth the amalgam surface. If the amalgam is only slightly tarnished or rough, the white stone can be the first abrasive to be used.

Burs of various shapes and sizes are used next to eliminate excesses or slight deficiencies and to reshape and define the anatomy (Fig. 35-65). The

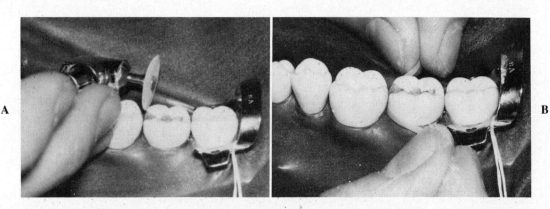

A   **B**

Fig. 35-64. Interproximal area being finished with, **A,** disk and, **B,** finishing strip.

burs used to finish amalgams are called finishing burs and differ from the cutting burs used to prepare teeth. Finishing burs have 18 to 20 cutting edges; cutting burs have fewer edges, which remove only a slight bit of amalgam or tooth structure. The finishing burs are designed to cut when they are rotated in a counterclockwise direction. Again, it is important to use light, short, intermittent strokes to reduce heat production.

A *small round bur* is used first to obtain or maintain the correct location and depth of the primary grooves. The clinician must use a fulcrum during this step, as always, and guide the bur along the groove; the bur is not rested on the tooth structure. The bur is moved back and forth along the grooves, and the primary grooves should join in the appropriate fossae (Fig. 35-66).

A *large round* or *pear-shaped bur* is used next to smooth the margins of the amalgam. The bur is rested on the tooth and amalgam and moved along the margin until the amalgam and tooth are flush. The bur is moved from tooth to amalgam, then from amalgam to tooth; progress should be checked with an explorer (Fig. 35-67).

A *large round* or *bud-shaped bur* is used to contour and shape the ridges and fossae (Fig. 35-68). One of two approaches can be used to finish the ridges and fossae. The bur can be moved back and forth over each individual ridge and into the respective fossa, or the buccal, then lingual, ridges can be finished. If the latter approach is used, the bur is guided as much as possible by the tooth and is moved back and forth along the entire buccal or lingual surface. The bur is raised and lowered to conform to the anatomy. In the first approach, the bur is moved back and forth over each ridge individually. In both of these methods, it is wise to also move the bur up and down the ridge a few times to cross-hatch the strokes and produce a smoother surface. The *flame-shaped bur* can also

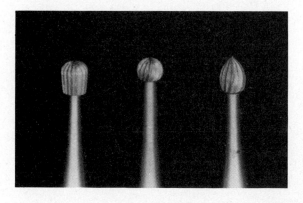

Fig. 35-65. Finishing burs. *From right to left:* Bud-shaped, round, and pear-shaped burs.

Fig. 35-66. Small round bur being used to shape groove anatomy.

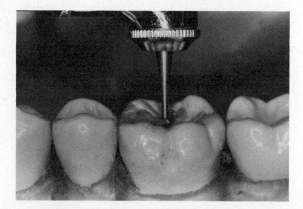

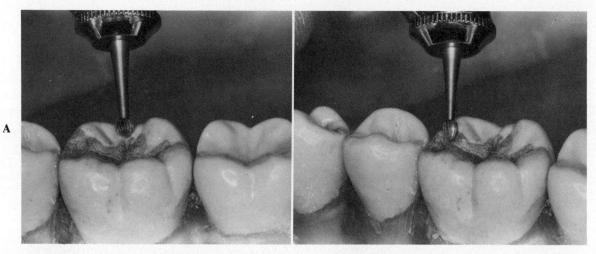

Fig. 35-67. **A,** Large round and, **B,** pear-shaped burs being used to smooth margins.

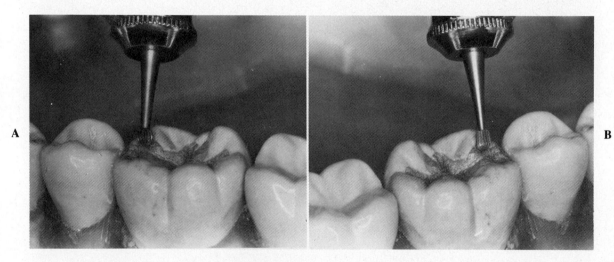

Fig. 35-68. **A,** Large round and, **B,** pear-shaped burs being used to contour and shape ridges and fossae.

be used for this step, but care must be used to avoid gouging the amalgam with its pointed tip.

The *small round bur* can be used once again, with a very light stroke, to redefine the groove if necessary. At the end of the bur step, the amalgam should have the desired contours and the surface should have a brushed appearance similar to the appearance of brushed jewelry.

Polishing the restoration with pumice

Pumice is used to remove the small scratches created by the burs (Fig. 35-69). Water is added to the pumice to form a wet slurry and is applied to the tooth with a bristle brush first and then with a rubber cup. The brush and cup are adapted to all areas of the occlusal surface, and the cup is adapted to the interproximal areas as described in Chapter 26. The brush and especially the cup create heat that can damage and weaken the amalgam and can damage the pulp of the tooth by the heat being conducted through the amalgam to the tooth. Obviously, the clinician must use a wet slurry of pumice and short, intermittent strokes to avoid damaging the tooth and/or restoration. The interproximal area is polished with pumice and dental tape. At the completion of this step, the amalgam should still have a brushed appearance similar to the appearance of brushed jewelry, but scratches from the bur should not be visible. The importance of this stage is usually overlooked by beginning clinicians. The pumice and brush should be used thoroughly, then the pumice and cup, and finally the pumice and dental tape. At the end of this stage the area should be thoroughly rinsed.

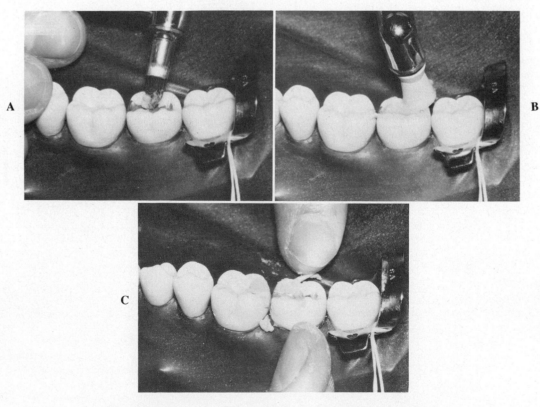

Fig. 35-69. Pumice being used with, **A,** brush, **B,** rubber cup, and, **C,** tape.

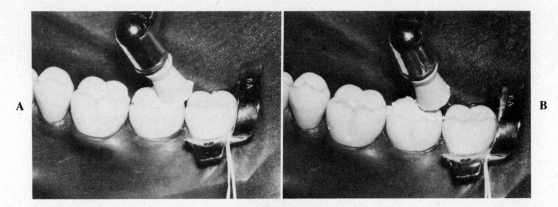

Fig. 35-70. **A,** Wet tin oxide with a cup being used and, **B,** dry tin oxide with a cup to achieve a shiny surface.

Polishing with tin oxide

A clean rubber cup is used with wet tin oxide and they dry tin oxide to polish the amalgam to achieve a shiny surface (Fig. 35-70). The cup and wet tin oxide are used first with short, intermittent strokes to reduce the amount of heat produced. The heat causes the mercury to rise to the surface and makes the restoration appear shiny. If the amalgam is overheated during this procedure, the mercury will rise to the surface and appear shiny initially but become cloudy later. If the amalgam is overheated, the pulp may be damaged. Wet tin oxide is also used with tape to polish the interproximal area to a high shine.

Dry tin oxide and a cup are used to create the final shine. *Extremely quick, intermittent* strokes are used during the procedure. If the clinician is working with an assistant, the assistant can direct a stream of cool air on the tooth while the pumice and tin oxide are being used.

The amalgam polish should be evaluated by both the clinician and the supervising dentist according to the criteria on p. 646.

Alternative procedures

Polishing can be achieved with the use of *chemically impregnated cups* and *points;* Brownie, Greenie, and Super-greenie (Shofu Co.) cups and points are used. The cups are adapted to the occlusal and interproximal areas, and the points are used on the occlusal areas. These cups and points are convenient and less messy than pumice, silex, and tin oxide, but they are more expensive. They can be used for a few restorations but wear down as they are used. The cups and points are formed onto a metal rod, so as they wear, the rod can become exposed and gouge the restoration. The clinician should watch for wear and change the cup or point in a timely fashion. The use of impregnated cups and points seems to provide a polished amalgam equal to one polished in the conventional manner (Reavis-Scruggs, 1982) (Fig. 35-71).

Finishing and polishing *Class I, III, and V* amalgam restorations is essentially the same, but modifications are made to accommodate the differences in anatomy. The Class I restoration is finished and polished in the same manner as the occlusal surface of the Class II restoration. The Class III amalgam is done like the Class II restoration, except it is the lingual surface that is done after the proximal one. The Class V restoration requires a little more modification. The green and white stones are used as needed, and a large round bur can be used to smooth the margins. A disk is used to further shape and smooth the restoration, followed by one of the polishing sequences (Fig. 35-72).

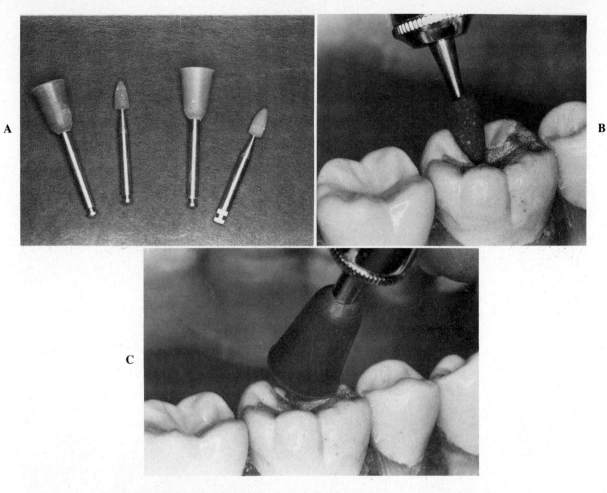

Fig. 35-71. **A,** Greenie and Brownine points and cups. **B,** Point and, **C,** cup adapted to tooth.

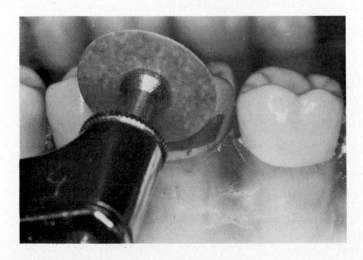

Fig. 35-72. Disk adapted to class V restoration.

Rubber dam placement and removal

Suggested check-off sheet

Mark **S** for satisfactory completion or **U** for unsatisfactory completion of each criterion in the appropriate space.

PERFORMANCE CRITERIA: Does the student

	FACULTY	STUDENT
1. Assemble the necessary armamentarium	___	___
2. Place the clamp properly		
a. Floss applied	___	___
b. All four prongs contacting tooth	___	___
c. Clamp stable	___	___
d. Clamp centered on tooth	___	___
e. Clamp does not impinge on gingiva	___	___
3. Properly punch the dam		
a. Correct number of holes	___	___
b. Position of holes modified for patient	___	___
4. Place the dam properly		
a. Dam stretched over clamp first	___	___
b. Most anterior tooth isolated and ligated	___	___
c. Frame placed	___	___
d. Dam carried through contact areas with tape	___	___
e. Frame readjusted	___	___
f. Clamp ligature pulled to outer surface	___	___
g. Dam tucked into sulcus around each tooth	___	___
h. Area rinsed and suctioned	___	___
5. Remove the dam properly		
a. Ligature on most anterior tooth cut	___	___
b. Interdental areas of dam pulled buccally and cut	___	___
c. Lingual portion of dam freed interdentally	___	___
d. Buccal portion of dam freed interdentally	___	___
e. Clamp ligature held and clamp, dam, and frame removed	___	___
f. Patient's mouth rinsed and suctioned	___	___
g. Dam and patient's mouth checked for rubber dam debris	___	___

Tofflemire matrix retainer and band placement and removal

Suggested check-off sheet

Mark **S** for satisfactory completion or **U** for unsatisfactory completion of each criterion in the appropriate space.

PERFORMANCE CRITERIA: Does the student	FACULTY	STUDENT
1. Assemble the necessary armamentarium		
2. Place the band in the retainer properly		
a. Occlusal opening of band faces curved portion of prongs		
b. Band held securely in retainer		
3. Place the band on the tooth properly		
a. Retainer on facial surface with knobs extending anteriorly		
b. Gingival portion of band around cervical area of tooth		
c. Retainer centered on buccal surface of tooth		
d. Band 1 to 2 mm above occlusal surface		
e. Band 1 to 2 mm below gingival margin		
f. Contact area burnished into band		
4. Place the wedge properly		
a. Inserted from lingual aspect		
b. Base of wedge placed against gingiva		
c. Wedge not extending into preparation		
d. Band held against tooth tightly		
5. Remove the retainer, band, and wedge properly		
a. Retainer removed		
b. Wedge removed		
c. Band removed from unrestored area		
d. Band removed from restored area from lingual to buccal aspect		
e. Restoration undamaged		

Zinc oxide–eugenol temporary restoration placement in a Class II preparation

---

Suggested check-off sheet

Mark **S** for satisfactory completion or **U** for unsatisfactory completion of each criterion in the appropriate space.

PERFORMANCE CRITERIA: Does the student	FACULTY	STUDENT
1. Assemble the necessary armamentarium		
2. Mix zinc oxide–eugenol to the proper consistency (according to the manufacturer's directions)		
3. Properly place the zinc oxide–eugenol restoration		
a. Zinc oxide–eugenol wiped into preparation		
b. Zinc oxide–eugenol packed into interproximal area and then into rest of preparation		
c. Preparation overfilled		
d. Excess zinc oxide–eugenol removed from matrix band with an explorer		
e. Matrix band removed		
4. Properly carve the zinc oxide–eugenol restoration		
a. Interproximal area carved with Hollenback carver		
b. Height of marginal ridge established with round end of large cleoid-discoid carver		
c. Margins cleared with Hollenback or pointed end of small cleoid-discoid carver		
d. Functional anatomy reproduced with Hollenback or cleoid-discoid carver		
e. Occlusion checked and carved as needed		
f. All margins sealed and flush		
g. Contact with adjacent tooth present		

Amalgam overhang removal (margination)

Suggested check-off sheet

Mark **S** for satisfactory completion or **U** for unsatisfactory completion of each criterion in the appropriate space.

PERFORMANCE CRITERIA: Does the student   FACULTY | STUDENT

1. Assemble the necessary armamentarium
2. Assess the overhang
3. Observe the order of instrumentation
   a. Amalgam knife
   b. Large files (e.g., Orban)
   c. Medium files (e.g., Hirshfeld)
   d. Fine file (e.g., Rhein No. 31/32)
   e. Universal curette
   f. Disks
   g. Finishing strips
   h. Dental tape with pumice
   i. Dental tape
4. Remove the overhang properly
   a. Area thoroughly lavaged
   b. Margins flush
   c. Amalgam smooth
   d. Contact present with adjacent tooth
   e. Interproximal contour of tooth reproduced
   f. Adjacent hard and soft tissues undamaged

Amalgam finishing and polishing

Suggested check-off sheet

Mark **S** for satisfactory completion or **U** for unsatisfactory completion of each criterion in the appropriate space.

PERFORMANCE CRITERIA: Does the student

	FACULTY	STUDENT
1. Assemble the necessary armamentarium		
2. Assess the amalgam		
3. Check the occlusion and make necessary modifications		
4. Isolate teeth		
5. Observe the order of instrumentation		
a. Disks		
b. Finishing strips		
c. Pear-shaped bur		
d. Bud- or flame-shaped bur		
e. Round bur		
f. Pumice with brush		
g. Pumice with rubber cup		
h. Pumice with floss or tape		
i. Wet tin oxide with rubber cup		
j. Wet tin oxide with floss or tape		
k. Dry tin oxide with rubber cup		
6. Finish and polish the amalgam restoration		
a. Lavage area after each abrasive		
b. Reproduce original contours of tooth		
c. All margins flush		
d. Amalgam smooth and shiny		
e. Remove dam and recheck occlusion		
f. Adjacent hard and soft tissues undamaged		

ACTIVITIES

1. Investigate the laws of the state to determine if dental hygienists are permitted to perform expanded duty procedures in the state.
2. Conduct a panel discussion with dentists, hygienists, assistants, and technicians on the topic, "Changing Roles of the Dental Auxiliary."
3. Conduct a survey of local dental hygienists to discover whether or not the hygienists would like their responsibilities to be expanded into the area of restorative dentistry. Conduct a similar survey on the role of dental assistants.
4. Perform as many of the restorative procedures as possible on typodonts and for patients.
5. Prepare a table clinic on alternative techniques for performing any of the restorative procedures.
6. Review the results of the Forsyth, Howard, Kentucky, and Iowa experimental programs using dental hygienists for restorative expanded functions.

REVIEW QUESTIONS

1. Briefly state the rationale for each of the following restorative procedures:
   a. Rubber dam
   b. Matrix band
   c. Temporary
   d. Overhang removal
   e. Amalgam polishing
2. State at least two contraindications to a margination procedure.
3. List the order of instrumentation for an amalgam finishing and polishing procedure.
4. Explain an overhang removal procedure to a patient.
5. State at least two conditions that would render a temporary restoration unacceptable.
6. Why must a contact area be burnished into a matrix band?

REFERENCES

Abrams, H., et al. 1978. Gingival sequela from a retained piece of rubber dam: report of a case. J. Ky. Dent. Assoc. **30:**21.

Abrams, R.A., et al. 1982. Dr. Sanford C. Barnum and the invention of the rubber dam. Gen. Dent. **30:**320.

ADA Council on Dental Materials, Instruments and Equipment and Council on Dental Therapeutics. 1983. J. Am. Dent. Assoc. **106:**519.

Axelsson, P. 1981. Concept and practice of plaque control. Pediatr. Dent. (Special Issue) **3:**101.

Ayers, W., Chin, M.M., and Johnson, C. 1977. Amalgam restoration. Seattle: University of Washington.

Berry, T.G., Spohn, E.E., and Halowski, W. 1975. Expanded duties. Lexington: University of Kentucky.

Charbeneau, G.T. 1964. An appraisal of finishing and polishing procedures for dental amalgam. J. Mich. State Dent. Assoc. **46:**135.

Charbeneau, G.T. 1965. Polishing amalgam restorations. J. Mich. State Dent. Assoc. **47:**320.

Charbeneau, G.T., et al. 1975. Principles and practice of operative dentistry. Philadelphia: Lea & Febiger.

Chasteen, J.E. 1978. Four-handed dentistry in clinical practice. St. Louis: The C.V. Mosby Co.

Cooley, R.L., et al. 1978. Heat generation during polishing of restorations. Quintessence Int. **9:**77.

Cooley, R.L. et al. 1982. Sterilization and disinfection of dental burs. Gen. Dent. **30:**508.

Corpron, R.E., et al. 1982. A clinical evaluation of polishing amalgams immediately after insertion: 18 month results. Pediatr. Dent. **4:**98.

Coxhead, L.J., et al. 1978. Amalgam overhangs—a radiographic study. N.Z. Dent. J. **74:**145.

Craig, R.G., editor. 1980. Restorative dental materials, ed. 6. St. Louis: The C.V. Mosby Co.

Craig, R.G., O'Brien, W.J., and Powers, J.M. 1983. Dental materials: properties and manipulation, ed. 3. St. Louis: The C.V. Mosby Co.

Creaven, P.J., et al. 1980. Surface roughness of two dental amalgams after various polishing techniques. J. Prosthet. Dent. **43:**289.

Cunningham, J. 1977. Finishing amalgam restorations: a comparison of techniques. Br. Dent. J. **142:**9.

Cunningham, P., et al. 1969. Control of the operating field by use of the rubber dam. Buffalo: State University of New York at Buffalo.

Dodson, L. 1976. Rubber dam. Seattle: University of Washington.

Eames, W.B., et al. 1966. Thermal response of amalgam to polishing instruments. J. Am. Dent. Assoc. **73:**111.

Gelsky, S.C. 1982. Overhanging amalgam restorations: their prevalence, ramifications, and irradication. Can. Dent. Hyg. **16:**19.

Gilmore, W.H., et al. 1982. Operative dentistry, ed. 4. St. Louis: The C.V. Mosby Co.

Gorzo, I., et al. 1979. Amalgam restorations, plaque removal, and periodontal health. J. Clin. Periodontol. **6:**98.

Greener, E.H. 1979. Amalgam—yesterday, today, and tomorrow. Oper. Dent. **4:**24.

Gullo, C.A., and Powell, R.N. 1979. The effect of placement of cervical margins of class II amalgam restorations on plaque accumulation and gingival health. J. Oral Rehabil. **6:**317.

Hakkarainen, K., and Ainamo, J. 1980. Influence of overhanging posterior tooth restorations on alveolar bone height in adults. J. Clin. Periodontol. **7:**114.

Highfield, J.E., and Powell, R.N. 1978. Effects of removal of posterior overhanging metallic margins of restorations upon the periodontal tissues. J. Clin. Periodontol. **5:**169.

Hobbs, E. 1976. Amalgam polish. Seattle: University of Washington.

Howard, W.W., and Moller, R.C. 1981. Atlas of operative dentistry, ed. 3. St. Louis: The C.V. Mosby Co.

Ireland, L. March 1962. The rubber dam: its advantages and application. Tex. Dent. J., p. 4.

Jeffcoat, M.K., et al. 1980. Alveolar bone destruction due to overhanging amalgams in periodontal disease. J. Periodontol. **51:**599.

Langslet, J. 1976. Margination—rationale and technique. Seattle: University of Washington.

Leon, A.R. 1977. The periodontium and restorative procedures: a critical review. J. Oral Rehabil. **4**:105.

Marshall, G.W., Jr., et al. 1980. Copper-rich and conventional amalgam restorations after clinical use. J. Am. Dent. Assoc. **100**:43.

Morgan, J. 1976. Matrix and wedge. Seattle: University of Washington.

Muhler, S. 1979. Amalgam polish module. Philadelphia: University of Pennsylvania.

Nevins, M. 1982. Interproximal periodontal disease—the embrasure as an etiologic factor. Int. J. Periodont. Restor. Dent. **2**:8.

Nitkin, D.A. 1979. Placing and polishing amalgam in one visit. Quintessence Int. **10**:23.

Reavis-Scruggs, R. 1982. Comparing amalgam finishing techniques by scanning electron microscopy. Dent. Hyg. **56**(9):30.

Restoration of cavity preparation with amalgam and tooth-colored materials. 1974. Washington, D.C.: U.S. Department of Health, Education, and Welfare.

Rodriguez-Ferrer, H.J., et al. 1980. Effect of gingival health of removing overhanging margins of interproximal subgingival amalgam restorations. J. Clin. Periodontol. **7**:457.

Rogo, E.S. 1983. Personal communication.

Schemlitzer, L.D., et al. 1982. A six month clinical evaluation of polishing techniques on the marginal integrity of a high copper alloy. J. Ind. Dent. Assoc. **61**:17.

Simon, W.J. 1978. Amalgam polishing by auxiliaries—a preventive measure. Dent. Surv. **54**(11):16.

Solow, R.A. 1981. Standard sequence for carving and finishing amalgam restorations. J. Prosthet. Dent. **46**:519.

Than, A., et al. 1982. Relationship between restorations and the level of the periodontal attachment. J. Clin. Periodontol. **9**:193.

Vale, J.D., and Caffesse, R.G. 1979. Removal of amalgam overhangs. J. Periodontol. **50**:245.

Weed-Fonner, L. 1981. Amalgam restoration: removing overhangs. RDH, **1**(5):32. (a)

Weed-Fonner, L. 1981. Amalgam restoration: removing overhangs. RDH, **1**(6):16. (b)

Woerth, J.K. 1981. Techniques for finishing and polishing amalgam restorations. Dent. Hyg. **55**(9):31.

PART FIVE

EVALUATION

Chapters 36 to 38 address the need to *evaluate* the success, or at least the outcomes, of practice. Success is defined as the success of therapy (in terms of both short- and long-term goals) for the individual patient considered and also as the relative success that the health care provider experiences as a result of his/her participation as a dental professional.

Evaluation is discussed as the final stage of the project development cycle, but since it is a cycle and since it almost always prompts ideas for change, evaluation may blend in with a new phase of assessment and its subsequent phases. Evaluation then becomes not the end but the beginning.

36 CASE DOCUMENTATION

OBJECTIVES: *The reader will be able to*

1. Discuss the value of case documentation in relation to record keeping.
2. Identify several ways case documentation can be used as an educational resource.
3. List the components of a case documentation.
4. Present a case documentation, using either a written or verbal format.

Case documentation refers to a thorough record of the patient's dental therapy. This record is both visual and written. The visual record is composed of intraoral photographs, radiographs, and study models. The written information includes examination notes, diagnostic chartings, and recordings of treatment. A documentation is comprehensive in that it is composed of initial assessment data, the treatment goals and plan, details of actual treatment, a record of the treatment outcome, and an evaluative summary of the therapy.

A lengthy record of each patient or each phase of care may not always be necessary. However, some patients with particular needs are well suited for case documentation. Patients who require extensive reconstruction therapy that includes home care instruction, initial hygiene periodontal preparation, and major restorative and periodontal procedures are candidates for documentation. With such cases, care is delivered in phases over an extended period of time. Thorough records of each phase that reflect the actual therapy are important for following care to completion. Occasionally a patient may expect an outcome that cannot be achieved. Records that document the steps of therapy may help the patient or other professionals evaluate the appropriateness of care.

Another patient may need to realize that even with impeccable home care procedures, fibrotic tissue from chronic inflammation will not change over several months. By documenting the condition, the decision for a minor surgical procedure can be made with the patient. A patient with a condition such as acute necrotizing ulcerative gingivitis, for which dental therapy will dramatically reduce the gingival conditions, is another type of case well suited for documentation.

A documentation of treatment enhances the accuracy of the patient's record. In retrospect, information on specific patient conditions and treatment procedures often lacks pertinent details.

In addition to improving record keeping, case documentation has several educational benefits.

For the clinician, the components of a documentation allow practice in almost all skill areas. Putting-it-all-together in such a way is helpful for the clinician (especially a student) in appreciating and evaluating total care for the patient.

For the patient, involvement in the case documentation creates a particular commitment to the goals of the treatment. The patient is motivated by participating in the data collection and seeing the results of therapy. At the completion of care, the patient takes pride in his/her role in the therapy and wants to maintain the successful outcome.

For colleagues and other patients, a documentation can be presented as an example from which to learn. Documentation of the success (or failure) of a particular treatment plan or mode of therapy is helpful to other clinicians. The comparison of actual cases is an excellent format for discussion and professional sharing.

For the lay person, the prospect of a significant amount of dentistry may be overwhelming. Examples of completed cases may be helpful in proposing or convincing a patient of the need for specific therapy. Seeing examples of the course of care for patients with similar problems may be reassuring to the patient anticipating similar therapy.

Showing patients the successful results of prevention-oriented dental therapy is one of the best motivators for preventive home care methods (Figs. 36-1 to 36-4).

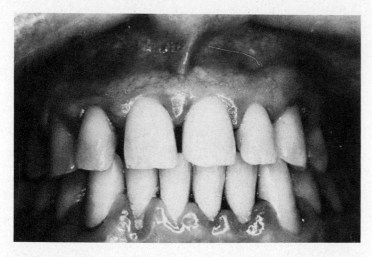

Fig. 36-1. Initial photograph. This 40-year-old man had multiple periodontal abscesses, one of which is clearly seen in mandibular right cuspid area. There are no systemic etiologic factors. Tissue bleeds readily and is swollen and edematous. Papillae are separated from lingual soft tissue. Maxillary and mandibular incisors are mobile, diastemas are present, and there is fremitus of anterior teeth in excursive movements. (From Corn, H., and Marks, M. 1978. Continuing Dental Education, University of Pennsylvania School of Dental Medicine **1:** No. 10.)

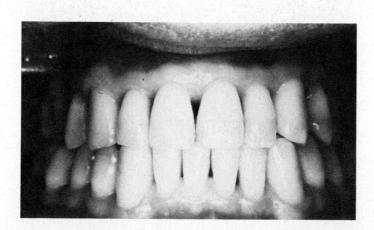

Fig. 36-2. This 12-year result clearly shows that reinforcement of plaque control procedures along with secondary preventive dentistry therapy has enabled patient to achieve this aesthetic result. Sequence of treatment was (1) successful completion of plaque control program and its reinforcement, (2) root scaling and root planing, (3) soft tissue curettage, (4) occlusal adjustment in centric relation, (5) minor tooth movement to retract maxillary anterior teeth, and (6) occlusal adjustment to gain group function in excursive movements and eliminate fremitus patterns. Result shows how stability of tooth position as well as a healthy gingival attachment can be achieved once dental disease has been arrested. (From Corn, H., and Marks, M. 1978. Continuing Dental Education, University of Pennsylvania School of Dental Medicine **1:** No. 10.)

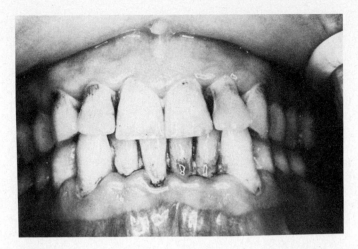

Fig. 36-3. This 50-year-old man had never been to a dentist and had no understanding of the benefits of preventive dentistry care. His treatment consisted of initial therapy and restoration of carious areas. (From Corn, H., and Marks, M. 1978. Continuing Dental Education, University of Pennsylvania School of Dental Medicine **1:** No. 10.)

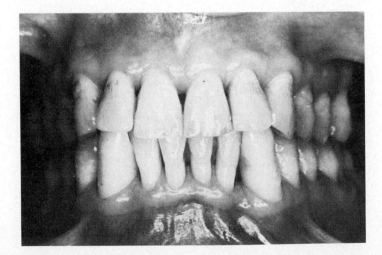

Fig. 36-4. Results of root scaling and root planing along with extensive soft tissue curettage have provided this 14-year postoperative result. It is important to ensure that patients not be discouraged at the initial examination, since it is likely that they are unaware of the benefits that preventive dentistry can provide. Secondary preventive procedures enabled this man to have renewed pride and enthusiasm for aesthetics that were achieved during periodontal therapy. (From Corn, H., and Marks, M. 1978. Continuing Dental Education, University of Pennsylvania School of Dental Medicine **1:** No. 10.)

DOCUMENTATION PROCEDURES

There is no doubt that documentation of care is time consuming. As a clinician approaches case documentation, the key word is *organization*.

The components of a case documentation are:
1. Review of the comprehensive health history
2. Initial clinical findings (intraoral and extraoral examination)
3. Chartings (periodontal survey, and indices—gingival, plaque, bleeding)
4. Radiographs
5. Diagnostic study casts
6. Photographs
7. Treatment considerations (goals, treatment plan)
8. Record of treatment
9. Posttreatment findings (review components 2 to 6)
10. Evaluation summary

The consistent quality of diagnostic aids is important. Periodontal records, radiographs, study models, and photographs are necessary to show changes in the patient's tissues as therapy progresses. Instruction for each of these procedures is given in earlier chapters.

Documentation involves making detailed notes of the dental appointment.

Sample chart note: 2/6/85—Prophylaxis with fluoride

A recording as general as this tells us very little about what actually occurred. A record entry noting the plaque index, results of a periodontal screening, indications of trouble spots in the dentition, the preventive education, the patient's response to care, the care rendered, and plans for future therapy documents the content of the appointment more specifically. Three months from the date of the appointment, the detailed chart notes will facilitate patient follow-up.

Documentation procedures are completed initially, during treatment, and after treatment. Prior planning with particular attention to the time needed to complete necessary documentation procedures is recommended to avoid frustration during each appointment or frustration with the results of poor documentation.

PRESENTION OF CASE DOCUMENTATION

The format for a case documentation presentation can be either written or verbal. A verbal presentation of case documentation is most common. One format for presentation is described; however, many formats are acceptable. The prospective audience, the facilities for presentation, and the purpose for the presentation will play a large part in determining the most appropriate format.

Patient assessment

Introduce the patient profile. Provide a summary of the health history, stating the chief complaint and the history of the present condition. Summarize the clinical findings and present pertinent information from the intraoral and extraoral examination. Show the initial intraoral photographs (slides), study casts, periodontal charting, indices, and radiographs. Describe the dental health education assessment. Use an order of presentation that emphasizes the important aspects of the individual case.

When extensive information is to be presented, a handout to complement the verbal presentation is helpful. The audience is able to take notes during the presentation so that important aspects of the presentation can be reviewed at a later time.

Patient planning

At this point, general concerns about the patient and reasons for selecting the case for documentation may be presented. State the goals of the treatment, and outline the proposed treatment schedule.

Implementation phase

Describe the treatment actually rendered at each appointment. Provide photographs and other indicators of ongoing care, such as periodontal indices. These aids support the treatment being described and allow the audience to follow the healing and restorative process.

Detailed slides of particular instrumentation procedures are excellent for educational purposes. A series illustrating ultrasonic scaling or soft tissue curettage procedures may illustrate a particular technique. This allows the presenter to discuss instrument selection, the choice of materials, or the sequence of therapy.

In this phase, implementation of the preventive education plan is presented. In what area was home care instruction given? What motivational appeal was used? How was the patient involved in learning? What positive reactions or roadblocks were encountered?

Treatment plans are often changed. Revisions are easily pointed out as the implementation phase is presented.

Posttreatment evaluation

This portion of the presentation allows for comparison of initial assessment data and follow-up data. Present the follow-up series of intraoral photographs, periodontal charting, indices, study models, and radiographs (if appropriate). When facilities allow, showing before and after slides simultaneously on two screens is effective.

Discuss or summarize the outcome in relation to the stated goals. If the outcome was not as anticipated, present the factors that may have influenced this. Alternative approaches to care may be included in the discussion also.

With the written presentation, the main consideration is organizing and including all the pertinent information. Present the patient with objective comments. Use information as it was found in chartings and as reflected by photographs, models, and radiographs. Detail the posttreatment data to demonstrate the effectiveness of the clinical course.

Judgments and evaluations are appropriate after the objective data are presented. Provide the rationale for therapy, amd summarize the treatment outcome in relation to expected goals.

SAMPLE

Case documentation

PATIENT PROFILE: Ms. Smith is a 23-year-old black woman. She lives in Philadelphia. She originally came to the dental school for pain in the maxillary left area. The patient presented with large occlusal caries in No. 16, which was eventually extracted.

CHIEF COMPLAINT: Ms. Smith came to the dental hygiene clinic because she felt her "gums were in bad shape."

PAST DENTAL HISTORY: The patient was seen by a private dentist about 4 years ago to have her teeth cleaned. She has not been to a dentist since except for the emergency care in which No. 16 was extracted.

MEDICAL HISTORY SUMMARY: Ms. Smith reports having had mumps and chickenpox when she was a child. No residual effects were reported. She had a cyst removed from her left cheek 2 years ago. This did not necessitate entering the hospital, as it was done on an outpatient basis. No complications were reported. The patient has broken her right leg and left arm in sports-related accidents. Both these accidents occurred more than 5 years ago, and the patient has recovered full function in both limbs.

The patient takes no prescribed medications at the current time. She does take a daily multivitamin. The patient does not take aspirin, because it upsets her stomach.

The patient's family history reveals that her father died of heart trouble when he was 82 years old. Her mother is alive and has high blood pressure. She has one sister who is alive and well. The patient is obese and follows a diet and exercise schedule prescribed by her physician. In the past 6 months she has lost 75 pounds.

We wish to thank Deborah Drazek, R.D.H., for permission to publish this case documentation with original photographs and study models. *Continued.*

SAMPLE
Case documentation—cont'd

REVIEW OF SYSTEMS:

HEENT: Wears glasses; recent sore throat

Skin, appendages: Reports her skin becomes dry when she diets

Bones, joints, muscles: Denies any related symptoms

CV: Denies chest pains, palpitations, syncope; blood pressure 130/86

Resp: Reports having bronchial trouble now and then, usually related to sore throats; quit smoking 2 months ago; denies excessive coughing

GI: When patient was taking liquid protein, she experienced gastrointestinal discomfort; no symptoms currently reported

GU: Drinking a great deal of water with the diet; states that this causes more frequent urination

Hemo: Denies excessive bruising or bleeding during extraction

Endo: Denies symptoms related to diabetes, thyroid disorder, and hormone function

CNS: Denies dizziness, restlessness, and hallucinations

CLINICAL FINDINGS:

Extraoral examination: The patient's facial symmetry, lips, TMJ, and larynx were within normal limits. Submandibular and posterior cervical lymph nodes were palpable.

Radiographic findings: Horizontal and vertical bone loss present between all mandibular anterior teeth. Radiographic calculus is apparent, especially on mandibular anterior teeth. Caries was detected on the distal of No. 29.

Intraoral examination: The patient presented with generalized periodontitis, most severe in the mandibular anterior area. The posterior pharyngeal wall appeared inflamed. Tonsils were present and appeared enlarged. Bilateral mandibular tori were present. Calculus was generalized throughout the mouth with the heaviest deposits located on the lower anterior teeth. The gingiva was inflamed and edematous with some suppuration evident in the lower anterior area. Except for the lower anterior section, the tissue was generally scalloped with normal pigmentation. Tooth No. 9 has mesioincisal fracture, and occlusal caries was detected on Nos. 2, 20, and 29 by exploration.

Periodontal examination: To document reduction in periodontal pocket depth, only the chartings of the maxillary left buccal and of the mandibular anterior facial are noted.

	9	10	11	12	13	14	15	16
Maxillary left	423	334	435	625	524	335	424	X

	323	335	544	535	534	533
Mandibular anterior	27	26	25	24	23	22

DENTAL HEALTH EDUCATION:

1. The patient brushed her teeth once a day but did not floss. A random scrubbing method was used for cleaning the teeth and gingiva.
2. Initial bleeding index: 22
3. Initial plaque index: 30 (on a 30-point scale)

INITIAL ASSESSMENT: See Figs. 36-5 to 36-8 for initial assessment.

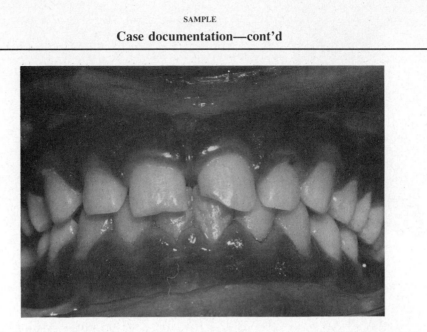

Fig. 36-5. Patient presented with generalized periodontitis more severe in lower anterior area. Gingiva is edematous with suppuration evident.

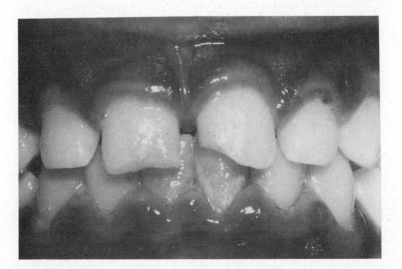

Fig. 36-6. Calculus is generalized but appears heaviest on facial and lingual aspects of mandibular anterior teeth. Several 4 to 5 mm pocket depths were noted on examination.

Continued.

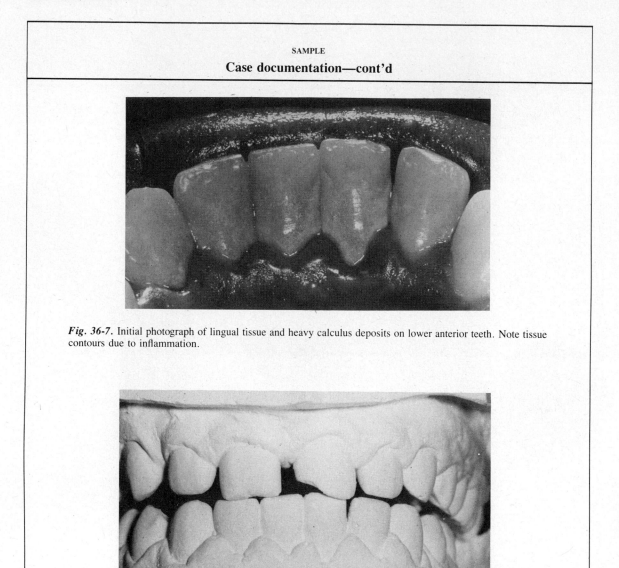

Fig. 36-7. Initial photograph of lingual tissue and heavy calculus deposits on lower anterior teeth. Note tissue contours due to inflammation.

Fig. 36-8. Close-up of initial study models indicates fractured maxillary central incisor and topography of gingival tissue.

Case documentation—cont'd

PLANNING:

Rationale for case selection: Due to the nature of the calculus deposits, the depth of the periodontal pockets, and the patient's willingness to improve her oral conditions, I feel this patient will benefit by participating in documentation procedures. I anticipate that with proper home care instruction and periodontal procedures including ultrasonic scaling, scaling and root planing, and soft tissue curettage, the patient's tissue will respond well.

Goals:

1. Improve the health status of the gingiva, teeth, and supporting ligaments, especially in the lower anterior area.
2. Remove all hard deposits so that the patient can effectively clean her own mouth.
3. Have the patient demonstrate how to correctly brush and floss to effectively remove plaque.
4. Reduce the depth of periodontal pockets.

Initial treatment plan:

Appointment 1: Medical history; intraoral, extraoral examination

Appointment 2: Complete series of radiographs; initial study casts

Appointment 3: Complete periodontal charting; initial series intraoral photographs

Appointment 4: Dental health education: emphasis on brushing technique; perform ultrasonic scaling for the entire mouth

Appointment 5: Dental health education: review brushing skills; emphasis on flossing techniques; complete mandibular scaling and root planing

Appointment 6: Dental health education: review flossing skills; assess for possible periodontal aids; complete maxillary scaling and root planing

Appointment 7: Dental health education: review all home care procedures; complete polishing and fluoride treatment; follow-up intraoral photographs

Appointment 8: Extension if necessary

IMPLEMENTATION: The treatment proceeded as planned. The patient was receptive to documentation procedures. No skill roadblocks were encountered with dental health education. The patient was able to demonstrate adequate skills with a modified sulcular brushing and loop flossing technique. The plaque index decreased steadily. Hygiene procedures were accomplished with a minimum of difficulty. Photographs were taken immediately after the ultrasonic scaling at appointment 4 (Figs. 36-9 and 36-10).

Continued.

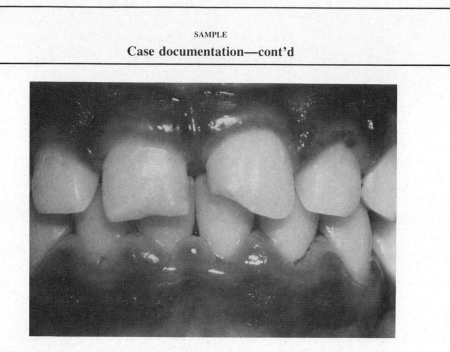

Fig. 36-9. Appointment 4. Following dental health education emphasizing brushing technique, entire mouth was ultrasonically scaled. Facial aspect of mandibular anterior teeth immediately following ultrasonic procedure.

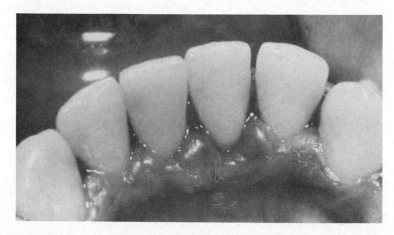

Fig. 36-10. Lingual aspect of mandibular anterior teeth following ultrasonic procedure. Compare with initial photograph, Fig. 36-7.

Case documentation—cont'd

Treatment revisions:

Appointment 7: Observed lower anterior tissues for possible curettage

Appointment 8: Reviewed dental health education and completed soft tissue curettage facial and lingual of Nos. 22 to 27; placed a periodontal pack

Appointment 9: Observed healing of lower anterior tissue; administered maxillary infiltration between Nos. 9 and 10, using approximately one-fourth Carpule (0.5 cc) or 14 mg mepivacaine (Carbocaine) 3% anesthetic solution; placed a composite resin on mesioincisal edge of No. 9

Appointment 10: Dental health education reinforcement; completed follow-up photographs and study models

Appointment 11: Follow-up periodontal charting; discussed recall and further restorative treatment needs

EVALUATION: Ms. Smith was treated in the dental hygiene clinic for a period of 2 months. The follow-up photographs and study models indicate that the tissue in the lower anterior area responded well to deposit removal and soft tissue curettage (Figs. 36-11 to 36-14). The patient can demonstrate an adequate technique for brushing and flossing. She effectively removes plaque and values her newly acquired skills and the appearance of her tissue. Continued home care has been reinforced to maintain this area. The final plaque index was 4, and the final bleeding index was 1. Following are the chartings of pocket depth after treatment in the areas originally noted.

Maxillary left	9	10	11	12	13	14	15	16
	323	333	323	413	313	325	323	X

Mandibular anterior	323	323	223	322	223	332
	27	26	25	24	23	22

The patient and I are pleased that our goals for this phase of treatment have been accomplished. Ms. Smith will continue with restorative treatment and will be seen for periodontal recall in 2 months.

Continued.

SAMPLE
Case documentation—cont'd

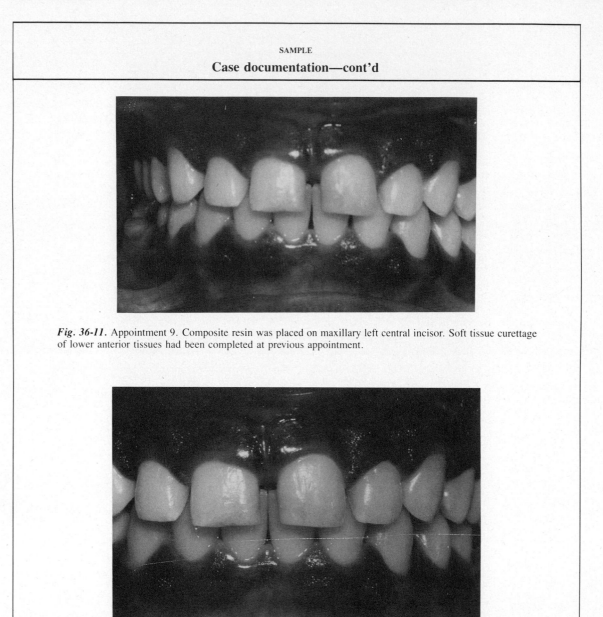

Fig. 36-11. Appointment 9. Composite resin was placed on maxillary left central incisor. Soft tissue curettage of lower anterior tissues had been completed at previous appointment.

Fig. 36-12. Ten days after curettage, healing process in lower anterior area is evident. Deepest pocket depth noted in this area was 3 mm.

Case documentation—cont'd

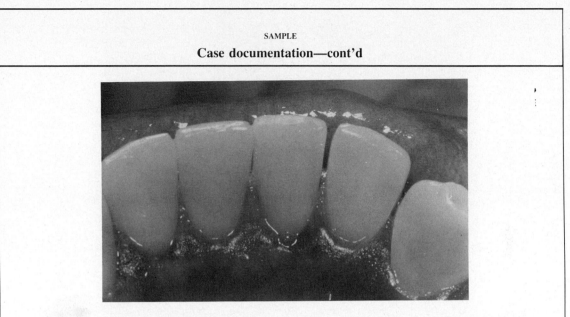

Fig. 36-13. Follow-up photograph of mandibular lingual anterior tissue reveals much improved gingival contour after deposit removal, root planing, and soft tissue curettage. Note papillae edge and stippled texture as compared with that in Fig. 36-7.

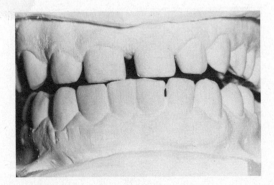

Fig. 36-14. Follow-up study models document healing process that occurred in mandibular anterior region and restoration of maxillary central incisor.

CONCLUSION

Student peers and professional colleagues enjoy learning from case documentations. This situation places the clinician/observer in a position to empathize with the care being delivered. Treatment options may be explored and discussed in an environment conducive to sharing past experiences and new ideas.

The clinician presenting is afforded the opportunity to display an aspect of his/her patient care. Fellow clinicians learn from observing the type and quality of care provided to the patient.

Practicing presenting a case documentation will be valuable experience as the student clinician enters the professional world. Maintaining standards for recording comprehensive quality care will become the responsibility of the clinician. Beyond this, sharing cases with others will be a primary area for professional contact and postgraduate education.

ACKNOWLEDGEMENT

The format for documentation in this chapter represents work developed by the health education, intraoral photography, and clinical faculty of the University of Pennsylvania Department of Dental Hygiene.

ACTIVITIES

1. Listen to case documentations presented by faculty, visiting clinicians, or more advanced students.
2. Create a format for presentation to suit specific clinic needs if necessary.
3. Prepare and present a case documentation.*†
4. According to class size, present documentations in groups of five or six. Select one documentation to be presented to the entire class and/or junior class.*†

REVIEW QUESTIONS

1. List the components of a case documentation.
2. Describe how case documentation:
   a. Enhances record keeping
   b. Can be used in patient education

---

*After the student has completed the necessary instruction on the components of a documentation, identify a patient (one or more) who presents conditions where observable tissue changes will occur. Because of the extent of procedures to be completed and the time required for follow-up, 10 weeks to a full semester may be necessary to complete the documentation.

†Evaluation. A case documentation presentation is designed primarily to demonstrate the effectiveness of performing a particular therapy. Although an aspect of the clinician's techniques and management skills will be inevitably demonstrated, a case documentation is not designed to measure the clinician's overall skills and abilities. Considering the scope of the documentation and the length of treatment, a variety of factors that may be out the the clinician's control may affect the outcome. In our experience, evaluation of the documentation presentation by providing feedback, suggestion, and support has been the most helpful and appropriate mechanism.

37 EVALUATING SUCCESS OF DENTAL HYGIENE CARE

OBJECTIVES: *The reader will be able to*

1. Explain how a philosophy of accountability for professional practice can affect a person's overall approach to providing care.
2. Identify several ways in which a dental hygienist can take account of the effectiveness of his/her professional practice, including:
   a. The degree to which prevention is emphasized in each day's routine
   b. The overall impact on health levels of the population group he/she serves
   c. The degree to which clinical protocols approximate nationally accepted standards
   d. Approach behaviors of patients to dental hygiene care
   e. Personal gratification and health
   f. Cost-effectiveness
3. Integrate mechanisms for personally evaluating the quality and effectiveness of care that he/she provides as a student and as a graduate clinician.
4. Share personal convictions regarding the goals of professional practice, personal goals regarding professional life, and the future outcomes of an "accountable" approach to health care delivery.

In an age of consumerism, consumers of goods and services (in this case, patients) believe they have a right to expect competent, quality care. Health care professions have made several attempts to reconcile their individual and collective responsibilities in assuring high-quality, available care with personal and professional goals that often include a sense of autonomy and authority. Although health professionals see themselves as serving people, the base tenet of *accountability* for care rendered has only recently been perceived as a major part of that service orientation. An increase in malpractice suits against health care providers and the increase in third-party payers during the 1970s in particular have increased the professions' inclinations toward reviewing and adopting systems that document the quality of care being provided.

Covering one's vulnerable areas is certainly one pragmatic reason for adopting a systematic approach to accountability. The prospect of defending one's reputation in court or of being denied reimbursement by a third-party payer for services provided because of suspected poor-quality care is unpleasant.

Emerging from the current debate regarding accountability is, however, a more palatable altruistic rationale for systematically evaluating the quality of care a health professional provides. A personal system that objectively evaluates the impact a person's efforts have in improving the quality of life his/her patients experience over short and long periods of time can add considerable personal gratification and meaning to the daily activities that may at times seem repetitious or even thankless. A sound system of accountability asks the overall questions: Why am I doing what I do? Am I contributing to society and making things better than they would be without me? Is what I do meaningful? How do I know the answers to these questions? Therefore, a system of *quality assurance* can be a means of reflection, of assessing sound data, and of discovering a comprehensive reward in clinical practice.

DEFINING GOALS

At the base of every system of accountability lies a series of goals, statements of what seems to matter in regard to achievement. These goals exist

665

whether or not they are ever written down or expressed aloud. The process of defining and actually writing out these personal goals or values can help clarify what needs to be evaluated to determine success or achievement. An exercise at the conclusion of this chapter provides one way in which these goals can be clarified and delineated for each individual.

Once a series of goals is defined, it is possible to project ways in which their achievement can be measured or at least examined. The following areas of evaluation are suggested for beginning a comprehensive program of self-evaluation.

PREVENTION ORIENTATION

Most of the literature that discusses the relative merits of prevention and treatment in irradicating disease supports prevention as the logical area of emphasis. Health care providers will forever be behind in keeping up with disease unless it can be prevented from occurring. Public health emphasizes prevention on a large scale. Clinical practice can emphasize it on a smaller scale.

If a clinician has established the value that preventing dental disease is a goal for professional practice, then the clinician may wish to document and evaluate the degree to which that orientation is apparent in daily practice. Some relatively simple measures can be recording and assessing the percentage of time spent in helping patients to care for themselves by plaque removal, routinely performing oral cancer self-examination, and adopting nutritional patterns that promote health. How many minutes per hour are spent educating the patient to prevent disease? Is time provided for measuring blood pressure to detect hypertension? Is the medical history updated at each visit? Are patients routinely evaluated for fluoride therapy and sealants?

If the vast percentage of the day is spent removing hard and soft deposits that reappear soon after the recall visit, has the clinician's goal of prevention been actualized or is it a value not yet integrated into behavior?

Impact on health levels

A more long-term measure of disease prevention is to evaluate the pattern of health needs each patient has had while receiving care. If prevention efforts are successful, disease prevalence should decrease in the clinician's patient population. If the primary etiologic factors in dental disease are avoided or controlled by the patient, the incidence of dental caries, periodontal disease, and oral cancer should decrease.

It may be useful to gather and retain the assessment data relative to plaque, gingival, and bleeding indices; calculus formation; caries rate; and any other indicators of health status. Annually a historic overview of the patient's progress in oral health will reveal whether the patient is developing little or no dental disease, showing a steady recurrence of problems, or is on a rapid downhill course to tissue destruction and tooth loss.

This overview can be accomplished at a recall visit when new assessment data are gathered. Sharing the findings with the patient can provide evidence of the effectiveness of the health partnership of clinician and patient. Observing health levels (or at least the absence of signs of disease) rise and remain high over the years provides a long-term evaluation of the quality of a preventive program.

COMPARISONS WITH NATIONAL STANDARDS

Regardless of whether the daily clinical procedures are prevention oriented or directed toward treating active disease to restore health, the health care provider may find it particularly helpful to compare his/her approaches to practice and specific procedures with those published as national standards.

Standards regarding acceptable treatment practices are (1) sometimes published by professional associations, (2) discussed and reported in journals and other professional literature, and (3) presented at professional meetings and continuing education sessions.

A significant form of self-evaluation is to systematically compare clinical protocols used in practice with those that have gained general acceptance. Such an evaluation process challenges one's modes of operation, conceptual base for practice, and belief systems. It also permits the individual to challenge the national standards, and it can stimulate inquiry into improved clinical practice and involve the clinician in research efforts to validate the efficacy of any ''accepted'' procedure.

One method is to join a professional study club or a peer group whose function it is to investigate, test, and validate clinical protocols and assist peers in the group in integrating the agreed-on procedures into their daily practices.

Being recognized as an open, up-to-date, competent clinician among peers can carry great personal reward and satisfaction.

APPROACH BEHAVIORS OF PATIENTS

It is a simple fact that regardless of the strength of a preventive program and the degree to which national protocols are challenged or observed, little overall success can be claimed by a clinician if the patient does not continue to seek care. If patients appear and disappear, there is some indication that the health care provider needs to assess the way patients are viewed in the overall health process. Is the patient a means to an end, whether it be clinical requirements or a reasonable income? Is the patient an object of care? Does the patient feel that the health care provider respects, values, and looks forward to seeing him/her?

If the treatment files show large numbers of long-term patients who have continued to seek care over the years, a relationship has developed that the patients see as helpful and worth maintaining.

The other point of view might be examined also. What are the approach behaviors of the clinician to patients? Does the health care provider have a preconceived notion of what a patient ought to be? Does the health care provider reject patients who do not meet the expected standards of behavior, or does the health care provider see each person as valuable and worthy of care regardless of initial compliance or noncompliance with the criteria for the "ideal" patient?

PERSONAL GRATIFICATION AND HEALTH

An annual physical can be a way of measuring success. If varicose veins; slumped shoulders; chronic headaches; regular use of drugs for indigestion, anxiety, insomnia, or "pep"; fatigue; and hostility are accurate descriptions of the health professional, the "health" professional may need to carefully examine the relationship of clinical practice to these problems. Successful practice should allow time for relaxation, pleasure, exercise, and a broadening understanding of life and the surrounding world, and it should be a source of pleasure rather than a daily drudgery. Physical and mental health reflect the degree to which the day's focus and activities stimulate gratification or anxiety.

The very process of evaluating annually the success of the preventive program, short- and long-term health progress of patients, compliance with accepted standards of practice, and approach behaviors of patients can produce a picture of gratification or dissatisfaction. One bottom line question is: Do the process and outcome of what I am doing with my life bring me gratification? If the answer is yes, the self-evaluation can bring a renewed spirit for the continuation of practice. If the answer is no, the clinician may need to identify what kind of change is necessary.

COST-EFFECTIVENESS

In an economy that is based on competition, one element that is not easily ignored is the evaluation of the cost-effectiveness of practice. Providing the highest quality health care services at a cost that is greater than the income generated from these services guarantees a short-lived practice. The basic costs of a health care facility (rent, insurance, utilities, supplies, salaries, etc.) must be covered by generated income. Therefore a complete evaluation of success should include an analysis of the ledger. A practice that does not break even or generate profit will need professional analysis of its operation and suggestions for change.

Cost-effectiveness implies more than generating sufficient income. Its primary connotation in terms of accountability to the profession and the public is the degree to which the expended health dollar actually improves health. Do patients pay money every 6 months for a slow immersion into advanced periodontal disease or eventual full mouth reconstruction, or does the money they pay ensure the restoration and maintenance of health over the years? The answer to this question brings the health care provider back to the evaluation of prevention effectiveness.

CONCLUSION

Each area of evaluation helps the health care provider assess his/her individual contribution to the quality of life—his/her own as well as that of each patient and thus of society. A well-planned, thoughtful approach to this process may make dental hygiene a truly rewarding career and a source of lifelong fulfillment, or it may be a means for

Defining and evaluating personal and professional goals

Use the following format for recording your response to questions 1 to 7.

Question

1	2	3	4	5	6	7
PROFESSIONAL GOALS:						

PERSONAL GOALS:

1. List each goal that is important for your sense of success (short- and long-term).
2. Rank each goal you have listed according to its relative importance and significance in your determination of success.
3. Give the earliest date you will be able to evaluate your progress toward each goal.
4. How will you know progress has been achieved (what is your measure)?
5. How will you know when each goal has actually been achieved?
6. When do you expect that each goal will be achieved?
7. What roadblocks to achievement of each goal can you identify? How can you reduce them?

planning career changes and personal growth in new areas.

A format that can be used for generating personal and professional goals and for displaying evaluation findings from the year(s) is suggested on pp. 668 and 669.

ACTIVITIES

1. Using the evaluation of success format presented on pp. 668 and 669, define personal and professional practice goals that when achieved or approximated are, in your opinion, signs of success. Then form groups of three to share those goals. Note similarities and differences in goals and values among the members of the small groups. Project ways in which these goals could be evaluated in practice on a regular, periodic basis.

2. Analyze the degree to which prevention-oriented procedures make up the clinical efforts in your daily practice as a student.

3. As a student, conduct a yearlong or a 1-semester system of accountability that measures the extent to which personal and professional goals are approximated or achieved.

REVIEW QUESTIONS

1. How can a philosophy of accountability of professional practice affect one's overall approach to providing care?

2. Identify six ways in which a health professional can measure effectiveness or success in practice.

3. What can a health care provider do if he/she sees little evidence of success or gratification in professional or personal life?

38 INTEGRATING DENTAL HYGIENE PROCEDURES INTO A PRACTICE SETTING

OBJECTIVES: *The reader will be able to*

1. Recognize the need to systematically apply the philosophy and procedures of dental hygiene care to a practice setting.
2. Identify strategies for integrating dental hygiene care into a practice setting in which:
   a. The practice has never had a dental hygienist on the team.
   b. The practice has had a hygienist for many years who has established well-accepted procedures for the practice.
   c. The practice has had a series of dental hygienists over the years who have integrated a variety of different approaches in varying degrees.
3. Set personal priorities for integrating various aspects of dental hygiene care into dental practice.

On graduation from a dental hygiene program, many clinicians seek their first employment in a private practice or group clinic situation. The recent graduate may encounter an ideal situation that allows the dental hygienist to apply the broadest scope of practice in a systematic manner to implement disease prevention and therapy. It is also quite possible that the clinical situation will not be ideal, but rather a shock in comparison with the clinical protocols followed in school. The dental hygienist may decide that the clinical situation needs vast amounts of improvement to meet even baseline needs. Or there may be only a few critical areas that appear to need revision but that seem firmly entrenched as the "accepted" way of doing things within the mainstream of activity. The employer may be receptive to change, but the rest of the dental team may be resistant. The opposite is also possible. Even in situations where everyone seems willing to accept suggestions for change, it may be wise to assess carefully how change should be suggested without disrupting the day-to-day activities of the team and without insulting those members who have functioned under the "unacceptable" protocols for some time.

CLINICAL SITUATIONS

To offer suggestions for addressing these possibilities, three scenarios or monologues are provided for review and discussion.

Although each of the three monologues is fictitious, together they represent the collective experiences and suggestions of dental hygienists who have returned to the educational environment to discuss their successes and their failures, their values and their commitment. A helpful sequel to this chapter may be to invite recent graduates and dental hygienists who have had years of experience, preferably in a variety of practice settings, to discuss what they encountered in dental hygiene practice and to answer questions regarding the implementation of dental hygiene care in dental practice.

Scenario 1: I remember the first weeks of practicing in the office of Dr. J. It felt so good to be out of school and really working in a dental practice as a dental hygienist. Dr. J. had given me a great deal of freedom to schedule my patients so that I could build up speed and ensure that each patient receive high-quality care. Quality was a very big item with Dr. J. I also had a great deal of freedom in selecting instruments, so one of my first official acts was to order eight new sets of scalers

671

and curettes so that I could improve on the few instruments that were left from the previous dental hygienist. The bill for the instruments was quite a shock to both the employer and to me, but Dr. J. seemed more than willing to go along with my suggestions as long as clean teeth and smooth roots could be accomplished.

For the first month Dr. J. checked every tooth surface with an explorer and a probe to find any remaining deposits. It reminded me a great deal of the early days in school, and I found myself praying that my clinical skill had developed sufficiently so that little if anything would be found. There were, of course, a few remaining pieces of calculus or root roughness found now and then, but it soon appeared that I had met the dentist's standards of excellence. Soon the careful checks of each surface were reduced to spot checks and a friendly conversation with the patient about the progress of care. Occasionally the patient was asked directly for his/her opinion as to whether I had done a good job.

The message became clear that the highest priority for this dentist was the clean tooth at the end of the dental hygiene appointment. As my speed picked up, I decided that instead of reducing the time of the dental hygiene appointments, I would begin to integrate other kinds of dental hygiene procedures into this new free time. I decided to polish all the amalgams over a series of recall visits so that eventually all the amalgams would be smooth and less likely to retain plaque and stain. I began to institute a much more thorough plaque control program, since the patients regularly returned with high plaque counts and seemed more willing to have me clean it off than to remove it themselves on a daily basis. I started teaching all the patients the oral cancer self-examination to round out the prevention program in the practice. I even dared to discuss the possibility of some heavy smokers reducing their use of tobacco to reverse some of the beginning signs of tissue change, such as nicotine stomatitis.

It never occured to me that the dentist might not agree that this series of decisions was appropriate or desirable. I had wanted to integrate this new approach as a sort of surprise for the dentist that would make for an even better feeling about my performance. I think what triggered the negative reaction was the complaint of a long-standing patient that he did not have time to sit around and practice flossing in a mirror or feeling the inside of his own cheeks. The patient hadn't seemed hostile during the appointment; I noticed nervousness but thought that was just because it was a new procedure. Anyway, the patient complained to the dentist, who wasn't fully aware of what I was doing. The dentist seemed to join sides with the patient and basically told me to cut out all that frivolous stuff and get back to scaling teeth. The dentist wanted to know whether I was charging the patients for all this ''prevention''; I had to tell the dentist I wasn't

because I hadn't wanted anything to block the patient's acceptance of the procedure.

That decision and my decision to forego discussion of my plans with the dentist were grave errors in this case. The dentist decided I was giving away my time that could be used to clean and plane teeth, which generated income for the office. The dentist also, it turned out, really didn't have much faith in prevention as a reasonable approach to dental disease. The philosophy that emerged in the somewhat heated discussion of how I was spending my time was that dental disease was basically inevitable, that all the dental health education in the world wouldn't reverse that trend, and that the most efficient way to spend time was to clean those teeth every 6 months. The final comment was that the practice could not afford to lose patients such as the one who had complained and that I was to cease and desist from my fancy prevention techniques and get back to basics.

Back to basics it was. My appointment times were reduced to 45 minutes per appointment. I was allowed to bring patients back for additional scaling or other technical procedures, but not for extensive plaque control. There was a lot less agitation in the office with this edict, but somehow I felt as though I had missed an opportunity to integrate some prevention into an otherwise (in my opinion) fine clinical practice by having made some critical mistakes in integrating the changes. The two basic mistakes seemed to be the unilateral decision I made to include those procedures and ignoring the possibility that the patients' and the dentist's philosophies might be quite different from mine. The other contributing factor I had ignored was the financial implications of my decision.

Confronting this same kind of situation, what do you think could have been done differently to make the change more positive? What do you think one can do now to help improve the situation? Would you continue in this practice?

Scenario 2: My first position as a dental hygienist was in a practice in which there had been an entire string of dental hygienists who had stayed for 1 or 2 years and then left. The dentist seemed quite accepting of the fact that no dental hygienist would ever have the commitment to stay and really develop within the dental team. It must have appeared that dental hygienists were born vagabonds who came and left after a short period of time. The dentist just wanted to have a dental hygienist to make sure that the recall program continued. The busy restorative schedule in the practice left no time for the dentist to perform routine prophylaxes.

A highlight of the practice was that I was involved in the initial examination of the patient. The dentist was quite willing to delegate the complete head and neck examination and the preparation of all dental chartings and radiographic series. All new patients were given a full 30-minute initial visit for the preparation of these assessment findings, which did not seem like much at first. As I was able to pick up speed, I realized that the time was ample as long as I was fairly efficient in my procedures. After having talked with some of my classmates who were expected to fit it all into 10 minutes, I began to see how "generous" this time allotment was. I really enjoyed performing the initial procedures as well as completing the recall scaling and polishing.

I had noticed at my interview that there was an autoclave in the laboratory but that only surgical instruments seemed to be prepared for that sterilization method. The tray of blue solution in the dental hygiene operatory was filled with explorers, scalers, and mirrors—a certain indication of the standard protocol for "sterilizing" instruments. I also had failed to see any oxygen supply in the office, and there was no fire extinguisher in the laboratory or anywhere, for that matter. I made a mental note to address these concerns early in my employment.

I had the notion that either I could just start using the autoclave to make my point as to how I wanted to sterilize my instruments or I could discuss the situation with the employer and with the other members of the dental team, especially those who were in charge of operating it for surgical instruments. I suppose in some instances I could have chosen the former option and just gone ahead, but something told me that I should discuss it with the people involved. I think it was the sense of ownership of the laboratory equipment I saw in the eyes of the dental assistant who prepared the instrument trays. This person apparently had never had anything to do with "hygiene instruments," and it appeared that there was a set schedule for using the autoclave.

My decision to discuss it was wise. I swallowed hard and used the cold disinfectant solution for the first morning of my employment there. I kept telling myself that this is the procedure used in many practices, and that I could reduce the number of microorganisms if I used fresh solution, few instruments, and an adequate soak time. I knew I was compromising my principles to use this technique, but I felt in the long run I could avoid many more opportunities for cross-contamination if I was able to reach my goal of using the autoclave for all my patients without alienating the staff. At lunchtime the dental assistant placed a batch of instruments into the autoclave, and we went to lunch. I asked the assistant if the dental hygienists had ever used the autoclave for their instruments. The answer was no. I then asked whether it would cause any problems if I used the autoclave. There was a skeptical look, but the reply was that as long as it didn't interfere with the regular schedule of use for dental instruments, there would be no problem.

We clarified what that schedule was. I made certain it was understood that I would be happy to autoclave my own instruments at other times, and the dental assistant agreed that there would be no major problem.

That afternoon, I continued to use the disinfecting solution, hoping it would be for the last time. I remember carefully questioning each patient regarding a history of hepatitis, as if this one day in my life would be my undoing. At the end of the day, I asked to speak with my employer. Dr. P expressed confidence in my work, which I appreciated, and said half-heartedly that it would be nice if I decided to stay for a while in the practice. Dr. P was surprised when I said that I looked forward to a long working relationship. I felt the beginning of closure in our conversation and decided to ask the big question: "Would you see any problems in my using the autoclave for sterilizing my instruments?" We had a brief discussion about how I would sharpen the instruments after autoclaving, since the sharpening stone would contaminate them again. I suggested the use of an autoclaved stone. Once that was settled, Dr. P frowned a bit and said that she really had no other qualms about using the autoclave for dental hygiene but that she wasn't sure how the dental assistant would respond to having a whole new batch of instruments to run several times per day, and she felt the dental assistant wanted control over the autoclave, since other people using it had seemed to increase the frequency of malfunction. I explained to Dr. P that I had sensed that problem and had discussed it with the dental assistant. I shared with Dr. P the fact that the dental assistant and I had agreed on a schedule and the fact that I could autoclave my own instruments. The next day the new system began, and the tray of blue solution was no longer used. Everything in the dental hygiene operatory could either be autoclaved or was disposable.

Several months later I brought up the issue about the oxygen and the fire extinguisher to the dentist. I felt it was important to move slowly with my suggestions, or the team might feel I was out to criticize and improve rather than to join what was already a solid dental team. The dentist responded fairly well to my suggestion that when funds were available we ought to purchase some emergency equipment—at least an oxygen unit and a fire extinguisher. Action wasn't immediate, but a few weeks later a purchase order for one item was sent in by the dentist. The second item was purchased 2 months later. We even had a session on how to use the equipment and set down some procedures in anticipation of an emergency situation. It seemed to me that I had been quite successful in bringing about meaningful change in the practice.

What I hadn't noticed was that a change had occurred in me as well. When I told Dr. P that I might want to have a long-standing relationship with the practice, I wasn't sure if I was being entirely truthful. Now that I have become a part of the practice and feel comfortable with the people I work with, I have decided that I really do want to remain in clinical practice with this team of people. I guess the proof of this is that I started working in that position 10 years ago, and I'm still there.

What would you have done in this situation?

Scenario 3: I was really lucky to find a practice in which the dentist was young and interested in adding a dental hygienist as the practice grew. I had all kinds of ideas about integrating dental hygiene into a clinical practice and really did not want to have to follow in the footsteps of a dental hygienist who had established all kinds of patterns and expectations over the years that might conflict with my ideas. I was certain that because the dentist was young, there would be great opportunity for innovation, especially in performing expanded functions such as local anesthesia and placement of restorations. I wanted to add myofunctional therapy and conduct a mini–research study of the efficacy of using a behavioral approach to modification of the swallowing habit. Somehow I felt that such therapy often failed because the educational techniques failed, and that this was true for dental health education in general. A small clinical study over many years could provide answers to those questions.

I remember having big plans and being excited about my new position. My first letdown was seeing the operatory in which I was to work. The equipment was ancient. There was an old belt-driven engine that squeaked relentlessly, an old cuspidor, and a bulb syringe and glass of water for irrigating the mouth. There was no high-speed evacuation and no stool to sit on. The comforting factor was that the dental chair had been partially converted from the old style to a lounge-type chair. However, I still had to pump it up with my foot and figure out all the levers for adjusting the back. My first reaction was one of grief and then of anger. The dentist had said he would equip an operatory for me, but I never thought it would be with this kind of equipment. I decided to confront Dr. W with the problem of my expectations versus his. At first, he was a bit defensive, saying he couldn't imagine how such equipment would be a problem. When I discussed how difficult it would be to work without evacuation, without a tri-syringe, and without a stool, he admitted that he simply could not go any deeper into debt to buy modern dental equipment. He wanted to add a dental hygienist to the team but couldn't add the luxury equipment that was necessary for ideal practice. What surprised me the most was how little he seemed to know about the needs of a dental hygienist in providing services for patients. The idea of

a high-speed evacuation system for dental hygiene care was a new one to him. Also, he hadn't seemed to generalize what he had learned about sit-down dentistry to dental hygiene. It seemed as though all the guidelines for efficient, relatively comfortable practice were not applicable to a dental hygienist.

Overcoming that first shock took quite a while. Plus there was the need to set up a reasonable recall system, to order appropriate supplies (sparingly to help balance the budget), to develop a system for appointing patients, and to set down even basic protocols regarding when a dental hygienist becomes involved in dental treatment. The dentist and I spent long hours discussing whether a dental hygienist *could* record the medical history and then we discussed whether a dental hygienist *should* record the medical history, even if the skill was well developed.

Procedure by procedure, we worked out the protocols. I was glad that I had a solid rationale for each of the procedures I was to perform and that I had good skills in performing them. Step by step, we integrated dental hygiene into the practice. It required almost 1 year to accomplish this. The actual procedures were moved into place very slowly. The dentist did not wish to rush into anything, and he was very concerned about the patients' acceptance of a dental hygienist. He personally had never had dental care from a dental hygienist.

Through all of these slow developments, I could see progress, but I couldn't help remembering my dream to use the expanded functions I had learned and to begin my small clinical study of myofunctional therapy.

I first discussed my hopes with the dentist after I had been there for 18 months. He did seem to trust me now. I decided to inquire about beginning the myofunctional therapy study first, since that would be slow to start and since he didn't seem to have much problem with detecting malocclusion and referring patients to orthodontists for care. I described what I wanted to do. The reply was a solid no. His rationale was basically that he didn't trust those kinds of efforts, that he had been taught in school that the only way to modify swallowing habits was with long-term orthodontic treatment, and that even then, the techniques seemed to fail. It became apparent that there was no point in discussing it as an appropriate project. Such an idea was ludicrous to Dr. W.

I returned to traditional practice for another few months and decided to approach the topic of giving my own anesthesia as needed prior to root planing and curettage. So far, the dentist had been performing the pain control procedures at the beginning of appointments where local anesthesia was indicated. I had learned and practiced local anesthesia in school and had received high praise from the dental hygiene faculty, the oral surgery faculty, and from periodontics faculty who had witnessed my technique and who had quizzed me on rationale, anatomy, pharmacology, and complications. I really knew my stuff. Again I tried to approach the topic as a suggestion for modification of my functions in the practice and pointed out to Dr. W that my performing the anesthesia procedure would make scheduling for his patients a good deal easier. He commented that it was really essential that a person who was specially trained be ready to respond to an emergency if local anesthesia procedures should trigger such an event. I pointed out to him that he routinely left patients who had received an injection to be monitored by a dental assistant and that the first few moments following an injection are those during which an untoward response such as a toxic or allergic reaction is most likely to occur. I told him about my background and my abilities and suggested that I would certainly be as able as the dental assistant to monitor signs and symptoms and that I had had a full course in emergency procedures, including CPR. My defense was offensive. There was no further discussion.

I retreated to traditional dental hygiene procedures. Fortunately, there was a great deal of diversity among the procedures I could perform, and I derived satisfaction from the manner in which I had been able to integrate so much into a practice, even if it had taken months and months to do so.

Based on the two previous reactions to my requests, I was, of course, hesitant to ask about restorative procedures. I wanted to be able to place the rubber dam and the matrix, place temporary restorations as needed, and place and carve amalgam and tooth-colored restorations. The dental practice was building, and the appointment book was filled for 3 weeks in advance. The practice was making a better income, and I was rewarded with new equipment for my operatory. I was asked to select the kind I wanted from three basic designs. Still, somehow I still wanted to be able to practice expanded functions. I kept thinking that if I could add restorative functions to my list of procedures, perhaps local anesthesia could be added eventually. When I inquired, I was informed that the dental assistant would be the one to perform those skills if the dentist ever decided to delegate them. Dr. W. did not feel it was within the scope of practice of the dental hygienist to become involved in restorative procedures. He felt it was imperative that the dental hygienist perform preventive procedures as was originally intended for the dental hygienist.

I am still practicing traditional dental hygiene in an efficient, well-designed, modern clinical practice in which dental hygiene procedures as they have been de-

fined for decades are valued and fully integrated into daily routines. I know I will probably never have the freedom to do the things I had hoped to do in research projects and with anesthesia and restorative procedures. If that day ever does arrive, it will have been so long since I used those skills that I will probably not be able to prove my ability. I have to make a decision regarding whether I should stay or try to find a position in which I can do what I really want to do. I keep remembering what my boss said regarding the matter of local anesthesia: "If you really want to do all these things, why don't you go to dental school?"

ACTIVITIES

1. Discuss each of the scenarios, analyzing the choice of actions the dental hygienist had in each of the situations and the appropriateness of the action selected. Focus on the likely outcomes of alternative choices of action. Place yourself in the position of the dentist in each case, and project how the dentist may be seeing the actions and attitudes of the dental hygienist.

2. Were the dentists in the scenarios male or female? Is it confusing to picture a dentist as a woman? Did you picture the dental hygienists to be women? Which one might have been a male hygienist? Why would you make that assumption? How does sex role bias affect the way we interpret and anticipate behavior, regardless of the professional role?

3. Set personal priorities for what you hope to accomplish and what you expect to find in the "ideal" dental practice. Share those expectations with a small group of classmates. Explain how you will make a choice regarding whether to try to change or to agree to live with less than ideal conditions. Ask others in the group how they would feel if they had a dental practice and you were to implement the approaches to change that you feel would work best in solving the less than ideal conditions.

4. Role play a variety of encounters with hypothetical employers and patients regarding attempts to change:
   a. Integration of preventive measures into a practice
   b. Integration of additional assessment procedures into the scope of practice of the dental hygienist
   c. Integration of expanded functions into the scope of practice of the dental hygienist
   d. Procedures regarding sterilization, instrument purchase, office cleanliness, and nonfunctional equipment

SUGGESTED RESPONSES

CHAPTER 1

1. The patient is viewed as a partner in care, involved extensively in decision making and in the self-care components necessary for health.
2. A faculty member has had an opportunity to compare expectations with reality and to develop an educational approach that blends the ideal with the real. Individual faculty members differ according to their clinical, conceptual, and futuristic perceptions of practice.
3. a. Dental practice acts define the scope and limitations of dental practice and dental hygiene practice in each jurisdiction (usually defined by state boundaries). In many instances they differ widely from one another, resulting in significantly different roles and responsibilities for dental hygienists, depending on the jurisdictions in which they reside.
   b. The practice acts often limit programs within their jurisdiction to include only those skills that are legally allowable for practice in that jurisdiction. Thus programs differ widely in the functions and responsibilities they may legally include.
4. Legalization of independent dental hygiene practice would allow entrepreneurial hygienists to open their own practices and perform the full array of legal dental hygiene services learned in dental hygiene school. It would open practice opportunities for hygienists currently unable to find work as employees in solo dental practices, where only 42% of dentists use dental hygiene services. It could perhaps extend dental hygiene, and eventually dental care, to a population group that currently does not seek care because of fear.

CHAPTER 2

1. Should. Turning the light on and off wears out the switch and causes the lamp to burn out more quickly.
2. a. Tilt chair back.
   b. Lower back of chair to supine position.
   c. Adjust headrest.
   d. Raise chair as necessary to proper height.
   e. Rotate chair if necessary.
3. To direct a stream of water; to direct a stream of air; and to spray air and water in an area
4. Become unscrewed and fall off

5. Most traditional dental hygiene functions require slow-speed torque; high speed will be less effective and could be dangerous.
6. The angle needs cleaning to remove abrasive and other foreign elements from the gears.
7. The clinician's feet are flat on the floor and thighs are parallel to the floor. The abdominal rest should fit snugly below the rib cage as the clinician inclines forward.
8. The assistant's eye level is approximately 5 inches above the clinician's eye level and thighs are parallel to the floor.
9. An oil soap to clean and soften the material
10. Ultrasonic cleaner (for removing debris) and autoclave and dry heat oven (for sterilizing)

CHAPTER 3

1. Except for surgeons, few other health professionals come in closer contact with patients for longer periods of time than the dental clinician. The oral cavity is abundant in organisms that are potentially pathogenic. The close physical contact with the patient, the nature of the work performed, and the instruments used all contribute to the clinician's susceptibility to infectious disease. The air, saliva, blood, and aerosols from instrumentation or breathing are potentially dangerous. The clinician must be aware of sources of infection and take precautions to protect himself/herself, the operatory environment, and patients from the spread of infectious organisms.
2. a. *Mycobacterium tuberculosis:* tuberculosis; indirect transmission from inanimate sources or respiratory droplets
   b. *Treponema pallidum:* syphilis; indirect contact, break in skin, or contact with lesion
   c. *Clostridium tetani:* tetanus; airborne transmission by means of dust-carried spores
   d. Respiratory virus (e.g., adenovirus): respiratory tract infection; respiratory droplet, aerosol
   e. Hepatitis B virus: serum hepatitis; oral or fecal route, saliva or respiratory droplets, or direct transmission by means of contact with contaminated blood
   f. Rubeola virus: measles; respiratory secretions, saliva, blood

3. a. True
    b. False
    c. True
    d. False
    e. True
    f. True
    g. True
    h. True
    i. False
    j. True
4. Sanitation: the mechanical and/or chemical cleaning of an object
    Disinfection: the destruction of bacteria and other microorganisms by means of chemicals or heat
    Sterilization: total destruction of all forms of microbial life
5. Start with an initial scrub that includes a thorough lathering of all surfaces using a brush, soap that may or may not contain an antiseptic, and copious amounts of running water; all jewelry should be removed; the initial scrub should be a series of three latherings, each followed by a thorough rinsing; the initial scrub should last 2 to 3 minutes.
6. Steam under pressure, dry heat, ethylene oxide gas, chemical vapor sterilizer, and chemical solutions (glutaraldehyde only)
7. Steam under pressure: 121° C (250° F) at 15 to 20 psi for 15 to 20 minutes
    Dry heat: 160° C (320° F) for a minimum of 1 hour
    Ethylene oxide gas: 49° C (120° F) for 2 to 3 hours *or* room temperature for 12 hours
    Chemical vapor sterilizer: 127° C (260° F) at 20 to 25 psi for 30 minutes
    Chemical solution (glutaraldehyde): room temperature for 6 3/4 to 10 hours, assuming that the chemical concentration is optimal and the instruments have been properly prepared
8. Tri-syringe: Sterilize tips if possible; wipe the unsterilized portion twice with an effective tuberculocidal disinfectant, using two separate gauze sponges.
    Handpiece: Sterilize if possible in the autoclave, chemical vapor sterilizer, or ethylene oxide sterilizer (depending on the manufacturer's instructions); if it cannot be sterilized by an approved method, it must be carefully scrubbed twice with a tuberculocidal disinfectant, using two separate gauze sponges.
9. The clinician should wear a mask under any of the following conditions: he/she has a contagious disease transmitted by saliva or respiratory droplets; the patient has a contagious disease transmitted by saliva or respiratory droplets; and/or he/she is operating or assisting in the use of the high-speed handpiece or ultrasonic scaler, from which there is a high level of aerosol production.

CHAPTER 4

1. The complete dental record is a medicolegal record that provides the information necessary to safely and knowledgeably treat a patient and provides protection for both the patient and the dental health care provider in a court of law.
2. a. Demographic data (name, address, and so on): to include the patient's identifying and emergency information
    b. Medical and dental histories: to identify the patient's past and present needs
    c. Examination findings: to identify the patient's present health status
    d. Treatment performed: to promote continuity of care and to protect the patient and the health care provider in a legal proceeding
    e. Fees charged and paid: as part of legal financial records
    f. Dates of all treatments: to promote continuity of care and to protect the patient and the health care provider in a legal proceeding
    g. Results of treatment: to provide follow-up, especially if the result was unexpected or unusual
    h. Radiographs: to provide a diagnostic aid to chartings, examinations, and tests
    i. Correspondence: to protect the patient and the health care provider in a legal proceeding
3. The primary difference is that the problem-oriented approach includes a problem list that is not included in the treatment-oriented approach.
4. The purpose of a chart audit is to ensure that the health care providers are maintaining complete, thorough, and accurate dental records.
5. A complete format would include the date, subjective findings, objective findings, medications administered, treatment, results, the patient's reactions, whether treatment is complete or incomplete, treatment to be performed at the next appointment, the amount of time before the next appointment, and the signature of the health care provider.

CHAPTER 5

1. To retract tissue, to reflect light, for indirect vision, and for transillumination
2. To detect root irregularities and hard deposits; to measure the depth of the gingival sulcus or periodontal pocket; to trace the topography of the soft tissue attachment to the tooth; and to measure recession, masticatory mucosa, and the size of lesions
3. To explore the teeth for caries; and to explore the teeth for irregularities such as calculus deposits, root roughness, anatomic defects, and margins of restorations
4. a. True
    b. False. If the first 1 to 2 mm is used, detection can

identify the specific location and less soft tissue trauma is likely to occur.
c. True
d. False. The terminal shank should be parallel to the long axis of the tooth.

5. | **Clinician position** | **Patient's head position** |
|---|---|

Right-handed

a. 11 o'clock	Straight
b. 9 o'clock	Away from clinician
c. 9 o'clock	Away from clinician
d. 11 o'clock	Toward clinician
e. 11 o'clock	Toward clinician
f. 9 o'clock	Away from clinician
g. 9 o'clock	Away from clinician

Left-handed

a. 1 o'clock	Straight
b. 3 o'clock	Toward clinician
c. 1 o'clock	Toward clinician
d. 3 o'clock	Away from clinician
e. 3 o'clock	Away from clinician
f. 1 o'clock	Toward clinician
g. 1 o'clock	Toward clinician

CHAPTER 6

1. d. Use of the clinician's fingernail to test instrument sharpness is a violation of acceptable methods of contamination control when used during patient treatment. Any of the other three methods would be preferable to this method.
2. a. False. The Arkansas stone is a natural stone.
   b. True. Cutting edges of good-quality stainless steel instruments are not dulled by steam sterilization (Parkes and Kolstad, 1981—see references for Chapter 6)
   c. False. Only the lower cutting edge of Gracey curettes is used for periodontal procedures. Therefore only that cutting edge should be sharpened.
3. b. The internal angle of 70 to 80 degrees forms a complementary angle with the sharpening stone, which is applied at 100 to 110 degrees.
4. Both the rounded toe and the rounded back of the curette design must be preserved during sharpening procedures.
5. a. Facial surface
6. b. Pressure is applied only to the downstroke to minimize formation of wire edges.

CHAPTER 7

1. If the hygienist ignores the patient's request to have her teeth polished, the patient will probably go elsewhere for the service or try it herself at home with a strong abrasive. If the hygienist is willing to simply polish at the first visit (after at least a medical history), there is a greater likelihood that the patient will return

for further care (as explained by the hygienist) *after* the big event. The mother of the groom wants white teeth now, not sore gums. In some instances in which no harm can result, a patient can be satisfied in this manner, with long-term positive results for both the hygienist and the patient.

2. It is difficult to determine whether the patient is dependent on the dentist, believing that he will retain his teeth as long as he returns periodically for care, or if he does not really care if he keeps his teeth but does not want to experience pain either (thus the necessity of dental visits). The hygienist might do well to point out the string of appointments for restorations and simply ask the patient if he expects to retain his teeth. Mentioning rather objectively that soon the restorative material will hold his teeth together and that soon after that the teeth will begin to give up may make an impression on the patient. Often a follow-up of, "If you decide you really *do* want to keep them, let me know. I think there might be a couple of things you can do to prevent losing them over a period of time," will move the patient to ask for help. The hygienist can always resort to blatant fear tactics to awaken such a patient, but usually they are less effective than a calm inquiry and suggestion. Different degrees of subtlety and different opening lines are appropriate for each person. There is no key phrase that works for all. In any case, the hygienist is unwise to proceed with a speech about flossing and diet. The patient will tune him/her out if possible.

3. Such a statement might imply a great deal of trust in the dental hygienist. It may also imply a dependency relationship in which the patient has transferred responsibility for oral health to the dental hygienist. Rarely do such patients have a thorough program of preventive self-care.

4. a. Excessive familiarity
   b. Professional closeness
   c. Professional closeness (but worthy of discussion)
   d. Professional aloofness

5. There are several possible actions, including refusing to provide care for the patient, having the patient sign a disclaimer for risks resulting from the omitted procedure, or working around the missing procedure until trust is increased and the need for the procedure becomes more apparent to the patient.

6. These are *possible* replies. The key to a *listening* response is that the *content* of the message is rephrased and the *affect* or emotion behind the statement is reflected.
   a. "It sounds like you're worried about what I'm going to see in there."
   b. "You don't feel as comfortable lying down for your dental work."

c. "You sound a little disturbed that you can feel this more than you could with other hygienists."

d. "You sound upset that the dentist has hired someone else to clean your teeth. You think the dentist is the person who should do it."

Each listening response enables the patient to confirm or correct the understanding the hygienist has of the patient's statement. Even more important, it allows the patient to say more, to elaborate on the problem or feeling, and to express wants, needs, or expectations.

7. a. While reassuring, it cuts off a message the patient is trying to give: there is some reason the hygienist will be unhappy. It may be very important for the patient to say it before the hygienist looks in. It also sounds like the patient may feel guilty. The patient may feel he/she is reporting in to the hygienist for judgment. A glib, nonlistening comment shuts off the patient's next statement and any exploring of what is behind the opening comment.

b. This, too, shuts off communication, because the hygienist is presenting a logical argument in favor of reclining chairs. The patient and the hygienist are both right, but the hygienist is actually denying the validity of the patient's statement by presenting his/her own and thus arguing.

c. Problem solving immediately after a comment closes off communication. The hygienist is closing out lots of information that the patient might have revealed if the hygienist had saved problem solving for later.

d. No matter how tempting it may be to lecture, the patient should be listened to *first* so that accurate perceptions are clear. Information to enlighten the misinformed should follow the reflection and listening. The patient then knows the hygienist understands, and he/she is more likely to listen.

CHAPTER 8

1. An appropriate response would be: "I realize this is time consuming, but it is important for us to discuss your general health before I check your teeth. Certain medical conditions and medications a patient may be taking may affect their dental treatment. For example, some patients with specific types of heart problems actually need to take an antibiotic before we treat them to prevent serious complications. The health history is the foundation for your total care. All this information is kept confidential. If some of the questions puzzle you, I'll be happy to explain why they are significant. My concern is that you receive safe and proper treatment. The few minutes we take at this point to get to know you and complete a thorough record are necessary to ensure that 'checking your teeth' stays as simple as it sounds."

2. All of the above (e) is the correct answer.

a. Rheumatic heart disease: Consult the physician to determine if damage to heart valves makes antibiotic premedication necessary.

b. History of myocardial infarction: Consult the physician to obtain a history of the most recent heart attack and to determine the severity of disease. The physician may advise on the patient's tolerance to stress and on the advisability of vasoconstrictors in local anesthetics.

c. Blood pressure reading of 160/100 (hypertension): Consult the physician to determine if medication is required for the patient.

d. Hemophilia: Consult the physician to determine the extent of the bleeding disorder, the need for transfusion before treatment, and other possible contraindications to treatment.

3. Antibiotic premedication is necessary for patients who report a history of (a) rheumatic heart fever with valve damage and/or (b) surgical replacement of a heart valve. Depending on the physician's consultation, the following conditions may also require antibiotic prophylaxis: (a) congenital heart defect repair and (b) pacemaker implant.

4. Communication principles:
Ask direct, but open questions.
Follow a logical order.
Guide, but do not dominate the interview.
Show support and empathy.
Reflect the patient's response to clarify meaning.
Avoid "yes" and "no" questions
Avoid "why" questions.
Use nonverbal signs to encourage patient response.
Ask probing questions concerning the topic at hand.
Close the interview with a summary.

5. As part of the review of a patient's health status, the dental hygienist must be aware of the medication a patient is taking. The *Physicians' Desk Reference* is helpful for identifying medication and providing information on drug composition, action, dosage, precautions, and side effects that may affect dental treatment.

CHAPTER 9

1. To gather assessment data for diagnosis and treatment planning; to provide early detection of disease, thus improving the prognosis for recovery; to detect contraindications to dental treatment; to provide baseline and continuing data of the patient's health status; and to provide descriptions of the patient's health status for use as legal records

2. Pulse, respiration rate, temperature, and blood pressure

3. a. Adult pulse: 60 to 80 beats per minute
b. Adult respiration rate: 14 to 20 breaths per minute

c. Adult temperature: 98.6° F (37° C)

d. Adult blood pressure: 120/80 mm Hg

e. Borderline temperature for fever: 99.6° F

f. Borderline blood pressure for hypertension: 160/95 mm Hg

4. a. Pulse rate: Rest the patient's arm in a comfortable position. Place the index and second fingers on the radial artery found on the thumb side of the wrist. Compress this area gently, and count the beats for 1 minute.

b. Blood pressure: Rest the patient's arm in a comfortable position. Roll up the patient's sleeve. Place the sphygmomanometer on the patient's arm about 1 inch above the bend in the arm. Feel the radial pulse, and inflate the cuff until the pulse is no longer felt. This provides an estimate of the systolic pressure. Release the air in the cuff. Let the patient's circulation return to normal. Inflate the cuff 20 to 30 mm Hg higher than that previously noted. Slowly deflate the cuff. Note the point at which the first sound is heard and the point at which the sound completely disappears. Record the first sound as systolic pressure and the last sound as diastolic pressure. Confirm this recording a second time. Remove the cuff.

5. a. Inspection: a visual examination of each of the structures before they are palpated for signs of abnormal color, texture, or consistency

b. Palpation: feeling or pressing on structures of the body: used for examining most intraoral and some extraoral structures

c. Auscultation: listening for sounds produced within the body: used for examining the temporomandibular joint and larynx

d. Percussion: striking tissues with the fingers or with an instrument to hear the resulting sounds and patient response; not previously described as a method used during the intraoral examination, but often used as a means of assessing pulpal disease in individual teeth

6. a. Submandibular lymph nodes: Standing behind the patient, push the soft tissues from one side of the submandibular area over to the other side; grasp these tissues with the cupped fingers of the hand, and roll tissues over bone of the mandible. Repeat for the other side.

b. Floor of the mouth: Place the fingers of one hand intraorally on the floor of the mouth and the fingers of the other hand extraorally beneath the same area. Use bimanual palpation to examine the entire floor area.

c. Buccal mucosa: Place one hand or several fingers intraorally and the other hand extraorally. Use bimanual palpation to examine the entire area from the labial mucosa back to the retromolar area.

7. To prevent the clinician from touching lesions in the mouth that might be contagious, such as syphilis; to prevent the clinician from contracting diseases transmittable through the bloodstream, such as hepatitis; to identify conditions that would contraindicate dental treatment for the patient's well-being, such as strep throat; and to prevent discomfort of the patient due to palpation of painful lesions such as ulcers

8. a. Auricular chain

b. Cervical chain

c. Occipital chain

d. Submandibular (posterior) and submental (anterior) chains

CHAPTER 10

1. Dental visits are often likely to create anxiety for patients. Patients who have a propensity for syncope (fainting) or other physical responses to anxiety are more likely to respond this way in the dental environment. Also, the drugs used in dentistry, including local anesthetics, may cause an emergency situation. The dental hygienist may be the first person to recognize and respond to the situation.

2. See Table 10-1 for a complete list. Make certain your list includes provision for the most common dental emergencies.

3. All emergency equipment should be readily available and functioning. Drugs maintained in the kit should be up to date. All members of the team should be able to recognize signs of patient distress, and they should be prepared to respond appropriately. Rehearsing the proper procedures for any kind of an emergency can be critically important if quick, responsible action is to occur. Emergencies can be prevented by the use of medical histories and fire and accident prevention devices and by careful monitoring of the patient.

4. a. Move instruments and other dental equipment away from the patient, place the patient in a full supine position (a patient in the late stages of pregnancy should be turned on her side), place a cool cloth on the patient's forehead, alert another team member, prepare an ammonia ampule for wafting under the patient's nose if he/she loses consciousness, and administer oxygen until the patient is recovered.

b. Place the patient in an upright position, send a team member to call for emergency assistance, administer oxygen, place a nitroglycerin tablet under the tongue, monitor vital signs, and begin CPR in the event of cardiac arrest. If the pain is associated with angina, the nitroglycerin will relieve the discomfort. If it is associated with heart failure or myocardial infarction, the pain will persist.

c. Place the patient in a supine position, and check

for vital signs. Begin CPR if breathing and a heart-beat are absent, and have a team member send for emergency assistance. If the patient is breathing and has a heartbeat, waft an ammonia ampule under his/her nose and administer oxygen. Continue monitoring vital signs until the patient is fully recovered. An awareness of the patient's medical history should help determine if there are causes other than syncope that could account for the loss of consciousness, such as hypoglycemia, hyperglycemia, cardiovascular problems, or acute adrenal insufficiency.

CHAPTER 11

1. Legal record of the patient's initial condition and changes in oral status over a period of time; helpful in preparing a treatment plan; useful in cross-checking financial records; and combines radiographic and clinical findings into a comprehensive record for diagnosis
2. a. Anatomic: most precise replica of tooth characteristic
   b. Geometric: stylized version of teeth and findings; usually makes charting neater and easier to read
   c. Numerically coded: provides a complete time line of oral conditions and changes on a single piece of paper

		Universal	Palmer's notation	International	Description
3.	a.	3	6⌋	16	Maxillary right first permanent molar
	b.	28	5⌉	45	Mandibular right second premolar
	c.	16	⌊8	28	Maxillary left third molar
	d.	n	⌈b	72	Mandibular left primary lateral
	e.	13	⌊5	25	Maxillary left second premolar

4. a. A, amalgam
   b. T, temporary
   c. TC, tooth-colored restoration
   d. FGC, full gold crown
   e. GF, gold foil
   f. C, caries
   g. SSC, stainless steel crown
   h. DGO, defective gold onlay
   i. RC, root canal
   j. PAP, periapical disease
5. a. Tooth anomaly: Mark with an asterisk, and describe the condition elsewhere on the page, preceded by the asterisk.
   b. Pontic: Mark the root as missing, fill in the crown with the appropriate restoration, and draw horizontal bars to connect it to the adjacent pontic or abutment.

c. Drifting: Draw a horizontal arrow parallel with and above the occlusal table, pointing in the direction of the drift.
d. Rotation: Begin an arrow on the proximal side of the proximal surface of the tooth that is rotated facially, and arc the arrow across the facial aspect of the tooth to suggest the direction of rotation.
e. Attrition: Draw a horizontal line through the facial view of the teeth to indicate the amount of tooth lost due to mastication.
f. Unerupted teeth: Circle.
g. Calculus: Draw in with a triangle, or include a written statement in the summary.
h. Overhang: Place an *O* in the appropriate box.
6. Retained root tip, unerupted teeth, bone loss, root canal filling, widened periodontol ligament space; loss of continuity of lamina dura, unerupted supernumerary teeth, periapical disease, and other disturbances of the hard tissues

CHAPTER 12

1. A calculus charting procedure assists beginning clinicians in identifying and classifying calculus as tactile sense and dexterity with instruments increase. It assists in developing abilities in differentiating between normal anatomy and calculus deposits. It provides valuable baseline data regarding a patient's oral conditions and is a useful tool in designing a treatment plan for dental hygiene care.
2. a. Ledge: a ring or part of a ring that encircles the tooth, projecting from the tooth toward the gingiva, thus appearing like a ledge. Such deposits are usually located subgingivally, although they may be visible above the margin of the gingiva if the tissue has receded.
   b. Veneer: veneer calculus, a thin sheet of burnished calculus that marks the location of a deposit incompletely removed by either an improperly adapted instrument or a dull instrument. The calculus is usually located subgingivally and is difficult to detect because it has been mechanically smoothed.
   c. Crustaceous: a chalky, white amorphous mass of calculus, usually appearing supragingivally on the lingual aspect of the mandibular anterior teeth and on the facial surfaces of the maxillary molars. It may be afforded some shape by the action of the tongue and the other musculature.
   d. Fingerlike projections: projections of calculus that dip into the pockets formed during the advancement of periodontal disease. They tend to cover large surface areas of the roots and are found almost exclusively subgingivally.
3. Although research continues into the etiology of periodontal disease, it is the general consensus that cal-

culus is a less important factor than plaque in the initiation and progression of periodontal disease. Calculus is usually covered with masses of microorganisms (plaque) that continuously irritate the tissues.

4. a. True
   b. True
   c. False. The outer portion is more porous.
   d. False. There are two: one associated with microorganisms and one that is not.
   e. True

CHAPTER 13

1. Acquired pellicle: a, f, h
   Materia alba: e, g
   Food debris: d, g
   Plaque: a, b, c, i
2. Calcification
3. Acid or low; decalcification of tooth structure or caries
4. a. Days 1 and 2: Microbial composition begins with gram-positive cocci.
   b. Days 3 and 4: Filamentous forms of organisms start to occur and eventually grow into the coccal layer and replace these initial organisms.
   c. Days 6 to 10: A more mixed bacterial flora begins to appear; plaque becomes more gram negative and contains anaerobic organisms.
   d. Days 8 to 10: Plaque weight is essentially maximized.
   e. Days 10 to 21: Inflammation of gingivae begins; plaque is composed of densely packed spirochetes and vibrios.
5. Enzymes (to dissolve the intermatrix substance that binds the bacteria); surface-active agents (to lower the ability of plaque to adhere to the tooth or pellicle); antibiotics (to destroy oral bacteria); antibacterial agents (to lower the number of bacteria; less potent than antibiotics); and flavor oils
6. Plaque thickness measurements, coronal extension of plaque or plaque area scoring systems, and plaque weight
7. Visual signs of inflammation (size, shape, texture, consistency); spontaneous bleeding (when probed or sprayed with compressed air)
8. The routine inclusion of indices in clinical practice provides baseline data for each patient, aids the health care provider in following a patient's progress or regression, and can generate valuable data regarding the overall success of the practice in minimizing or eradicating dental disease. If such data follow unchanging criteria and are performed by one clinician or by clinicians carefully following the same standardized procedures, valid epidemiologic information about the practice's population can be provided. Finally, the indices are valuable tools for patient mo-

tivation in assuming greater personal responsibility for lowering plaque levels and thus dental disease.

CHAPTER 14

1. Establish baseline data on the patient; aid in establishing a diagnosis; serve as a resource during treatment planning; aid in implementation of the treatment plan; as a reference for evaluating treatment success; as a source of legal evidence; and in forensic dentistry
2. The amount of masticatory mucosa on the buccal surface of the tooth minus the buccal pocket depth of the same tooth equals the amount of attached gingiva.
3. Overangulate. The consequence of overangulating in a given area is that the reading may be slightly higher than the actual pocket depth. This would alert the hygienist or dentist to a potential problem area before it existed to that degree. If the probe is underangulated, the clinician runs the risk of assuming that an area is healthier than it actually is, and it may be overlooked in the dentist's diagnosis and treatment plan. Which would be worse for the patient?
4. No. Pocket depths are essentially meaningless unless the height of the gingival margin is also known. The depth of the pocket must be viewed in the context of whether or not there has been abnormal enlargement of the tissues or apical migration of the junctional epithelium. Without this context, the clinician would not know whether a 3 mm pocket could be interpreted as normal, the result of gingival inflammation, or the result of periodontal destruction.
5. a. False. The probe should be adapted as close to parallel as possible as long as the clinician is certain that the tip is closely adapted to the tooth; the parallel relationship will exist for buccal and lingual adaptation, but the probe should be angled slightly for best assessment of the interproximal areas.
   b. False. In situations in which calculus prevents the clinician from adapting the probe to the base of the sulcus or pocket, it is often necessary to perform some scaling before accurate pocket depths can be determined.
   c. False. Although there are six prescribed areas where pocket readings are taken, it is the deepest point within each area that is recorded. This may not necessarily occur at exactly the same point on every tooth; in fact, it is unlikely that that would be true. In addition, if two distinctly separate vertical defects are detected within the same area of the tooth, the clinician may choose to include an extra reading to further define the boney morphology around that tooth.

CHAPTER 15

1. Permanent records, diagnostic aid, educational aid, and fabrication of temporary appliances
2. Water-to-powder ratio, water temperature, and method of manipulation
3. The tray should be large enough to permit ¼ inch (6 mm) of alginate to flow between the tray and oral structures without impinging on the soft tissues and without causing pain.
4. Fill the tray to the level of the beading wax; smooth alginate with wet fingers; retract one cheek with the fingers; retract the other cheek with the side of the tray as it is being inserted; loosen the cheek and insert the other side of the tray; center the tray; place the posterior border of the tray first, and then the rest of the tray; muscle mold; and hold the tray gently.
5. Muscle molding is forming pliable materials (i.e., alginate) to conform to the muscle attachments of the soft tissues to include the muscle attachments in the cast for diagnostic and fabrication purposes.
6. The clinician can try to divert the patient's attention, reassure the patient, and/or ask the patient to breathe through the nose. If the patient reports a history of a gagging problem, the clinician can ask the patient to hold an ice cube in the mouth before inserting the tray or rinse the mouth with an anesthetic mouthwash.
7. Distortion and/or ripping of the alginate
8. To permit the dental personnel to correctly relate the mandibular cast to the maxillary cast during the trimming procedure
9. Initially, the gypsum is flowed into the tray in small increments to coat the tooth surfaces, and the excess is allowed to run out of the impression tray. Gradually, larger increments are added and flowed around the impression.
10. Compare your drawing with Fig. 15-28.

CHAPTER 16

1. Any four of the following: diagnostic aid, treatment planning, case presentation, case documentation, education/motivation, and instruction/peer review
2. Single-lens–reflex camera body, 100 mm automatic short-mount lens or 100 mm macrolens, fully automatic bellows, electronic point-source flash attachment, rotating bracket for flash, proper color correction filters, and pistol grip and cable release
3. a. 9
   b. 10
   c. 5
   d. 2
   e. 1
   f. 8
   g. 7
   h. 6
   i. 4
   j. 3
4. a. Wet the cheek retractor.
   b. Ask the patient to relax the lips and open the mouth slightly.
   c. Place the rim of the retractor onto the edge of the lower lip.
   d. Rotate the handle of the retractor until it is parallel to the corner of the mouth.
   e. Instruct the patient to bite down. Pull the retractors out laterally and forward.
5. a. Mandibular anterior lingual: a lingual view of the mandibular anterior teeth and gingiva from the distal of the right cuspid to the distal of the left cuspid
   b. Buccal of right side: a direct buccal view of the right maxillary and mandibular teeth in occlusion from the distal of the right cuspid to the retromolar or maxillary tuberosity area
   c. Anterior direct: a direct view of the maxillary and mandibular teeth in occlusion from the distal of the right cuspid to the distal of the left cuspid
   d. Maxillary occlusal: a view of the maxillary occlusal surfaces and palatal tissues

CHAPTER 17

1. Education of the public and of private patients in dental health has always been part of the profession of dental hygiene. Because of the nature of the work the clinician performs (monitoring the health of the oral tissues, cleaning the teeth, and providing periodontal or restorative therapy), he/she is in an excellent position to educate the patient as to the causes of dental disease and the steps necessary to avoid disease. Considering the number of patients with periodontal disease, preventive education is perhaps the hygienist's most important role.
2. Dental plaque has been identified as an important factor in inflammatory gingival disease. The relationship of oral hygiene and plaque has led scientists to conclude that controlling or disorganizing dental plaque is the answer to preventing dental disease at the current time.
3. An individualized approach to preventive education is valuable because the patient easily sees his/her role. The patient is involved in decisions about goals and has an opportunity to feel commitment to a plan designed particularly for him/her. By personalizing the dental health education plan, the hygienist finds that instruction is less likely to become routine from patient to patient.
4. a. Small step size allows the rate of instruction to not overwhelm the patient.
   b. Active participation allows the patient to become

involved and practice using the new concepts or skills.

   c. Immediate feedback provides the patient with cues and encouragement about performance so that corrections can be made or reinforcement can be given early in practice.

   d. Self-pacing gives the learner a significant role in determining what instruction will be given and when.

5. a. Skill does not seem to be the problem, so do not bore the patient.

   b. This is a bit extreme at this point in treatment.

   c. The best response. Most likely the patient is having a difficult time understanding or accepting the need for improved home care. Perhaps he/she is having difficulties adjusting to new routines, and a few words of encouragement or helpful suggestions are all that is needed.

   d. You've given up too soon if you consider yourself a preventive educator.

6. a. Short-term; security
   b. Long-term; social
   c. Short-term; security
   d. Long-term; esteem

7. Disagree. A specific technique is less important than the degree of thoroughness in cleaning. Many brushing techniques are adequate. Brushing can be performed several times a day, but unless the bacterial plaque is thoroughly and consistently disorganized, disease will continue. Also, regular interproximal cleaning must be performed in addition to following a brushing routine.

8. Keeping the tissue in tone is an important consideration. The patient may find the use of an interdental stimulator such as the periodontal aid, wood wedge, rubber tip, or oral irrigator helpful. For the bridge, a floss threader will be necessary to clean under the bridge and to floss the abutment teeth. The oral irrigator can flush food debris from this area also. Yarn may be suggested for polishing the last tooth in the arch adjacent to the removable partial denture if regular floss is not cleaning thoroughly. Variable-diameter floss (which incorporates the threader, yarn, and regular floss) and an oral irrigator for flushing and stimulation may be the aids of choice. Selecting the aid the patient is most comfortable using is most important.

9. a. A disclosing agent is needed to identify the plaque and to evaluate areas missed in cleaning. It is probably the only way to ensure thoroughness in the initial preventive program.

   b. Brushing in a random or haphazard fashion rarely results in thoroughness. Establishing a habit of brushing in sequence is a mechanism for ensuring that all areas are attended to.

   c. Because of the anatomic limitations of this area, the usual application of the brush is difficult. The patient needs particular instruction in this area.

   d. The tongue and soft tissue collect bacterial plaque and decomposing food particles. Tissue regeneration accounts for sloughing of dead cell layers also. Although the saliva functions to rinse the oral cavity, brushing or scraping the tissues enhances the cleanliness of the mouth.

CHAPTER 18

1. The nature of the patient's condition; a suggested plan of treatment; discussion of likely outcomes of treatment; risks involved in treatment; the likely outcome of not proceeding with care; and alternative treatment approaches

2. Technical assault

3. The final treatment plan is more likely to be acceptable to the patient, and it will reflect a blending of the needs as seen by the patient and the dental hygienist, which will facilitate a partnership relationship and will increase the probability of cooperation in care and the achievement of health goals.

4. Emergency

5. The dental hygienist should perform thorough, reliable assessments; draw preliminary conclusions from the data, including proposed treatment and scheduling; use the dentist as a resource and arbiter of decisions regarding the patient's status and proper treatment; and follow through with high-quality care, providing status reports as care progresses.

CHAPTER 19

1. The guided self-assessment exercise is designed to help the patient become familiar with the normal structures of the oral cavity and the current conditions of his/her mouth.

2. Some patients may be embarrassed or fearful of the self-assessment exercise. Others may think that they already know all that is necessary and may desire to leave the rest of the care to the dental team. As with most other types of personalized instruction, patient involvement will differ in each case. The hygienist needs to remain sensitive to the patient's value system.

3. a. Knowledge of the appropriate dental terminology creates a more comfortable environment in which the patient can discuss his/her dental concerns and understand his/her treatment needs.

   b. When the patient has an appreciation of the anatomic structures in his/her mouth, conditions can be described more appropriately, and changes from the normal can be recognized more readily.

   c. and d. The awareness of dental plaque and the signs of inflammation will be building blocks for other aspects of preventive education.

4. Oral cancer caused an estimated 9200 deaths in 1983. Many of those deaths could have been prevented by early detection and treatment. One way of promoting early cancer detection is through teaching patients to examine their own mouths, faces, and necks.
5. Face, neck, lips, cheeks, roof of mouth, gums, tongue, and floor of mouth
6. To teach the patient how to examine and palpate each of the areas included in the examination; to foster independence in the patient; and to motivate the patient to want to perform the examination periodically

CHAPTER 20
1. Carbohydrates, fats, and proteins
2. Any of the three nutrients consumed in excess can cause weight gain. Their total contribution to daily caloric intake determines fat deposition (if it is in excess of expended calories) or fat utilization (if it is less than expended calories).
3. a. 6
   b. 7
   c. 5
   d. 9
   e. 10
   f. 14
   g. 11
   h. 13
   i. 1
   j. 4
   k. 3
   l. 12
   m. 2
4. Often the patient is fully aware of what he/she *ought* to include in the daily diet. Information about what to do and what not to do may not be what is needed. After the patient demonstrates his/her level of knowledge about diet and nutrition, it is easier to decide what kind of information still needs to be provided in the follow-up discussion. The self-assessment process itself may cause the patient to develop a need to know or a need to change.
5. The RDA's and the four food groups provide a guideline or standard for evaluating the appropriateness and healthfulness of a person's diet. If these guidelines are generally followed or met, all essential nutrients should be provided in the diet. With these guidelines, missing elements in a person's diet can be readily identified and suggestions for change can be made.
6. Plaque provides a matrix for absorbing fermentable carbohydrates, which are converted by bacteria into acid, which demineralizes the tooth structure. Plaque promotes smooth-surface caries, providing an attachment to the teeth that maintains acid contact.
7. Saturated and unsaturated fats; salt-cured, smoked, and salt-pickled foods; alcohol; and food contaminants, including additives. Alcohol in combination with tobacco promotes oral cancer.
8. Vegetables, especially raw vegetables (lettuce, celery) and cruciferous vegetables, in particular (cabbage, cauliflower, brussels sprouts, broccoli)

CHAPTER 21
1. When calculus is located with a cutting instrument, increased horizontal or lateral pressure against the tooth is used to engage the blade next to the deposit so that it is removed with a working stroke. For calculus removal, the blade must be angled to the tooth to ensure that the cutting edge can be engaged effectively and to reduce tissue damage by the unused blade.
2. a. True
   b. False. It is used with a push stroke on the proximal surfaces of anterior teeth with the shank perpendicular to the long axis of the tooth.
   c. True
   d. True
   e. False. The size, shape, and length of the shank and blade dictate where the various universal curettes may be used.
   f. False. The sickle scaler is best reserved for supragingival calculus and for calculus that is barely below the margin of the gingiva.
   g. False. All plaque and endotoxin must be removed from the root surface, or the disease will continue to advance subclinically.
3. Exploring; observing signs of continued inflammation in localized areas; and air directed on the teeth and into the sulcus

CHAPTER 22
1. a. While there are many other criteria used in patient selection for ultrasonics, the presence of large amounts of deposits is the primary factor.
2. Severe diabetes
3. No. Ultrasonic scaling devices should not be used for children (young, growing tissues).
4. a. The clinician and the assistant should wear face masks and protective lenses. The patient should wear protective lenses.
   b. Immediately following the procedure, the area should be thoroughly wiped with a disinfectant.
   c. A laminar air flow system should be used to reduce the numbers of airborne microorganisms.
   d. Patients known to have virulent pathogens such as hepatitis viruses or tuberculosis mycobacteria should not have ultrasonics used at all.
5. Ultrasonic instruments use high-frequency sound waves to fracture deposits from teeth and to cavitate the accompanying water supply to mechanically flush the area.
6. e, c, d, g, b, a, f

7. Decreased; increased
8. Chisel, beaver tail, universal curette style, and periodontal probe style
9. All of the statements are *true*.

CHAPTER 23

1. a. In scaling, a variety of instruments are used, including scalers, hoes, chisels, files, curettes, and ultrasonic instruments; root planing requires the use of fine curettes with small blades and shank designs that facilitate access to any area. Examples of these are the Gracey curettes.
   b. Root planing requires many more strokes over an area than scaling.
   c. Root planing is best accomplished when a variety of different stroke directions overlap onto the same area; hand scaling is usually accomplished with several strokes in a single optimal direction.
   d. Scaling often requires heavy lateral pressure during the working stroke; root planing starts with moderate, even pressure, which is decreased as the surface becomes harder and smoother.
2. a. Gracey curettes generally have a smaller blade size than universal curettes.
   b. Gracey curettes have offset cutting edges, with one located lower than the other; cutting edges are parallel on the universal curette blade. Both edges of a universal curette are used; only the lower edge of the Gracey curette is used.
   c. The universal curette has a simple shank design, facilitating its use throughout the mouth; Gracey shanks are designed so that each is optimally used in specific areas of the mouth.
3. Tactile sensations reveal that the root is regular, smooth, and hard; audio clues reveal a high squeaky pitch or no sound at all during working strokes; visual clues reveal a homogeneous, shiny, tooth-colored surface; and tissue resolution reveals shrinkage of pocket depth, normal architecture, and no sulcular bleeding.
4. a. If these are the sole criteria, more tooth structure may be removed than is necessary. Hardness is deceptive because you can plane well into healthy dentin without detecting a significant change in hardness. Not all teeth will achieve glasslike smoothness, so using these criteria may be misleading.
   b. The differences between diseased cementum, healthy cementum, and healthy dentin are not clinically significant; even an experienced clinician cannot always detect the differences between them through tactile evaluation.

CHAPTER 24

1. a. Soft tissue curettage: the use of the sharp blade of a curette to remove diseased tissue from the soft tissue pocket wall, thus converting a chronic inflammatory wound into a surgical wound to promote healing of the area
   b. Coincidental curettage: the inadvertent scraping of the cutting edge of an instrument against the soft tissue wall of a pocket or sulcus while the working edge is engaged in scaling or root planing
2. Shrinkage is the only predictable result of this procedure.
3. False. If the procedure is done thoroughly and correctly, the underlying subsulcular connective tissue that is diseased and part or all of the junctional epithelium will also be removed.
4. Since it is stated that the lack of healing cannot be attributed to poor plaque control, then it may be because of incomplete removal of diseased tissue during the curettage, excessive trauma to the tissues during curettage, or incomplete root planing and submarginal plaque control.
5. a. Indication
   b. Contraindication
   c. Indication
   d. Contraindication
   e. Indication
   f. Contraindication
   g. Contraindication
   h. Contraindication
6. a, c, and d

CHAPTER 25

1. A periodontal dressing protects the area from irritants, protects newly exposed root surfaces, stabilizes mobile teeth, protects sutures, maintains the position of repositioned tissue, and helps control bleeding.
2. Either one can be used, depending on clinician preference. The eugenol pack is believed by some practitioners to soothe the tissues; other practitioners believe that eugenol irritates the tissues. Other factors to be considered are storage time, mixing time, consistency of the pack, and ease of manipulation of each material.
3. Refer to Fig. 25-15 for the suggested response.
4. If the sutures were tied on the facial surface, then the lingual pack should be removed first. The sutures can be cut on the lingual portion, and then they can be removed from the buccal portion at the same time the pack is removed. The clinician must be sure *never* to pull the knot through the tissue.

CHAPTER 26

1. a. Concern about tooth appearance
   b. Associated with or embedded in deposits associated with caries and gingival diseases
2. a. Exogenous: stains that originate outside the tooth
   b. Endogenous: stains that develop within the tooth
   c. Extrinsic: exogenous stain on the exterior of the tooth; removable by the patient or professional
   d. Intrinsic: within the tooth structure; not removable by the patient or by basic polishing or scaling
3. a. The prevention-oriented classification was developed to enable the dental professional to better understand the prevention of stain and to correlate this with the medical bases for development of tooth abnormalities and discolorations.
   b. Both classify extrinsic stains similarly.
4. It removes and prevents formation of stains and/or discolorants (pellicle).
5. Essentially the same abrasives are used in both; higher concentrations are present in professional products.
6. Abrasive hardness, particle size, shape, concentration, and the pressure and speed used
7. Operate at a low speed (minimal speed at which the attachment can be applied to the tooth without stalling); use *light, intermittent* pressure on the tooth; and use sufficient amounts of abrasive to minimize direct contact of rubber and brush with the tooth
8. Portability, provides gentle massage, can reach surfaces obscured by malposed teeth, generates minimal frictional heat, generates minimal noise, and is easily cleaned and sterilized
9. It is slow and tedious and requires considerable hand effort.
10. The presence of stains that cannot be readily removed by the patient
11. Air pressure and water force a slurry of sodium bicarbonate against the tooth structure, loosening stain and polishing the tooth.

CHAPTER 27

1. Removable appliances must be cleaned to remove plaque, materia alba, and food debris, and to lessen the likelihood of irritating the soft tissues.
2. Full denture: The denture can be cleaned with an abrasive paste, powder, or soap, and a denture brush. All areas of the denture should be brushed. Occasionally it can be soaked for 15 minutes in a solution of Clorox and Calgonite. Overdenture: This is cleaned in the same manner as a full denture, but the indentations for teeth must be cleaned with a cotton-tipped applicator.
   Orthodontic appliance: The appliance is cleaned with a toothbrush and paste. All surfaces should be brushed.

3. The patient should be informed that it is not enough; brushing daily is advised.

CHAPTER 28

1. a. Overbite: the vertical distance that the maxillary teeth overlap the mandibular teeth
   b. Occlusal trauma: forces that cause damage to the supporting structures
   c. Occlusal traumatism: Damage due to abnormally arranged forces
2. Tooth position, tooth-to-tooth habits, foreign object-to-teeth habits, oral musculature habits, and iatrogenic factors
3. Subjective: aching muscles, teeth that move, pain when biting, or pain with temperature changes. The patient may report grinding or clenching teeth or a habit of holding a pipe with the teeth or chewing or sucking a foreign object.
   Clinical: mobility; wear patterns; changes in tooth position; poorly contoured restorations; plunger cusps; severe overbite or overjet; overdevelopment of the muscles of mastication; clicking, pain, or improper movement of the temporomandibular joint; and tooth sensitivity.
   Radiographic: widened periodontal ligament space, necrosis of the periodontal ligament, cemental tears, loss of the lamina dura, bone resorption, and root resorption.
4. a. False. There must be damage to the supporting structures caused by occlusal trauma for the condition to be considered occlusal traumatism.
   b. False. Occlusal trauma does not cause periodontal pockets. Periodontitis is an inflammatory disease that affects the supporting structure; occlusal traumatism is a *non*inflammatory disease that affects the supporting structure.
   c. True in most cases.

CHAPTER 29

1. a. Parts per million
   b. Hydroxyapatite
   c. Fluoroapatite
   d. Decayed, missing, and filled surfaces
   e. Decayed and filled teeth
   f. Sodium monofluorophosphate
2. a. 1 ppmF
   b. 1000 ppmF
   c. 12,300 or 12,500 ppmF
3. To improve crystallinity; to make the enamel more stable; to increase resistance to acid; to promote remineralization; and to inhibit plaque organisms from adhering and from producing acid
4. a. None
   b. Water, tablets, toothpastes, and professional fluoride treatments

c. Water, tablets, toothpastes, professional fluoride treatments, and rinses

d. Same as c

e. Same as c

5. a. Sodium fluoride is available in solution form and is applied at four consecutive appointments, 1 week apart, at ages 3, 7, 11, and 13.

b. Acidulated phosphate fluoride is available in solution and in gel forms and is applied semiannually from age 2 through age 15 or 16, or until the caries rate is under control.

c. Stannous fluoride is applied as a solution semiannually from age 2 until the caries rate is under control.

6. Although the prophylaxis might serve to remove the unreactive outer layer of enamel and expose a more reactive layer to the fluoride, it is at the same time removing the most concentrated fluoride layer from the tooth. Removal of plaque and acquired pellicle is not necessary for fluoride effectiveness.

7. See the check-off sheet (p. 518) for each step.

8. c. All teeth to be treated must be covered by the fluoride gel or solution before the 4-minute timing begins.

9. Adults: 5 to 10 g
Children: 32 mg/kg body weight
The amount of fluoride gel or solution applied is somewhere in the range of 125 to 200 mg.

10. d. All three are acceptable antidotes for acute fluoride poisoning. Seek immediate emergency care if symptoms persist or if the amount ingested is more than 3.5 mg/kg body weight, or is unknown.

CHAPTER 30

1. Previous methods to prevent pit and fissure caries included (1) smoothing out the anatomic contours to make the surface less retentive and (2) conservatively restoring the surfaces. The time spent and the loss of tooth structure associated with both of these methods outweighed their benefits. Various medicaments and cements have been used to close the occlusal anatomy, but the materials usually failed to hold up. Systemic fluorides are relatively unsuccessful because they act to reduce caries on proximal and smooth surfaces most significantly and less so on occlusal surfaces. Today's sealant materials have had a significant impact on preventing pit and fissure caries. Through improved materials and processes, the problems of material retention and wear have been greatly reduced. Single applications of sealant have been shown to reduce occlusal caries greater than 80% during the first year in experimental studies. Compared with previous methods for pit and fissure caries prevention, sealants seem very successful.

2. This patient is at a caries-prone age and shows a history of restorations in commonly susceptible teeth. The patient's susceptibility may be exaggerated, since she previously lived in a nonfluoridated area. Clinically, the patient presents with good home care and a good preventive attitude reinforced by the parents. The newly erupted teeth are sound, and radiographic data reveal that there are no interproximal caries. These factors indicate that the patient is a good candidate for sealant protection. In a consultation between the hygienist, dentist, patient, and family, information about the sealant procedure, the benefits, risks, and responsibilities should be discussed and a decision made. (We would elect to seal teeth No. 18 and No. 31 and recommend that the patient return when teeth No. 2 and No. 15 erupt if this occurs prior to the next regularly scheduled visit.)

3. Steps in the sealant application procedure: (1) remove hard and soft deposits; (2) polish with pumice; (3) rinse thoroughly; (4) isolate and dry teeth; (5) condition the teeth; (6) rinse and examine (recondition if necessary); (7) reisolate and dry teeth; (8) apply sealant; (9) polymerize sealant; and (10) rinse and examine.

CHAPTER 31

1. Areas where the dentin is exposed, primarily as a result of enamel and/or cementum being eroded or planed away

2. Root surface scaling, gingival surgery (causing gingival or root exposure recession), cavity preparation, and placement of crowns

3. Mechanical, thermal, and chemical

4. Depositing or precipitating insoluble materials at nerve endings (Tomes' fibers); denaturing nerve endings; stimulating secondary dentin formation; and reducing pulp hyperemia

5. a. False; two have been accepted
b. True
c. True
d. True

6. a. Differences: Fluoride is applied more frequently; can be burnished on very sensitive areas.
b. Similarities: Teeth should be clean (scaled and polished) and dry prior to application. The same preparations can be used. If the entire mouth is treated, the same mode of application (tray, painted on dried teeth) can be used.

CHAPTER 32

1. The hygienist should participate in a formal local anesthesia course that provides in-depth information about nerve anatomy, the chemistry and pharmacology of local anesthetics, the modes of actions of each, medical complications, and treatment of the compli-

cations. The course should also include a laboratory portion that teaches the techniques of administering local anesthetics.
2. Refer to Fig. 32-1.
3. a. Hard tissue: second and third molars and the first molar, excluding the mesiobuccal root and the associated supporting structures; soft tissue: overlying facial tissue
   b. Hard tissue: none; soft tissue: palatal tissue from the margin of the gingiva to the midline and from the distal aspect of the posterior-most molar to the cuspid
   c. Hard tissue: none; soft tissue: buccal tissue of mandibular molars
   d. Hard tissue: premolars, cuspid, incisors, and associated supporting structures of the maxilla; soft tissue: tissue overlying facial tissues and the lip
4. a. Mental, long buccal, and lingual
   b. Posterior superior alveolar, infiltration over the mesiobuccal root of the first molar, or middle superior alveolar; a greater palatine if the patient's palate is sensitive to the clamp
   c. Mandibular facial infiltration in the area of the central incisor

CHAPTER 33

1. Conscious sedation refers to a state of relaxation or central nervous system depression in which the patient remains conscious at all times. A conscious patient is defined as one who is capable of rational response to command and has all protective reflexes, such as maintenance of an airway and the cough reflex, intact.
2. a. Inorganic inhalation agent, sweet smelling, and nonflammable
   b. Has a low blood gas solubility as compared with oxygen
   c. Eliminated unchanged by the lungs
   d. A mildly potent anesthetic when administered with oxygen
   e. Affects the person's psychologic reaction to pain perception
3. a. The patient with emphysema has a compromised respiratory system. Various concentrations of oxygen may decrease this person's ability to function. Expiration is difficult and may affect elimination of nitrous oxide from the bloodstream.
   b. Generally, the patient with an upper respiratory tract infection is experiencing difficulty in breathing through the nose. Since this is necessary to permit effective inhalation sedation, the patient will not benefit from the procedure.
4. $\dfrac{4}{4+6} = \dfrac{4}{10} = 40\%$

This is higher than the recommended optimal level for sedation (30% to 35%). Although patient responses vary, close observation is necessary to avoid an adverse response to too high a concentration. Although nitrous oxide and oxygen conscious sedation raises the pain threshold, the body perceives the pain and reacts to it. In the case of a tooth extraction, local or regional anesthesia is necessary.
5. Any three of the following: the patient appears lethargic, falls asleep, begins to perspire, complains of nausea, moves in an uncoordinated fashion, becomes uncooperative, and/or reports dreaming. See Table 33-1 for other responses.

CHAPTER 34

1. False. An attempt should be made to provide some service for the child, even if it is just counting teeth with a mouth mirror. The child may be more willing to cooperate if all procedures are carefully explained in simple terms that attract the patient rather than create fear.
2. Carefully explain each procedure, perhaps showing how pieces of equipment to be used function. Child patients may be allowed to manipulate some of the simpler pieces of equipment such as the air-water spray or the dental chair. A child may be allowed to feel the rubber cup. Encourage the patient to ask questions regarding the care he/she will receive so that he/she does not build up unnecessary fears.
3. For the patient who is visually handicapped, the hygienist can communicate by way of the other functioning senses. If the patient can hear, describe the procedures to be performed. Let the patient touch the equipment and hear it work before an intraoral procedure is attempted. Guide the patient with a gentle touch, and support his/her cooperation. Verbally introduce each step of care. Concerning home care techniques, allow the patient to feel the method for brush and floss manipulation, in addition to feeling it intraorally. Repeat each step of instruction as necessary. Emphasize the feel of clean, plaque-free teeth.
4. a. An appointment routine helps the patient anticipate a familiar experience. This helps put the patient at ease in the dental environment.
   b. Most patients accept dentistry best when they are rested and well-nourished. A midmorning appointment is most likely to catch both the patient and the clinician in a receptive mood for treatment.
5. Implements for delivery of safe dental care: physical restraints, mouth props (bite blocks), steel mirrors, rubber dam application, instruments secured with floss, and thimbles modified for finger protection.
6. Assessments should be made to determine the pa-

tient's sensory abilities and ability to communicate before treatment begins so that appropriate modifications can be made. Manipulation of tissue should be kept to a minimum to avoid unnecessary trauma and resultant slower healing. Medical history assessments should be thorough, since complicated medical histories may be encountered when older patients are treated. Appropriate modification based on medical histories should be made.

7. At age 6 months if the child has a developmental disorder or if the parents have poor oral health; other children should be seen between the ages of 18 and 24 months.

8. Only if stains are present. Preferred practice is to have the child (or parent) deplaque the teeth with a brush and fluoride paste, practicing proper technique and checking results with a disclosant. Topical fluoride can then be applied.

9. Depending on the limitation and the patient's ability to use his/her hand, wrist, and fingers, a brush could be modified by heating the plastic handle to turn the brush head in a way that would be more useful. The brush handle could be enlarged or elongated by attaching the brush to an object such as a ball or a wooden dowel. If the patient has head and neck mobility, an electric toothbrush could be mounted on a surface so that the patient could place his/her mouth on the brush and move his/her head position. It is important to evaluate the patient's abilities before helping select or create a modified tool.

10. The answer should include at least three of the following responses:
    a. Inform the patient when dentistry should be provided and what to avoid (radiographs, medications, treatment in the first and third trimesters).
    b. Dispel any myths the patient may have about dentistry and pregnancy.
    c. Stress the need for plaque control to prevent gingival inflammation.
    d. Stress the need for a balanced diet and nutrient supplements.
    e. Explain the role of sugar and decay—baby bottle syndrome.
    f. Discuss fluorides, the development of teeth, and/or eruption dates.

11. Dental services are necessary to ensure that the oral cavity is as healthy as possible before cancer treatment. This includes prophylactic services, home care instruction, periodontal treatment, extractions, impressions and models of oral tissues, and restoration of caries and of teeth that may support a future oral prosthesis. Cancer therapy will alter the saliva and increase the tendency toward caries and the patient's susceptibility to infection. Soft tissues and periodontal conditions will be greatly aggra-

vated during treatment. Dental complications will be reduced if the patient is in good dental health and is motivated about continuous dental care throughout therapy and after recovery. To provide the most comprehensive care for the patient, the hospital staff and dental staff should work together.

CHAPTER 35

1. a. A rubber dam is used to isolate the teeth being treated from the oral cavity. The dam provides the patient protection and allows the clinician to place a high-quality restoration.
   b. The matrix band and wedge provides the clinician with a surface against which to pack the restorative material. The wedge prevents the restorative material from forming an overhang.
   c. A temporary restoration maintains a traumatized tooth that may have been traumatized in function until the tooth can be permanently restored. Some zinc oxide–eugenol materials soothe the pulp of the tooth.
   d. Overhangs can be an irritant just as calculus can be an irritant that is plaque retentive. When an overhang is removed, the patient is provided with a smooth, non-plaque-retentive interproximal surface.
   e. Amalgam polishing provides a smooth, non-plaque-retentive restoration with an increased life expectancy.

2. An open margin, large deficiency, open contact, caries on another surface, a large overhang that should be replaced, and other such complications

3. Disks and finishing strips for the interproximal area; burs (pear shaped, bud or flame shaped round); a brush, rubber cup, and tape with pumice; rubber cup and tape with wet tin oxide; and a rubber cup with dry tin oxide

4. An overhang is an extension of the silver filling away from the tooth. This extension irritates the gum and allows plaque to accumulate in the area. An overhang may be caused by a number of factors, but it is important to have the area smoothed so you will be able to keep the area clean. Does this sound like a reasonable procedure to you?

5. An open contact, open margin, extremely deficient margin, low marginal ridge, margins that are not sealed, and other such conditions

6. A restoration must contact the adjacent tooth of the original tooth contacted, so that the restored tooth does not drift. The burnished area permits the clinician to pack the restorative material into the area more effectively.

CHAPTER 36

1. Components of a case documentation: health history review, initial clinical findings, chartings, radiographs, study casts, photographs, treatment plan, record of actual treatment, posttreatment findings, and evaluation summary

2. a. Case documentation enhances record keeping by ensuring that accurate data are available for the clinician to follow the patient's care. Documentation of before-and-after treatment establishes the initial condition and treatment outcome. Such information may be useful and necessary for reference and comparison at a later date.

   b. Participating in case documentation procedures is motivating for the patient as he/she is able to realize the changes that have occurred throughout the course of treatment. Examples of other patient documentations demonstrate potential modes of therapy and may aid the patient in making a decision for personal treatment.

CHAPTER 37

1. A system of accountability defines goals that can provide a direction or a target for the daily activities of practice. Such a system can add meaning to a lifetime of clinical practice. Accountability can also develop a support system for encounters with malpractice or third-party payer investigations.

2. The degree to which prevention is emphasized in each day's routine (i.e., the amount of time or effort spent on prevention and preventive educational activities); the overall impact on health levels of the population (maintenance, improvement, or loss of health over time); the degree to which clinical protocols approximate nationally accepted standards, through comparison with published protocols, reviews of the literature, and participation in peer group study clubs; approach behaviors of patients to dental hygiene care through the development of a long-term patient population; personal gratification and health; and cost-effectiveness.

3. Decide to live with the dissatisfaction or develop a plan for change

INDEX

A

A-type calculus, 199
Abrasion, charting of, 189
Abrasive instruments for amalgam finishing and polishing, 634, 634p
Abrasiveness of toothpaste, 468, 468t
Abrasives, 469
Abutment teeth, 187
Accepted Dental Therapeutics, 444, 508
Access problems in root planing, 423-424, 424p
Accessories, photographic, 277-279, 278-283p
Accident prevention, 174
Accountability for care and cost, 665-667
Acellular cementum, 422
Acid conditioning for occlusal sealing, 522-523, 527p, 530p
Acid demineralization, 423
Acid etching with sealants, 523, 527p
Acidulated phosphate fluoride, 504-506
Acquired immune deficiency syndrome, 31-32
Acquired pellicle and plaque, 205
Acrylic facing, 186
Acrylic testing stick, 96-97, 96p
Acute adrenal insufficiency, 171
Acute necrotizing ulcerative gingivitis, 218-219
 and curettage, 431
 and root planing, 426
 and ultrasonics, 394, 395
Acycloguanosine and herpes, 31
Adaptation
 of instruments, 86, 86i, 87-92p, 378-379, 380i, 382p, 385, 385p, 416, 417-419p, 436-438, 437-438p
 of periodontal dressing, 451, 451-452p
 of rubber cup, 474, 474i
Addison's disease and sedation, 564
ADHA; *see* American Dental Hygienists' Association
Adjunct explorers, 92
Adjunct instruments, 387-389, 387-389i, 387-389p
Aerosols in disease transmission, 24, 33, 51-53
 from ultrasonics, 396
Age of patient
 and cancer, 352
 and conscious sedation, 564
AHA; *see* American Hospital Association
AIDS; *see* Acquired immune deficiency syndrome
Aim toothpaste, 468, 505

Air contamination, 51, 396
Air-water syringe 13-15, 14p; *see also* Tri-syringe
Alcohol, isopropyl, 36
Alert, medical, 57-58
Alginate, 242p, 247p; *see also* Study models
Allergic reaction to anesthesia, 173, 547
Allergy
 to dentures, 477-478
 in health history, 128
 to rubber dam, 598
Altered consciousness as emergency, 173
Alumina compounds, 468
Alveolar concentration of nitrous oxide, 566
Alveolar ridges, 158, 159p
Amalgam files, 629-632, 631i, 631p
Amalgam knife, 629, 630p, 631i
Amalgam overhang removal, 628-633, 628i, 630-631p, 633p
Amalgam restorations, 186
 finishing and polishing of, 633-639, 634-641p
American Academy of Pediatrics, on effects of anesthetics, 568
American Dental Association
 Accepted Dental Therapeutics, 444, 508
 accepted fluoride dentifrices, 505t
 on desensitizing toothpastes, 537
 report on hygiene graduates, 6
American Dental Hygienists' Association, practice site definition, 6
American Dental Society of Anesthesiology, Inc., 562
American Heart Association, prophylactic regimen for dental procedures, 119
American Hospital Association
 health history questionnaire, 121-122i
American Medical Association, Journal of; *see Journal of the American Medical Association*
American Society of Anesthesiologists, on effects of anesthesia, 568
Amide anesthetics, 544-545, 557
Amine-accelerated BIS-GMA, 529
Analgesia machinery, 566, 567p
Analysis form, occlusal, 493i
Anatomic charting, 178i, 179
Anatomy
 in local anesthesia, 553
 occlusal, 488
Anchor tooth, 606p
Anemia, 129
Anesthesia
 local, 541-557, 546-549t, 547-548i, 550-556p
 for curettage, 435-436

Illustration is indicated by *i*, photograph by *p*, and table by *t*, following page numbers.

Anesthesia—cont'd
  local—cont'd
    for probing, 231-232
    reaction to, 173-174
    for root planing, 415-416
  topical, 541-544, 558*p*
Anesthetic agents and components, 544
Angle's classifications of occlusion, 485-487, 485-487*i*
Angulation, instrument, 382, 383-384*i*, 383*p; see also* Instrumentation
Animal tests of fluoride, 502
Anomalies, developmental, charting of, 189
Anorexia nervosa, 160-161
"Anterior" explorer exercises, 90-91
Anterior lingual brushing, 308-309, 309*p*
Anterior photographic views, 286-287
Antibacterial agents
  in periodontal dressings, 446
  and plaque, 207
Antibacterial effects of fluoride, 501
Antibiotic therapy, 30
  contraindications for ultrasonics, 395
  and plaque, 207
Antiplaque agents, 296
Antiseptic solution, 37, 555
ANUG; *see* Acute necrotizing ulcerative gingivitis
Aperture setting, 276-277
APF; *see* Acidulated phosphate fluoride
Appliances
  care of removable, 477-482, 478-482*p*
  fabrication of temporary, 240
Appointment, dental hygiene, 8-9
Appointment plan, 334-335, 336-343*i*
  for patient with special needs, 575
Appraisal, general, 137-138
Approach behaviors of patients and clinicians, 667
Aqua-fresh toothpaste, 467-468, 505
Armamentarium
  for amalgam overhang removal, 629-632, 629-631*p*
  for amalgam polishing, 634, 634*p*
  for anesthesia, 553-557, 553-554*p*
  for curettage, 436
  for matrix band system, 615*p*
  for root planing, 413-416, 415*p*
  for rubber dam placement and removal, 598-599, 599*p*
  for study models, 241-244, 242-243*p*
  for zinc oxide–eugenol temporary restoration, 623-628, 623*p*
Arnim, S.S., and discovery of disclosant, 306
Arterial blood pressure; *see* Blood pressure
Articulating paper, 495, 495-496*p*
Articulator, 240*i*
ASA number, 276
Ascorbic acid; *see* Vitamins
Asepsis, 23, 32, 555
Aspartane, 366

Assessment; *see also* Self-assessment
  in case documentation, 654
  in dental hygiene appointment, 9
  of health status, 301-303
  of restoration for finishing and polishing, 635
Assistant
  chairside, position of, 72-73, 72*p*, 73*i*
  for rubber dam placement, 599
Associate degree programs, 6
Asthma
  as emergency, 172
  and sedation, 563-564
Attrition, tooth, charting of, 189
Audio evaluation for root planing, 420
Audit form sample, 61*i*
Auricular lymph nodes, 149
Auscultation in examination, 137
Autoclaving, 37-40
  bags for, 43-44, 44*p*
  effect of, on instruments, 18-19*p*
  trays for, 39*p*
Autogenous infection, 26
Automatic toothbrush, 319, 324*p*

B

BIS-GMA; *see* Bisphenol A-glycidyl methacrylate, 528-529
Bisphenol A-glycidyl methacrylate, 528-529
Black, G.V., restoration classification system, 182, 184-185*i*
Black-line stain, 466
Blanket as emergency supply, 166
Bleaching of teeth, 470
Bleeding, 297*p*
  in curettage evaluation, 439
  in gingival assessment, 211, 211*t*, 226
  and periodontal dressing, 450-451
  and probe sensitivity, 231
  and root planing, 424-425
Blind patient, 574-575
Block anesthesia, 548
Blood, clotting of
  after curettage, 439
  and root planing, 426
  and vitamin K, 364
Blood diseases, 129-130
Blood donation and disease, 28
Blood pressure, 139-140, 140*i*, 143*i*, 143*p*
  in emergency, 165-166
  positional low, 142
Blood tests
  and hepatitis, 28-29
  and syphilis, 30
Blood vessel avoidance with injection, 553
Bloodstream and disease transmission, 23-24, 32
"Bobbing" with instruments, 85-86, 87

Body communication, 123
Boiling water in disinfection, 36
Bonding mechanism of occlusal sealants, 523-528
Bone formation, 363-364
Bone level, 223
Boney defects, 223
Boney structures, examination of, 152
Boxing study models, 256, 258p
Brand name and generic name of drug, 132
Bridges, fixed, 186
Brush use in polishing, 472p, 473-474
Brushing, 308-312, 308-309i, 309p, 311i; *see also* Toothbrush
Buccal mucosa, 155-156, 156p
Buccal photographic views, 288-289
Buccal pocket walls, curettage of, 436
Bud-shaped burs, 637, 637p
Bullae, 147
Bulimia, 160-161
Bunsen burner maintenance, 37
Burnished calculus, 197
Burnishing of matrix band, 618-620, 619p

C

Calcium, 364
    in calculus, 198
    and vitamin D, 363
Calcium carbonate, 469
    in toothpaste, 467
Calcium pyrophosphate, 468
Calculus, 196-202, 379i, 389-390, 391
    charting of, 193, 199, 200-201i, 202t
    and disease, 198
    and plaque, 205-206
    and probe reading, 232, 232i
    radiographs of, 193, 193i
    scoring of, 202, 202t
Calibrated probe, 66-67, 227-228; *see also* Periodontal probe
Caloric intake, 362-363
Calories, nutrient source of, 362-363
Camera loading, 284
Camera systems, selection of, 272-276
Cancer
    and anesthesia, 568
    detection of, 136
    and diet, 366-367
    oral, 352-359, 355-358p
    self-examination for, 352-359, 355-358p
    therapy and dental care, 585-588
Carbocaine, 545, 545t
Carbohydrates, 362, 365
Carcinoma, squamous cell, 352
Cardiac arrest, 173
Cardiac arrhythmia, 127, 546
Cardiopulmonary resuscitation, 164, 168-170t, 173

Care; *see also* Treatment
    modified for patient with special needs, 574-595, 576-583p, 590-591p
    refusal of, 334
Career motivation, 3, 109, 113
Caries
    charting of, 189
    index of, 503
    and nutrition, 364-366
    pathogenesis of, 502
    and plaque, 205-206
    scoring of, 503
Carious lesions, radiographs of, 192
Carnegie Commission (1970) and Council (1976) recommen-dations for dentistry, 5
Cart, modular, 18, 18p
Cartridge, 553, 554p
Carving of restoration, 624-628, 626-627p
Case documentation, 651-664, 652-653p, 655-656i, 657-658p, 659i, 660p, 661i, 662-663p
    sample, 655-659i
Case presentation, 110-111
Cast trimming, 259
    check-off sheet for, 268i
CEJ; *see* Cementoenamel junction
Cementoenamel junction, 86-87, 218, 224-225
Cementum, periodontal disease effect on, 421-422
Central nitrous oxide and oxygen system, 565-566, 565-566p
Centric occlusion and relation, 489-490, 490t, 494-495, 495p
Certificate programs, 6
Cervical-enamel projections, 223
Chairside assistant, position of, 72-73, 72p, 73i
Change agent, dental hygienist as, 671
Chart; *see* Dental record
Charting, 177-194, 182-183i
    oral, 193-194
    preappointment, 222-224
    in treatment plan, 330
Charting forms, 178-180i
Charting symbols, 178i, 182-183i
Chayes-Siemon apparatus, 539
Cheek in cancer self-examination, 356, 356p
Cheek retractors, 278-279, 279-283p
Chemical curettage, 441
Chemical denture cleaners, 478
Chemical disinfection and sterilization, 33-34, 35t
Chemical stimulation of hypersensitivity, 536
Chemically impregnated cups and points, 640, 641p
Chemocaries, 586-587
Chemotherapy, 586-587
Child abuse or neglect, 161
Child patient, 589-591, 590-591p
    injection of, 557
Chisel, 388, 388p, 388t
Circular compression, 147, 148-151p

Circumferential stroke; *see* Stroke patterns

Circumvallate papillae, 158

Citanest, 545, 545*t*

Clamps for rubber dam placement, 599, 605-608*p*, 613-614*p*, 614*i*

Classification
    of caries and restoration, 184-185*i*
    of occlusion, 485-487, 485-487*i*

Cleaning
    of instruments before sterilization, 36-42
    interproximal, 312-317, 312*p*, 314-325*p*
    of removable appliances, 477-482
    and sanitation, 32-33
    of teeth, 307-327

Cleansing tools, 318-325

Clinical caries index, 503

Clinical evaluation of sealants, 522-523

Clinical examination, 224-234

"Clinical" pocket depth, 231

Clinical situations, scenarios of, 671-675

Clinical trials of fluoride, 502-503

Clinician position, 72-74, 72*p*, 73*i*, 153

Close-up toothpaste, 468

Closing of occlusal anatomy, 522

Clothing and contamination, 50

Coe-Pack Hard and Fast Set periodontal dressings, 446

Cognitive factors in pain reaction, 542-543

Coincidental curettage, 379*i*, 424

Col area, 229

Cold sterilization, 36

Colgate toothpaste, 467, 505

College pliers, 457*p*

Color assessment of gingiva, 225

Color coding
    of nitrous oxide and oxygen equipment, 566
    of nutritional self-assessment, 368-369

Communications
    in questionnaire/interview, 120-122
    with patient with special needs, 574-575

Communications ability and sedation, 563-564

Community fluoridation, 504

Community health planning, plaque scoring in, 207

Complicating factors in root planing, 423-425

Comprehensive charting, 177-181, 178-180*i*

Comprehensive health history; *see* Health history

Compressed air
    in evaluation, 389
    in polishing, 472

Computers in dentistry, 60

Concentration of anesthetic agents, 545, 545*t*

Concise White Sealant and Enamel Bond, 529; *see also* Bisphenol A-glycidyl methacrylate

Condensing of zinc oxide–eugenol, 624, 625*p*

Conditioning of enamel, 527*p*, 529-530, 530*p; see also* Sealants

Confidentiality, patient, and dental record, 56

Congenital defect
    of heart, 126
    and tooth staining, 465

Congenital malformation and anesthesia, 568

Congestive heart failure, 127

Conscious sedation, 542
    with nitrous oxide and oxygen, 561-572, 563*t*, 564-570*p*

Conscious state, 561-562

Consciousness, altered, as emergency, 173

Consent, informed, 57, 333

Constructive dependence on provider of care, 113

Consumer
    patient as, 295
    and provider accountability, 667

Contact inhibition of epithelium overgrowth, 432-433

Contagious diseases, 128-129

Contamination
    of air, 396
    chain of, 48
    control of, 32-53
    from nitrous oxide, 568-569
    from ultrasonics, 396

Continuity of medical-dental care, 118-120

Contour
    of crown and plaque, 223
    of gingiva, 225-226
    of matrix band, 618, 618-619*p*
    of wedge, 621*p*

Contra-angled explorer, 90

Contraindications
    to conscious sedation, 563-564
    to curettage, 431-433
    to dental treatment, 136
    to occlusal sealing, 528, 528*t*
    to root planing, 425-426
    to ultrasonic scaling, 395-396

Control
    of dental disease, 295-327
    of pain, 541-544, 561-562

Controls
    of dental chair, 12-13
    of tri-syringe, 13
    of ultrasonics, 397-398, 397*p*

Coronal plaque, 205

Coronary artery disease, 126

Coronary thrombosis, 126

Corrosion products on amalgams, 633

Corticosteroids
    as contraindication to ultrasonics, 395
    for hypersensitivity, 539
    and sedation, 564

Cosmetic effect of prophylaxis, 378

Cosmetic procedures, 470

Cost of disposable supplies, 43

Cost-effectiveness, 667

Cost estimate, 333
Cotton rolls in fluoride application, 515-517, 516*p*
Cotton pliers, 457*p*
Counseling, nutritional, 361-362, 365-367
CPR; *see* Cardiopulmonary resuscitation
Craig-Marton toothpaste, 467
Cranial nerve, 548
Crest toothpaste, 468, 505
Criminal act as emergency, 174
Cross-contamination, 17-18, 24, 42, 244-245; *see also* Contamination
Crowns, 186
  abnormal morphology of, 223
  and intrinsic staining, 470
  and plaque retention, 145
Cup, rubber, adaptation; *see* Rubber cup adaptation
Curettage, 430-441, 433-434*i*, 437-438*p*
  coincidental, 379*i*, 424
  effectiveness of, 440
  healing following, 439
  with ultrasonics, 406
Curette, 97-98, 98*i*
  for curettage, 436-439, 437-438*p*
  for margination, 629-632, 630*p*
  and periodontal pack, 456-459, 457*p*
  for root planing, 413-416, 415*p*, 417-419*p*
  for scaling, 382-386, 382-384*i*, 383*p*
  universal, 382-387, 385*p*; *see also* Universal curette
Curricula, dental hygienist and assistant, 5
Cuspidor, 13-15, 14*p*
Cutting instruments, care of, 18
Cuttle disk, 632
Cyanoacrylate periodontal packs, 446
Cyclamates, 366

D

Deaf patient, 574-575
Decalcification, charting of, 189
Decay resistance and fluoride, 364
Decision making in care planning, 110-111
DEJ; *see* Dentoenamel junction
Delton, 529; *see also* Bisphenol A-glycidyl methacrylate
Demographic information in patient record, 57
Denquel toothpaste, 537
Dental aerosols; *see* Aerosols
Dental caries; *see also* Caries
  nutritional basis of, 364, 365-366
Dental chair, 11-13, 12*p*
  as contamination site, 48-49
Dental disease, elimination of, 8
Dental floss; *see* Floss
Dental history, 57
Dental hygiene care
  evaluation of, 665-670
  scope of, 8, 344

Dental lounge chair, 11-13, 12-13*p*
Dental morphology and sensitivity, 536
Dental plaque; *see* Plaque
Dental practice act, 8
  and study models, 240
Dental record, 56-62
  audit form, 61*i*
Dental stains, 464-471, 466-467*t*, 470*t*
Dental tape, 312
  in amalgam polishing, 436-437, 437*p*
  in margination, 633
Dental team, positioning of, 72-83
Dental unit, 13-17
Dentifrices and stain; *see also* Toothpastes
  fluoride, 505-506, 505*t*
Dentin, 422
  removal of, 292-293
Dentist, consultation with, in matrix band placement, 618
Dentoenamel junction, sensitivity in, 536
Denture brushes, 479, 479*p*
Denture cleaning, 478-481
Denture plaque, 477
Deposits
  complete removal of, 389-390
  soft, 204-205
Depth of field, 276
Dermal pH and microorganisms, 24
Desensitizing toothpastes, 537
Design of instruments, 67-68
Developmental defects and tooth stain, 465
DFS; *see* DMFS caries index
DFT; *see* DMFS caries index
Diabetes, 127
  as contraindication to curettage, 432
  as contraindication to ultrasonics, 295
  as emergency, 171
Diagnosis
  legal limits in, 344
  medical, 119
  periodontal, 221
  study models in, 239-240
Diametric index for nitrous oxide and oxygen connection, 566
Diastema, 222-223
Diastolic pressure, 139-140, 140*i*
Dibasic calcium phosphate, 467
Dibasic sodium citrate, 537
Diet in general and oral health, 361-364
Digital palpation, 147
Dilute acids, 479
Disclosants and polishing, 475
Disclosing agents, 210-211
  in home care, 306-307
Disease
  and calculus, 197-198
  control of dental, planning for, 295, 327

Disease—cont'd
    detection of, 136
    oral, and plaque, 205-206, 206*i*
    transmission of, 22-31, 50
Disinfection, 32-37
Disks, finishing, 632-633, 641*p*
Disposable supplies for asepsis, 42-43
Distal inclination, 190
Distopalatal groove, 223
DMFS caries index, 503
DMFT; *see* DMFS caries index
Documentation
    case, 651-664, 652-653*p*, 655-656*i*, 657-658*p*, 659*i*, 660*p*,
        661*i*, 662-663*p*
        sample of, 655-659*i*
    dental record as, 58-59
    intraoral photography in, 272
Dosage
    of anesthetics, 545-546, 546*t*
    of fluoride, 500, 517
    of vitamins, 363-365, 370-371*t*
Double-ended instruments, 67*p*, 68
Double-pour method of study models, 257
Down's syndrome and hepatitis, 28
Dressings, periodontal, cyanoacrylate, 446
Drifting of teeth, 190
Drugs
    action of, 132-133
    classification of, 132
    as cause of stain, 467
    for emergency, 166*t*
Dry foil, 453, 453*p*, 457*p*
Dry heat sterilization, 38, 40-41
Dull instruments, identification of, 95-97, 96*i*, 96*p*
Dummy tooth, 187
Dynamic individual occlusion concept, 484

E

Ear examination, 146
Economics of prevention, 297
Education in dental hygiene profession, 4-6
Educational resource
    case documentation as, 651-654
    photography as, 272
    study model as, 240
Educator, hygienist's role as, 295-296, 378
Efficiency
    in instrumentation, 72
    of sharp instruments, 95
Elderly patients, 592-595
Embolism, 118
Emergency drugs, 166*t*
Emergency procedures, 164-175
Emergency signs, 168-170*t*
Emergency supplies and equipment, 166-167

Emergency treatment, priority of, 165-166
Emotional factors in pain reaction, 543
Emotional stress in periodontal disease, 217
Employment opportunities, 8
Enamel
    etching of, 527*p*, 529-530, 529-530*p*
    fluoride in, 500-501, 501*t*
    impact of occlusal sealing on, 523, 527*p*
Endotoxin and gingivitis, 411
Engine-driven polishing, 472-475, 472*p*, 474*i*
Enlargement, gingival, 232-233, 232*i*
Environment of care for patient with special needs, 575-580
Environmental contamination from nitrous oxide, 568-569
Environmental factors
    in occlusion, 488
    in tooth stain, 466
Enzymes, 479
    and plaque, 207
Epidemiologic studies, plaque scoring in, 207-208
Epilepsy, 128
Epinephrine, 545, 545*t*
Epithelium
    inflammation of, 432-434, 433-434*i*
    junctional, removal of, 433*p*
Epoxylite 9075, 529; *see also* Bisphenol A-glycidyl
Equipment
    for emergency, 166-167
    as contamination site, 49-50
    general care of, 20
    for nitrous oxide and oxygen, 564-569, 564-568*p*
    portable, 580
    ultrasonic, 397-401, 397-401*p*
Erosion, 147
    charting of, 189
Erythrosine, 210-211
Esteem and prevention, 199-200
Ester anesthetics, 544-545, 557
Estimates of cost and time, 331, 332*i*, 333, 336-339*i*
Etching for sealant bonding, 527*p*, 529-530, 529-530*p*
Ethyl aminobenzoate, 557, 559
Ethylene oxide gas sterilization, 38, 41
Etiologic factors in occlusal trauma, 491
Etiology of tooth hypersensitivity, 535-536
Eugenol and noneugenol periodontal packs, 444-447, 447*p*,
        455-456, 455*p*
Eugenol temporary restoration, zinc oxide–, 623-628, 625-627*p*
    check-off sheet for, 644*i*
Evacuation, 11-12
Evaluation
    of care outcomes, 661-664
    of case documentation, 655
    of curettage, 439-440
    and dental hygiene appointment, 9
    of dental hygiene care, 635-670
    of occlusion, 635

Evaluation—cont'd
of periodontal dressing, 453
of root planing, 420-423
of stain, 470-471, 470*t*
of treatment, periodontal chart in, 221
Examination
clinical, 224-234
and nutritional patterns, 367
instruments of, 63-67
intraoral and extraoral, 135-160
oral, for elderly, 593
periodontal, 220-221
and treatment plan, 331
Excavator spoon, 618, 619*i*
Exercise(s)
with instruments, 84-92, 86*i*, 87-92*p*
in positioning, 73, 84-85
Expanded functions, 6-8, 7*t*, 598
Exploratory stroke, 90-91, 378, 381*p*
Explorer, 64-65*p*, 65-67, 104
and calculus, 201*i*
contra-angled, compared with sickle scaler, 381*p*
exercises with, 86-92, 87-92*p*
in root planing, 415-416
Extraction and radiation therapy, 588
Extraoral examination, 144-153
Extraoral palpation, 147-152, 148-151*p*
Extrinsic stains, 466-469, 466-467*t*
professional treatment of, 468-469
Exudate, inflammatory, 226-227
Eye examination, 146
Eyeglasses, protective, 52-53

F

F-stop, 276-277
Face mask, 52
Facial examination and inspection, 146
for cancer, 354, 355*p*
Facial photographic views, 286
Factors in cancer, 353
Fail-safe systems for nitrous oxide, 566
Family medical/dental history, 125
Fats and cancer, 367
Fatigue, hand, effect of ultrasonics on, 394
Fear of dental care, 589
Feedback and prevention implementations, 302
Field anesthesia, 548
Files, 388-389, 388*i*, 389*t*
for overhang removal, 629-632, 631*i*, 631*p*
in root planing, 414
Filiform papillae, 156
Film characteristics for intraoral photography, 276-277, 284
Financial incentives for prevention, 300-301
Financial records, 57, 60, 62, 177
Fine scaling, 410-413; *see also* Scaling

Finger rest, 68-70, 69-70*p*, 86, 90-91, 378, 390-391, 390-391*p*
Finger-wrapping of floss, 312-313, 312*p*, 314*p*
Finishing
of amalgam restorations, 633-639, 634-641*p*
check-off sheet for, 646*i*
versus polishing, 636
of study models, 266
Finishing burs, 636-639, 637-638*p*
Finishing disks and strips, 632-633, 633*p*, 641*p*
Fire prevention, 174
First aid, 164-165, 168-170*t*
First-time patients, 588-592
Fissures, 522-523, 524-527*p*
sealants for, 528-529
Fixed bridges, 187
Flame-shaped burs, 637-639
Flash unit, 275-276; *see also* Intraoral photography
Flavor oils and plaque, 207
Floor of mouth
in cancer self-examination, 356, 357*p*
palpation of, 156-157, 156*p*
Floss
and rubber dam placement, 599, 607-610*p*
variable-diameter, 318, 321*p*
Floss holder, 318, 322*p*
Floss threader, 318, 320*p*
Flossing, 313, 314-317*p*, 316*i*
to tuck rubber dam, 609-611
Flow meter for nitrous oxide, 366, 367*p*
Fluoride
for desensitization, 538
and radiation therapy, 587
Fluoride cups, 473
Fluoride therapy, 296, 364, 499-519, 500-502*i*, 504-506*t*,
511*p*, 513-516*p*
check-off sheet for, 518*i*
Fluoride toxicity, 245
Fluoroapatite, 500-501
Fluorosis, 500*t*
Flush valve, 568
Food debris and plaque, 205
Food groups, 369-370, 369*t*
Food stain, 467
Foot controls, 15-16, 397
Forceps
for rubber dam placement, 599, 605*p*, 613*p*
and sterile instrument transfer, 43, 45-46, 45*p*
Forensic dentistry, periodontal chart in, 221
Formalin, 538
Fraser-Sweatman analgesic machine, 567*p*
Friction from abrasives, 469
Fulcrum; *see also* Finger rest
alternative placement of, 390-391, 390-391*p*
for injection, 555, 556*p*
Functions, dental, expanded and traditional, 4-5

Fungicides, 34
Fungiform papillae, 157
Furcation, 227*i*, 234-235, 234*i*

G

Garner clamps, 516-517, 517*p*, 529, 529*p*
Garnet disk, 632
Gauze
    for flossing, 318, 322*p*
    and periodontal dressing, 455
Gel, fluoride, 507, 510
General anesthesia, 542
General appraisal in clinical examination, 137-138
General physical evaluation, 135-161
Generic and brand name of drug, 132
Genetic factors
    in occlusion, 487-488
    in tooth stain, 465
Geometric charting, 179, 179*i*
Germicides, 34
Gingival assessment, 218*t*, 224-227, 225*i*
Gingival Bleeding Index, 211
Gingival cleft, 316*p*
Gingival crevicular fluid, 226-227
Gingival and subgingival curettage, 431
Gingival enlargement and recession, 232-233
Gingival inflammation indices, 211-214, 211-214*i*
Gingival infection as contraindication to ultrasonics, 395
Gingival tissue, effect of amalgam overhang on, 629
Gingivitis and calculus, 198
Gingivitis Index, Suomi and Barbano, 212*t*
Gingivostomatitis, herpetic, 30
Gland examination findings, 152
Gleem toothpaste, 468
Gloves and contamination, 47
Glutaraldehyde and disinfection, 36, 38, 41-42
Goal setting, 665-666, 668-669*i*
Gold crown, 186
Gold foil, 186
Gold inlay and onlay, 186
Gold restorations, 186
Gracey curette, 98, 98*i; see also* Curette
    for curettage, 436-438, 437-438*i*
    for root planing, 414-416, 415*p*, 417-419*p*
Gram-negative bacteria, 433
Granulomatous tissue, 30, 433
Graphic representation, 178*i*, 182-183*i*
Grasp, instrument, 68, 69-70*p*, 74*p*, 90-91, 378
Green stain, 466
Gum in cancer self-examination, 356, 357*p*
Gummas, 30
Gypsum products in study models, 243-244, 254-257*p*

H

Habit and prevention, 301
Hair inspection, 146

"Halo" and ultrasonic tip, 398, 399*p*
Halothane and nitrous oxide, 562
Hand instruments, 18
Hand scaling, 377-391; *see also* Scaling
Handicapped patients; *see also* Special needs, patients with
    periodontal disease in, 581
Handle, instrument, 67, 67*p*
Handpiece, 15-16
    and contamination, 48-49
    for polishing, 472-473, 472*p*
    ultrasonic, 398, 398*p*
Handwashing, 46-47
Hard palate palpation, 156-157, 157*p*
Head and neck examination, 135-160
Headrest, 13*p*
Healing
    after curettage, 439
    in elderly, 594
Health care planning, regional and national, 5-7
Health conditions, undiagnosed, 119
Health goals in treatment plan, 330
Health hazards with study models, 244-245
Health history, 28, 30, 117-133
    baseline data in, 137-138
    and chemotherapy, 586-587
    clinical examination and, 224
    of elderly patient, 592-593
    and local anesthesia, 546-547
Health levels and dental hygiene care, 666
Health manpower, 5-6
Health status of patient, 123-130, 124*i*, 136
    and treatment plan, 330
Heart defects and disorders, 126-127
Heart failure, 172-173
Heat from polishing friction, 473-474
Heat disinfection, 33, 36-37
Heat-sensitive symbols and autoclave, 39*p*, 40
Heat sterilization, 37-46
Heimlich maneuver, 171-172
Hemiplegics, transfer technique for, 575, 576-577*p*
Hemophilia and disease transmission, 28
Hemorrhagic disorders, 129
    from chemotherapy, 586
Hepatitis, 128-129
    A and B virus, 27-29, 27*t*
    and acquired immune deficiency syndrome, 31-32
    instrument sterilization and, 43
Hereditary factors in tooth stain, 465
Herpes simplex, 30-31
High-speed handpiece, 15-16
High-volume suction, 15
History, medical, 546-547; *see also* Health history
Hoe, use of, 387-388, 387*i*, 387*t*
    in root planing, 414
Home care, 214, 467-468; *see also* Prevention
    assessment of, 301-302

Home care—cont'd
of child patient, 589-591
following curettage, 439
for handicapped patients, 581-582
and stain, 467-468
for tooth sensitivity, 537
Horizontal stroke; *see* Stroke patterns
Hormonal deficiencies as contraindication to curettage, 433
Horseshoe-shaped headrest, 13
Hospitalized patients, 592-595
Hot oil instrument disinfection, 36-37
Human needs, Maslow's hierarchy of, 299-300
Hydrochloride salt solution in local anesthetics, 544
Hydrophilic group in local anesthetics, 544
Hydroxyapatite, 500
Hyperemia, 536
Hyperglycemia, 171-172
Hypersensitivity and fluoride therapy, 536, 538-539
Hypertension, 127, 140-144, 546
Hyperventilation, 172
Hypocalcification, 189
Hypodermic needles and syringes, 42; *see also* Syringes
Hypoglycemia, 171
Hypoxia, 571

I

I-type fissure, 523, 526*p*
Iatrogenic factors in occlusion, 491
IM; *see* Intramuscular injection
Immunity, 24, 28
Impacted teeth, charting of, 222
Impression check-off sheets, 266-267
Impression taking, 246, 248-250*p*
Impression tray, 243, 243*p*, 248-250*p*
Incisive papilla, 157
Incursions, pathologic, 466
Independent practice, 8
Index, stain, 470-471, 470*t*
Index systems for nitrous oxide and oxygen connection, 566
Indications
for curettage, 431-433, 433-434*i*
for occlusal sealing, 528, 528*t*
Indices
of clinical caries, 503
of plaque, 204-215
Indirect lighting, 153
Individualized care, 581-582
Infection, 24-26
Infectious diseases, 27-31, 128-129
Infectious hepatitis; *see* Hepatitis
Infiltration anesthesia, 435, 548
Inflammation, 297*p*
and chemotherapy, 586
and curettage, 430-433, 433-434*i*
and root planing, 426
treatment of, 230

Informed consent, 57, 333
Inhalation sedation; *see* Conscious sedation
Injection
placement of, 550-552*p*
in relation to nerves and tissues, 548*i*, 549*t*
Ink and record permanence, 58
Inlay, gold, 186
Innervation by trigeminal nerve, 548*i*
Inorganic nutritional elements, 364
Inspection in examination, 137
Instruments
adaptation of, 86, 86*i*, 87-92*p*, 378-379, 380*i*, 382*p*, 385, 385*p*, 416, 417-419*p*, 436-438, 437-438*p*
anterior, 90-91
design of, 67-68, 68*p*, 97-98, 97-98*i*
disinfection of, 33-34
disposable, 42-43
double-ended, 67*p*
exercises with, 68-71, 85-92
hand, 63-68
paired, 68*p*
sharpening of, 95-106, 96-99*i*, 99-105*p*, 105*i*
sterilization of; *see* Sterilization
storage of, 17-18, 43-45
transfer of, and sterilization, 45-46
ultrasonic, 394-395, 397-405
wrapping of, for sterilization, 43-45, 44*p*
"Instrumentate," 85
Instrumentation, 63-72, 69-71*p*, 76-83*p*, 229*i*, 232-234*i*
for curettage, 436-439, 436-438*p*
for fine scaling, 412-413
for polishing, 475
for root planing, 412-413, 416-423, 417-419*p*
for scaling, 378-391, 379-380*i*, 381*p*, 382-384*i*, 383*p*, 387-388*i*, 387-391*p*
for tooth sensitivity, 537
for ultrasonics, 402
Insulin shock, 171
Insurance; *see* Third-party insurers
Interdental papillae curettage, 437-438, 438*p*
Intermediate linkage in local anesthetics, 544
International numbering system, 181, 181*t*
Interocclusal record, 252, 253*p*
Interproximal area, finishing of, 636, 636*p*
Interproximal brush, 319, 324*p*
Interproximal cleaning, 312-327, 312*p*, 314-325*p*
Interview, health history, 120, 123
Interviewing, 123
Intramuscular injection, 166, 168-170*t*, 171-174
Intraoral examination, 153-159
of occlusion, 494-495, 494-497*p*
Intraoral mirrors, 279-283, 280-283*p*
Intraoral photography, 271-290
checklist for, 290*i*
Intraoral pigmentation, 155
Intravenous injection, 166, 168-170*t*, 171-175

Intrinsic stain, 469-470
Iodine
  in diet, 364
  as disinfectant, 36
Iodophors and disinfection, 36
Ionizing radiation, 587-588
Iontophoresis, 538-539
Iron in diet, 264
Irrigation, 13, 426
Isopropyl alcohol, 36
IV; *see* Intravenous injection

J

Jewelry and contamination, 51
Journal of the American Medical Association, on congenital
    defects, 466
Junctional epithelium, 430-431, 438

K

Keratosis, 157
Kerr Pit and Fissure Sealant, 529; *see also* Bisphenol A-glycidyl
    methacrylate
Kidney disease, 128

L

Labial inclination, 190
Labial mucosa, 154-155, 155*p*
Laboratory tests
  of fluoride, 501-502
  results of, 56
Larynx, 152, 152*p*
Lateral excursion, 490, 495-496*p*
"Laughing gas"; *see* Nitrous oxide and oxygen conscious se-
    dation
Lavage, water, and ultrasonics, 309, 406
Lead lining and radiographs, 18
Leather products, maintenance of, 20
Lee Seal, 529; *see also* Bisphenol A-glycidyl methacrylate
Left-handed clinician position, 74*p*, 75*t*, 80-83*p*
Legal contract, treatment plan as, 330
Legal evidence, periodontal chart as, 221
Legal limits, 8
  in diagnosis and treatment planning, 344
Legal record, history as, 120, 137
Lemonstron apparatus, 539
Lens aperture setting, 276-277
Lesions, descriptions of, 146-147
Leukemia, 129
Levonordefrin, 545, 545*t*
Liability, legal, 333
Lidocaine, 545, 545*t*, 557, 559
Life support in emergencies, 164-174, 168-170*t*
Light reflection on sharp instrument, 96-97, 97*i*
Lighting, 16-17, 73-74, 74*i*
  in intraoral examination, 153

Lighting—cont'd
  for intraoral photography, 274-275
  in self-examination, 349*p*
Lingual frenum, 156, 348*t*
Lingual inclination, 190
Lingual photographic views, 287-288
Lingual pocket walls, curettage of, 436
Lingual vein, 156
Linkage, intermediate, 544
Lip examination 146, 154
  in cancer self-examination, 356, 356*p*
Lipids, 362-363
Lipophilic group in local anesthetics, 544
Listening, 112-113
Listerine toothpaste, 467
Liver dysfunction and local anesthetic, 546-547
Local anesthesia, 541-557, 546-549*t*, 547-548*i*, 550-556*p*
Löe and Silness Gingival Index, 211-212, 212*t*
Lubricant, rubber dam, 604, 604*p*, 606
Lubrication of handpieces, 16
Lymph nodes
  examination findings, 152
  palpation of, 148*p*, 149, 150-151

M

Macleans toothpaste, 467-468, 505
Maintenance
  of equipment, 11-20
  and replacement of emergency supplies, 166-167
Malocclusion; *see* Occlusion
Malposed teeth, charting of, 189-190, 222
Management of time, 331-332, 332*i*
Mandible, palpation of, 147-148, 148*p*
Mandibular opening, maximum, 494, 494*p*
Mandibular fluoride tray, 514, 515*p*
Mandibular photographic view, 287-288
Mandibular reconstruction from cancer surgery, 585
Manual palpation, 147-160, 148-151*p*, 155-160*p*
Margin
  evaluation of, 635*p*
  open, 632
  overhanging, 189
Marginal gingiva, curettage of, 438
Margination, 628-633, 628*i*, 630-631*p*, 633*p*
  check-off sheet for, 645*i*
Mask, oxygen, 166
Maslow's hierarchy of human needs, 299-300
Masseter muscle, palpation of, 149-150
Massler PMA index, 211
Master's degree programs, 6
Masticatory mucosa, 233
Materia alba and plaque, 205
Matrix band, *see* Tofflemire matrix band and retainer system
Mattress suture, simple, 459
Maxillary fluoride tray, 514, 515*p*

Maxillary impression and model, 250-251p
Maxillary photographic views, 287
Mean alveolar concentration, 562
Mechanical bonding, 523
Mechanical denture cleaning 478
Mechanical polishing devices, 471-475, 471-473p, 474i
Mechanical stimulation of hypersensitivity, 536
Mechanisms
    of sensitivity, 536
    of fluoride action, 500-501
Medial palatal raphe, 157
Medical alert in patient record, 57-58
Medical classification, 130, 130t
Medical conditions, undiagnosed, 119
Medical and dental care continuity, 117-120
Medical factors in curettage, 431-433
Medical history
    in case documentation, 56-57
    and conscious sedation, 563-564
    and curettage, 435
    of elderly, 592-593
    and emergency, 164
    and local anesthesia, 547-548
Medical release letter, 130-132, 131i
Medically compromising conditions, 126-130
Medication
    with anesthetics, 546-547
    antihypertensive, 142
    in health history, 117-118, 125
    and nutrition, 368
Medicolegal records, 56-58
Meds; see Medication
Megavitamin dosage, 363-365
Mentalis muscle, palpation of, 147
Mepivacaine, 545, 545t
Mercury vapor for amalgam overhang, 632
Mesial inclination, 190
Metabolizing plaque, 205
Metallic stain, 467
Metastasis as contraindication to ultrasonics, 395
Methacrylic periodontal dressings, 446
Microbial plaque formation, 296
Microflora, 23-27
Microorganisms, 23t
    control of, 32-53
    and equipment, 13, 16
Microscope
    for instrument evaluation, 96-97, 97i
    and prevention, 326
Microscopy for periodontal evaluation, 234-235
Mineralization, 199
Minerals in diet, 364, 371t
Mirror, 63-64, 228, 415-436
    exercises with, 84-85
    intraoral, 279-283, 280-283p
    in self-examination, 349p

Miscarriage from anesthesia, 568
Missing teeth
    in radiographs, 189, 190i
    on periodontal chart, 222
Mixed dentition and occlusion, 489
Mobile cart, 19p
Mobility of teeth, measurement of, 233-234
Model trimmer, 244
Models, study; see Study models
Modified care of patient with special needs, 574-595
Modified Navy Plaque index, 208, 209i
Modified pen grasp, 69p; see also Pen grasp
Modified toothbrush, 319, 325p
Modular cart, 18, 18p
Moist heat sterilization 37-46
Monitoring
    of conscious sedation, 570-571
    of sterilization, 40
Monofluorophosphates, 505
Morphology, root, 413
Motion management in instrumentation, 72
Motivation
    of hygienist, 109
    of patient, 299-301, 378
Motor-driven polishing, 473
Mouth in cancer self-examination, 356, 357p
Mouth mirror; see Mirror
Mouth props, 580-581, 581p
Mouth rinses, fluoride, 505, 506t
Mouthwashes and contamination, 52
Mucositis and cancer therapy, 586-588
Mucous protection, 24
Multijointed headrest, 13
Muscle examination findings, 152
Muscle molding
    for alginate impression, 246
    of periodontal dressing, 452, 452i
Muscular anatomy in local anesthetic, 548
Myocardial infarction and sedation, 563-564

N

Naber's probe, 234
Names of teeth in self-assessment, 349-350
Nasal masks for conscious sedation, 567-568
Nasal obstruction and sedation, 563-564
National Academy of Science Committee on Diet, Nutrition,
    and Cancer, 366-367
National Academy of Science, on Recommended Daily Dietary
    Allowances, 370, 371t
National health insurance, 8
National Institute of Dental Research fluoride studies, 499
National standards of dental hygiene care, 666-667
Nausea
    with conscious sedation, 571-572
    and pregnant patient, 584-585

Neck
   in cancer self-examination, 354, 355*p*
   examination of, 146
Needle, 553-554*p*
Neural anatomy in local anesthetics, 548-549, 548*i*, 549*t*
Newman, Irene, 295-296
Nitrous oxide and oxygen conscious sedation, 561-572, 563*t*, 564-570*p*
   contamination from nosepiece with, 50
   gagging on, 562-563
   potency of, compared with halothane, 562
"No oral hygiene procedure" plaque study, 206-207
Nodules, 146
Nonmineralized deposits, 204-211
Norepinephrine, 545, 545*t*
Nose examination, 146
Novocaine; *see* Procaine
Numbers, tooth, 181, 181*t*
Numeric charting, 179, 180*i*
Nutritional assessment, 361-373
   of elderly, 593
Nutritional deficiencies as contraindication to curettage, 433
Nutritional disorders, 160
   and radiation therapy, 587
Nutritional self-assessment, 361-373, 369*t*, 370-371*t*
Nuva-Cote and Nuva-seal PA, 529; *see also* Bisphenol A-glycidyl methacrylate

O

Oblique stroke; *see* Stroke patterns
Obturation of occlusal anatomy, 522
Occipital lymph nodes, 149
Occlusal analysis, 493-494, 493*i*
Occlusal anatomy, 483, 485-490
Occlusal brushing, 309, 309*p*
Occlusal sealants, 522-533, 524-527*p*, 528*t*, 529-532*p*
Occlusal screening, 491-492, 492*i*
Occlusal surface, finishing of, 636-637
Occlusal trauma, 220, 490-491
Occlusal view, 228*i*
   photographic, 287-288
Occlusion, 483-498, 485-488*i*, 494-497*p*
   and restoration, 624-628
Ocular keratitis, 30
O'Leary Plaque Control Record, 208-210, 210*i*
Onlay, gold, 186
Open contact, 634
"Open flap" conditions, 425-426
Open margin, 632
Operation of equipment, 11-20
Oral cancer, 352-359, 355-358*p*
Oral charting, 193-194
Oral condition, self-assessment of, 345-359
Oral examination; *see also* Examination
   and syphilis, 30
   tray setup for, 144*i*

Oral herpes; *see* Herpes
Oral Hygiene Index, 202
Oral irrigator, 319, 325*p*
Oral prophylaxis; *see* Prophylaxis
Orange stain, 466
Orangewood points, 471
Orangewood stick, 47
Organization of dental records, 57-58
Orthodontic appliance cleaning, 482, 482*p*
Orthodontic concept of occlusion, 484
Osseous anatomy, 548
Osteomyelitis as contraindication to ultrasonics, 395
Osteoradionecrosis, 588
"Other-oriented" career motivation, 109
Oven, dry heat, 40-41
Overbite, 487, 487*i*
Overdenture cleaning, 480-481*p*, 481
Overhang, amalgam, removal of, 628-633, 628*i*, 630-631*p*, 633*p*
Overhanging margins
   charting of, 187
   radiographs of, 191-192
Overhead light
   maintenance of, 16-17
   placement of, 74, 74*p*
Overjet, 485, 487*i*
Overlapping stroke pattern, 86
   in root planing, 416
Oxidizing denture cleaners, 478
Oxygen
   in emergency, 166-167
   and nitrous oxide sedation, 561-572, 563*t*, 564-570*p*

P

Pacemaker and ultrasonics, 295
Pain control, 541-559, 546*t*, 547-548*i*, 549*t*, 550-556*p*
   for elderly patient, 594
   and perception, reaction, and reaction thresholds, 541-543
     with nitrous oxide and oxygen, 561
Paired explorer; *see also* Explorer
   exercises with, 86-90
Paired instruments, 67*p*, 68
Palatal foveae, 157
Palatal rugae, 157
Palatal photographic views, 287-288
Palate
   examination of, 157
   self-assessment of, 349
Palatine uvula, 157
Palm-up position, 85
Palmer's notation, 181, 181*t*
Palpation in examination, 147-160, 148-151*p*, 155-160*p*
Papillary Bleeding Index, 213, 213*t*, 214*i*
Paraplegics, transfer techniques for, 576-580, 576-580*p*
Parent with child as first-time patient, 589

Parenteral disease transmission, 28
Parotid gland, palpation of, 149, 149*p*
Partial denture cleaning, 481, 481*p*
Partner in care concept, 109-112
Paste, noneugenol, 447-448*p*
Pathogenesis of caries, 502
Pathogenic incursion, 466
Pathogenic organisms, 25-27
Pathogens, bacterial and viral, 25-26*t*
Pathologic factors in occlusion, 488
Patient
    assessment of, in case documentation, 654
    care, acceptance and refusal of, 334
    confidentiality of, and dental record, 56
    consideration of, in examination, 145
    education, 295-296, 306-307*p*, 435-436, 475, 584-585
        for elderly, 593
    expectations of, and dental records, 56
    involvement of, in care, 213-214
    instructions to
        for denture cleaning, 480
        for periodontal dressing, 454*i*, 455
    motivation of, 299-301, 372-373, 435-436, 584-585, 588
    as "partner in care," 109-112, 477
    perceptions of, 109-115
        in occlusal trauma, 491
    planning in case documentation, 654
    position
        for elderly, 593-594
        for handicapped, 582-584, 582-583*p*
        for pregnant patient, 584
    preparation of
        for curettage, 435-436
        for fluoride therapy, 509-510
        for periodontal dressing, 446-447
        for rubber dam, 602
        for ultrasonics, 396
    privacy of, 145
    profile of, 123, 124*i*
    with special needs, 160-161, 574-595, 576-583*p*, 590-591*p*
Patient-centered care, 3, 111
PDR; *see Physician's Desk Reference*
Pear-shaped burs, 637, 637-638*p*
Pearl Drops toothpaste, 467
Pedodontic charting, 179, 194
Peer review, 137
Pen grasp, 68, 69-70*p*, 74*p*, 90-91, 378
Percussion in examination, 137
Periapical conditions, radiographs of, 193, 193*i*, 223
Pericoronitis, 222
Periodontal aid, 319, 323*p*
Periodontal care, 377-427, 483-498
Periodontal charting, 220-224, 227*i*
    and curettage, 435

Periodontal disease, 217-220
    effect of, on cementum, 421-422
    and plaque, 410-411
Periodontal Disease Index, 202
Periodontal dressings, 439, 443-459, 446*t*, 447-455*p*
    placement of, 450-451, 450-451*p*
    removal of, 456-459, 456-458*p*
        checklist for, 458*i*
Periodontal examination, 219-220
    microscopy, dark-field, in, 235-236
Periodontal findings in radiographs, 192-193
Periodontal packs; *see* Periodontal dressings
Periodontal pocket, 66
Periodontal probe, 65-67, 66-67*p*, 436; *see also* Probe
    ultrasonic tip of, 401-402, 401*p*, 405*p*
Periodontal probing, 227-235
Periodontal procedures with ultrasonics, 407
Periodontal surgery, 233
Periodontitis, 198, 219-229, 230
Peripac periodontal dressings, 446, 453
Permanent dentition and occlusion, 489
Personal injury emergency, 174
Petroleum jelly, 602
pH, dermal, and microorganisms, 24
Pharmacologic terms, 132
Pharynx examination, 157, 157*p*
Phillips toothpaste, 467
Philosophy of prevention, 298
Phosphorus, 364
Photographic accessories, 277-279, 278-283*p*
Photography, 56, 271-290
Photomicrographs of fissures, 524-527*p*
Physical evaluation, 135-144
Physician care and treatment, 330-331
Physician's Desk Reference, 132-133
Physiologic factors in occlusion, 488
Pigmentation, intraoral, 155
Pin index for nitrous connection, 566
Pipe cleaner, 319, 323*p*
Pit and fissure sealants, 522-533, 524-527*p*, 528*t*, 529-532*p*
Plak-lite, 211
Planing; *see* Root planing
Planning
    of appointments, 334-335, 336-343*i*
    of control and prevention, 295-327
    and dental hygiene appointment, 9
    of national health care, 5-7
    patient involvement in, 110-112
Plaque, 204-211
    agents against, 295
    and calculus, 199
    control of, 296-298, 298*p*
    and diet, 366
    fluoride and, 501, 508
    indices, 208-211, 209-210*i*

Plaque—cont'd
  and periodontal disease, 410-411
  removal of, 298*p*
    with child, 591
  retentive area for, 629
  scoring of, 208-211, 209*i*
  staining of, with disclosant, 200, 210-211
  weight, 211
Plaque Thickness Index, 204*t*, 208
Plica fimbriata and lingualis, 156
PMA gingival index, 211
Pocket
  depth of, 228-229*i*, 229-231, 232-233*i*, 430-431, 433-434*i*
  formation of, 297*p*
  treatment of, 230
Pocket wall, curettage of, 436-437, 437*p*
Podshadley and Haley plaque scoring index, 208, 209*i*
Poisoning from fluoride, 517
Polishing
  of amalgam restorations, 639-640
  and desensitizing, 538
  devices for, 471-473, 471-473*p*
  versus finishing, 636
  of study models, 266
  of teeth, 464-475, 471-473*p*, 474*i*
Polymerization, 532-533, 532*p*
Pontics, 187
Pontocaine, 544-545, 545*t*, 557-559
Porcelain, charting of, 186
Portable equipment for patient with special needs, 580
Porte polisher, 471-472, 471*p*
Position
  of dental chair, 11-13, 12-13*p*
  of dental team, 63, 72-92
  of handicapped patient, 582-584, 582-583*p*
  of clinician, 72-74, 72*p*, 73*i*, 153
    and patient, 153, 154
  of pregnant patient, 584
Positional low blood pressure, 142
Posterior photographic views, 288-289
Postsedation effects, 572
Posture of clinician, 17
Potassium ferrocyanide, 538
Potency of anesthetics, 545, 545*t*, 562
Pouring study models, 252-257
Practice acts, 598
Practice roles, 6-8
Pregnancy, 584-585
  fluoride supplements during, 585
  and sedation, 563-564
Premedication for examination, 224
Preparation
  of child patient, 592
  of clamps for rubber dam, 601*i*, 604-606, 605-606*p*
  for desensitizing, 538

Preparation—cont'd
  for emergencies, 174-175
  of rubber dam, 603-604, 603*i*, 603-604*p*
  for self-assessment, guided, 346, 347*p*
  for study models, 245-246
  for ultrasonics, 396
Presentation
  case, 333-334, 336-343*p*, 654-655
  of study models, 266
Pressure gauges of nitrous oxide and oxygen tanks, 565*p*
Prevention, 298-299, 467-468
  assessment in, 301-302, 303*i*
  education in, 301-306
  evaluation of, 306, 306*i*
  implementation of, 302, 305*i*
  literature on, 326
  motivation for, 299
  orientation on, 666
  philosophy of, 298
  planning for, 302, 304*i*
  of plaque, 296-298, 297-298*p*
  priority of, in treatment plan, 331
  of tooth stain, 467-468, 468*t*
Prilocaine, 545, 545*t*
Primary dentition and occlusion, 488-489
Primary provider, emergency role of dental hygienist as, 164-165
Priority assignment in treatment planning, 331, 332*i*
Privacy of patient, 145
Probe, 64-67, 415; *see also* Periodontal probe
  for charting, 227-228
  exercises with, 85-86, 86*i*
Problem-oriented records, 59-60, 60*t*
Procaine, 544-545, 545*t*
Professional closeness to patient, 113-114
Progress notes in patient record, 58-59
Prophylactic regimen for dental procedures, American Heart Association, 119
Prophylaxis, 377-378
  and fluoride therapy, 509-510
Prophylaxis angle, 16, 472-473, 472*p*
Prophylaxis paste, 468-469
Prophy-Jet, 473
Propoxycaine, 544-545, 545*t*
Prosthetic concept of balanced occlusion, 484
Prosthetics and cancer therapy, 585-586
Protect desensitizing dentifrice, 537
Protective apparel, 30-32, 52-53
  with ultrasonics, 396
Proteins, 362
Protrusive excursion, 490, 497*p*
Psychologic effects of nitrous oxide, 568-569
Psychosomatic pain control, 542, 543-544
Pulmonary disease and sedation, 563-564
Pulp, bleaching and, 470

Pulse, 138-139, 144-145, 145*p*
Pumice, 469, 633, 639, 639*p*
Pustules, 147

Q

Quadrant numbering, 181
Quadriplegic, transfer techniques for, 576-580, 577-580*p*
Quality assurance and accountability, 665
Questionnaire
   health history, 120-122, 122*i*
   nutritional, 368-369
Quigley and Hein Plaque Scoring Index, 208

R

Race and cancer, 352-353
Radiation therapy, 587-588
Radiographic charting, 179, 190-194, 191*i*, 193-194*i*
Radiographs
   in case documentation, 56
   in dental record, 56
   and occlusion, 528
   and periodontal diagnosis, 222-224
   and pregnant patient, 584
Ravocaine; *see* Propoxycaine
RDAs, *see* Recommended Dietary Allowance
Recommended Dietary Allowances, 369-370, 370-371*t*
Reconstruction and cancer surgery, 585
Record
   dental, 56-62
     organization and style of, 57-59
   study models in, 238-239
Record audits, 60-62
Record keeping, photographic, 283
Referral for nutritional counseling, 373
Refusal of care, 69
   by patient, 71
Regulators for nitrous oxide and oxygen, 565, 565-566*p*
Relaxation techniques and pain control, 544
Release, medical, 130-132, 131*i*
Remineralization, 523
Research; *see also* Studies
   on calculus, 198-199
   on curettage, 431-433, 440-441
   on dental disease, 296
   on desensitizing products, 537-538
   on fluoride, 499-503
   on healing after root planing and curettage, 430-431
   on nitrous oxide and oxygen conscious sedation, 568-569
   occlusal sealants, 522-523
   on periodontal dressings, 443-444
   plaque scoring in, 208
   prophylaxis and disease, 377-378
   on root planing, 421-423
   on tooth polishing, 464-465
   on ultrasonics, 394, 406-407

Reservoir bag, 568
Resident and transient bacteria on skin, 46-47
Respiration rate, 139
Respiratory infection, 22-27
   and sedation, 563-564
Restorations
   carving of, 620
   charting of, 182-187, 183*i*
   evaluation of, 628-629
   finishing and polishing of amalgam, 633-639, 634-641*p*
   marking of, 182-186
   matrix bands in placement of, 614-622
   overhang, 628-629
   radiographs of, 189-191, 190*i*
   and stain, 467
Restraints and handicapped patients, 580-581
Retainer and band system, Tofflemire matrix, 614-622
Retardation of patient and sedation, 563
Retention of patient records, 58
Retractors, cheek, 64-65, 278-279, 278-283*p*
Review of systems, 125, 330
Rheostat foot pedal, 15-16*p*
Rheumatic fever and heart disease, 126
Right-handed clinician position, 72-83, 72*p*, 73*i*, 74*p*, 75*t*, 76-79*p*
Ring headrest, 13
Rinse, 15, 426
   and fluoride, 505
   and periodontal dressing, 455
Role of dental hygienist, 6-8
Role playing in positioning exercises, 84
Rolling stroke brushing, 308-309, 309*i*
Root morphology, 413
   abnormal, 223
Root planing, 413-427, 415*p*, 417-419*p*, 424
   compared with fine scaling, 412-413
   before curettage, 435
   and desensitizing, 538
Root structure and ultrasonics, 394, 406-407
ROS; *see* Review of systems
Rotary engine equipment, 15-16
Rotation of dental chair, 12
Round burs, 637, 637*p*, 639
"Routine" care, 335
Rubber cup adaptation
   for amalgam polishing, 640, 640-641*p*
   for teeth polishing, 474, 474*i*
Rubber dam,
   in amalgam finishing and polishing, 635-636
   placement and removal of, 599-614, 599-600*p*, 601*i*, 602-614*p*, 603-604*i*, 611-614
     check-off sheet for, 642*i*
   and polishing, 635-636
   and occlusal sealing, 529-533, 529-532*p*
   tucking of, 609-610, 610*p*

Rubber tip, 319, 324*p*
Rust from autoclaving, 43

S

Safe-plaque, 205
Saliva
  and calculus, 198-199
  and disease, 23-24
  and probing, 232
Saliva ejector, 228
Salt and cancer, 367
Sample case documentation, 655-661
Sanguinaria (sanguinarine), 296
Sanitation, 32, 33
Satisfaction, patient, 111-112
SBI; *see* Sulcular Bleeding Index
Scaler, 379-380*i*, 380-382*p*
Scaling, 377-391, 410-413; *see also* Prophylaxis
  and desensitizing, 538
  and root planing, 410-413
  topical anesthetics for, 558-559
  with ultrasonics, 410-413
Scavenging nasal mask, 568, 568*p*
School-based clinic, 4, 5*p*
Scope of practice, 8, 344
Scoring
  of calculus, 202, 202*t*
  of clinical caries, 503
  of plaque, 208-211, 209*i*
  of stains, 470, 470*t*
Screening, occlusal, 491-492, 492*i*
Screening, cursory, in intraoral examination, 154, 154*p*
Scrub brush method, 310
Scrubbing of hands, 46-47
Sealants, 187-189, 296, 522-533
Secondary teeth and occlusion, 489
Sedation, conscious; *see* Nitrous oxide and oxygen conscious sedation
"Seesaw" motion in flossing, 313
"Selective polishing," 464
Self-assessment, 145
  nutritional, 361-373, 369*t*, 370-371*t*
  of oral condition, 345-351, 347-350*p*
Self-reliance of patient, 113
Sensitivity
  to periodontal dressing, 444
  potassium ferrocyanide for, 538
  from probe, 231
  after root planing, 425
Sensodyne desensitizing dentifrice, 537
Septic environment, 32
Sequence
  of amalgam finishing and polishing, 634
  of examination, 147-160
  of scaling, 386-387
  of self-assessment, 346-351

Serum hepatitis, 28-29
Settings for hygiene practice, 6
Sex and cancer, 352-353
Shank of instrument, 67
Sharpening of instruments, 95-106; *see also* Instruments
  skills in, and root planing, 421
Sharpening machines, 98, 103-104
Sharpening stone, 99-105, 99-105*p*
Short-mount lens, 273
Shutter speed, 276
Sickle scaler, 97, 97*i*, 380-381, 380*i*, 381*p*
Silicate and silica in toothpaste, 468
Silicate cement coloration, 470
Silness and Löe Plaque Thickness Index, 204*t*, 208
Silver nitrate, 538
Single-lens reflex cameras, 273-274, 273-274*p*
Single-pour method for study models, 256, 256*p*
Sink, 17
Slide evaluation, 289
Sliding board transfer technique, 579-580*p*, 580
Sling sutures, 459-462, 459-460*i*, 461-462*p*
Smoking and periodontal disease, 217
Smoking and stain, 467, 467*t*
Sodium fluorescein, 211
Sodium fluoride, 504-506, 538-539
Sodium hypochlorite, 36, 441
Soft deposits, 204-205
Soft palate examination, 157
Soft-textured brush, 308*i*
Soft tissue
  curettage of, 430-441, 433-434*i*, 437-438*p*
  in gingival assessment, 227
  in root planing, 426-427
  in self-assessment, 227, 349-350*p*
Solution, fluoride, 516-518, 518*i*
Special needs, patients with, 574-595, 576-583*p*, 590-591*p*
  identification of, 160-161
Sphygmomanometer, 142-144, 144*p*
Splatter, 51-53
Splints, 187
Spoon excavator, 619-620, 620*p*
Sporicides, 34
Stainless steel, care of, 20
Stains, 464-471, 466-467*t*, 470*t*
Standards of dental hygiene care, 666-667
Stannous fluoride, 504-506
  in desensitizing, 539
Steam sterilization; *see* Autoclaving
Sterilization, 32, 37-46
  equipment for, maintenance of, 19-20
  methods of, compared, 38*t*
Sternocleidomastoid muscle, palpation of, 150, 151*p*
Stethoscope and blood pressure, 142-144, 143*i*
Stillman's brushing method, 310, 311*i*
Stimuli of hypersensitivity, 536

Stomatitis from chemotherapy, 586
Stool, placement of, 17
Storage, 17-18
    of bags for sterilization, 43-45
    of photographic supplies, 283
Storage tanks for nitrous oxide and oxygen, 564-566, 564*p*
Strips, finishing, 632-633, 633*p*
Stroke count in hand scrubbing, 46
Stroke patterns
    in curettage, 436-438, 437-438*p*
    in root planing, 416, 417*i*, 417-418*p*
    in scaling, 378-380, 381*p*, 383*p*, 384*i*, 385*p*
    with ultrasonics, 401-402, 403-405*p*
Strontium chloride, 537
Studies; *see also* Research
    on anesthesia and clinician, 568-569
    clinical
        on "no oral hygiene," 129
    on sealants, 522-523
Study casts; *see* Study models
Study models, 238-268, 239-241*p*, 247*i*, 252-255*p*, 260*p*, 264-265*p*
    in case documentation, 658*p*, 663*p*
    in dental record, 56
    pouring of, 252-255, 253-254*p*
Styrofoam impression trays, 243
Subcutaneous injection, 165
Subgingival calculus, 197, 197*i*, 202*t*
Subgingival and gingival curettage, 431
Subgingival plaque, 205
Subgingival scaling, 382, 383*p*
Sublingual caruncle and folds, 156
Submandibular and submental palpation, 150, 150*p*
Submarginal; *see* Subgingival entries
Submental region examination, 150, 150*p*
Suction, 15
    in emergency, 166
Sugar and sugar substitutes, 366
Sulcular bleeding, 236
Sulcular Bleeding Index, 211, 211*t*
Sulcus measurement, 86, 229-231; *see also* Pocket
"Sunshine" vitamin, 363
Suomi, D., and Barbano, J., Gingivitis Index, 212*t*
Super-heated steam; *see* Autoclaving
Superfloss; *see* Floss
Supernumerary teeth
    on radiographs, 188-189
    on periodontal chart, 222
Supervised neglect, 113
Supine positioning, 11-12, 12*p*, 42*p*
Supplies
    disposable, 42-43
    for emergency, 166-167
Supragingival calculus, 196-197, 202*t*
Supragingival plaque, 205

Supramarginal; *see* Supragingival entries
Surface-active agents and plaque, 207
Surface disinfection, 34-36
Surface texture assessment of gingiva, 236
Surgery, periodontal, 233
Surgical valve replacement, 126
Suture removal, 459-462, 459-460*i*, 460-461*p*
Sweat glands and microorganisms, 24
Symbolic factors in pain reaction, 543
Symbols, charting, 178*i*, 182-183*i*
Syncope, 167-171
Syphilis, 30
Syringe, 553, 554*p*, 556*p*
    in emergency injection, 166
Systemic fluoride, 503-504
Systolic pressure, 139-140, 140*i*

T

Tactile sense
    in curettage, 437
    in root planing, 420-421
    and sharp instruments, 95
Tarnish on amalgams, 633
Tartar and plaque, 205-206
Taste buds, 349
Taste loss in elderly, 593
Teaching approach to cancer self-examination, 353-354
Technical assault, 333-334
Teeth
    abutment of, 187
    bleaching of, 470
    brushing of, 467-468, 468*t*
    capping of, 470
    cleaning of, 377-378, 467-468
    crowning of, 470
    foils and plaque study of, 206
    formation of, 362-364
    hypersensitivity of, 535-539
    loss of, in elderly, 593
    mobility of, 233-234
    numbering of, 181, 181*t*
    polishing of, 464-475, 471-473*p*, 474*i*
    position and occlusion of, 485-489
    staining of, 465-469
Temperature
    sensitivity to, following root planing, 425
    technique for taking, 139
    of water with ultrasonics, 406
Temporalis muscle, palpation of, 150
Temporary restorations, 187
    zinc oxide–eugenol, 623-628, 625-627*p*
Terminal plane, 488-489, 488*i*
Terminal tooth, 606
Temporomandibular joint, 483
    assessment of, 491-493
    palpation of, 148-149, 148*p*

Terminal shank, 67*t*, 68

Test organism in sterilization, 40

Tetracaine, 544-545, 545*t*, 557-559

Texture of food, 371

Therapeutic agents causing stain, 467

Therapy, fluoride, 499-519

Thermal stimulation of hypersensitivity, 536

Thermodent desensitizing dentifrice, 537

Third-party insurers

    accountability to, 365-367

    examination records and, 137

    prevention and, 300-301

    record audit by, 61, 61*i*

Three-quarter gold crown, 186

Thyroid gland, palpation of, 151, 151*p*

Time considerations with ultrasonics, 394, 395

Time estimates in case presentation, 331, 332*i*, 334-335, 336-339*i*

Time

    management of, 153, 331

    and motion efficiency, 50

    perception of, altered by sedation, 562-563

Tin oxide for polishing, 633, 640, 640*p*

Tinnitus from ultrasonics, 396

Tissue

    and cancer therapy, 586

    descriptive terminology for, 146

    irritation of, from topical anesthetics, 557

    management of, 439

    retraction of, 153, 154*p*

Tissue tag removal, 438

Tobacco stains, 467, 467*t*

Tofflemire matrix band and retainer system, 614-617, 615*p*, 616*i*, 617*p*

    check-off sheet for, 643*i*

    placement of, 617-621, 619-621*p*

    removal of, 620-623, 622-623*p*

Tongue

    cleaning of, 309

    examination and palpation of, 157-158, 157-159*p*

    in self-examination, 348*p*, 349

        for cancer, 356, 357, 358*p*

Tongue blade in examination, 154, 154*p*

Tooth; *see* Teeth

Toothbrush, 307-308, 307*p*

    automatic, 319, 324*p*

    modified, 319, 325*p*

Tooth-colored restorations, 187

Topical anesthesia, 541-544, 555, 556*p*, 558*p*

Topically applied fluoride, 500-502, 504-507, 506*t*, 511-513, 517*i*, 518

Toxic reaction to anesthesia, 173

Toxicity

    of anesthesia, 545-546, 546*t*, 556

    of fluoride, 517

Toxicity—cont'd

    and gas sterilization, 41

    of mercury vapor, 632

    of vitamins, 364-365

Tranquilizers and hyperventilation, 122

Transfer techniques for patients with special needs, 575-580, 576-580*p*

Transient and resident bacteria on skin, 46-47

Transillumination, 84

Transmission of disease, 22-32

Trauma

    from dentures, 477-478

    occlusal, 490-491

Traumatism, 490-491

Tray

    impression, 243, 243*p*, 248-250*p*

    packaging of, for procedures, 43-45

    selection of, for fluoride, 510-512, 511*p*, 514*p*

    setup of

        for anesthesia injection, 144*i*, 553*i*

        and asepsis, 44-45

        for fluoride, 513*p*

        for periodontal dressing, 456*p*

        for self-assessment exercise, 347*p*

Tray systems, 17

Treatment

    goals of, 333

    of hypersensitivity, 536-539

    outcome of documented, 655

    plan for, 119, 330-331

        legal limits in, 344

        in patient record, 57

        periodontal examination in, 221

        photography in, 272

        for ultrasonics, 401-402

        worksheet for, 332*i*

    record of, in case documentation, 654

Treatment-oriented records, 59-60, 60*t*

Tribasic calcium phosphate, 467

Trigeminal nerve, 548*i*, 548*t*

Trimmer, model, 244

Trimming study model, 259-265, 259-265*p*, 268*i*

Trimming check-off sheet, 268

Tri-syringe, 13-15, 14*p*, 228

    and contamination, 49

Trust in patient-provider relationship, 113-115

Tuberculosis, 29-30

Tumor, 147

Typodont and rubber dam, 610*i*

U

Ulcer, 147

Ultra-Brite toothpaste, 468

Ultrasonic equipment, maintenance of, 18-19*p*

Ultrasonic procedures, 393-407, 397-401*t*, 403-405*t*

Ultrasonic scalers for amalgam overhang, 632
Ultraviolet polymerization, 533-534, 533*p*
Uncontrollable patient, 582-584, 582-583*p*
Undiagnosed health conditions, 119
Unerupted teeth, radiographs of, 189
Uniform clothing and contamination, 50
Unit controls and contamination, 34
Universal curette, 97-98, 98*i*, 382-387, 385*p; see also* Curette
    in root planing, 417-419*p*
    ultrasonic tip, 401-402, 401*p*, 404*p*
Universal matrix bands, 617
Universal tooth numbering system, 181, 181*t*
Updating patient's record, 130
Uptake of fluoride, 504
Urban areas and incidence of tuberculosis, 29-30

V

V-type fissure, 523, 524-525*p*
Vaccine for hepatitis, 29
Vascular anatomy in local anesthesia, 548-549
Vasoconstrictors, 545, 545*t*
Veneer, 197
Venereal disease, 129; *see also* Syphilis
Vertical stroke; *see* Stroke patterns
Verucides, 34
Vesicles, 147
Vibration, transmission of, 86
Vibrator for study models, 244
Viewbox, 18
Views of study models, 239
Viral hepatitis; *see* Hepatitis
Viral pathogens, orally transmittable, 26*t*
Viricides, 34
Vision enhancement
    instruments for, 63-65
    position for, 76-78*p*
Visual evaluation of root planing, 420, 424*p*
Visual inspection, 145-167
Vital signs
    in clinical examination, 138-144
    during emergency, 165-166, 168-170*t*
Vitamins, 361-364, 370-371*t*
Vomiting during conscious sedation, 571-572

W

"Walking" of probe, 85-86, 228
Wall alarm for conscious sedation system, 566*p*
Water
    in diet, 364
    with ultrasonics, 397-398, 397-400*p*
Water pressure polishing, 473
Water supply
    and contamination, 49, 436
    fluoridation of, 500, 500*t*, 503-504, 504*t*
Wedge, 319, 324*p*, 616*i*, 617-620, 619-621*p*
Weight-sensitive cup, 15
Wizard rubber dam holder, 599, 602*p*
Woodbury rubber dam holder, 599, 602*p*
Wooden point (porte) polisher, 471-472
Worksheet, treatment planning, 332*i*
Working stroke, 379-380, 381*p*
World Health Organization, 204
Wrist rock, 68-71, 70-71*p*, 86-87, 90-91

X

X-ray unit, 19-20*p*
    contamination of, 50
Xylocaine; *see* Lidocaine
Yarn for flossing, 318, 322*p*

Y

Young's frame rubber dam holder, 599, 602*p*, 607-608*p*

Z

Zamet on effectiveness of curettage, 440
Zerfing chisel ultrasonic tip, 400*p*, 401-402
Zinc chloride
    in desensitizing, 538
    in obduration, 522
Zinc oxide–eugenol and noneugenol dressings, 444-448, 445*t*, 447-449*p*, 455-456, 455*p*
Zinc oxide–eugenol temporary restoration, 623-628, 625-627*p*
    check-off sheet for, 644*i*